Biopsy Pathology
of the Bronchi

BIOPSY PATHOLOGY SERIES

General Editors

Professor Leonard S. Gottlieb, MD, MPH
Mallory Institute of Pathology
Boston, USA

Professor A. Munro Neville, MD, PhD, MRC Path
Ludwig Institute for Cancer Research,
Zurich, Switzerland

Professor F. Walker, MD, PhD
Department of Pathology,
University of Aberdeen, UK

Biopsy Pathology of the Bronchi

ELIZABETH M. McDOWELL,

B Vet Med, PhD (Cantab)

*Professor of Pathology, University of Maryland
School of Medicine, Baltimore, Maryland, USA*

and

THEODORE F. BEALS

MD

*Assistant Professor of Pathology
University of Michigan School of Medicine
Director of Clinical Electron Microscopy Program
Veterans Administration Medical Center, Ann Arbor, Michigan, USA*

SPRINGER-SCIENCE+BUSINESS MEDIA, B.V.

Originally published by Chapman and Hall in 1986
Softcover reprint of the hardcover 1st edition 1986

ISBN 978-0-412-24080-5

British Library Cataloguing in Publication Data

McDowell, Elizabeth M.
　　Biopsy pathology of the bronchi.—(Biopsy pathology series)
　　1. Bronchi—Diseases—Diagnosis　2. Biopsy
　　I. Title II. Beals, Theodore F.　　III. Series
　　616.2'30758'028　　RC778

ISBN 978-0-412-24080-5　　　ISBN 978-1-4899-3398-0 (eBook)
DOI 10.1007/978-1-4899-3398-0

Contents

Contents   vii

Preface

Biopsy Pathology of the Bronchi is intended to provide the practicing pathologist with a convenient source of diagnostic information, combined with pertinent clinical patterns and a background of histogenesis. It is hoped that the book will facilitate the accuracy of diagnosis, minimize pitfalls of interpretation and assist in the rapid evaluation of acute and chronic bronchial lesions, including neoplasms. Biopsy is taken in the widest sense and the book includes discussions on cytology, microbiopsies (fine needle aspiration biopsies, curette samples, and biopsies obtained by microforceps) and macrobiopsies, obtained at the time of surgery. Part I of the book deals with the procurement and preparation of bronchial specimens and includes a chapter on fetal development and structure of the normal adult epithelium. In Part II, the histopathology of numerous bronchial diseases are described in detail. Emphasis is placed on the diagnostic features of human lesions which are illustrated by numerous high quality light and electron micrographs. Understanding normal bronchial structure, cell kinetics, and modulations of phenotypic expression provide insight into many pathological processes. Therefore, although emphasis is placed on the diagnostic features of human disease, the histopathology of corresponding lesions in experimental animals is discussed where this provides information helpful in the interpretation of the human lesions.

Elizabeth M. McDowell
Baltimore

Theodore F. Beals
Ann Arbor

1985

Acknowledgments

We give thanks to friends and colleagues who reviewed one or more chapters for us during the writing of this book. We are grateful for their constructive criticisms and comments. Our thanks extend to Björn Afzeluis, Oscar Auerbach, Stephen Chensue, Barry Gusterson, Leopold Koss, Stephen Kunkel, Pat Mastin, Philip Pratt, Victor Roggli, Geno Saccomanno, John Shelburne, Leslie Sobin, Sergei Sorokin and Lee Weatherbee.

We also extend our thanks to Andrew Flint and Bernard Naylor for contributing specimen slides for photography; to Bryan Corrin, Geno Saccomanno, and Julia Polak for providing photomicrographs; and to Douglas Henderson for permission to use tabular material. We also thank Daniel S. Cutler for the three dimensional drawing of a cilium.

We thank Sandra Minton for her help in copy editing and for implementing the telecommunications of the typescript. Finally, our warmest thanks go to Donna Erb for typing the entire manuscript and for seeing us to completion through multiple drafts and rewrites.

Part one:
General considerations

1 Introduction

This book is concerned with pathological lesions of the bronchi and the tissues which immediately surround them. Bronchi are defined as those tubes which lie proximal to the last plate of cartilage along an airway (Chapter 3). Pathological lesions associated with bronchioles, alveoli and other elements of the peripheral lung are not considered in this text. As a general rule the book will discuss those lesions which are within the reach of the fiberoptic bronchoscope.

In this chapter the techniques available for procurement of bronchial biopsies are described. In practice, cytological specimens are nearly always obtained simultaneously, and their procurement will be discussed briefly as well. Furthermore, although the rest of the book is directed specifically to pathology of the bronchi, fine needle aspiration, open lung biopsy and mediastinoscopy are also described briefly, so as to provide the full range of specimen procurement options available and to address the question of their most appropriate use.

1.1 The bronchial tree

The pattern of branching of the bronchi from the trachea outward into the lung parenchyma is more or less constant in different people. It is important to understand this pattern of branching since most pulmonary lesions are focal in nature, that is they occur in only one particular region of the lung. The positioning of a lesion by means of physical signs, x-ray imaging and now with the aid of computed tomography, requires an understanding of the bronchial pattern. Communication with others about the anatomical location of specific disease requires a common nomenclature. With the widespread use of flexible bronchoscopy, a thorough knowledge of the bronchial tree is essential to the bronchoscopists as they search for and localize lesions within the lungs as far distally as the subsegmental bronchi. Careful attention to the specifics of the nomenclature is necessary for the pathologist as well, to insure the correct labeling of specimens and to eliminate ambiguity in reports. Although some variation from the common pattern is seen, a standard system of naming the bronchi to the segmental level is commonly used (Table 1.1). This system uses positional names as well as numerical designations. Fig. 1.1 is a drawing of the most common patterns of branching with the numerical designations for the segmental bronchi as given in Table 1.1. This is an anterior view. The segmental bronchi are labeled 1 through 10 for each of the lungs. Subsegmental designation by lower case letters is also used. As an example, it is therefore possible to label a lesion: endobronchial mass at the bifurcation of the Right B3a and B3b, which would be at the subsegmental carina between the apical and posterior subdivisions of the anterior segmental bronchus of the right upper lobe.

1.2   Bronchoscopic specimens

The rigid bronchoscope was introduced at the turn of the century chiefly as an instrument to aid in the retrieval of aspirated foreign objects. It is a metal tube usually 7 mm in diameter and 40 cm long. Pediatric and various models for special purposes vary in size, generally smaller in diameter and length. Current models include a variety of accessories which allow illumination and magnified visualization of the airways as well as aspiration of secretions, biopsy, brushing, electrobiopsy and cautery. The patient breathes through the tube during examination. As can be imagined the greatest difficulty is that the instrument cannot be made to conform to the angles of the airways, and although flexible biopsy forceps and means to direct the illumination to the sides are available, the airways must be aligned to insert the bronchoscope.

With the development of fiberoptics, this limitation was greatly minimized and Ikeda's introduction of the flexible bronchofiberscope has revolutionized the inspection and sampling of the pulmonary airways (Ikeda *et al.*, 1968). Current instruments allow controlled flexion and

Table 1.1 Bronchial tree

RIGHT	LEFT
Upper lobe	Upper lobe
1. Apical segment	1, 2. Apical-posterior segment
2. Posterior segment	3. Anterior segment
3. Anterior segment	4. Superior lingular segment
Middle lobe	5. Inferior lingular segment
4. Lateral segment	Lower lobe
5. Medial segment	6. Superior segment
Lower lobe	7, 8. Anteromedial basal segment
6. Superior segment	9. Lateral basal segment
7. Medial basal segment	10. Posterior basal segment
8. Anterior basal segment	
9. Lateral basal segment	
10. Posterior basal segment	

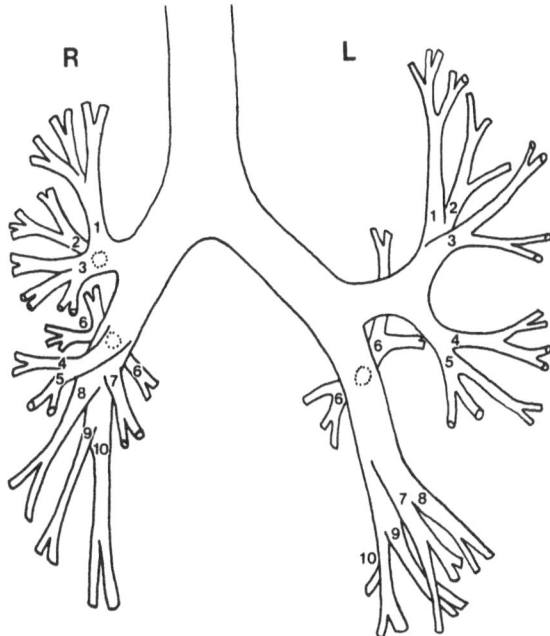

Fig. 1.1 Bronchial pattern of branching as viewed from the anterior. The trachea divides into right and left main bronchi. The right main bronchus gives rise to the bronchus to the upper lobe and continues as the intermediate bronchus. After dividing to provide the bronchus to the middle lobe the intermediate bronchus continues as the inferior bronchus to the right lower lobe. The left main bronchus divides into superior and inferior bronchi. The superior bronchus then divides into an upper divisional bronchus and the lingular bronchus. The inferior bronchus supplies the left lower lobe. Segmental branches are numbered and named according to the system listed in Table 1.1.

extension of the tip of the probe and a flexible main portion which will follow the guided tip as the bronchoscopist advances the scope into predetermined bronchial segments. The range of directional change is controlled by combinations of flexion/extension of the tip and rotation of the entire instrument. The lumen of the bronchus in front of the advancing bronchoscope is illuminated by a light source which is transmitted to the tip of the scope through a bundle of optical fibers. The image, through an angle of about 70°, is likewise transmitted through another bundle of fibers to an ocular which is held in the hand of the bronchoscopist. There is a slight magnification of the mucosa as seen through the ocular.

In general, ventilation during flexible bronchoscopy is accomplished in the airway around the probe. Usually one channel is provided for instilling rinsing solutions, suctioning secretions and introduction of forceps, brushes, needles or coagulation electrodes. Various forceps are available for grasping objects, as well as for taking the biopsy specimen. There is some variation in configuration, size and optical properties from the several manufacturers. Fig. 1.2a shows a standard instrument with two types of biopsy forceps and a brush. Fig. 1.2b is a close-up of the tip in a flexed position showing the extent to which the instrument can be manipulated as various bronchi are approached.

Introduction of the bronchofiberscope into the lower airways can be accomplished by transnasal or transoral approaches. The transoral approach can be directly into the oropharynx or by insertion through an endotracheal tube or a rigid bronchoscope. In the United States the most common approach is transnasal (Sackner, 1975; Harrell, 1978). However, a transoral approach is described by various authors (Zavala, 1975; Sanderson and McDougall, 1978; Oho and Ameniya, 1980). The choice appears to be largely related to training. A high intensity light source is attached to the instrument: this is about the only limitation to its freedom of movement, and examination can be at the patient's bedside. Most procedures, however, are performed in specially designed bronchoscopy units. Fluoroscopy is a significant adjunct and is necessary when the abnormality is focal and more peripherally located. Local anesthesia is usually all that is necessary (Newton and Edwards, 1979). However, for extended examinations such as those needed to localize malignancy in patients with positive sputum cytology and roentgenographic occult lesions, general anesthesia may be necessary (Tahir, 1972; Sanderson et al., 1974).

The principal advantage of the flexible fiberoptic bronchoscope is the ability to reach, visualize and sample abnormality in selected subsegmental bronchi. There is generally high acceptance by the patient; the procedure can be quick and leads to few complications in the hands of an experienced bronchoscopist (Dull, 1980). The procedure has been proven effective in establishing the diagnosis of pulmonary lesions including infections, particularly mycotic (Wallace et al., 1981), bronchogenic neoplasms including early nonvisualized carcinomas (Sanderson et al., 1974; Hayata et al., 1982), metastatic carcinoma to the lung (Mohsenifar et al., 1978),

---

Fig. 1.2 (a) Fiberoptic bronchoscope. One of the commonly used fiberoptic bronchoscopes. The ocular for viewing is on the right at the top. Extending directly down is the fiberoptic bundle from the accessory light supply. The opening to the channel for inserting instruments is the small hole to the left of the ocular. Control for flexion and extension of the tip is situated just above the flattened handle, within reach of the operator's thumb. The flexible portion of the bronchoscope, which extends into the patient, is marked with white bands to indicate the depth of insertion. Two types of biopsy forceps and a bronchial brush are included to show their relative size. (b) Close-up of the tip of the fiberoptic bronchoscope in a partially flexed position. Two types of biopsy forceps and a bronchial brush are also shown at the same magnification.

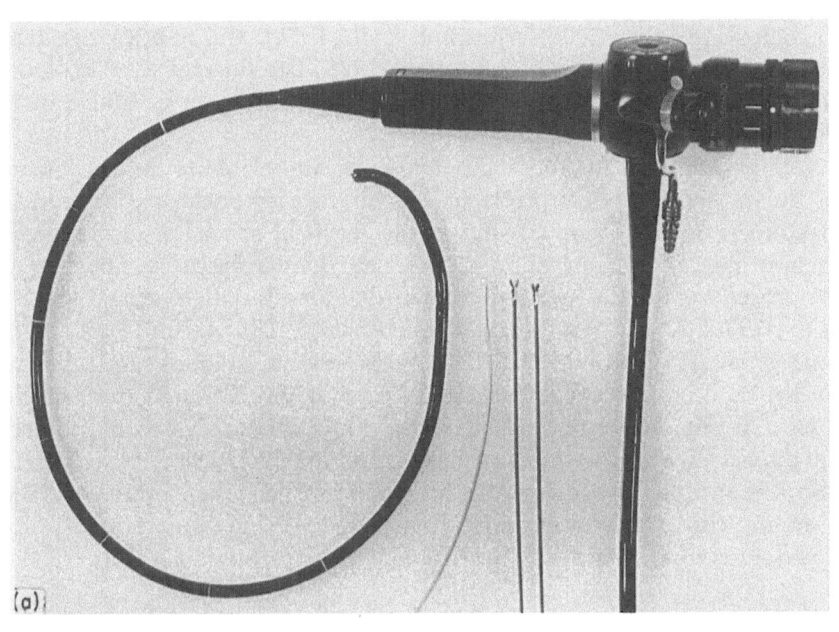

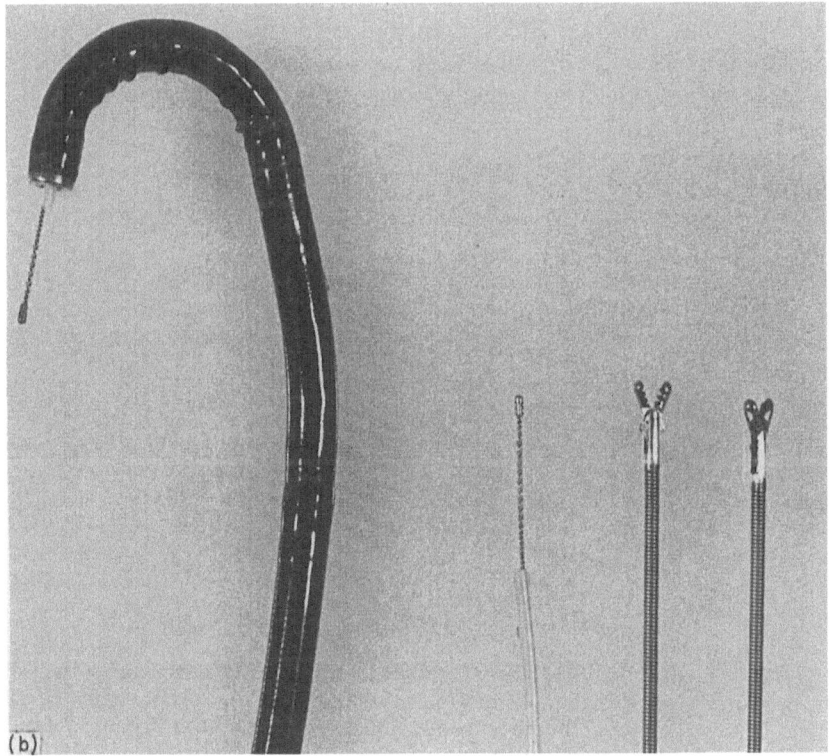

sarcoidosis (Koontz, 1978; Whitcomb *et al.*, 1978), and to a lesser extent diffuse infiltrative diseases (Anderson, 1978; Dreisin *et al.*, 1978). Most would consider it a necessary procedure in the staging of lung cancer (Robbins *et al.*, 1979).

Complications of fiberoptic bronchoscopy are related to the anesthetic, to the presence of the probe in the airways (bronchospasm, cardiac arrythmias and hypoxemia), and to the result of specimen procurement (hemorrhage and pneumothorax). There are deaths directly attributable to the procedure, usually resulting from cardiac arrests or hemorrhage (Suratt *et al.*, 1976; Zavala, 1978a; Wlademir *et al.*, 1978; Dreisin *et al.*, 1978; Luck *et al.*, 1978; Khan, 1978). The rates of complications are less than for the rigid bronchoscope (Lukomsky *et al.*, 1981). For a comprehensive review of bronchoscopy the contributions to a symposium on the subject are published with co-editors Anderson and Faber (1978). Sackner (1975) also has an excellent review. In the remaining sections of this book the term bronchoscopy will mean fiberoptic bronchoscopy unless specifically noted otherwise.

1.2.1   Endobronchial biopsy

Most biopsies obtained during bronchoscopy are from endobronchial lesions. Biopsy is with one of several forceps designed to obtain samples of these lesions which are usually visible to the bronchoscopist. Fig. 1.3

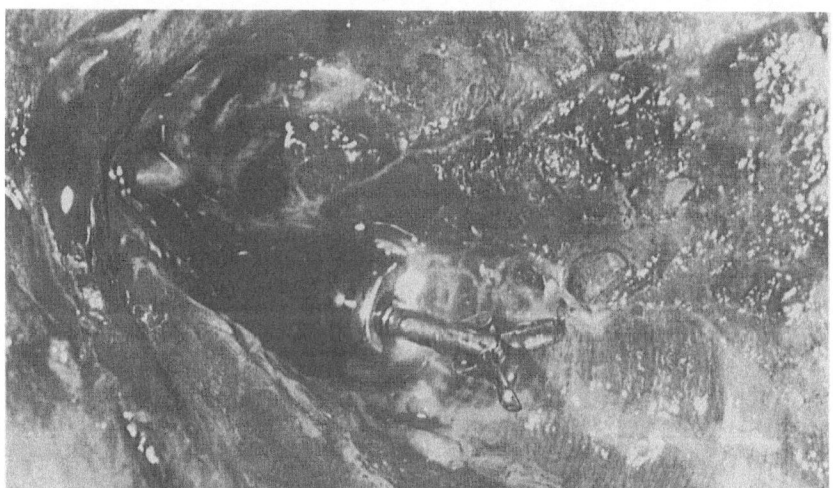

Fig. 1.3 View of the tip of the bronchoscope within a segmental bronchus. The biopsy forceps are extending from the instrument channel. This particular instrument has two fiberoptic bundles for illumination, one on each side of the main channel, visible here as bright spots.

shows a bronchoscope positioned to the level of a subsegmental bronchus. Light from two fiberoptic bundles illuminates the lumen of the bronchus distal to the tip while the biopsy forceps are advanced. The diagnostic yield in these cases is very high particularly when the lesion is neoplastic (Rudd *et al.*, 1982). There is a reduced diagnostic yield on peripheral nodules which require fluoroscopic guidance to insure that the sample is from the lesion (Cortese and McDougall, 1979). The yield is greater with nodules larger than 2 cm in diameter (Radke *et al.*, 1979) and with multiple biopsies (Popovich *et al.*, 1982). There is mechanical distortion of the specimen resulting from the pinching effects of the forceps (Fig. 1.4). These are not 'cutting' in the usual sense; rather the specimen is grasped

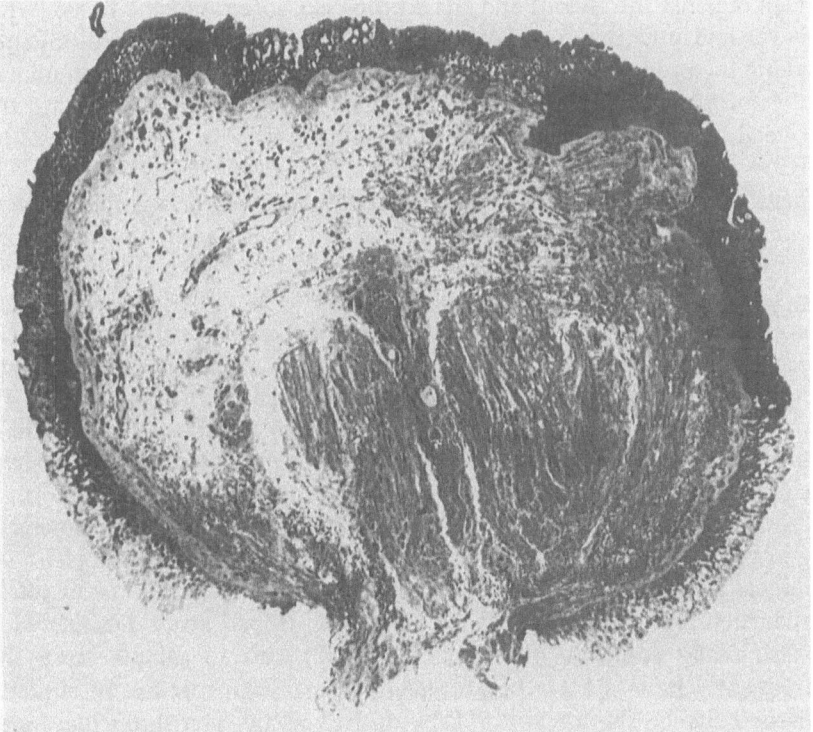

Fig. 1.4 An example of the mechanical distortion caused by the pinching action of the forceps. Respiratory epithelium covers the specimen even into the pinched portion. What appears as a mass in the middle of the specimen is smooth muscle in the lamina propria which is bent back on itself to form a mass rather than the normal flat layer. The pinched portion resembling the neck of a narrow-mouthed vase marks the position of the forcep ends. Notice that rather than cutting the tissue off at this place there is additional tissue which has been torn from the bronchus as the grasping forceps are pulled back. (Epon/Araldite section stained with toluidine blue.)

and torn from the surrounding tissue. Some forceps have holes cut into each of the grasping cups designed to minimize the crushing effect when the specimen is squeezed between the closing cups. It is necessary to withdraw the forceps with the grasped biopsy fragment, and to push the fragment from the cups into an appropriate receptacle (Chapter 2 discusses the proper handling of the specimens). The forceps must then be cleaned and reinserted through the channel of the bronchoscope for the next biopsy. The easiest biopsy is taken from the saddle of a carina, by advancing the open forceps to straddle the bifurcation, and then by grasping and tearing away the tissue. Lesions along the wall of the bronchus are more difficult to acquire. Two techniques are used to collect these lesions. The tip can be flexed so that it pushes against the lateral wall (against the lesion) and the forceps closed around the tissue, which is pushed into the cups. Alternatively, the open forceps are advanced along the bronchial wall which causes a mound of tissue to accumulate in the forcep cup which is pressed against the wall. The forceps are then closed around this 'mass'. Biopsy specimens vary in size from less than 0.5 mm to 5 mm. Size is somewhat limited by the diameter of the instrumentation channel of the bronchoscope which is 2 mm in many commonly used models. Larger pieces can be dragged from the biopsy site by complete withdrawal of the bronchoscope with the forceps and grasped tissue protruding from the tip. This is not a very satisfactory approach because further examination means reinserting the broncho-scope. The smallest specimens are usually from attempts to sample sessile lesions of the bronchus which are difficult to grasp with the forceps. This difficulty is made worse as the bronchoscope is advanced into smaller bronchi where it is virtually impossible to aim the forceps at the wall, since the bronchus simply moves as the tip is flexed. Carina and exophytic lesions are most easily grasped by the forceps. The largest specimens are generally from large (often occluding) friable masses which present easy targets for the forceps. Since the forceps are not designed to cut off the specimen these larger specimens are simply ripped away. Lesions which extrinsically compress the bronchi are difficult to sample since they frequently have a layer of normal or at least nonspecifically abnormal tissue between the forceps and the desired tissue. Transbronchial biopsy or brushing into these masses through tears in the mucosa made with forceps are more successful.

1.2.2   Transbronchial biopsy

The use of transbronchial biopsies, in which the lesion is peribronchial or in lung parenchyma proper, are the subject of continued debate. These specimens are usually taken without endoscopic visualization of abnormality and usually with fluoroscopic localization (Zavala, 1978b). The greatest yields are in diffuse diseases, particularly sarcoidosis, metastatic neoplasms and opportunistic infections (Ellis, 1978; Jenkins *et al.*, 1979; Poe *et al.*, 1979; Haponik *et al.*, 1982).

Particular attention has been addressed to the use of transbronchial biopsy in the immunosuppressed host with progressing pulmonary disease (Cunningham *et al.*, 1977; Katzenstein and Askin, 1980) and in the patient with chronic infiltrative disease (Wall *et al.*, 1981). Increased numbers of biopsies enhance the diagnostic yield (Roethe *et al.*, 1980). Most investigators suggest that transbronchial biopsy with its reduced morbidity, mortality and greater patient acceptance compared with thoracotomy (Section 1.4) is a worthwhile procedure in the evaluation of these patients, particularly when the disease is progressing. The consensus is that if a transbronchial specimen is either nonspecific or nondiagnostic in these patients, an open biopsy should be obtained (Katzenstein and Askin, 1980; Wall *et al.*, 1981; Haponick *et al.*, 1982). Most bronchoscopists would include brushing as an adjunct to biopsy particularly in more peripheral lesions (Section 1.2.3). To obtain tissue the opened forceps are pushed against the bronchial wall and closed while maintaining pressure, so as to force the forceps through the wall into the adjacent parenchyma. The tissue is then torn free and withdrawn through the channel of the bronchoscope.

There is an increased incidence of pneumothorax, hemorrhage and deaths from transbronchial compared to endobronchial biopsies (Anderson *et al.*, 1973; Herf and Suratt, 1978; Anderson, 1978).

1.2.3 Cytology specimens

The cytopathologic evaluation of sputum is a proven noninvasive procedure for detection of malignancy in the airways. Specimens are also frequently collected for cytologic examination at the time of bronchoscopic examination. These include bronchial washings, brushings, lavages and needle aspirates.

(a) Sputum

The specimen should be collected from a deep cough when first waking in the morning. If three such specimens, collected on different days, are examined, it has been shown that 90% of the cases which would ultimately be diagnostic are positive in these specimens (Koss *et al.*, 1964; Erozan and Frost, 1970). Since alveolar macrophages are found in secretions of the distal bronchi, whether the patient is normal or has pulmonary disease, the presence of these cells in sputa is considered an indication that the smear contains cells from the bronchi and not saliva or upper airway secretions. Since the usual reason for examining sputa cytologically is to screen for malignant cells in the lower airways, the presence of alveolar macrophages is used as the criteria of adequacy of the specimen. Although sputa without alveolar macrophages are not adequate for the evaluation of bronchogenic carcinoma, these specimens should always be examined, since malignancies in the oral cavity, pharynx and larynx can also be detected in these specimens. Diagnostic yields of sputum cytology are variable depending on collection and preparation techniques, experience of the cytopathologist and type and location of the malignancy. Sixty to seventy per cent of bronchogenic carcinomas can be diagnosed by sputum cytologic evaluation. The several studies on the early detection of bronchogenic carcinoma indicate that sputum cytologic examination is capable of detecting nonsymptomatic, radiologically occult bronchogenic carcinoma (Pearson et al., 1967; Melamed et al., 1977; Woolner, 1981). Proximal epidermoid (squamous) carcinomas are most readily detected but all forms of benign and malignant bronchogenic neoplasms as well as metastatic malignancies have been diagnosed with cytological preparations. Deep mycoses can be detected in sputa. The common micro-organisms which colonize the upper airways contaminate sputa and the clinical relevance of their presence is questionable.

(b)   Bronchial washings

During the course of the examination secretions are collected from the bronchi and are usually submitted for microbiological culture and cytologic examination, as bronchial washings. These specimens tend to be more or less contaminated with micro-organisms and exfoliated cells from throughout the bronchial tree, but are somewhat more specific than sputa.

(c)   Bronchial brushings

A variety of brushes is available for mechanically removing cells from the bronchi and lesions within lung (Figs 1.5, 1.6). They can be passed directly down the access channel in the bronchoscope, or more commonly passed within an outer plastic sheath so as to minimize contamination both of the brush and the channel. Disposable brushes are now available which make multiple selective brushings practical (Woolner, 1981). Brushings are particularly rewarding when the lesion is proximal and not endoscopically visible (Cortese and McDougall, 1979; Woolner, 1981) and when the lesion is so distal that it is not accessible to the biopsy forceps (Ellis, 1975; Ono et al., 1981; Popovich et al., 1982). Most investigators conclude

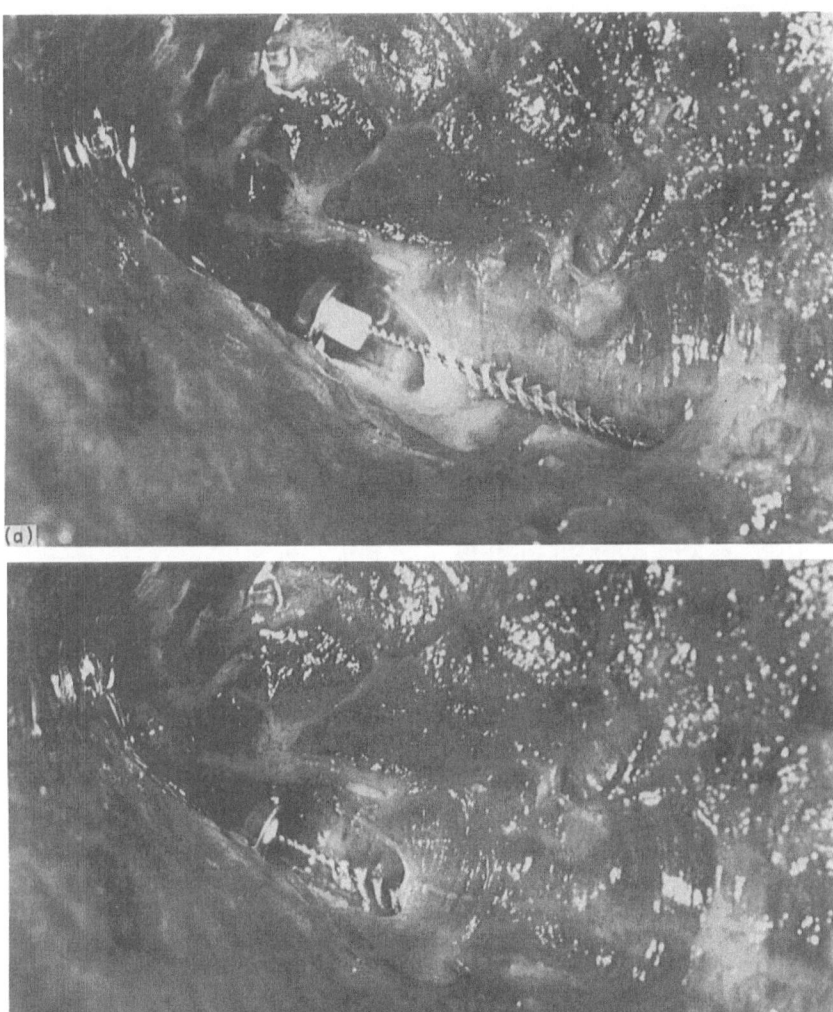

Fig. 1.5 Bronchial brushing. The bronchoscopic brush extends from the tip of the fiberoptic instrument. The plastic sheath, which is used to enclose the brush as it is inserted and withdrawn through the channel of the bronchoscope, can be seen extending from the port. The brush can be used (a) to abrade the surface of lesions visible through the bronchoscope (b) extended with the twisted guide wire into lesions beyond the reach of the bronchoscope or forceps. Once beyond the view of the bronchoscope, accurate positioning of the brush requires fluoroscopic guidance.

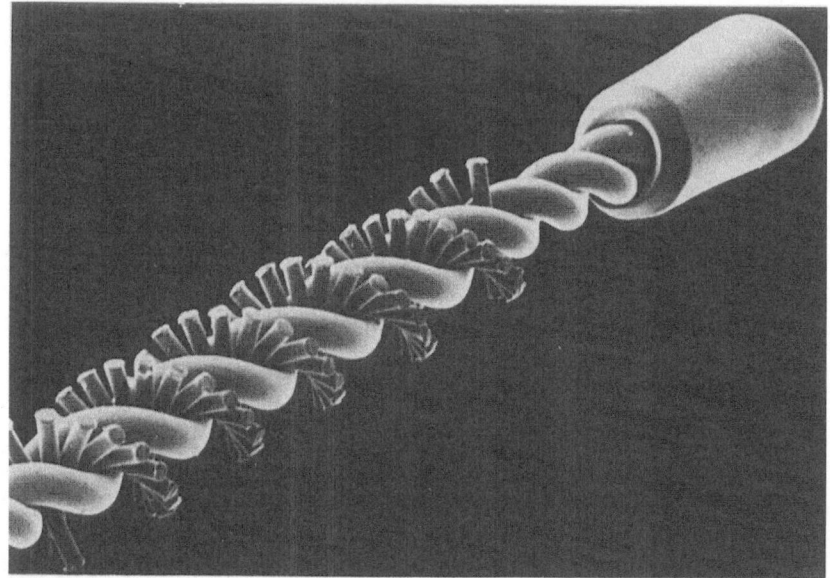

Fig. 1.6 One of the several types of bronchial brushes designed to abrade cells from pulmonary lesions and produce smears for cytologic examination. (Scanning electron micrograph: horizontal field width = 8 mm.)

that bronchial biopsy and brushing are complementary and advocate using both procedures. In a recent study in which catheter aspirates were evaluated as a means of detecting bronchogenic carcinoma, 91% of the neoplasms were diagnosed by brushing, 88% by catheter aspirate and 60% by biopsy (Muers *et al.*, 1982). Bronchial brushing of distal lesions is accompanied by an increased incidence of pneumothorax and parenchymal hemorrhage.

(d) Bronchial lavage

This involves the instillation of physiologic solutions into the distal bronchi and aspiration of the fluid with bronchoalveolar secretions and cells. The specimen is analyzed biochemically, immunologically and by cell counts with differential. The cell counts are made by automatic equipment and air-dried smears are examined with hematologic stains to distinguish the various leukocytes. This technique is being used to better understand the physiologic changes which occur in the lung, as well as during pulmonary disease. Of particular interest have been changes which occur in sarcoidosis and diffuse interstitial disease. To date there are very few clinical applications (Smith, 1981). However, sporadic reports of specific diagnoses have appeared, including histoplasmosis (Finley *et al.*, 1967), pneumocystis pneumonia (Kelley et al., 1978), and alveolar cell carcinoma (Dobbins et al., 1973). An excellent review by Dr Hunninghake and colleagues (Hunninghake et al., 1979) provides additional information and has a very extensive list of references.

(e)   Transbronchial fine needle aspiration

This is another technique with limited diagnostic experience (Buirski et al., 1981; Wang et al., 1981). The lesion is approached with the broncho-scope and a needle is advanced into the lesion under fluoroscopic guid-ance. Aspirated cells are prepared as smears for cytologic examination. The principal application has been with small neoplasms which are beyond the reach of the biopsy forceps or brush but visible radiologically. Me-diastinal adenopathy is within the reach of this technique. There is too little experience with bronchial lavage and transbronchial needle aspira-tion to comment on complications beyond those of the bronchoscopy itself.

1.3   Transthoracic fine needle aspiration

Fine needle aspiration is not a new procedure but it has been reintroduced after extensive experience in Scandinavia (Johansson and Zajicek, 1963; Zajicek, 1965; Nordenström, 1967). A needle (20 to 24 gauge) is introduced into the lesion through the thoracic wall and cells are aspirated into the needle with suction applied with a large syringe. The suction is reduced and the needle withdrawn. The specimen, which consists of a very small drop of tissue fluid, cells and debris, is then sprayed from the needle or dropped onto a glass microscope slide and fixed in alcohol for cytologic staining or air dried for hematologic stains. Exact positioning of the needle is facilitated by fluoroscopy (Sargent et al., 1974; Kaminski, 1981) or by ultrasound (Izumi et al., 1982), which is more useful for pleural-based lesions. Nodular lesions which are large enough to be detected radiograph-ically can be successfully sampled. The greatest diagnostic yield is with peripheral nodules where it is more successful in diagnosing malignancies than transbronchial biopsy or bronchoscopic brushing (Anderson et al., 1973; Zavala, 1978a; Stringfield, 1979). Its diagnostic yield is less with infectious disease (Greenman et al., 1975; Zavala and Schoell, 1981). It is less accurate in correctly diagnosing the cell type of malignancies than bronchoscopy (Rudd et al., 1982) which is probably related to the fact that the cells sampled by fine needle aspiration tend to be more disorganized than in bronchoscopic biopsies and are more often from deeper into a malignant nodule where the cells are frequently degenerated or dead. When the nodule is cavitary it is important to attempt to aim the needle tangentially into the edge of the lesion rather than into the central cavity which may lack diagnostic material. One disadvantage of needle aspiration is the reduced confidence of the specific localization of the lesion in the lung. In the case of operable lesions this could be a handicap and the better localization obtained with bronchoscopy may be required. Specimens for microbiologic and viral culture can be obtained by rinsing the needle with sterile saline. The absence of abnormal cells is difficult to interpret in smears from transthoracic fine needle aspirates particularly with small localized lesions.

Pneumothorax and hemorrhage are the chief complications of fine needle aspiration (Sinner, 1976) and the risk of pneumothorax exceeds that for bronchoscopic transbronchial biopsies or brushings. Ten to twenty per cent of patients will need chest tube drainage to resolve the pneumothorax. Two more serious complications, air embolism (Westcott, 1973) and seeding of the malignant cells along the needle tract, have not been reported with the use of thin needles, 20–24 gauge (Sinner and Zajicek, 1976; Zajicek, 1979), although one example of malignant spread in the chest wall following thin needle aspiration may have been the result of seeding (Kaminsky, 1982).

1.4 Open biopsy

Surgical biopsy (open biopsy) through thoracotomy has the greatest diagnostic yield and is the most specific of the approaches to pulmonary disease (Anderson *et al.*, 1973; Greenman *et al.*, 1975; Ray *et al.*, 1976; Burt *et al.*, 1981). In diffuse pulmonary disease the increased yield and in particular the increased size of the specimen provided by open lung biopsy makes it the procedure of choice (Carrington and Gaensler, 1978; Leight and Michaelis, 1978; Gaensler and Carrington, 1980). Because most surgeons prefer general anesthesia for open biopsy there is an increased risk and morbidity. Therefore, the usual approach is to proceed, as rapidly as the clinical situation warrants, from the least invasive (sputum cytology) through the more invasive bronchoscopic and transthoracic needle approaches. If a specific diagnosis which will allow appropriate treatment is not obtained, one should proceed to open biopsy (Anderson *et al.*, 1973; Leight and Michaelis, 1978; Rossiter *et al.*, 1979; Toledo-Pereyra *et al.*, 1980). The free margin of the lingula and the middle lobe should be avoided even though they are anatomically easily accessible because of an increased incidence of nonspecific chronic inflammatory changes at these sites. When the pathological process is diffuse the surgeon should not biopsy the portion of lung with the most severe changes but should select an abnormal area with evidence of active disease, since the most severely damaged lung may have only end-stage changes, often

Table 1.2 Techniques for obtaining specimens

Technique	Principal uses	Advantages	Limitations
Sputum cytology	Detection of proximal neoplasms and screening of high risk patients	Noninvasive	Not site specific
Bronchoscopy:			
Endobronchial biopsy	Visible endobronchial lesions to the level of subsegmental bronchi	Site specific	Small size of specimens
Transbronchial biopsy	Focal peribronchial lesions	Less invasive than open	Small size of specimens
Bronchial brushings	Adjunct to biopsy for visible superficial lesions, lesions beyond the reach of the forceps and in localizing occult endobronchial neoplasms	Site specific	Small disrupted specimens
Bronchial washings	Adjunct to biopsy and brushings	No additional risk	Not site specific
Bronchial lavage	Inflammatory lesions		Little clinical experience
Transbronchial needle aspiration	Peribronchial masses and infections deep within lung parenchyma	Minimal risk	Little clinical experience
Transthoracic fine needle aspiration	Peripheral neoplastic masses and nonresectable neoplasm not within reach of bronchoscope	Minimal risk	Disrupted intercellular relationships
Mediastinoscopy	Mediastinal lymphadenopathy and staging of bronchogenic carcinoma	Minimal risk	Accessibility of lesion
Open lung biopsy	When other techniques are not definitive	Nearly always adequate tissue for diagnosis	Risk to the patient

nonspecific in character. The reported mortality rate due to thoracotomy and biopsy itself is 0.3–0.4% (Ray *et al.*, 1976; Gaensler and Carrington, 1980).

Thoracoscopic biopsy is another approach to diffuse lung disease. This differs from open biopsy in that an endoscope is used under local anesthesia, to enter the pleural space through a small incision in the thoracic wall. Multiple biopsies can be obtained. Equivalent diagnostic yields to open biopsy with less risk to the patient are reported (Dijkman *et al.*, 1982; Boutin *et al.*, 1982).

Mediastinoscopy allows access to the lymph nodes and masses in the superior mediastinum through an incision in the thoracic wall using some type of endoscope. This is particularly useful in granulomatous diseases and is often used prior to thoracotomy as a means of assessing operability of bronchogenic carcinomas.

Table 1.2 is a summary of the available techniques for obtaining specimens from bronchial and peribronchial lesions. Experience has shown that the greatest success in establishing a clinically relevant diagnosis of lung disease with the least risk to the patient requires consultation and cooperation between the physician in charge of the patient, the pulmonary specialist, the thoracic surgeon and the pathologist. The best approach and method of handling the specimen are related to the nature of the suspected disease and the clinical status of the patient. The time required for consultation, particularly with the pathologist, is usually well spent and may avoid excessive delay in initiating appropriate therapy and unnecessary hardship for the patient. The pathologist must understand the clinical situation when deciding on appropriate special procedures (discussed in the next chapter) and when interpreting the specimens. Inconsistencies between the clinical pattern and the findings from the biopsy also require consultation between the pathologist and the clinicians and may determine that additional specimens are necessary before a meaningful diagnosis can be determined. The pathologist who renders diagnoses without all the pertinent clinical information and the clinician who feels that the pathologist should make an 'objective' diagnosis, that is, without any knowledge of the patient's condition, are hopefully relics of the past and have no place in the current practice of medicine.

References

Anderson, H.A. (1978), Transbronchoscopic lung biopsy for diffuse pulmonary disease. Results in 939 patients. *Chest*, **73**, 734–6.

Anderson, H.A. and Faber, L.P. (1978), Diagnostic and therapeutic applications of the bronchoscope. Partial Proceedings of World Conference on Bronchoscopy. *Chest*, **73**, 685–778.

Anderson, H.A., Miller, W.E. and Bernatz, P.E. (1973), Lung biopsy: transbronchoscopic, percutaneous open. *Surg. Clin. No. Am.*, **53**, 785–93.

Boutin, C., Viallat, J.R., Cargnino, P. and Rey, F. (1982), Thoracoscopic lung biopsy: experimental and clinical preliminary study. *Chest*, **82**, 44–8.

Buirski, G., Calverley, P.M.A., Douglas, N.J., Lamb, D., McIntyre, M., Sudlow, M.F. and White, H. (1981), Bronchial needle aspiration in the diagnosis of bronchial carcinoma. *Thorax*, **36**, 508–11.

Burt, M.E., Flye, M.W., Webber, B.L. and Wesley, R.A. (1981), Prospective evaluation of aspiration needle, cutting needle, transbronchial and open lung biopsy in patients with pulmonary infiltrates. *Ann. Thorac. Surg.*, **32**, 146–53.

Carrington, C.B. and Gaensler, E.A. (1978), Clinical-pathologic approach to diffuse infiltrative lung disease. In *The Lung. Structure, Function and Disease* (eds W.M. Thurlbeck and M.R. Abell), Williams & Wilkins, Baltimore, pp. 58–87.

Cortese, D.A. and McDougall, J.C. (1979), Biopsy and brushing of peripheral lung cancer with fluoroscopic guidance. *Chest*, **75**, 141–5.

Cunningham, J.H., Zavala, D.C., Corry, R.J. and Keim, L.W. (1977), Trephine air drill, bronchial brush and fiberoptic transbronchial lung biopsies in immunosuppressed patients. *Am. Rev. Respir. Dis.*, **115**, 213–20.

Dijkman, J.H., van der Meer, J.W.M., Bakker, W., Wever, A.M.J. and van der Broek, P.J. (1982), Transpleural lung biopsy by the thoracoscopic route in patients with diffuse interstitial pulmonary disease. *Chest*, **82**, 76–83.

Dobbins, P.K., Swenson, E.W., Hackett, R.L. and Coalson, J.J. (1973), Alveolar cell carcinoma. Diagnosis by lobar lavage. *Am. Rev. Respir. Dis.*, **107**, 665–9.

Dreisin, R.B., Albert, R.K., Talley, P.A., Krygger, M.H., Scoggin, C.H. and Zwillich, C.W. (1978), Flexible fiberoptic bronchoscopy in the teaching hospital. Yield and complications. *Chest*, **74**, 144–9.

Dull, W.L. (1980), Flexible fiberoptic bronchoscopy: an analysis of proficiency. *Chest*, **77**, 65–7.

Ellis, J.H., Jr. (1975), Transbronchial lung biopsy via the fiberoptic bronchoscope. Experience with 107 consecutive cases and comparison with bronchial brushing. *Chest*, **68**, 524–32.

Ellis, J.H., Jr. (1978), Diagnosis of opportunistic infections using the flexible fiberoptic bronchoscope. *Chest*, **73**, 713–15.

Erozan, Y.S. and Frost, J.K. (1970), Cytopathologic diagnosis of cancer in pulmonary material: a critical histopathologic correlation. *Acta Cytol.*, **14**, 560–5.

Finley, T.N., Swenson, E.W., Curran, W.S., Huber, G.L. and Ladman, A.J. (1967), Bronchopulmonary lavage in normal subjects and patients with obstructive lung disease. *Ann. Int. Med.*, **66**, 651–8.

Gaensler, E.A. and Carrington, C.B. (1980), Open biopsy for chronic diffuse infiltrative lung disease: clinical, roentgenographic and physiological correlations in 502 patients. *Ann. Thorac. Surg.*, **30**, 411–26.

Greenman, R.L., Goddall, P.T. and King, D. (1975), Lung biopsy in immunocompromised hosts. *Am. J. Med.*, **59**, 488–96.

Haponik, E.F., Summer, W.R., Terry, P.B. and Wang, K.P. (1982), Clinical decision making with transbronchial lung biopsies. The value of nonspecific histologic examination. *Am. Rev. Respir. Dis.*, **125**, 524–9.

Harrell, J.H., II (1978), Transnasal approach for fiberoptic bronchoscopy. *Chest*, **73**, 704–6.

Hayata, Y., Kato, H., Konata, C., Ono, J., Matsushima, Y., Yoneyama, K. and Nishimiya, K. (1982), Fiberoptic bronchoscopic laser photoradiation for tumor localization in lung cancer. *Chest*, **82**, 10–14.

Herf, S.M. and Suratt, P.M. (1978), Complications of transbronchial lung biopsies. *Chest*, **73**, 759–60.

Hunninghake, G.W., Gadek, J.E., Kawanami, O., Ferrans, V.J. and Crystal, R.G.

(1979), Inflammatory and immune processes in the human lung in health and disease: evaluation by bronchoalveolar lavage. *Am. J. Pathol.*, **97**, 149–90.

Ikeda, S., Yanai, N. and Ishikawa, S. (1968), Flexible bronchofiberscope. *Keio J. Med.*, **17**, 1–16.

Izumi, S., Tamaki, S., Natori, H. and Kira, S. (1982), Ultrasonically guided aspiration needle biopsy in disease of the chest. *Am. Rev. Respir. Dis.*, **125**, 460–4.

Jenkins, R., Myerowitz, R.L., Kavic, T. and Slasky, S. (1979), Diagnostic yield of transbronchoscopic biopsies. *Am. J. Clin. Pathol.*, **72**, 926–30.

Johansson, B. and Zajicek, J. (1963), Sampling of cell material from human tumours by aspiration biopsy. *Nature*, **200**, 1333–4.

Kaminsky, D.B. (1981), In *Aspiration Biopsy for the Community Hospital*, Masson, New York.

Kaminsky, D.B. (1982), Personal communication.

Katzenstein, A.-L.A. and Askin, F.B. (1980), Interpretation and significance of pathologic findings in transbronchial lung biopsy. *Am. J. Surg. Pathol.*, **4**, 223–34.

Kelley, J., Landis, J.N., Davis, G.S., Trainer, T.D., Jakab, G.J. and Green, G.M. (1978), Diagnosis of pneumonia due to pneumocystis by subsegmental pulmonary lavage via the fiberoptic bronchoscope. *Chest*, **74**, 24–8.

Khan, M.A. (1978), Fiberoptic bronchoscopy revisited. *Chest*, **74**, 119–20.

Koontz, C.H. (1978), Lung biopsy in sarcoidosis. *Chest*, **74**, 120–1.

Koss, L.G., Melamed, M.R. and Goodner, J.T. (1964), Pulmonary cytology--a brief survey of diagnostic results from July 1st, 1952 until December 31st, 1960. *Acta Cytol.*, **8**, 104–13.

Leight, G.S., Jr. and Michaelis, L.L. (1978), Open lung biopsy for the diagnosis of acute, diffuse pulmonary infiltrates in the immunosuppressed patient. *Chest*, **73**, 477–82.

Luck, J.C., Messeder, O.H., Rubenstein, M.J., Morrissey, W.L. and Engel, T.R. (1978), Arrhythmias from fiberoptic bronchoscopy. *Chest*, **74**, 139–43.

Lukomsky, G.I., Ovchinnikov, A.A. and Bilal, A. (1981), Complications of bronchoscopy: comparison of rigid bronchoscopy under general anesthesia and flexible fiberoptic bronchoscopy under topical anesthesia. *Chest*, **79**, 316–21.

Melamed, M., Flehinger, B., Miller, D., Osborne, R., Zaman, M., McGinnis, C. and Martini, N. (1977), Preliminary report of the lung cancer detection program in New York. *Cancer*, **39**, 369–82.

Mohsenifar, Z., Chopra, S.K. and Simmons, D.H. (1978), Diagnostic value of fiberoptic bronchoscopy in metastatic pulmonary tumors. *Chest*, **74**, 369–71.

Muers, M.F., Boddington, M.M., Cole, M., Murphy, D. and Spriggs, A.I. (1982), Cytological sampling of fiberoptic bronchoscopy: comparison of catheter aspirates and brush biopsies. *Thorax*, **37**, 457–61.

Newton, D.A.G. and Edwards, G.F. (1979), Route of introduction and method of anesthesia for fiberoptic bronchoscopy. *Chest*, **75**, 650.

Nordenström, B. (1967), Transthoracic needle biopsy. *New Engl. J. Med.*, **276**, 1081–2.

Oho, K. and Amemiya, R. (1980), In *Practical Fiberoptic Bronchoscopy*, Igaku-Shoin, Tokyo.

Ono, R., Loke, J. and Ikeda, S. (1981), Bronchofiberscopy with curette biopsy and bronchography in the evaluation of peripheral lung lesions. *Chest*, **79**, 162–6.

Pearson, F.G., Thompson, D.W. and Delarue, N.C. (1967), Experience with cytologic detection, localization and treatment of radiographically undemonstrable bronchial carcinoma. *J. Thorac. Cardiovasc. Surg.*, **54**, 371–82.

Poe, R.H., Utell, M.J., Israel, R.H., Hall, W.J. and Eshleman, J.D. (1979), Sensitivity and specificity of the nonspecific transbronchial lung biopsy. *Am. Rev. Respir. Dis.*, **119**, 25–31.

Popovich, J., Jr., Kvale, P.A., Eichenhorn, M.S., Radke, J.R., Ohorodnik, J.M. and Fine, G. (1982), Diagnostic accuracy of multiple biopsies from flexible fiberoptic bronchoscopy. A comparison of central versus peripheral carcinoma. *Am. Rev. Respir. Dis.*, **125**, 521–3.

Radke, J.R., Conway, W.A., Eyler, W.R. and Kvale, P.A. (1979), Diagnostic accuracy in peripheral lung lesions. Factors predicting success with flexible fiberoptic bronchoscopy. *Chest*, **76**, 176–9.

Ray, J.F.M., Lawton, B.R., Myers, W.O., Toyama, W.M., Reyes, C.N., Emannel, D.A., Burns, J.L., Pederson, D.P., Dovenbarger, W.V., Wenzel, F.J. and Sautter, R.D. (1976), Open pulmonary biopsy. Nineteen years experience with 416 consecutive operations. *Chest*, **69**, 43–7.

Robbins, H.M., Morrison, D.A., Sweet, M.E., Solomon, D.A. and Goldman, A.L. (1979), Biopsy of the main carina. Staging lung cancer with the fiberoptic bronchoscope. *Chest*, **75**, 484–6.

Roethe, R.A., Fuller, P.B., Byrd, R.B. and Hafermann, D.R. (1980), Transbronchoscopic lung biopsy in sarcoidosis. Optimal number and sites for diagnosis. *Chest*, **77**, 400–2.

Rossiter, S.J., Miller, D.C., Churg, A.M., Carrington, C.B. and Mark, J.B.D. (1979), Lung biopsy in the immunosuppressed patient. Is it really beneficial? *J. Thorac. Cardiovasc. Surg.*, **77**, 338–45.

Rudd, R.M., Gellert, A.R., Boldy, D., Studdy, P.R., Pearson, M.C., Geddes, D.M. and Sinha, G. (1982), Bronchoscopic and percutaneous aspiration biopsy in the diagnosis of bronchial carcinoma cell type. *Thorax*, **37**, 462–5.

Sackner, M.A. (1975), Bronchofiberscopy. *Am. Rev. Respir. Dis.*, **111**, 62–88.

Sanderson, D.R., Fontana, R.S., Woolner, L.B., Bernatz, P.E. and Payne, W.S. (1974), Bronchoscopic localization of radiographically occult lung cancer. *Chest*, **65**, 608–12.

Sanderson, D.R. and McDougall, J.C. (1978), Transoral bronchofiberoscopy. *Chest*, **73**, 701–3.

Sargent, E.N., Turner, A.F., Gordonson, J., Schwinn, C.P. and Pashky, O. (1974), Percutaneous pulmonary needle biopsy. Report of 350 patients. *Am. J. Roentgenol. Rad. Therapy Nuclear Med.*, **122**, 758–68.

Sinner, W.N. (1976), Complications of percutaneous transthoracic needle aspiration biopsy. *Acta Radiol. Diag.*, **17**, 813–28.

Sinner, W.N. and Zajicek, J. (1976), Implantation metastasis after percutaneous transthoracic needle aspiration biopsy. *Acta Radiol. Diag.*, **17**, 473–80.

Smith, L.J. (1981), Bronchoalveolar lavage today. *Chest*, **80**, 251–2.

Stringfield, J.T., III (1979), Fiberoptic bronchoscopy. Some questions. *Chest*, **76**, 121.

Suratt, P.M., Smiddy, J.F. and Gruber, B. (1976), Deaths and complications associated with fiberoptic bronchoscopy. *Chest*, **69**, 747–51.

Tahir, A.H. (1972), General anesthesia for bronchofiberscopy. *Anesthesiol.*, **37**, 564–6.

Toledo-Pereyra, L.H., DeMeester, T.R., Kinealey, A., MacMahon, H., Churg, A. and Golomb, H. (1980), The benefits of open lung biopsy in patients with previous non-diagnostic transbronchial lung biopsy. A guide to appropriate therapy. *Chest*, **77**, 647–50.

Wall, C.P., Gaensler, E.A., Carrington, C.B. and Hayes, J.A. (1981), Comparison of transbronchial and open biopsies in chronic infiltrative lung disease. *Am. Rev.*

Respir. Dis., **123**, 280–5.

Wallace, J.M., Catanzaro, A., Moser, K.M. and Harrell, J.H., II (1981), Flexible fiberoptic bronchoscopy for diagnosing pulmonary coccidioidomycosis. *Am. Rev. Respir. Dis.*, **123**, 286–90.

Wang, K.P., Marsh, B.R., Summer, W.R., Terry, P.B., Erozan, Y.S. and Baker, R.R. (1981), Transbronchial needle aspiration for diagnosis of lung cancer. *Chest*, **80**, 48–50.

Westcott, J.L. (1973), Air embolism complicating percutaneous needle biopsy of the lung. *Chest*, **63**, 108–10.

Whitcomb, M.E., Domby, W.R., Hawley, P.C. and Kataria, Y.P. (1978), The role of fiberoptic bronchoscopy in the diagnosis of sarcoidosis. *Chest*, **74**, 205–8.

Wlademir, P., Jr., Kovnat, D.M. and Snider, G.L. (1978), A prospective cooperative study of complications following flexible fiberoptic bronchoscopy. *Chest*, **73**, 813–16.

Woolner, L.B. (1981), Recent advances in pulmonary cytology: early detection and localization of occult lung cancer in symptomless males. In *Advances in Clinical Cytology* (eds L.G. Koss and D.V. Coleman), Butterworths, London, pp. 95–135.

Zajicek, J. (1965), Sampling of cells from human tumours by aspiration biopsy for diagnosis and research. *Europ. J. Cancer*, **1**, 253–8.

Zajicek, J. (1979), The aspiration biopsy smear. In *Diagnostic Cytology and its Histopathologic Bases*, 3rd edn (ed. L.G. Koss), Lippincott, Philadelphia, pp. 1009–11.

Zavala, D.C. (1975), Diagnostic fiberoptic bronchoscopy. Techniques and results of biopsy in 600 patients. *Chest*, **68**, 12–19.

Zavala, D.C. (1978a), Complications following fiberoptic bronchoscopy. The 'good news' and the 'bad news'. *Chest*, **73**, 783–5.

Zavala, D.C. (1978b), Transbronchial biopsy in diffuse lung disease. *Chest*, **73**, 727–33.

Zavala, D.C. and Schoell, J.E. (1981), Ultrathin needle aspiration of the lung in infectious and malignant disease. *Am. Rev. Respir. Dis.*, **123**, 125–31.

2 Preparation of specimens

2.1 How should the biopsy be fixed?

Careful handling of the biopsy specimen and a basic understanding of the preparative procedures that will be used are essential for optimal preservation of chemical composition and hence morphological detail of the tissue. Pathologists are becoming increasingly aware that routine light microscopic examination of histological sections, or of cytological preparations of exfoliated cells, is often inadequate to make a definitive diagnosis. Additional approaches such as immunocytochemistry and electron microscopy are powerful tools which are being used with increasing frequency, not only for research but also for diagnostic purposes. Since most bronchial biopsies are very small it would be ideal if a fixative-embedding combination was available that would render tissues suitable for sectioning for both light and electron microscopy, as well as permitting routine and special light microscopical stains including immunocytochemistry, as well as those stains required for electron microscopy. So far a fixative-embedding combination suitable for all methodologies for use on a routine everyday basis has not been forthcoming, although it is likely that such methodologies will be developed in the future.

When ancillary approaches are anticipated in addition to routine light microscopy, the pathologist must make a careful decision at the time the specimen is processed. If there is enough biopsy material from a given lesion to allow several tissue blocks to be processed in the various different ways that are most suitable for the particular methodologies contemplated, the separate pieces can be handled individually.

Appropriate preparation is the cornerstone for any histological, cytochemical or immunocytochemical study and if several methodologies are planned it is unlikely that any one method will be ideal for all of them. Therefore, if the specimen is abundant it can be divided into several parts. One part can be stored unfixed in liquid nitrogen and the remaining parts can each be fixed in a different fixative. Phosphate buffered formaldehyde (Carson *et al.*, 1973) is recommended for routine light microscopy but if demonstration of antigens by immunocytochemistry is desired, alternative fixatives may be more satisfactory. Different fixative solutions exhibit markedly different effects on immunoreactivity and no one fixative is ideal for demonstration of all antigens. Although buffered formaldehyde, with or without low concentration of glutaraldehyde, is satisfactory for demonstration of many antigens, antigenicity may be diminished or even inactivated, especially if the glutaraldehyde concentration exceeds 1%. Greater immunoreactivity may be preserved by coagulative fixation with 100% ethanol or by fixatives containing picric acid or heavy metals (Banks, 1979; Mukai and Rosai, 1980; Montero, 1981). Detailed accounts of different fixatives suitable for immunocytochemistry are given by Brandzaeg (1982) and Grzanna (1982). Glutaraldehyde at 3% concentration or mixtures of formaldehyde and glutaraldehyde are the fixatives of choice for electron microscopy.

Although potentially rewarding, fixing the specimen in several different fixatives is cumbersome and consumes valuable technical time. Furthermore, the biopsy specimen is often so small that only one or two pieces are available. Moreover, the specific lesion may be represented in only one, or a portion of one, of these pieces. In these cases the tissue must be prepared in such a way that most or all of the techniques required can be performed on one tissue block. There is clearly a need for simplified methods of tissue preparation and some compromise measures are available, as described in Section 2.2.

Nearly all cytology specimens should be fixed in alcohol. These include sputa, bronchial washings and brushings, lavages and fine needle aspirates. Ethanol, in concentrations of 70–95%, gives the preferred nuclear and cytoplasmic characteristics (Keebler and Reagan, 1975), although methanol, isopropanol and gin have been proposed as alternatives. Specific fixation procedures for cytology specimens are given in detail in Section 2.4.

2.2   Practical fixatives for combined light and electron microscopy

The rapidly increasing use of immunoperoxidase techniques at the light microscopic level and the value of the electron microscope in diagnostic problems require that routine fixation practices provide tissues suitably prepared for all contingencies, even after prolonged storage of the tissues in the fixative solution at room temperature.

Until recently it was a widely accepted practice to prepare tissue specifically for electron microscopic study, when this approach was contemplated. Implicit was the myth that if tissue was not removed extremely rapidly from the body, chopped into minute pieces and fixed immediately in chilled fixative, it would render little or no scientific information. Although the delay between removal of tissue and fixation should be as short as possible, the urgency for instant fixation is less than is often

supposed. For example, liver held for 3 hours at room temperature prior
to fixation was almost indistinguishable from that fixed immediately
(Rømert and Matthiessen, 1981), and even after 10 hours the fine structure
was surprisingly well preserved (Ito, 1962). In fact, liver and kidney kept
at 20°C for 24 hours revealed comparatively slight alterations in all of the
organelles (Ericsson et al., 1967). However, marked autolytic changes
occur rapidly if tissues are kept at 37°C (Trump et al., 1962; Bassi and
Bernelli-Zazzera, 1964; Trump et al., 1965; Osvaldo et al., 1965; Latta et
al., 1965). Thus, the rate of autolytic change decreases as the temperature
approaches the freezing point of water, and whenever possible tissues
should be stored at 4°C after removal from the body if fixation has to be
delayed for any reason. Tissues must also be prevented from drying and
on no account should tissues be frozen prior to fixation.

It is well known that glutaraldehyde has superior cross-linking properties compared to formaldehyde (Bowes and Cater, 1965) and great advances were made when Sabatini and co-workers recommended glutaraldehyde as the primary fixative for ultrastructural studies (Sabatini et al.,
1963, 1964). Glutaraldehyde has been advocated by some for light microscopy, but it has major disadvantages. This fixative penetrates very
slowly into tissue, approximately 0.7 mm in 3 hours, leaving the central
area unfixed for long periods of time (Hayat, 1981a). If the specimen is
large, this will allow autolysis to occur (Ericsson and Biberfeld, 1967;
Chambers et al., 1968). Glutaraldehyde-fixed tissues embedded in paraffin
are frequently brittle and harder to section than specimens fixed in
formaldehyde. In addition, the periodic acid-Schiff (PAS) reaction can be
obscured by false staining introduced by free aldehyde groups when
glutaraldehyde is used at or above a 2% concentration. Special procedures
such as dimedone blocking are required prior to PAS staining to prevent
this artefact (Chayen et al., 1969). Furthermore, eosinophilia is enhanced
with hematoxylin and eosin (H&E) staining, causing sections to appear
overstained. Glutaraldehyde in concentrations above 1% has further disadvantages. Because of the avidity with which this fixative cross links
proteins, the activity of some enzymes is destroyed and antigenicity is
diminished, thereby compromising some enzymatic and immunocytochemical studies.

Formaldehyde is suitable for preservation of the activity of many
antigens (Falini and Taylor, 1983) but commercial formaldehyde, as used
in routine histology laboratories has been contraindicated as a fixative for
ultrastructural studies because it contains 12–15% methanol, which potentially can act as a coagulative fixative and a protein denaturant (Pease,
1964). Instead, solutions of paraformaldehyde in appropriate buffers have
been recommended (Lynn et al., 1966; Carson et al., 1972). These solutions
are expensive and cumbersome to prepare and are unstable with storage.

A re-evaluation of fixation by commercial formaldehyde (containing methanol) by Carson *et al.* (1973) showed that 4% commercial formaldehyde (4F) in a modified Millonig's phosphate buffer provided acceptable fixation for ultrastructural studies. Paraformaldehyde fixation was *not* superior. The recommended phosphate buffered 4F fixative is quite adequate for electron microscopy, and ultrastructural preservation remains satisfactory after prolonged storage in fixative at room temperature. Even better ultrastructural preservation can be achieved by using a mixture of 4% formaldehyde and 1% glutaraldehyde (4F-1G) (McDowell and Trump, 1976; McDowell, 1978). Both fixatives (4F and 4F-1G) will give easy and satisfactory preservation for routine automated histological processing, yet still permit demonstration of many antigenic moieties present in bronchial and bronchial-related tissues. Details of preparation and use of these fixatives are given below.

The low concentration of glutaraldehyde (1%) does not appear to diminish antigenicity appreciably more than 4F alone, and in our hands, results with 4F and 4F-1G fixatives have been comparable for several antigens. However, if immunocytochemical studies are to be used to demonstrate an antigen such as keratin protein that is known to be particularly sensitive to aldehyde fixation, it is important that a piece of tissue be fixed in ethanol or another suitable fixative for light microscopic study. Unfortunately, tissue fixed in this way is often quite unsuitable for electron microscopy. Further comments on fixation for electron microscopy and immunocytochemistry are given by Bullock (1984).

2.2.1   *4% phosphate buffered formaldehyde (4F) (Carson et al., 1973)*

1.86 g $NaH_2PO_4.H_2O$
0.42 g NaOH
90 ml water
10 ml 40% commercial formaldehyde

The final pH should be 7.2. The osmolality of the buffer alone, *exclusive of the formaldehyde*, is 290 mosm, which is near to that of plasma and is considerably higher than that of the buffer used in conventional neutral formalin which is still used in many laboratories.

No special techniques need be adopted when fixing specimens for combined light and electron microscopy using this fixative. Tissue sections are fixed by immersion at room temperature and should not exceed 4 mm in thickness. The minimum fixation time recommended is 6 hours. If ultrastructural studies are planned in advance, it is advisable to fix 1 mm thick slices of tissue for electron microscopy and larger pieces for routine light microscopy. However, satisfactory ultrastructural preservation occurs at the periphery of larger tissue blocks, and 1 mm slices may be shaved from a surface that was initially exposed to the fixative and prepared for electron microscopy.

Ultrastructural preservation appears unchanged after storage of tissues in this fixative in air-tight containers at room temperature for many years. However, storage of formaldehyde-fixed specimens in 70% ethanol is unsatisfactory; after 8 weeks of storage membranes appear focally discontinuous and indistinct at the ultrastructural level. Another disadvantage of storage in ethanol is that eosinophilia is much enhanced with time and H&E-stained paraffin sections of alcohol-stored tissues are displeasing.

2.2.2   4% formaldehyde-1% glutaraldehyde (4F-1G) (McDowell and Trump, 1976)

1.16 g $NaH_2PO_4.H_2O$
0.27 g NaOH
88 ml H_2O
10 ml 40% formaldehyde
2 ml 50% glutaraldehyde

The final pH should be 7.2. The osmolality of the buffer alone, *exclusive of the aldehydes*, is 176 mosm.

Although this fixative gives superior ultrastructural preservation, some precautions are necessary. The fixative is *not* stable at room temperature. Over a period of 4 to 8 weeks the pH falls 0.2–0.3 units and the solution becomes cloudy due to formation of a precipitate. If used at this stage, the fixative gives satisfactory results for light microscopy. There is some deterioration of ultrastructural preservation. To prevent this, the fixative should be made up weekly, if stored at room temperature. If stored at 4°C it is stable for approximately 3 months. Once the tissue is fixed it can be stored in the same fixative at room temperature for many years without detrimental effects.

Glutaraldehyde is a larger molecule than formaldehyde and does not penetrate tissues as deeply or as rapidly as formaldehyde. Thus, in 24 hours the glutaraldehyde component penetrates only 1.8 mm, whereas formaldehyde penetrates some 6 mm. In addition, the overall depth of penetration of the aldehyde mixture is less than with formaldehyde alone. Therefore, when using 4F-1G, tissue blocks should not be more than 3 mm thick so that the whole block will be penetrated evenly by both aldehydes. The minimum fixation time recommended is 6 hours. Eosinophilia is enhanced to a pleasing degree in H&E-stained sections when compared with formaldehyde fixation alone. If larger tissue blocks are used (up to 1 cm thick), only the outer shell will be fixed by both aldehydes, whereas the center will be fixed by formaldehyde alone. If ultrastructural studies are planned in advance, it is advisable to fix slices only 1 mm thick. If larger tissue blocks are being used, the outer 0.5 mm may be shaved from the surface.

Cells suspended in fluids, such as sputa, bronchial washings and lavages are fixed very rapidly in either of these fixatives (4F and 4F-1G) and are preserved satisfactorily for combined light and electron microscopic study (see Section 2.4 for further processing of these specimens). It should be remembered, however, that these fixatives will alter the cytological appearance of the cells and alcoholic fixation is necessary to properly evaluate specimens for cytopathology.

There is no doubt that the overall quality of routine light microscopy will be increased by the use of either 4F or 4F-1G fixatives. Many of the problems assumed to be the result of autolysis may result from poor fixation as occurs with unbuffered or insufficiently buffered fixatives. The commonly used neutral buffered formalin is quite hypotonic in ions other than formaldehyde which is osmotically inactive (Carson et al., 1973).

2.3   Preparation of specimens for light microscopic histopathology

Sections cut from tissue embedded in paraffin are generally all that is required for light microscopic examination of the bronchial biopsy. Occasionally in older patients some of the cartilage may be partially calcified. Very brief decalcification should be used when this is discovered. Without decalcification the paraffin-embedded material will cut very poorly and the sections will be difficult to evaluate. This is less of a problem when embedding in plastic (Section 2.3.2). For very small specimens trimming is best done using a dissecting microscope (Section 2.5.1). The specimen should be wetted with fixative all the time during trimming and should never be allowed to dry out. Correct orientation of the specimen is important, so that histological sections include epithelium cut parallel to the long axes of the columnar cells and at right angles to the basal lamina. When the biopsy is small, with no tissue to spare, the pathologist may prefer to orient the tissue personally in the embedding medium. The mucosal surface can be seen as a smooth, often glistening face of the specimen, whereas the deeper tissues are usually pinched and irregular (see Chapter 1; Fig. 1.4).

2.3.1   Embedding in paraffin

Different Autotechnicon schedules have been tested to determine which give the best results for preparation of paraffin sections fixed 4F-1G. Good results have been obtained with a schedule utilizing alcohol and xylene; the paraffin-embedded tissues are easy to cut and free from knife chatter. The following schedule has proven satisfactory: 70% ethanol (2–3 hours); 95% ethanol (3 changes, 30 minutes each); 100% ethanol (1 change,

30 minutes); 100% ethanol (2 changes, 1 hour each); xylene (2 changes, 1 hour each). In all cases embedding is completed in two changes of paraffin (about 1 hour each at 60°C). Intermittently poor quality blocks occur if processed using an alcohol-acetone-xylene schedule. Splitting of the sections, knife chatter, and some tissue shrinkage have been seen with this sequence. If this occurs, collection of the paraffin sections onto iced water rather than warm water may minimize the effect.

2.3.2   Embedding in glycol methacrylate

When a special need arises high resolution light microscopy can be achieved using tissues dehydrated in an alcohol series and embedded in glycol methacrylate (Ruddell, 1967a, b; Sorokin and Hoyt, 1978). Two-micron thick sections, cut with glass knives, can be stained with most of the routine and special stains, including immunoperoxidase methods, that are commonly applied to paraffin sections (Kennedy and Little, 1974; Bennett et al., 1976; Brinn and Pickett, 1979; Sorokin et al., 1981; Moosavi et al., 1981). The sections are very informative because of the high resolution they afford (Fig. 2.1).

2.3.3   Routine and special stains

Hematoxylin and eosin stains, as well as Alcian blue (pH 2.5)-PAS (AB-PAS) stains with and without diastase digestion (Mowry and Winkler, 1956), should be prepared routinely on all biopsy tissues. If the biopsy is small, such as a needle biopsy, it is recommended that step sections be made through the entire tissue. Every third slide is stained with H&E for initial screening. The remaining slides can be used for AB-PAS stains and for additional special stains which might be required. Such stains would include stains for fungi or acid-fast organisms if a granuloma is present or suspected, stains for dense-cored endocrine granules if a carcinoid, small cell carcinoma or atypical endocrine tumor is suspected and any immunoperoxidase staining that is deemed appropriate. Further details relating to the use of special stains will be given throughout the book in the relevant text.

2.3.4   Immunoperoxidase techniques

The application of immunoperoxidase methods, due largely to original contributions from Nakane and Pierce (1966), Avrameas (1969) and Sternberger et al. (1970), added new and expanding dimensions to diagnostic pathology. The basic methods and their more recent variants are now used extensively in surgical pathology because of the permanence of the preparations and the opportunity afforded to perform routine and

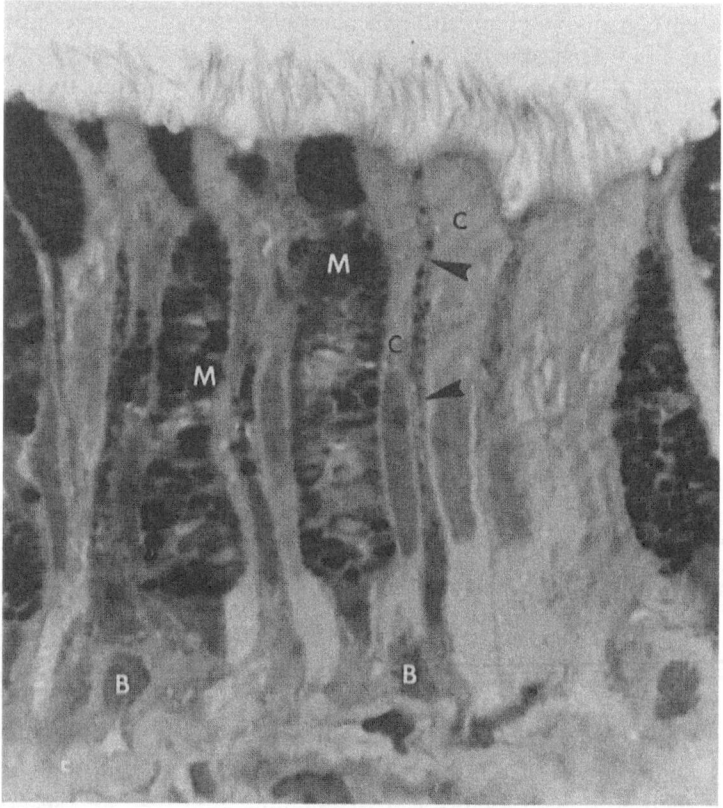

Fig. 2.1 High resolution light micrograph of pseudostratified human bronchial epithelium. Columnar mucous cells (M) and ciliated cells (C) reach from basement membrane to lumen, whereas short basal cells (B) do not. Some mucous cells are distended with secretions (goblet cells) but others are not, and the cells are slender (arrows). 2 μm-thick glycol methacrylate section stained with PAS-lead hematoxylin. (× 1700)

special stains on adjacent sections of the same specimen. Basic immunoperoxidase methods include direct and indirect peroxidase-labeled antibody methods, the labeled antigen method, the enzyme bridge procedure and the peroxidase-antiperoxidase (PAP) immune complex method. The PAP technique is particularly popular since it does not involve chemical manipulation and has great sensitivity. In these methods, peroxidase is localized at the site of the antigen by an antigen-antibody reaction. Peroxidase localization is visualized by developing the sections with a chromogenic hydrogen donor, usually diaminobenzidine, in the presence of hydrogen peroxide. Diaminobenzidine may be carcinogenic and should be handled with precaution in a hood.

Other approaches fast gaining in popularity include the protein

A-immunoenzymatic techniques, hapten-coupled antibodies for immu-noenzymatic staining, the biotin-avidin method and double immunoen-zymatic techniques. The various techniques and their pitfalls, control procedures, and applications in pathology have been reviewed extensively in scientific journals (Taylor, 1978; Heyderman, 1979; Sternberger, 1979; De Lellis *et al.*, 1979; Mukai and Rosai, 1980; Taylor and Kledzik, 1981; Montero, 1981; Pinkus, 1982; Falini and Taylor, 1983; Lewis *et al.*, 1983) and in specialized texts (Bullock and Petrusz, 1982, 1983; Polak and Van Noorden, 1983).

Most cytoplasmic antigens can be demonstrated in paraffin embedded specimens, assuming that the antigen was sufficient in amount and not rendered inactive by fixation. However, if the antigen was in small amount, weakly antigenic or soluble, or rendered inactive by fixation, briefly fixed or even unfixed frozen cryostat sections will be necessary (Grzanna, 1982; Falini and Taylor, 1983).

Using these methods, many cell products can be demonstrated in routinely fixed, paraffin- or glycol-methacrylate-embedded tissues, many years after their obtainment. The only limit to the applicability of im-munoperoxidase techniques seems to be the availability of specific antisera and the antigenic preservation following fixation. Inappropriate fixation does diminish antigenicity (Sections 2.1 and 2.2) but the techniques are very sensitive and usually allow satisfactory demonstration of an increas-ing library of antigens.

Furthermore, many of these techniques have been modified so that they can be used at ultrastructural level. For transmission electron microscopy (TEM) the techniques include post-embedding peroxidase methods (Or-dronneau, 1982), the avidin-biotin peroxidase method (Childs, 1983) and methods which employ colloidal gold as a marker (Roth, 1982, 1983). Immunocytochemical methods have also been modified for scanning electron microscopy (SEM) (Hartman and Nakane, 1983; Molday, 1983).

2.3.5   *Frozen sections and touch preparations*

Under special circumstances it may be desirable to obtain immediate light microscopic examination of specimens. Cryostat-cut sections allow eval-uation of tissue within minutes. The specimen must be received fresh since fixed tissues do not freeze well and are difficult to keep from washing off the microscope slide during processing. It is preferable to keep the specimen from drying by wrapping it in a sterile saline-wetted gauze. After gross examination the specimen is rapidly frozen and mounted on a metal chuck in the cryostat. Sections are cut while frozen. They thaw as they are picked up on the surface of a standard microscope slide. The sections mounted on the slide are then rapidly fixed and stained according to the dictates of the particular case.

Touch preparations are often prepared from fresh specimens as a means of providing rapid evaluation of suspected lymphomas and leukemic infiltrates. They have been proposed as a rapid technique for the diagnosis of pneumocystis pneumonia (Section 2.4.3). A freshly cut surface of the specimen is lightly touched to the surface of a microscope slide, leaving a residuum of cells. The best preparations are obtained when this process is repeated numerous times over the surface of the slide. Once stained, the best areas can be selected and examined. For Wright-Giemsa staining the preparations are air dried. Chemical fixation may be used for special purposes.

2.4 Preparation of specimens for light microscopic cytopathology

The judgement required for cytodiagnosis depends on consistent preservation and staining of the cells. Alcoholic fixation and a series of stains assembled by Papanicolaou (1942) are the nearly universal choice of cytopathologists. The alcoholic fixation is either by immersion of the smeared specimen on a microscope slide into 70–95% ethanol or by spraying the smeared specimen with an aerosol containing ethanol with various additives designed to increase the adherence of cells to the slide. Spray fixatives specifically manufactured for cytology slide preparation are commercially available. For many years some laboratories have used a commercial hair spray which was considerably less expensive than sprays sold specifically for cytologic fixation. However, the ingredients of that hair spray have been changed and it is now unsuitable as a fixative.

Papanicolaou's original stain procedure has been modified over the years by himself (1954) and others (Miller and Woolner, 1976; Bales and Durfee, 1979; Johnston and Frable, 1979). Some cytology laboratories use slight modifications for different types of specimens or techniques used in preparing the slides. If the reader is interested in the full range of such modifications, the handbook published by the American Society of Clinical Pathologists is recommended (Keebler and Reagan, 1975).

2.4.1 *Sputum*

Two different techniques for preparing sputum specimens are widely used. Fresh material can be spread directly onto the glass microscope slide and fixed by immersion in ethanol (Miller and Woolner, 1976; Bales and Durfee, 1979; Johnston and Frable, 1979). Alternatively, and when the smear cannot be prepared within a few hours after the sputum is collected, the specimen is immediately fixed by mixing with a solution of ethanol and polyethylene glycol (Saccomanno *et al.*, 1963). Such prefixed sputa are mechanically liquefied and the cells concentrated with centrifugation prior to preparing the smear. The liquefaction is usually accomplished with a high speed food liquefier (Keebler and Reagan, 1975; Miller and Woolner, 1976; Johnston and Frable, 1979). Either of these two techniques are used effectively in preparing smears of excellent quality.

Fresh sputa give excellent cell preservation and it is possible for the technologist who is preparing the smear to select portions of the submitted specimen which are more likely to contain pertinent cells, such as rust-tinted or more mucoid areas, avoiding the more liquid saliva. The prefixed technique, which has come to be called the Saccomanno technique, gives a greater yield of cells on the slide and a more uniform distribution of cells. Furthermore, mucin is eliminated as an interfering background. Although the basic distinction between the two techniques is whether the specimen is received in a fresh (unfixed) or fixed condition, some laboratories use the Saccomanno technique with fresh sputa.

2.4.2 Bronchoscopic specimens

Material for cytologic examination obtained during bronchoscopy include bronchial washings, bronchial brushings, bronchial lavage and transbronchial needle aspirates.

(a)   Bronchial washings

These are usually handled like sputa, although centrifugation at 2000 rpm for 10 minutes allows the removal of excess liquid used in rinsing the bronchi. The Saccomanno technique is widely used with bronchial washings because of the increased yield of cells.

(b)   Bronchial brushings

These are smeared directly onto glass microscope slides at the time they are obtained. They are best preserved with a spray fixative to reduce the chance of air drying, which introduces severe artefacts that make the smear difficult if not impossible to interpret accurately. When disposable brushes are used they can be clipped from the guide wire and placed in a small volume of saline. The brush is vigorously shaken in the solution and the cells collected for cytologic examination by cytocentrifugation (Marsan et al., 1982) or by filtration (Schwinn and Ferguson, 1976). The brush can then be placed in a combined light and electron microscopic fixative (Section 2.2) and stored. If it is determined at a later time that the lesion could be better defined with ultrastructural characteristics, the cells and fragments of tissue which are trapped among the bristles of the brush can be teased free and processed for ultrastructural examination (Section 2.5).

(c)   Bronchial lavage

is useful in a quantitative evaluation of the alveolar inflammatory cell infiltrate in diffuse disease of the lung (Hunninghake *et al.*, 1979). The investigative emphasis of this technique is most concerned with the biochemical analysis of the fluids obtained. Most studies have also evaluated the cell content, usually with an automatic cell counter. However, air-dried smears of the centrifuged pellet stained with the Wright-Giemsa stain and smears made for cytologic examination are also helpful. Cytologic smears are handled like bronchial washings.

(d)   Transbronchial fine needle aspirates

These are prepared at the bronchoscopy site by squirting the small amount of aspirated material directly onto glass microscope slides and immediately spray fixing or by immersing in alcohol. The fine aerosol which is usually formed from the small amount of material as it is sprayed onto the slide gives a satisfactory thin spread of cells for examination. However, if the specimen is bloody or unusually abundant it is necessary to spread the cells over the glass surface to give a clear view of the cells. There are two ways to accomplish this. One way is similar to the technique used for making hematology smears of blood. With this technique drying occurs very rapidly and the specimen must be fixed instantly. Some workers prefer to spread the cells more gently so as to do as little damage as possible and spread the drop of material by placing a second slide over the first slide, at right angles. The specimen spreads between the two surfaces forming a large splotch. The two slides are then separated, avoiding lateral motion, by pulling them apart vertically. Both slides are then fixed immediately. In some institutions, particularly when the procedure is done on an outpatient basis, the pathologist is requested to examine the aspirate immediately to determine if the lesion was adequately sampled. A more rapid Papanicolaou procedure is then used (Kaminsky, 1981). Alternatively, the fixed smears are processed by the usual cytologic technique. The needle and the syringe used in the aspiration should be rinsed with saline. In this way, many cells and even microbiopsies which would otherwise have been discarded can be retrieved. The saline is centrifuged and the pellet fixed and embedded in epoxy resins as if for electron microscopy. One micron thick (semithin) sections, stained with toluidine blue, are cut for examination in the light microscope (Section 2.5.3). The enhanced cellular detail resulting from post-fixation in osmium tetroxide, the plastic embedding, and the thinness of these sections can be very helpful in arriving at a specific diagnosis. In addition, if electron microscopic examination is judged to be necessary to establish the diagnosis, appropriately prepared material is available for thin sectioning (Beals, 1983).

2.4.3 Special techniques

Sputa and bronchial lavage or washings can be examined for the presence of asbestos bodies (ferruginous bodies) by direct inspection of the smears prepared for cytologic examination, but more satisfactory yields are obtained by digestion and concentration of the specimen (Smith and Naylor, 1972). Prefixed or fresh material is digested with full-strength commercial bleach. The greater the volume of deep cough material digested the greater the yield, and several hundred milliliters of sputum can be collected for this purpose. The time necessary for complete digestion varies with the specimen and is accelerated with agitation, but several hours is generally adequate. After digestion the material is centrifuged at 800 rpm for 5–10 minutes and the supernatant decanted off. The sediment, which includes any asbestos bodies and other inorganic particles, is then clarified by repeated extractions with an equal mixture of chloroform and 50% aqueous ethanol. The bodies are collected after each step with centrifugation. The final sediment, which will usually be invisible to the unaided eye, is resuspended in a small volume of 100% ethanol and pipetted onto a microscope slide for inspection in the light microscope. Alternatively, the last sediment can be resuspended in 100% ethanol and the bodies collected on a filter, which is then placed on a glass slide and dissolved by adding a layer of chloroform on top of the filter. When the chloroform evaporates, the filter will resolidify, leaving the asbestos bodies on the surface of the slide. The slide is then wetted with xylene and coverslipped with a suitable mounting medium. Staining is not necessary because the asbestos bodies have an inherent golden-brown color due to the iron-containing material which has encrusted the asbestos fibers.

Papanicolaou-stained smears demonstrate the nuclear and cytoplasmic inclusion bodies of viral infections very satisfactorily. Furthermore, most pathogenic fungi are clearly stained in Papanicolaou preparations and their distinctive morphologies are easily recognized without the aid of special stains. On the other hand, *Pneumocystis carinii* is remarkably difficult to detect in Papanicolaou- or H&E-stained biopsy material (Kim and Hughes, 1973). The organisms stain pink with a variable intensity and are difficult to distinguish from background debris. Air-dried smears or touch preparations stained with toluidine blue according to the procedure of Chalvardjian and Grawe (1963) demonstrate the micro-organisms very well. Methenamine silver (Repsher *et al.*, 1972; Churukian and Schenk, 1977), cresyl violet (Bowling *et al.*, 1973) and toluidine blue (Pritchett *et al.*, 1977) stains have all been advocated to facilitate detection of this parasite. *Pneumocystis carinii* is essentially never discovered as an incidental finding, and the pathologist who receives a specific request to examine the specimen for pneumocystis is alerted to use the special stains.

Sputa, bronchial washings and lavages can be centrifuged and fixed with 4F as a pellet for embedding in paraffin. This is a routine procedure in some cytology laboratories. Our experience is that the paucity of diagnostically relevant cells results in very little additional information for considerable extra technical effort. In the usual malignant sputum there may be only 1–10 cells per smear which are diagnostically significant, with several hundred totally nonspecific cells. In sectioned material from cell blocks this ratio becomes even worse. Such cell blocks, however, could be used for immunoperoxidase labeling. Information is more readily available by direct application of the immunoperoxidase technique to cell smears and imprints. The techniques are straightforward and provide high sensitivity and good morphology (Nadji, 1980; Coleman et al., 1981).

2.5　General principles of processing tissue for electron microscopy

2.5.1　Trimming the tissues

In the case of a small bronchial biopsy, a portion of it may be processed directly for electron microscopy and further trimming is not necessary. Inspection of the biopsy under a stereoscopic dissecting microscope is very helpful in selecting pieces for electron microscopy. If relatively large pieces of tissue, such as a tumor, were originally fixed by immersion in 4F or 4F-1G, the specimen must be trimmed and thin slices must be shaved from the outer surfaces prior to post-fixation in osmium tetroxide and subsequent processing for electron microscopy. However, if 1 mm thick slices are fixed initially, it is sufficient to dice these slices into 1 mm cubes or smaller pieces. Osmium tetroxide penetrates very slowly into tissues, approximately 0.6 mm during the first hour. Obviously, processing time will be reduced if very small tissue pieces are utilized.

2.5.2　Use of specimen previously embedded in paraffin for ultrastructural study

Sometimes the need arises to examine the biopsy ultrastructurally, but all of the tissue has been embedded in paraffin. In these cases the specimen can be deparaffinized and prepared for electron microscopy (Hübner, 1966; Rossi et al., 1970; Zeitoun and Lehy, 1970; Zimmerman et al., 1972). A small piece of tissue is cut from the particular portion of the paraffin block which contains the lesion in question. Since fixation is better at the edges of the block (areas first exposed to the fixative), these are preferred areas from which to select the lesion if it is present throughout the block. The paraffin is dissolved and removed by immersion in two changes of xylene, 15 minutes each. The tissue is then rehydrated in decreasing concentrations of ethanol starting with 100% (two changes), 95%, 70%, and 35%. The remaining alcohol is removed in changes of a suitable buffer solution. The tissue is then post-fixed in osmium tetroxide, dehydrated in alcohol and embedded in plastic for TEM (Section 2.5.3) or prepared for SEM (Section 2.5.4). Methods are also available for retrieving paraffin-embedded tissue sections from the microscope slides (Rossi *et al.*, 1970; Zeitoun and Lehy, 1970). Similar techniques are available for retrieval of material from cytology smears (Beals, 1983). These specimens allow the diagnosis of gross ultrastructural abnormalities which are well below the resolution limit of the light microscope. However, membrane clarity is lost and cytoplasmic membranes of the endoplasmic reticulum, mitochondria and nuclei acquire a 'ghost-like' appearance, particularly if the specimen was originally fixed in 4F. Membrane preservation is better if the specimen was fixed in 4F-1G or glutaraldehyde. Nevertheless, other features such as heterochromatin, nucleoli, microtubules, microfilaments, ribosomes, lysosomes, autophagic vacuoles, and intercellular junctions are relatively well preserved and in carcinoid and small cell carcinomas the dense cored granules are still recognizable even in 4F-fixed specimens, although the limiting membrane is lost (Fig. 2.2). Viral particles and some other specific inclusions may also be recognized in these preparations.

2.5.3   *Preparation for transmission electron microscopy (TEM)*

Before post-fixation in osmium tetroxide, the tissue must be washed to rid the tissue of aldehydes, which may react and cause precipitation with osmium. If it is intended to stain the tissue *en bloc* with uranyl acetate after osmication (see below), it is essential that the tissues be washed thoroughly prior to osmication in a buffer that will not cause precipitation of salts by interaction of buffer components with uranyl acetate. Uranyl salts will precipitate with phosphate buffers; thus, tissues fixed as advocated above (4F and 4F-1G) must be washed in a suitable buffer. In our hands sodium cacodylate is quite satisfactory. However, Hayat (1981b) states that uranyl reacts strongly with both cacodylate and phosphate buffers, causing precipitation of electron-dense salts in the tissues. In view of this warning, veronal acetate-HCl buffer may be preferable. If processing time is not important, tissues can be left in the buffer for 24 hours up to several days before post-fixation. If time is important, the tissues should be washed rapidly and thoroughly in three changes of buffer, at least 15 minutes in each rinse, prior to post-fixation.

It is commonplace to post-fix in osmium tetroxide. Although this step is not absolutely essential, osmium fixation stabilizes lipids including membrane lipids and acts as an electron-dense stain. Osmium-fixed tissues have heightened contrast compared with those fixed only in aldehydes. The osmium is dissolved in a buffer such as cacodylate-HCl, s-collidine-HCl or veronal acetate-HCl.

After post-fixation in osmium the tissue blocks may be stained *en bloc* with uranyl acetate, prior to dehydration (Farquhar and Palade, 1965).

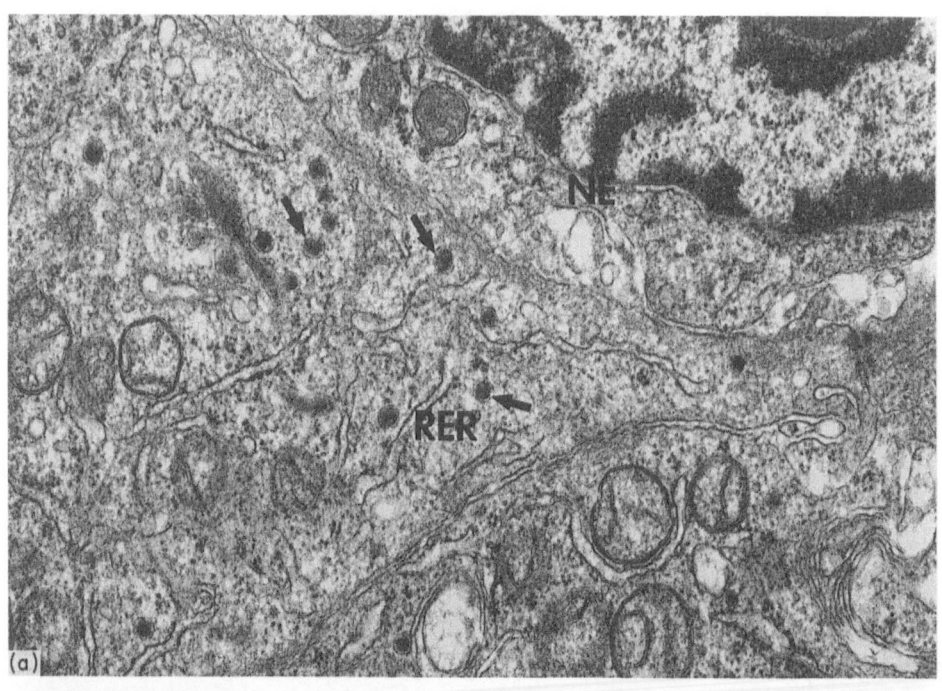

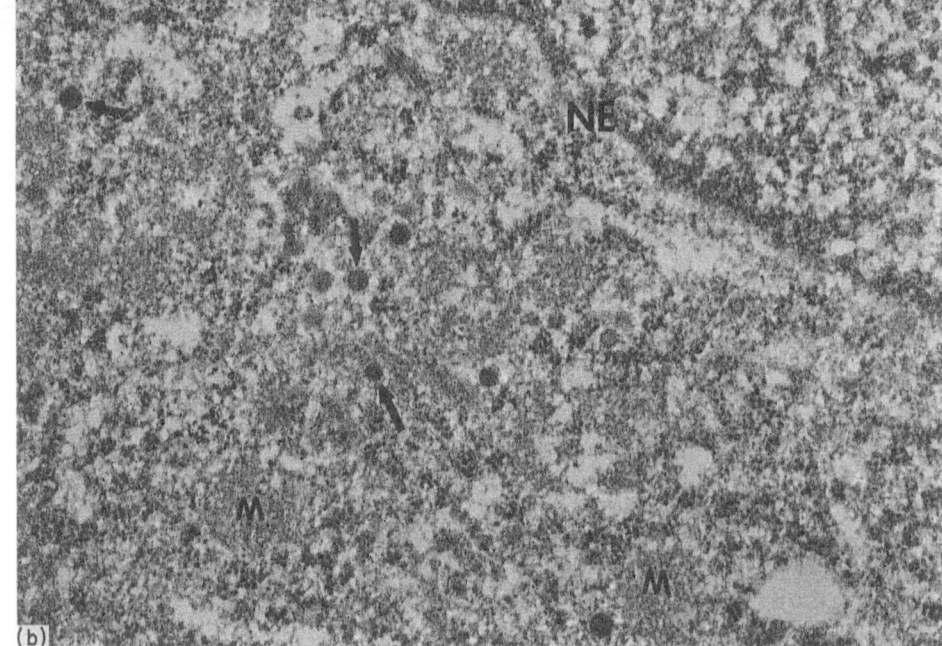

This results in increased contrast of proteins, nucleic acids, and cytoplasmic membranes. The amount of phospholipid-phosphorus extracted during dehydration is much reduced if tissues are prestabilized by uranyl acetate, which acts both as a stain and as a fixative. However, *en bloc* staining in aqueous uranyl acetate, which has an acid pH, may cause glycogen to become electron lucent. This can be avoided by the addition of 0.5 M potassium ferricyanide to the osmium tetroxide fixative solution (Cohen *et al.*, 1977).

When epoxy resins are used for embedment, dehydration of the tissue is necessary because these resins are immiscible with water. Ethanol is commonly used as the dehydrating agent. The tissues are transferred through a graded alcohol series and brought to 100% ethanol. Absolute ethanol is miscible with the solvent propylene oxide, which is miscible with epoxy resins such as Epon or Araldite, the final embedding medium. All embedding should be done in a fume hood. There are a variety of plastic embedding mixtures with various reported advantages. Depending upon the type of resin, polymerization can be effected either by heating or by ultraviolet radiation. These variations are adequately discussed in several texts on electron microscopy techniques (see the end of this section for references).

Semithin sections (0.5 to 1.0 μm thick) of the plastic-embedded material, usually cut with glass knives and stained with toluidine blue (Trump *et al.*, 1961), are invaluable for surveying the specimens. It is essential that semithin sections be examined by light microscopy before making the decision as to which portion of the block(s) should be sectioned for ultrastructural examination. This also allows orientation and correlation of the light microscopic and ultrastructural features of the specimen. The detail seen by light microscopy in semithin sections far exceeds that obtained from 5–10 μm thick paraffin sections as routinely prepared in the histology laboratory. The resolution is equivalent and perhaps superior to that achieved in aldehyde-fixed sections embedded in glycol methacrylate because of post-fixation of the tissues by osmium and uranyl salts which stabilize the membranes. However, the number of special stains that can be applied to epoxy-embedded sections is limited, and often

Fig. 2.2 Electron micrographs of a bronchial carcinoid tumor. (a) This specimen was fixed in 3% glutaraldehyde and prepared specifically for TEM. Note the clarity of the cytoplasmic membranes including the nuclear envelope (NE), rough endoplasmic reticulum (RER) and mitochondrial membranes. Membranes also surround the characteristic dense-cored granules (arrows). ($\times$ 25 000) (b) This specimen was originally fixed in 4% formaldehyde and embedded in paraffin. Later a small piece was deparaffinized, post-fixed in OsO_4 and prepared for TEM. The cytoplasmic membranes are lost, including those of the nuclear envelope (NE), rough endoplasmic reticulum and mitochondria (M). However, the dense cores of the characteristic granules (arrows) are clearly recognizable, although their limiting membranes are lost. ($\times$ 30 000)

special procedures to make the plastic permeable are necessary prior to staining (Burns, 1978; Litwin and Kasprzyk, 1980; Hall *et al.*, 1982).

Prior to cutting the thin sections it is necessary to trim the blocks into small trapezoid shapes. Selective trimming is essential to assure that the area of interest will be included in the section. Thin sections, approximately 60 nm thick, are cut and mounted onto copper grids. The sections are stained with electron-dense metals prior to being examined in the electron microscope. It is common to double stain the sections, first with uranyl salts and then with lead salts, in order to obtain maximum contrast. However, if *en bloc* staining with uranyl acetate has been employed, it is often sufficient to stain the mounted sections with a lead stain only. Many uranyl and lead stain recipes are available; a choice of any particular method is often a matter of personal preference. Further details of ultra-structural technique are available in several books (Pease, 1964; Glauert, 1975; Meek, 1977; Hayat, 1981b).

2.5.4   *Preparation of material for scanning electron microscopy (SEM)*

For special purposes it may be considered advantageous to examine biopsy or other specimens by SEM. This is rarely necessary for diagnostic purposes but is often of research or teaching interest. SEM is becoming increasingly popular because of the ease of preparation of the specimens, the increased size of specimen which can be examined, the dramatic three dimensional image and the detail it provides of the surface features of cells. The microscope produces images with a magnification range between × 20 and × 200 000. Fig. 2.3 is an SEM image of bronchial mucosa which shows how effectively this microscope demonstrates relationships between components of a specimen.

Specimens are prepared as described for TEM, including post-fixation in osmium tetroxide. Some trimming may be necessary for large specimens because of the difficulty of complete dehydration. However, most instruments are capable of mounting specimens several centimeters in diameter. Dehydration in a graded series of alcohols is followed by either freeze drying (de Harven *et al.*, 1977; Hayat, 1978a) or critical point drying (Cohen, 1979), insuring that the specimens are dried without subjecting them to the distortion of surface tension pressure. The specimens are attached to stubs with glue or adhesive tape and grounded with a rim of silver or graphite paint, and the entire specimen is coated with gold or gold palladium in a vacuum evaporator or DC sputter coater (Hayat, 1978b; Postek *et al.*, 1980). Further details of preparation of the respiratory tract for SEM and a review of the surface morphology of the airways of man and animals are found in the review by Andrews (1979). Specimens which have been prepared for and examined in the SEM can later be reprocessed for TEM by placing the specimen in propylene oxide and

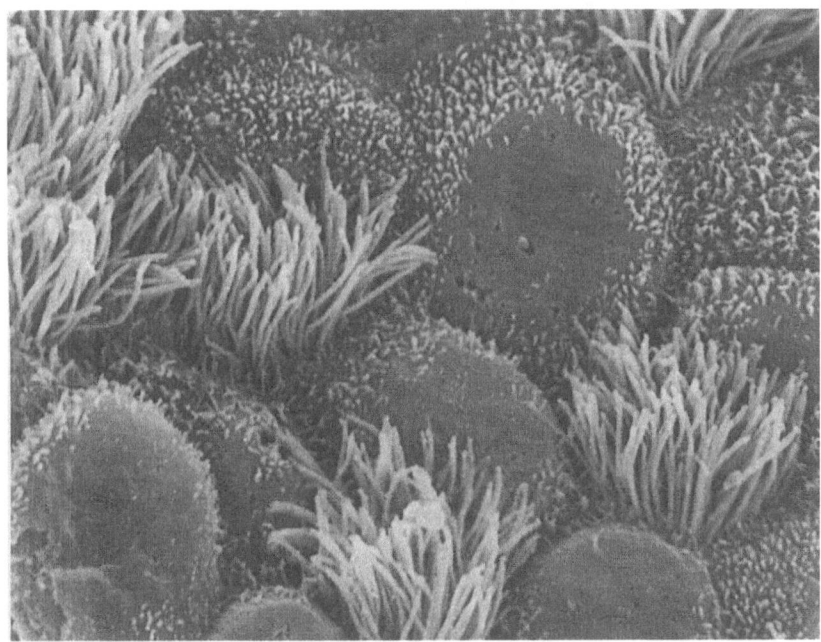

Fig. 2.3 Luminal surface of bronchial epithelium. Both ciliated cells and nonciliated (mucous) cells are seen. Some nonciliated cells have a central smooth area devoid of microvilli, a change which precedes release of mucin. The ciliated cells have microvilli mixed among the long and thicker cilia. (Scanning electron micrograph: horizontal field width = 30 μm.)

proceeding with the plastic embedding procedures described above (Section 2.5.3).

Free floating cells or clusters of cells as found in bronchial washings and lavages are especially well suited for SEM because they have extensive natural surfaces (Fig. 2.4). They are obtained fresh, centrifuged and rinsed in buffer to reduce soluble materials such as protein, which when fixed would obscure the cell surfaces. The cells are then fixed in glutaraldehyde or in 4F-1G. If preferred, cells can be fixed while still in their natural fluids by mixing the fluid with an equal volume of twice concentrated fixation solution. Prefixed cells can be collected on glass or plastic substrates which have been coated with poly-L-lysine (Mazia *et al.*, 1975; Sanders *et al.*, 1975; Domagala and Koss, 1981). Unfixed cells can be collected on filters and then fixed in place. Nuclepore® filters provide a more pleasing background because they have a smooth surface with circular holes. The other commonly available filters have a mesh composition. Unfixed cells collected on filters become adherent with glutaraldehyde fixation. Post-fixation in osmium tetroxide, dehydration in alcohol, drying and conductive coating are as described above (Beals, 1983).

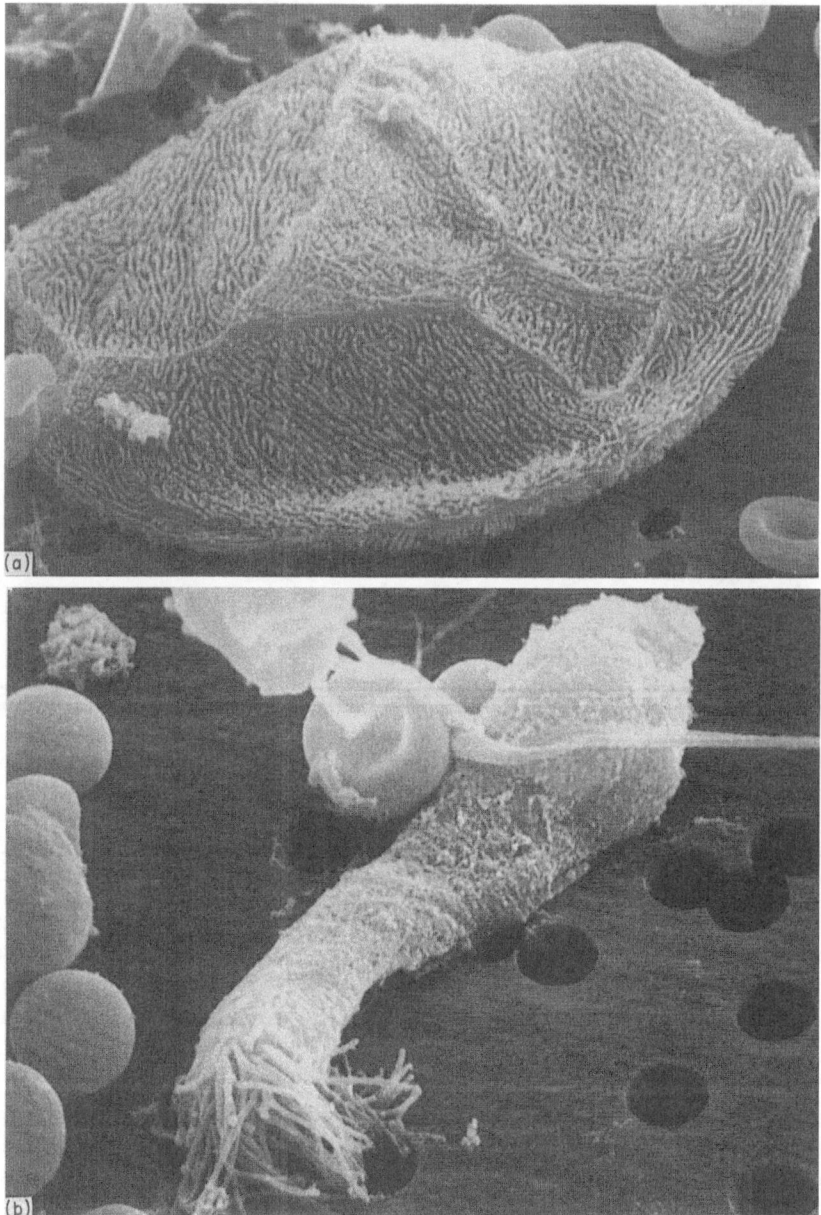

References

Andrews, P.M. (1979), The respiratory system. In *Biomedical Research Applications of Scanning Electron Microscopy*, Vol. 1 (eds G.M. Hodges and R.C. Hallowes), Academic Press, New York, pp. 177–202.

Avrameas, S. (1969), Coupling of enzymes to proteins with glutaraldehyde. Use of the conjugates for the detection of antigens and antibodies. *Immunochem.*, **6**, 43–52.

Bales, C.E. and Durfee, G.R. (1979), Cytologic techniques. In *Diagnostic Cytology and its Histopathologic Bases*, 3rd edn (ed. L.G. Koss), J.B. Lippincott, Philadelphia, pp. 1187–1266.

Banks, P.M. (1979), Diagnostic applications of an immunoperoxidase method in hematopathology. *J. Histochem. Cytochem.*, **27**, 1192–4.

Bassi, M. and Bernelli-Zazzera, A. (1964), Ultrastructural cytoplasmic changes of liver cells after reversible and irreversible ischemia. *Exp. Mol. Path.*, **3**, 332–50.

Beals, T.F. (1983), Cytology and electron microscopy, Chapter 4 in *Diagnostic Electron Microscopy*, Vol. 4 (eds B.F. Trump and R.T. Jones), Wiley, New York, pp. 179–225.

Bennett, H.S., Wyrick, A.D., Lee, S.W. and McNeil, J.H. (1976), Science and art in preparing tissues embedded in plastic for light microscopy with special reference to glycol methacrylate, glass knives, and simple stains. *Stain Technol.*, **51**, 71–95.

Bowes, J.H. and Cater, C.W. (1965), Cross linking of collagen. *J. Appl. Chem. (London)*, **15**, 296–304.

Bowling, M.C., Smith, I.M. and Wescott, S.L. (1973), A rapid staining procedure for *Pneumocystis carinii*. *Am. J. Med. Tech.*, **39**, 267–8.

Brandtzaeg, P. (1982), Tissue preparation methods for immunohistochemistry. In *Techniques in Immunocytochemistry*, Vol. 1 (eds G.R. Bullock and P. Petrusz), Academic Press, New York, pp. 1–75.

Brinn, N. and Pickett, P. (1979), Glycol methacrylate for routine special stains, histochemistry, enzyme histochemistry and immunohistochemistry: a simplified cold method for surgical biopsy tissue. *J. Histotechnol.*, **2**, 125–30.

Bullock, G.R. (1984), The current status of fixation for electron microscopy. A review. *J. Microscopy*, **133**, 1–15.

Bullock, G.R. and Petrusz, P. (1982), In *Techniques in Immunocytochemistry*, Vol. 1, Academic Press, New York, pp. 1–306.

Bullock, G.R. and Petrusz, P. (1983), In *Techniques in Immunocytochemistry*, Vol. 2, Academic Press, New York, pp. 1–290.

Fig. 2.4 Cells from bronchial washings. (a) An individual exfoliated metaplastic (squamous) cell. The pattern of microridges on the upper surface is somewhat different within each of the eight facets. The facets reflect how this cell interfaced with neighboring cells *in vivo*. The upper surface of this cell is natural now that the overlying cells have exfoliated. Several red blood cells are handy as indicators of size. (Scanning electron micrograph: horizontal field width = 50 μm.) (b) An individual ciliated bronchial epithelial cell. Only the ciliated surface is natural; the sides of the columnar cell have been torn free from their natural attachments with adjacent cells. Large numbers of these cells individually or in small groups are common in bronchial washings and must be the result of trauma to the mucosa by the bronchoscopy. (Scanning electron micrograph: horizontal field width = 30 μm.)

Burns, W.A. (1978), Thick sections: techniques and applications. In *Diagnostic Electron Microscopy*, Vol. 1 (eds B.F. Trump and R.T. Jones), Wiley, New York, pp. 141–66.

Carson, F.L., Lynn, J.A. and Martin, J.H. (1972), Ultrastructural effect of various buffers, osmolality, and temperature on paraformaldehyde fixation of the formed elements of blood and bone marrow. *Texas Reports Biol. Med.*, **30**, 125–42.

Carson, F.L., Martin, J.H. and Lynn, J.A. (1973), Formalin fixation for electron microscopy. A re-evaluation. *Am. J. Clin. Path.*, **59**, 365–73.

Chalvardjian, A.M. and Grawe, L.A. (1963), A new procedure for the identification of *Pneumocystis carinii* cysts in tissue sections and smears. *J. Clin. Pathol.*, **16**, 383–4.

Chambers, R.W., Bowling, M.C. and Grimley, P.M. (1968), Glutaraldehyde fixation in routine histopathology. *Arch. Path.*, **85**, 18–30.

Chayen, J, Bitensky, L., Butcher, R. and Poulter, L. (1969), In *A Guide to Practical Histochemistry*, J.B. Lippincott, Philadelphia, p. 77.

Childs, G.V. (1983), The application of the avidin-biotin peroxidase complex technique to the localization of anterior pituitary hormones on plastic sections and cell monolayers. In *Techniques in Immunocytochemistry*, Vol. 2 (eds G.R. Bullock and P. Petrusz), Academic Press, New York, pp. 85–102.

Churukian, C.J. and Schenk, E.A. (1977), Rapid Grocott's methenamine-silver nitrate method for fungi and *Pneumocystis carinii*. (Letter to the Editor) *Am. J. Clin. Path.*, **68**, 427–8.

Cohen, A.L. (1979), Critical point drying – principles and procedures. *Scanning Electron Microscopy*, **1979/II**, 303–24.

Cohen, G.M., Siegel, A.J. and Fermin, C.D. (1977), Procedure for contrasting glycogen in the embryonic chick's ear. In *Proceedings EMSA*, Claitor's, Baton Rouge, pp. 546–9.

Coleman, D.V., To, A., Ormerod, M.G. and Dearnaley, D.P. (1981), Immunoperoxidase staining in tumor marker distribution studies in cytologic specimens. *Acta Cytol.*, **25**, 205–6.

de Harven, E., Lampen, N. and Pla, D. (1977), Alternatives to critical point drying. *Scanning Electron Microscopy*, **1977/I**, 519–24.

De Lellis, R.A., Sternberger, L.A., Mann, R.B., Banks, P.M. and Nakane, P.K. (1979), Immunoperoxidase technics in diagnostic pathology. *Am. J. Clin. Path.*, **71**, 483–8.

Domagala, W. and Koss, L.G. (1981), Configurations of surfaces of cells in effusions by scanning electron microscopy. In *Advances in Clinical Cytology* (eds L.G. Koss and D.V. Coleman), Butterworths, London, pp. 270–4.

Ericsson, J.L.E. and Biberfeld, P. (1967), Studies on aldehyde fixation. Fixation rates and their relation to fine structure and some histochemical reactions in liver. *Lab. Invest.*, **17**, 281–98.

Ericsson, J.L.E., Biberfeld, P. and Seljelid, R. (1967), Electron microscopic and cytochemical studies of acid phosphatase and aryl sulfatase during autolysis. *Acta Path. Microbiol. Scand.*, **70**, 215–28.

Falini, B. and Taylor, C.R. (1983), New developments in immunoperoxidase techniques and their application. *Arch. Pathol. Lab. Med.*, **107**, 105–17.

Farquhar, M.G. and Palade, G.E. (1965), Cell junctions in amphibian skin. *J. Cell Biol.*, **26**, 263–91.

Glauert, A.M. (1975), *Practical Methods in Electron Microscopy*, North Holland American Elsevier, New York.

Grzanna, R. (1982), Light microscopic immunocytochemistry with fixed, unembedded tissues. In *Techniques in Immunocytochemistry*, Vol. 1 (eds. G.R. Bullock and P. Petrusz), Academic Press, New York, pp. 183–204.

Hall, P., Smith, R.D. and Gormley, B.M. (1982), 'Routine' stains on osmicated resin embedded hepatic tissue. *Pathology*, **14**, 73–4.

Hartman, A.L. and Nakane, P.K. (1983), Immunological methods in scanning electron microscopy using peroxidase. In *Techniques in Immunocytochemistry*, Vol. 2 (eds G.R. Bullock and P. Petrusz), Academic Press, New York, pp. 103–16.

Hayat, M.A. (1978a), Drying. In *Introduction to Biological Scanning Electron Microscopy*, University Park Press, Baltimore, pp. 131–66.

Hayat, M.A. (1978b), Specimen coating. In *Introduction to Biological Scanning Electron Microscopy*, University Park Press, Baltimore, pp. 219–38.

Hayat, M.A. (1981a), Glutaraldehyde. In *Fixation for Electron Microscopy*, Academic Press, New York, pp. 66–129.

Hayat, M.A. (1981b), *Principles and Techniques of Electron Microscopy. Biological Applications*, Vol. 1, 2nd edn, University Park Press, Baltimore.

Heyderman, E. (1979), Immunoperoxidase technique in histopathology: applications, methods and controls. *J. Clin. Path.*, **32**, 971–8.

Hübner, G. (1966), Electron microscopy of formalin-fixed human tissue. *J. Histochem. Cytochem.*, **14**, 757–8.

Hunninghake, G.W., Gadek, J.E., Kawanami, O., Ferrans, V.J. and Crystal, R.G. (1979), Inflammatory and immune processes in the human lung in health and disease: evaluation by bronchoalveolar lavage. *Am. J. Pathol.*, **97**, 149–206.

Ito, S. (1962), Light and electron microscopic study of membranous cytoplasmic organelles. In *The Interpretation of Ultrastructure*, Symposia of the International Society for Cell Biology, Vol. 1 (ed. R.J.C. Harris), Academic Press, New York, p. 129.

Johnston, W.W. and Frable, W.J. (1979), In *Diagnostic Respiratory Cytopathology*, Masson, New York, pp. 5–18.

Kaminsky, D.B. (1981), In *Aspiration Biopsy for the Community Hospital*, Masson, New York, pp. 10–15.

Keebler, C.M. and Reagan, J.W. (1975), *A Manual of Cytotechnology*, 4th edn, American Society of Clinical Pathologists, Chicago.

Kennedy, A.R. and Little, J.B. (1974), Staining of glutaraldehyde fixed, glycol methacrylate embedded hamster lungs. *Amer. J. Med. Tech.*, **40**, 411–15.

Kim, H. and Hughes, W.T. (1973), Comparison of methods for identification of *Pneumocystis carinii* in pulmonary aspirates. *Am. J. Clin. Pathol.*, **60**, 462–6.

Latta, H., Osvaldo, L., Jackson, J.D. and Cook, M.L. (1965), Changes in renal cortical tubules during autolysis. Electron microscopic observations. *Lab. Invest.*, **14**, 635–57.

Lewis, R.E., Johnson, W.W. and Cruse, J.M. (1983), Pitfalls and caveats in the methodology for immunoperoxidase staining in surgical pathologic diagnosis. *Surv. Synth. Path. Res.*, **1**, 134–52.

Litwin, J.A. and Kasprzyk, J.M. (1980), Alcian blue staining of semithin Epon sections for light microscopy. *Acta Histochem.*, **67**, 265–71.

Lynn, J.A., Martin, J.H. and Race, G.J. (1966), Recent improvements of histologic technics for the combined light and electron microscopic examination of surgical specimens. *Am. J. Clin. Path.*, **45**, 704–13.

Marsan, C., Pasteur, X., Alepee, B., Laurent, J., Accard, J., Cava, E., Eloit, P. and Maoret, J.J. (1982), Automatic cytopathologic diagnosis of bronchial carcinoma.

I. Cytocentrifugation of bronchial brushings for image analysis. *Acta Cytol.*, **26**, 545–50.

Mazia, D., Schatten, G. and Sale, W. (1975), Adhesion of cells to surfaces coated with polylysine: application to electron microscopy. *J. Cell Biol.*, **66**, 198–200.

McDowell, E.M. (1978), Fixation and processing. In *Diagnostic Electron Microscopy* (eds B.F. Trump and R.T. Jones), Wiley, New York, pp. 113–39.

McDowell, E.M. and Trump, B.F. (1976), Histologic fixatives suitable for diagnostic light and electron microscopy. *Arch. Path. Lab. Med.*, **100**, 405–14.

Meek, G.A. (1977), *Practical Electron Microscopy for Biologists*, 2nd edn, Wiley, New York.

Miller, F. and Woolner, L.B. (1976), Specimen preparation for material from the respiratory tract. In *Compendium on Diagnostic Cytology*, 4th edn (eds G.L. Wied and J.W. Reagan), International Society of Cytology, Chicago, pp. 275–98.

Molday, R.S. (1983), Labelling of cell surface antigens for SEM. In *Techniques in Immunocytochemistry*, Vol. 2 (eds G.R. Bullock and P. Petrusz), Academic Press, New York, pp. 117–54.

Montero, C. (1981), Immunocytochemical methods and their achievements in pathology. In *Cell Markers*, Vol. 10, *Methods and Achievements in Experimental Pathology* (eds G. Jasmin and M. Cantin), Karger, Basel, pp. 1–36.

Moosavi, H., Lichtman, M.A., Donnelly, J.A. and Churukian, C.J. (1981), Plastic-embedded human marrow biopsy specimens. Improved histochemical methods. *Arch. Pathol. Lab. Med.*, **105**, 269–73.

Mowry, R.W. and Winkler, C.H. (1956), The coloration of acidic carbohydrates of bacteria and fungi in tissue sections with special reference to capsules of *Cryptococcus neoformans*, pneumococci and staphylococci. *Amer. J. Path.*, **32**, 628–9.

Mukai, K. and Rosai, J. (1980), Applications of immunoperoxidase techniques in surgical pathology. In *Progress in Surgical Pathology*, Vol. 1 (eds C.M. Fenoglio and M. Wolff), Masson, New York, pp. 15–49.

Nadji, M. (1980), The potential value of immunoperoxidase techniques in diagnostic cytology. *Acta Cytol.*, **24**, 442–7.

Nakane, P.K. and Pierce, G.B. (1966), Enzyme-labeled antibodies. Preparation and application for the localization of antigens. *J. Histochem. Cytochem.*, **14**, 929–31.

Ordronneau, P. (1982), Post-embedding unlabeled antibody techniques for electron microscopy. In *Techniques in Immunocytochemistry*, Vol. 1 (eds G.R. Bullock and P. Petrusz), Academic Press, New York, pp. 269–81.

Osvaldo, L., Jackson, J.D., Cook, M.L. and Latta, H. (1965), Reactions of kidney cells during autolysis. Light microscopic observations. *Lab. Invest.*, **14**, 603–22.

Papanicolaou, G.N. (1942), A new procedure for staining vaginal smears. *Science*, **95**, 438–9.

Papanicolaou, G.N. (1954), *Atlas of Exfoliative Cytology*, Harvard University Press, Cambridge.

Pease, D.C. (1964), *Histological Techniques for Electron Microscopy*, 2nd edn, Academic Press, New York.

Pinkus, G. (1982), Diagnostic immunocytochemistry of paraffin-embedded tissues. *Human Path.*, **13**, 411–15.

Polak, J.M. and Van Noorden, S. (1983), In *Immunocytochemistry. Practical Applications in Pathology and Biology*, Wright, Bristol, pp. 1–396.

Postek, M.T., Howard, K.S., Johnson, A.H. and McMichael, K.L. (1980), In *Scanning Electron Microscopy. A Student's Handbook*, Ladd Industry, pp. 154–66.

Pritchett, P.S., Murad, T.M. and Webster, M.J. (1977), Identification of *Pneumocystis carinii* infection in cytology specimens. (Abstract) *Acta Cytol.*, **21**, 784–5.

Repsher, L.H., Schröter, G. and Hammond, W.S. (1972), Diagnosis of *Pneumocystis carinii* pneumonitis by means of endobronchial brush biopsy. *New Engl. J. Med.*, 287, 340–1.

Rømert, P. and Matthiessen, M.E. (1981), Swelling of mitochondria in immersion-fixed liver tissue. Effect of various fixatives and of delayed fixation. *Acta Anat.*, 109, 332–8.

Rossi, G.L., Luginbühl, H. and Probst, D. (1970), A method for ultrastructural study of lesions found in conventional histological sections. *Virch. Arch. Path. Anat. Abt. A*, 350, 216–24.

Roth, J. (1982), The protein A-gold (pAg) technique – a qualitative and quantitative approach for antigen localization on thin sections. In *Techniques in Immunocytochemistry*, Vol. 1 (eds G.R. Bullock and P. Petrusz), Academic Press, New York, pp. 107–33.

Roth, J. (1983), The colloidal gold marker system for light and electron microscopic cytochemistry. In *Techniques in Immunocytochemistry*, Vol. 2 (eds G.R. Bullock and P. Petrusz), Academic Press, New York, pp. 217–84.

Ruddell, C.L. (1967a), Hydroxyethyl methacrylate combined with polyethylene glycol 400 and water; an embedding medium for routine 1–2 micron sectioning. *Stain Tech.*, 42, 119–23.

Ruddell, C.L. (1967b), Embedding media for 1–2 micron sectioning. 2. Hydroxyethyl methacrylate combined with 2-butoxyethanol. *Stain Tech.*, 42, 253–5.

Sabatini, D.D., Bensch, K. and Barrnett, R.J. (1963), Cytochemistry and electron microscopy. The preservation of cellular ultrastructure and enzymatic activity by aldehyde fixation. *J. Cell Biol.*, 17, 19–58.

Sabatini, D.D., Miller, F. and Barrnett, R.J. (1964), Aldehyde fixation for morphological and enzyme histochemical studies with the electron microscope. *J. Histochem. Cytochem.*, 12, 57–71.

Saccomanno, G., Saunders, R.P., Ellis, H., Archer, V.E., Wood, B.G. and Beckler, P.A. (1963), Concentration of carcinoma or atypical cells in sputum. *Acta Cytol.*, 7, 305–10.

Sanders, S.K., Alexander, E.L. and Braylan, R.C. (1975), A high-yield technique for preparing cells fixed in suspension for scanning electron microscopy. *J. Cell Biol.*, 67, 476–80.

Schwinn, C.P. and Ferguson, R. (1976), Cytopreparatory techniques. In *Compendium on Diagnostic Cytology*, 4th edn (eds G.L. Wied, L.G. Koss and J.W. Reagan), International Society of Cytology, Chicago, pp. 360–9.

Smith, M.J. and Naylor, B. (1972), A method for extracting ferruginous bodies from sputum and pulmonary tissue. *Am. J. Clin. Pathol.*, 58, 250–4.

Sorokin, S.P. and Hoyt, R.F. (1978), PAS-lead hematoxylin as a stain for small-granule endocrine cell populations in the lungs, other pharyngeal derivatives and the gut. *Anat. Record*, 192, 245–59.

Sorokin, S.P., Hoyt, R.F. and McDowell, E.M. (1981), An unusual bronchial carcinoid tumor analyzed by conjunctive staining. *Human Pathol.*, 12, 302–13.

Sternberger, L.A. (1979), *Immunocytochemistry*, 2nd edn, Wiley, New York.

Sternberger, L.A., Hardy, P.H., Cuculis, J.J. and Meyer, H.G. (1970), The unlabeled antibody enzyme method of immunohistochemistry. *J. Histochem. Cytochem.*, 18, 315–33.

Taylor, C.R. (1978), Immunoperoxidase techniques. Practical and theoretical aspects. *Arch. Path. Lab. Med.*, 102, 113–21.

Taylor, C.R. and Kledzik, G. (1981), Immunohistologic techniques in surgical pathology – a spectrum of 'new' special stains. *Human Path.*, 12, 590–6.

Trump, B.F., Goldblatt, P.J. and Stowell, R.E. (1962), An electron microscopic study of early cytoplasmic alterations in hepatic parenchymal cells of mouse liver during necrosis *in vitro* (autolysis). *Lab. Invest.*, **11**, 986–1015.

Trump, B.F., Goldblatt, P.J. and Stowell, R.E. (1965), Studies on necrosis of mouse liver *in vitro*. Ultrastructural alterations in the mitochondria of hepatic parenchymal cells. *Lab. Invest.*, **14**, 343–71.

Trump, B.F., Smuckler, E.A. and Benditt, E.P. (1961), A method for staining epoxy sections for light microscopy. *J. Ultrastruct. Res.*, **5**, 343–8.

Zeitoun, P. and Lehy, T. (1970), Utilization of paraffin-embedded material for electron microscopy. Study of an A_2-cell type microadenoma of the endocrine pancreas. *Lab. Invest.*, **23**, 52–7.

Zimmerman, L.E., Font, R.L., Ts'o, M.O.M. and Fine, B.S. (1972), Application of electron microscopy to histopathologic diagnosis. *Trans. Am. Acad. Opthamol. Otol.*, **76**, 101–7.

3 The bronchial airways

3.1 Embryogenesis

3.1.1 Overview

Knowledge of bronchial development is important to understanding many pathological processes of the adult organ. Development has been studied extensively in the human and the following brief summary highlights some of the key events.

Intrauterine growth of the lungs is commonly divided into four stages: the *embryonic period*, when the lung is first delimited and the primitive bronchi and their divisions are established; the *glandular period*, which involves the dichotomous branching and multiplication of divisions of the bronchial tree; the *canalicular period*, when more distally located respiratory portions of the lung are formed; and finally the *saccular period*, when the alveolar ducts and alveoli are established.

The *embryonic period* extends to 7 weeks of gestation. The epithelial lining of the lung, from larynx to the most distal alveoli, arises from endoderm. The lung bud appears 26 days following ovulation as a ventral groove in the floor of the gut, caudal to the pharyngeal pouches. The larynx and trachea grow caudally as a ventral diverticulum of endoderm, separated from the foregut by an ingrowth of primitive mesodermal elements. The caudal end of the trachea divides around 4 weeks into two bronchial buds which form the major bronchi. Further growth of the bronchi is asymmetric, the right side exceeding the left side. By 5 weeks the lobar bronchi are present and by 6 weeks the segmental bronchi are formed. Each bronchus is associated with a mass of mesodermal elements. These bronchial-associated masses will later form the individual lobes of the lung.

The *glandular period* extends through 16 weeks of gestation and the bronchial tubes, enmeshed in connective tissue, take on a glandular appearance, each tube being lined by a simple columnar epithelium (Fig. 3.1). Growth is very rapid between 10 and 16 weeks so that by the end of this period most of the bronchial tree is formed. Thus, while airway size continues to increase during later times, the pattern of bronchial branching does not. The *canalicular period* follows, during which the epithelial cells become specialized and the mesodermal tissues become highly vascularized. At this time, 17 weeks onwards, the respiratory

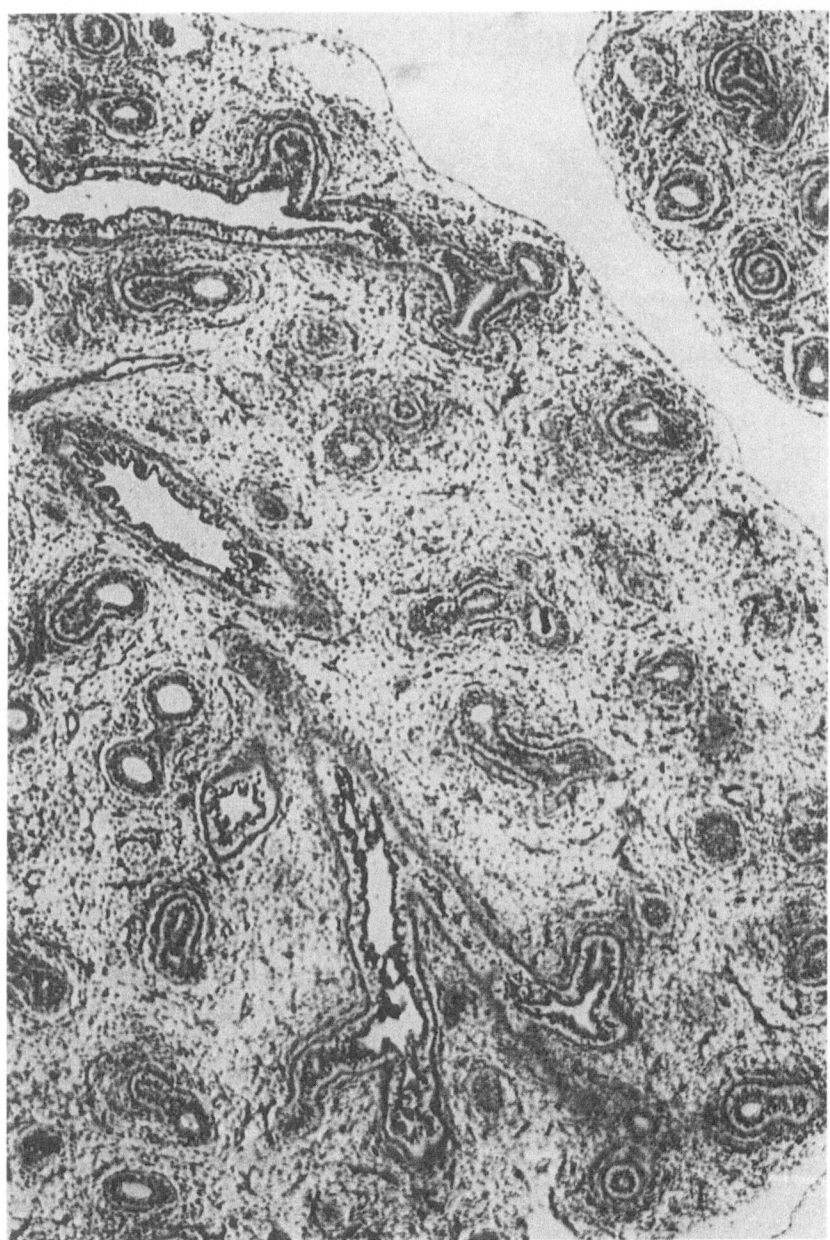

Fig. 3.1 Low power light micrograph of lung from 10-week-old fetus. The bronchial tubules, enmeshed in connective tissue, have a glandular appearance and are lined by primitive columnar cells. The branching growth pattern of the developing bronchial tree is evident. (Paraffin section stained with hematoxylin and eosin: × 120.)

bronchioles develop and the alveoli become less compact. The *saccular period* starts around 6 months gestation and the rudimentary alveolar ducts become established; however, most of the alveoli develop after birth (Boyden, 1977).

3.1.2 Early development

At the earliest recognizable stage the developing lung consists of a system of branching tubules lined by a single layer of unspecialized columnar epithelial cells which rest on a thin basal lamina. In paraffin sections the bronchial tubules may appear to be lined by stratified epithelium, but this appearance is due to tangential cuts of branching tubules (Conen and Balis, 1969). The tubules are never solid and even at the earliest times a central lumen can be recognized (Campiche *et al.*, 1963). The unspecialized columnar cells contain variable amounts of endoplasmic reticulum, and masses of glycogen fill the basal cytoplasm (Fig. 3.2a, b, c). Glycogen is abundant until about the fourth month (Boyden, 1977). Glycogen is absent from normal adult epithelial cells but is commonly seen in neoplastic lesions. This is discussed in Chapters 9 and 10.

3.1.3 Differentiation

Throughout the developmental process interactions between mesodermal and endodermal elements are essential for induction of ordered growth (Sorokin, 1965; Taderera, 1967; Wessells, 1970; Masters, 1976). At first all connective tissue and epithelial cells appear unspecialized. However, towards the end of the glandular period and throughout the canalicular period, cell specialization occurs in the epithelium and in the surrounding mesoderm. Differentiation of epithelium and mesoderm spreads in a wavelength fashion down the airways from the trachea to the terminal buds. The connective tissue condenses around the branching tubes, and collagen, elastic tissues, cartilage, smooth muscle, vascular channels, lymphatics and fatty tissues emerge (Emery, 1969; Bucher, 1969).

(a) Specialization of surface epithelium

The primitive bronchial epithelium is composed of unspecialized cells whereas, in the adult epithelium, basal cells, mucous cells, ciliated cells and dense-core granulated (endocrine) cells are arranged in a pseudostratified configuration (Section 3.2.3). How and when do these changes come about? Surprisingly little is known of the kinetics in the early stages of development, although it seems likely that the columnar cells of the primitive epithelium are the 'stem cells' from which specialized cell types initially arise. Mitotic figures are common and the first specialized cells

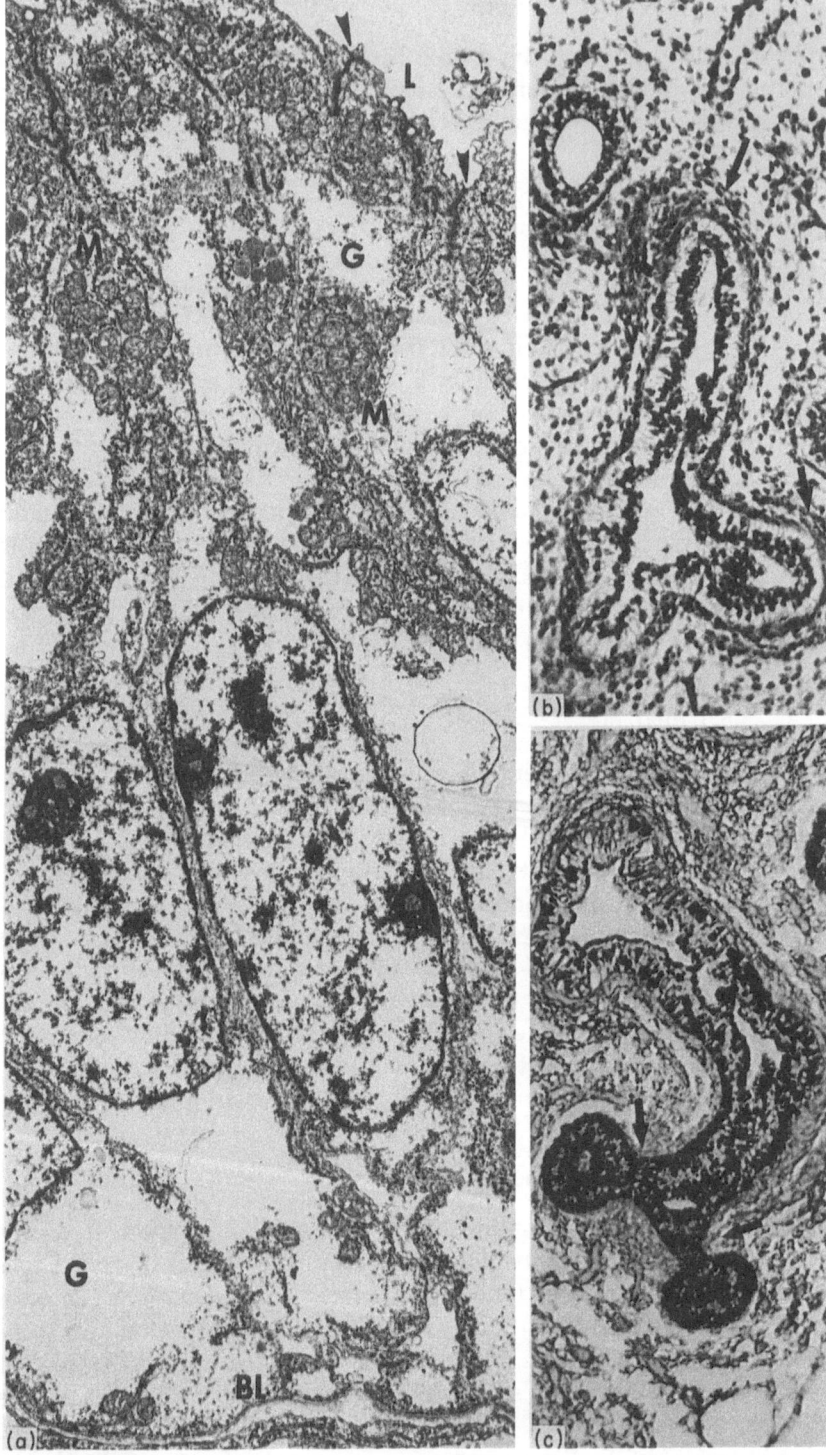

(a)

(b)

(c)

arise by differentiation of the progeny of the primitive cells. In a recent study of bronchial development, Sorokin *et al.* (1982) described the sequence of genesis of specialized cells during development of fetal rabbit lung. Prior to cell specialization glycogen storage was uniform throughout the primitive columnar cells. Dense-core granulated cells were the first specialized cells to be recognized and their emergence was preceded by glycogen depletion in single cells and in groups of cells, preferentially located at bronchial bifurcations. At a later stage, glycogen depletion was more widespread and heralded specialization of mucous cells and ciliated cells. Glycogen depletion occurs in epithelial cells at the onset of differentiation and corresponds to a shift in metabolism towards an aerobic respiration (Sorokin, 1965).

Starting at 10 weeks in the human fetus, cells that differ from the primitive columnar cells can be recognized (Jeffery and Reid, 1977a). Some of these are short cells that do not reach to the lumen and their appearance converts the epithelium from one that is simple columnar to one that is pseudostratified. Cells which do not reach to the lumen include so-called basal cells and some dense-core granulated cells; the latter are observed in human tracheas before the appearance of mucous cells (Cutz *et al.*, 1975). Superficial columnar cells containing a few PAS-positive droplets are seen at 10 weeks, and columnar cells secreting acidic glycoproteins are well established by 13 weeks gestation (Bucher and Reid, 1961; de Haller, 1969). Ciliated cells are first seen in the human trachea and main bronchi at 10 weeks and more peripherally by 13 weeks (Bucher and Reid, 1961). It is not known at what stage of development the adult structure is attained in man (Jeffery and Reid, 1977a). The events that occur during specialization of mucus-secreting cells and ciliated cells have not been studied in the human fetus at the ultrastructural level; however, a detailed study of ciliogenesis, as it occurs during fetal development of the rat, has been made by Sorokin (1968).

In a study of developing airways in fetal lambs, the primitive cells were shown to be joined apically by tight junctions. These junctions had associated gap junctions during the glandular and canalicular periods, times when cell specialization was occurring. Gap junctions allow for electrical coupling between adjacent cells and permit intercellular

---

Fig. 3.2 (a) Low power electron micrograph of bronchial tubule from 10-week-old fetus. The primitive columnar epithelial cells rest on the basal lamina (BL) and reach to the lumen (L). The cells are joined apically (arrowheads). Numerous mitochondria are present (M) and the cells contain pools of glycogen (G) (× 5000). (b) Same specimen as in Fig. 3.2a. Condensations of mesodermal elements (arrows) are closely associated with a branching bronchial tubule. The epithelial lining is simple columnar. (Paraffin section stained with hematoxylin and eosin: × 230.) (c) Same specimen as in Fig. 3.2a. Glycogen is abundant in the cells especially at loci of branching growth activity (arrows). (Paraffin section stained with PAS: × 230.)

metabolic exchanges. Gap junctions were absent during the alveolar phase of development when cellular differentiation was established (Schneeberger *et al.*, 1978).

(b)   Formation of bronchial glands

In the adult, mucus glycoproteins are secreted by cells of the surface epithelium and by multicellular tubulo-acinar glands in the submucosa. These glands lie beneath the mucous membrane, often extending to the outer side of the cartilage. In humans the first signs of glandular development in the bronchi occur at 9 weeks' gestation (Sorokin, 1960). The first hints of formation are the appearance of aggregates of cells with dark nuclei within the surface epithelium. The basement membrane is deflected downwards and the glandular bud grows down into the subepithelial layers to give rise to a primitive tubular gland (Bucher and Reid, 1961). This process has recently been studied in other mammals by combined light and electron microscopy and prolific formation of simple branched tubules lined by cuboidal mucus-secreting cells was described. Many of the secretory cells were seen in mitosis (Smolich *et al.*, 1978). In the human, development progresses through 12 and 13 weeks so that by 14 weeks the tubular glands are well developed (Bucher and Reid, 1961; Tos, 1968).

3.2   The adult bronchial tree

3.2.1   *General structure*

The trachea and bronchi are a continuous system of air-conducting tubes. The larynx opens into the trachea, which divides at the carina into two main bronchi. These follow a short extrapulmonary course and enter the hilum of their respective lungs together with the main pulmonary vessels and nerves. The main bronchi divide into five lobar bronchi, two on the left and three on the right (Chapter 1). Further details of the complex anatomy of the human conducting airways lie outside the scope of this book, and interested readers are referred to specialized texts for detailed descriptions of the multiple branchings of the bronchial tree (Boyden, 1955; von Hayek, 1960; Nagaishi, 1972).

3.2.2   *The bronchial wall*

The wall of the conducting airways is composed of three major elements: the lining epithelium (surface and glandular), connective tissue, and the muscularis (Fig. 3.3).

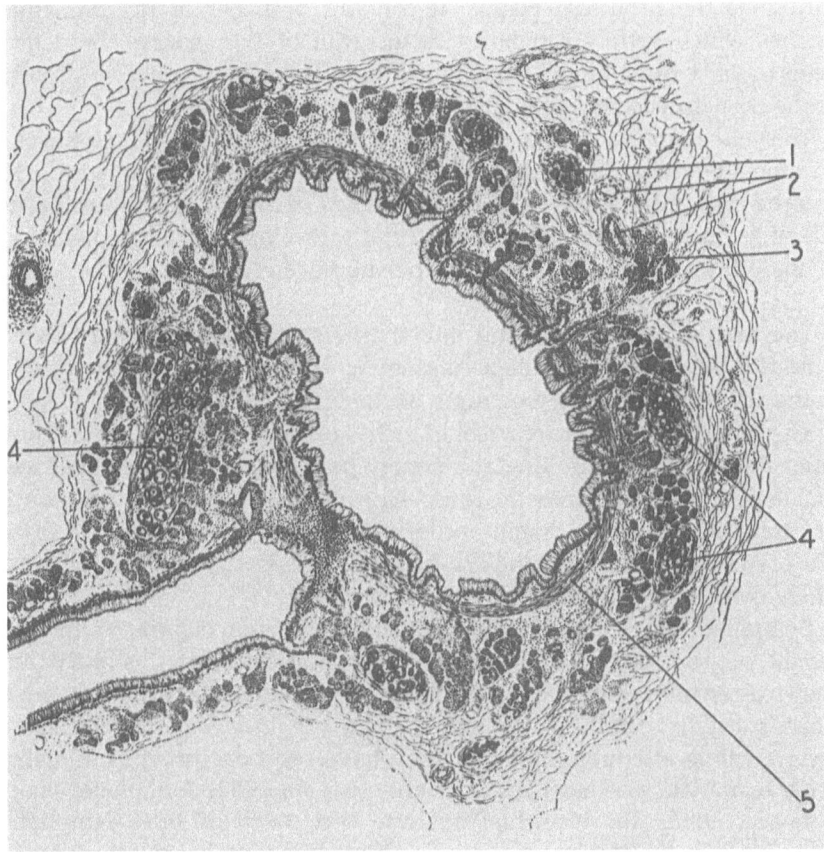

Fig. 3.3 Transverse section through a medium-sized bronchus: (1) section of a ganglion and its accompanying nerve (2) sections of the bronchial artery (3) gland with its duct opening into the lumen of the bronchus (4) sections of cartilage (5) smooth muscle. Reproduced with permission from Miller (1947).

The *mucosa* consists of the epithelial lining, the supporting basal lamina and a rather cellular underlying lamina propria composed of elastic fibers, collagen fibers, vascular and lymphatic channels, and nerves. Elastic fibers are oriented predominantly in a longitudinal direction and form a loose continuous network of elongated meshes. The elastic fibers become condensed into an elastic membrane that demarcates the lamina propria from the submucosa.

The *submucosa* is composed largely of collagen fibers. It has a loose lamellar construction and permits sliding of the mucous membrane against the layers below. The submucosa is thickest in the large bronchi, where it surrounds the bronchial glands. It contains branches of the bronchial arteries which supply capillaries to the wall of the airways. Bronchial veins traverse the submucosa near the hilum. The submucosa thins distally as the bronchi become smaller.

The *muscularis* is a layer of smooth muscle lying between the submucosa and the adventitia. The muscularis is most extensive in the large bronchi and the muscle fibers attach to the open ends of the C-shaped cartilagenous rings. In smaller bronchi the muscularis develops into a complete ring of smooth muscle located between the submucosa and the cartilage (Fig. 3.3).

The mucosa, submucosa and muscularis are surrounded by a fibrous *adventitia* in which the cartilage rings are embedded. Bronchial arteries lie in the adventitia running the length of the bronchial tree.

The bronchial arteries are small branches of the descending aorta. They enter the hilum of each lung and supply branches to the bronchial tree. Smaller branches penetrate the muscularis into the submucosa. A network of capillaries lies in the lamina propria of the mucosa. Venous plexuses are present deep to the capillary bed on both sides of the muscularis. These connect with the bronchopulmonary veins.

Lymphoid follicles are found focally along the bronchial tree within the lamina propria. Little is known of their function, although it is likely that they play an important role in host defense. Morphologically they resemble Peyer's patches of the intestine. To date the bronchial follicles have received little attention, although they have been described in humans, other mammals, and chickens (McDermott *et al.*, 1982). Lymphatic channels accompany the bronchial tree and a network of small lymphatic vessels lies in the lamina propria. The bronchial lymphatics interconnect with lymphatics from the visceral pleura at the hilum, where they drain into the tracheobronchial lymph nodes.

The bronchi are innervated from branches of the vagus nerve and from the cervical sympathetic ganglia. These neural pathways influence the beating of cilia, secretion of mucus and epithelial permeability, as well as their classical actions on the vasculature and smooth muscle. Stimulation of the vagus nerve causes discharge of secretions from the bronchial glands and contraction of the muscularis. Sympathetic stimulation inhibits the vagus and causes the bronchi to dilate. The nerves which enter the lung form two plexi, one in the adventitia and one which lies superficial to the cartilage ring. The lamina propria has a rich innervation with bundles of myelinated and unmyelinated fibers. Intraepithelial nerves have been found in the main stem extrapulmonary bronchi and the trachea (Jeffery, 1982).

The bronchial airways vary in width and length throughout the lungs and the structure of the bronchial wall varies according to the size of the tubes. As the lumen narrows, so the bronchial wall becomes thinner. The structure of the bronchial wall was described in considerable detail by von Hayek (1960). He differentiated three structural types of bronchi according to their size: large, medium and small. Of course there is no sharp line of demarcation between these rather arbitrary divisions. The small bronchi pass into the bronchioles, which in turn pass into the alveoli. As mentioned at the beginning of Chapter 1, this book does not describe the normal or abnormal respiratory tract distal to the smallest branches of the bronchi, i.e. those tubes which lie proximal to the last plate of cartilage (see below).

The structure of the walls of the large bronchi resembles that of the trachea. The larger airways are supported by C-shaped cartilagenous plates which are open posteriorly. Cartilage is abundant and muscle fibers are attached to the open ends of the C-shaped rings so that the posterior gap is filled to form the membranous part (*pars membranacea*). Cartilage is irregular in medium-sized bronchi but the muscularis is well developed. The medium-sized bronchi are especially rich in glands. The small bronchi have few glands and are characterized by a rich venous plexus located between the muscularis and the fibrous cartilage-containing adventitia.

Jeffery and Reid (1977a) have suggested that airways should be designated by structure and position along their pathway, rather than by size. They advocate the following definition of bronchi based on the presence and distribution of cartilage. Accordingly bronchi are defined as those air tubes which lie proximal to the last plate of cartilage along an airway. The most proximal generations can be considered as 'large bronchi'. Cartilage is so abundant in their walls that some cartilage will always be included in any cross-section. 'Small bronchi' lie between the fifth and fifteenth generations, where cartilage is sparse, so that many cross-sections will not include cartilage.

Dense bands of elastic fibers are collected at the posterior membranous part of the large bronchi. The elastic fibers run in longitudinal bundles the entire length of the airways from the trachea to the smallest bronchial tubes, where they continue into the spiral elastic fibers of the alveolar ducts and alveolar wall. The elastic fibers fan out distally so that they exist beneath the epithelial lining around the entire circumference of the smaller bronchial tubes. These bundles of elastic fibers account for the longitudinal mucosal corrugations of the membranous part of the trachea and large bronchi (Miller, 1947; Monkhouse and Whimster, 1976). In the medium and small bronchi, where the C-shaped rings give way to a mosaic of cartilage plates, the longitudinal corrugations become evenly spaced around the inside of the tube. The function of the longitudinal folds is not known.

3.2.3 Surface epithelium

The delicate epithelial lining of the bronchial airways serves many functions, one of which is to provide a mucociliary escalator which effects the removal of particulates and noxious substances to the larynx so that they can be expectorated or swallowed. Inhaled gases are absorbed into the bronchial secretions and are similarly removed. Bronchial secretions from the surface and glandular epithelium include mucus, muramidase (lysozyme), and secretory IgA. The epithelial lining of the adult is composed largely of four types of epithelial cells (see below), but cells of the immune series such as lymphocytes and mast cells may migrate within the epithelium. A higher proportion of mast cells is found in the distal airway epithelium of smokers than in nonsmokers (Lamb and Lumsden, 1982). There are also a few nerve terminals which may initiate reflex action in response to chemical and/or mechanical stimuli (Jeffery, 1982).

The baseline for defining the 'normal' state stems from comparative evaluation of what is known of the structure of the epithelium in developing fetuses, neonates and young animals free of respiratory disease and from what is known of the reaction of the adult epithelium to injury. The epithelia of neonates and of young animals that have not been exposed to irritants show a pseudostratified architecture. This means that the bases of all cell types rest upon the basement membrane, but only the apical surfaces of columnar mucous, ciliated, and some dense-core granulated cells reach to the airway. The apices of the short basal cells do not reach to the airway. Thus, in normal pseudostratified epithelium, the basal cells do not form a continuous cell layer but are separated by the basal cytoplasm of the columnar cells which rest upon the basement membrane (Figs 2.1, 3.4). This architecture is seldom seen in adult human bronchi and many specimens show varying degrees of basal cell hyperplasia, mucous cell hyperplasia, stratification, and/or epidermoid (squamous) metaplasia, at least in focal areas (Chapter 9). It remains uncertain how many, if any, of the columnar cells actually rest upon the basement membrane in such specimens, because basal cells appear to be contiguous,

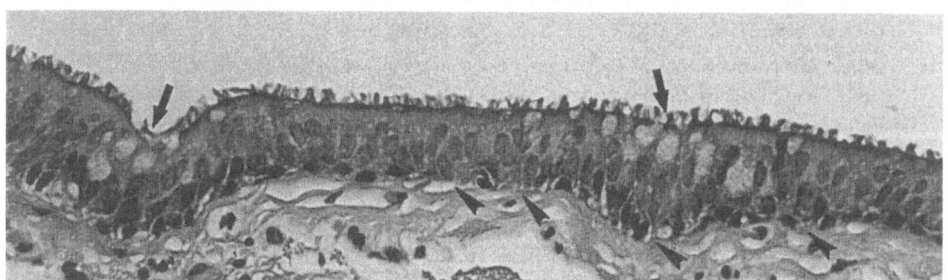

Fig. 3.4 Pseudostratified appearance of normal bronchial epithelium. Note that the small dense-stained basal cells do not form a continuous cell layer but are separated by the columnar cells (mucous and ciliated) which rest on the basement membrane (arrowheads). Some of the mucous cells are distended with secretions (arrows). (Paraffin section stained with hematoxylin and eosin: × 250.)

forming a complete cell layer. This departure from a pseudostratified architecture presumably reflects minimal change from normal. It is interesting to note that implants of human epithelium maintained subcutaneously in athymic nude mice for several months reverted to the pseudostratified form in the sheltered environment afforded by this host (Valerio et al., 1981).

Only four epithelial cell types are recognized with certainty in the surface epithelium of adult human bronchi. These are columnar *mucous cells* and *ciliated cells* that do reach to the airway lumen, *dense-core granulated cells*, some of which reach the lumen, and *basal cells* that do not reach to the bronchial lumen. In addition, a few immature *preciliated cells* are seen.

Mucous cells demonstrate an abundant electron-dense cytoplasm when they are not distended with secretion product (Fig. 3.5a). The Golgi apparatus and rough endoplasmic reticulum are very well developed. Mucus is synthesized in the endoplasmic reticulum and Golgi apparatus and is stored in the apical cytoplasm in membrane-bounded granules. The granules are distributed between the Golgi apparatus and the cell apex. The mucosubstances are electron lucent but sometimes an electron-dense core is present. When the cells contain few granules, the apical cell surfaces tend to be rather flat, but the apical surface may bulge into the lumen when mucus is abundant, causing distention of the cytoplasm, typical of classical 'goblet cells' (Fig. 3.5b). Thus, depending on the amount of secretion stored within the cell, *mucous cells* appear morphologically different (Figs 2.1, 3.5a, b). The mucous granules coalesce when the secretion is abundant (Fig. 3.5b). When mucous cells contain minimal amounts of secretion they can be easily overlooked in paraffin sections stained with hematoxylin and eosin (Fig. 3.6a). This is well demonstrated when an adjacent section is stained with Alcian blue-PAS (Fig. 3.6b). On the other hand, if the cells contain abundant mucus secretion, they are plump and swollen and are easily recognized, even in sections stained with hematoxylin and eosin (Fig. 3.4).

Most mucous cells of the surface epithelium secrete acidic mucosubstances. These can be PAS reactive or PAS unreactive. Sulphomucins stain blue and sialomucins stain purple with Alcian blue (AB)(pH 2.5)-PAS because the former are PAS unreactive and the latter are PAS reactive (blue plus magenta colors purple). A few surface cells secrete only neutral mucosubstances. These cells stain magenta with the AB-PAS stain; that is, their mucosubstances are PAS reactive but do not stain with Alcian blue.

A few tonofilament bundles may be seen in normal mucous cells, consistent with the presence of keratin proteins (Schlegel et al., 1980; Mitchell and Gusterson, 1982). Furthermore, monoclonal antibodies can

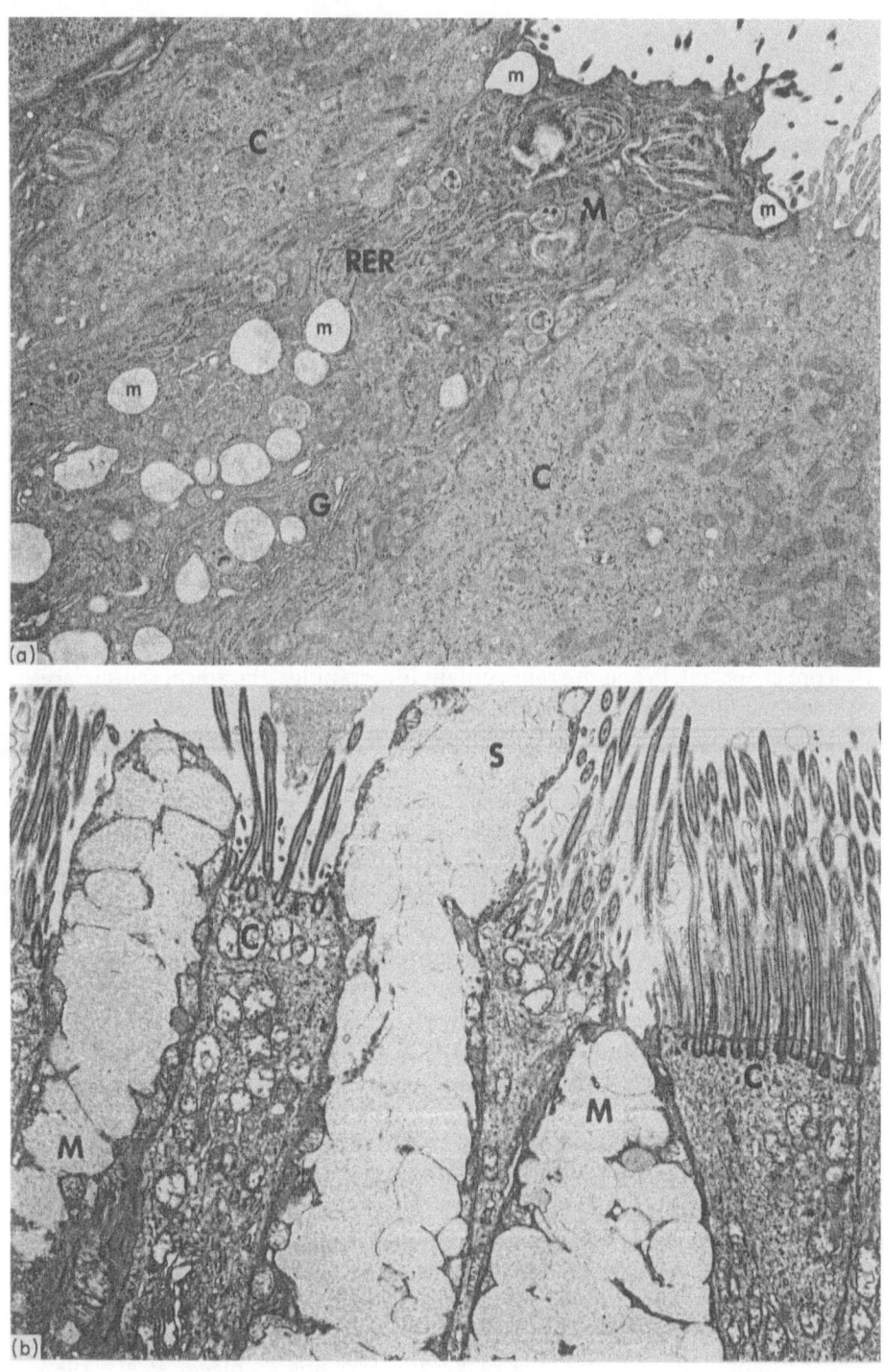

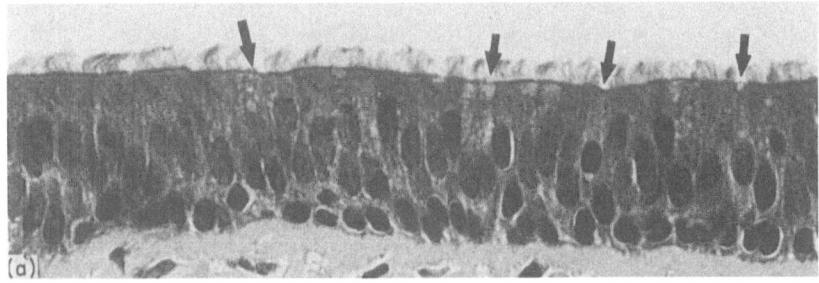

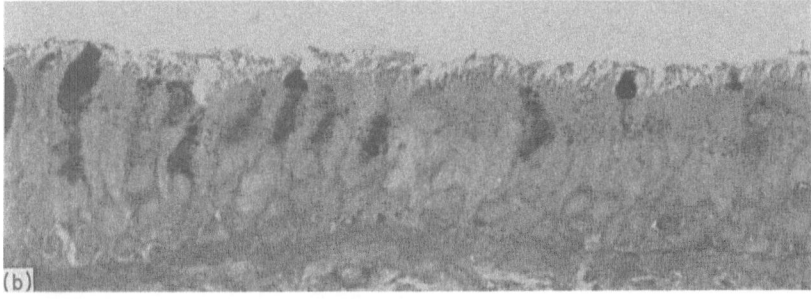

Fig. 3.6 (a) Pseudostratified mucociliary epithelium. Most columnar cells appear to be ciliated; however, close examination shows several nonciliated mucous cells (arrows). (Paraffin section stained with hematoxylin and eosin: × 500.) (b) When an adjacent section is stained with Alcian blue-PAS, mucous cells are more easily seen. Some mucous cells contain abundant secretions, whereas others contain only a few small granules. Compare with equivalent ultrastructures, Figs 3.5a, b. (Paraffin section stained with Alcian blue-PAS: × 500.)

discriminate between the keratin in mucous and ciliated cells from that in basal cells (Ramaekers *et al.*, 1983; Blobel *et al.*, 1984).

Ciliated cells (Figs 3.5b, 3.7a) have been described in detail in man and animals, and they appear to be quite similar in all species studied (Jeffery and Reid, 1977b; Breeze and Wheeldon, 1977). Ciliated cells are columnar, characterized by a fringe of apical cilia which readily allows discrimination from mucous cells by light microscopy (Fig. 3.6a). The cytoplasm is electron lucent, and the microvilli, which project from the cell apices between the cilia, are long and slender (Fig. 3.7a). The proportion of ciliated cells and the density and lengths of the cilia decrease from proximal to more distal

---

Fig. 3.5 (a) Mucous cell (M), flanked by paler ciliated cells (C). The mucous cell has abundant cytoplasm; the Golgi apparatus (G) and rough endoplasmic reticulum (RER) are well developed. Mucous granules (m) are dispersed. (Electron micrograph: × 10 000.) (b) Mucous cells (M), flanked by ciliated cells (C). The mucous cells are distended with multiple coalescent mucous granules. This morphology is typical of 'goblet' cells. The mucous cell at center is discharging its secretion (S). Following discharge this cell would resemble the mucous cell in Fig. 3.5a. (Electron micrograph: × 5000.)

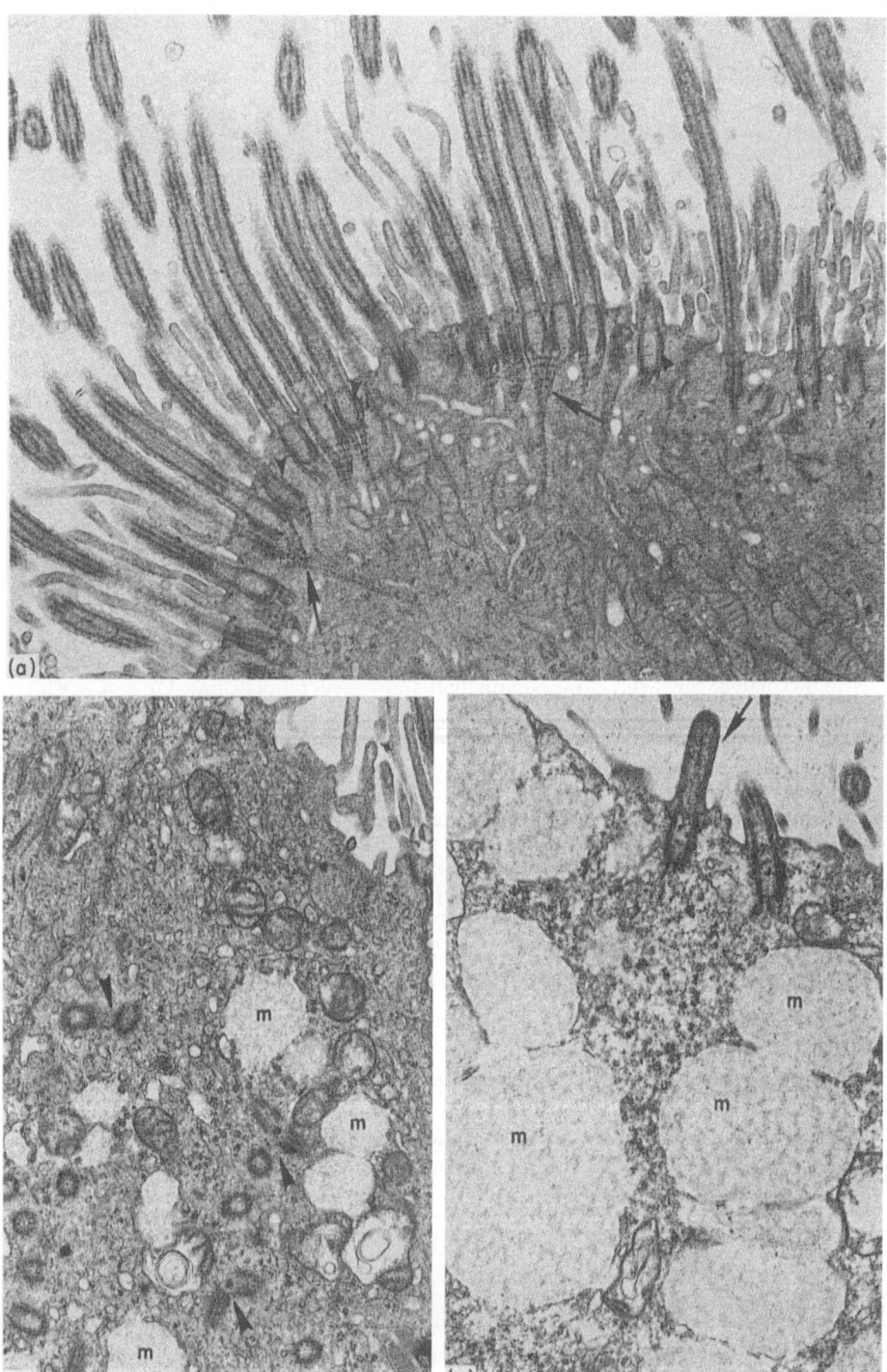

airways, which implies that rates of mucociliary clearance are slower in the smaller peripheral airways than in the major bronchi (Sturgess, 1979).

Details of ciliary structure are given in Chapter 7. All cilia in one field beat in the same direction, but those in neighboring fields beat in slightly different directions (Van As and Webster, 1972). The collective directions of the beats are up the airways, and the tips of the cilia contact the mucus and claw it forward. The mucus coating the airways is usually considered as a two-phase system in which a viscoelastic gel of mucus floats on a watery, less viscous sol phase. The cilia beat in the sol phase and their tips interact with the bottom of the gel, propelling the mucus cephalad (Sleigh, 1981).

Preciliated cells (Fig. 3.7b) are immature ciliated cells. They are rarely seen in normal adult bronchi. Preciliated cells become very numerous during epithelial regeneration immediately prior to restoration of the mucociliary state (Chapter 9). Their low numbers in normal epithelium reflect a low mitotic rate of progenitor cells, yet of sufficient magnitude to replace effete ciliated cells. Preciliated cells are nonciliated columnar cells characterized by an abundant pale electron-lucent cytoplasm. The apical membrane bears long slender microvilli similar to those seen in mature ciliated cells. Preciliated cells show signs of ciliary development in their apical cytoplasm, first in the form of aggregates of fibrogranular material and later as multiple basal bodies (Fig. 3.7b), which line up perpendicular below the apical membrane to form the ciliary basal bodies. A single cilium develops from each of the newly formed basal bodies. The process of ciliogenesis *per se* is the same in the fetus as in the adult (reviewed by Jeffery and Reid, 1977a). The apical cytoplasm of preciliated cells often contains mucous granules, presumably carried over from division of the parent mucous cell (see Chapter 9). Preciliated cells mature into ciliated cells, and cells which bear budding cilia and contain mucous granules in their apical cytoplasm are occasionally seen (Fig. 3.7c).

Basal cells (Fig. 3.8a) are small pyramidal cells that are attached to the basal lamina by well-developed hemidesmosomes. They are overlaid by columnar ciliated and mucous cells (Fig. 3.4). The cytoplasm of basal cells is moderately electron dense and the nuclear-cytoplasmic ratio is high

---

Fig. 3.7 (a) Ciliated cell. Numerous cilia and long slender microvilli project from the apical cell membrane. The basal bodies of the cilia (arrowheads) are firmly attached within the apical cytoplasm by striated rootlets (arrows). (Electron micrograph: × 16 000.) (b) Preciliated cell. Developing basal bodies (arrowheads) are scattered throughout the apical cytoplasm. Mucous granules (m) are also present. The cell bears apical microvilli, similar to those seen in mature ciliated cells. Compare with similar cell in regenerating hamster trachea (Fig. 9.6). (Electron micrograph: × 13 000.) (c) Maturation of preciliated cell to a ciliated cell; a cilium is growing out from the basal body (arrow). The formation of new ciliated cells is described in Chapter 9. (Electron micrograph: × 17 000.)

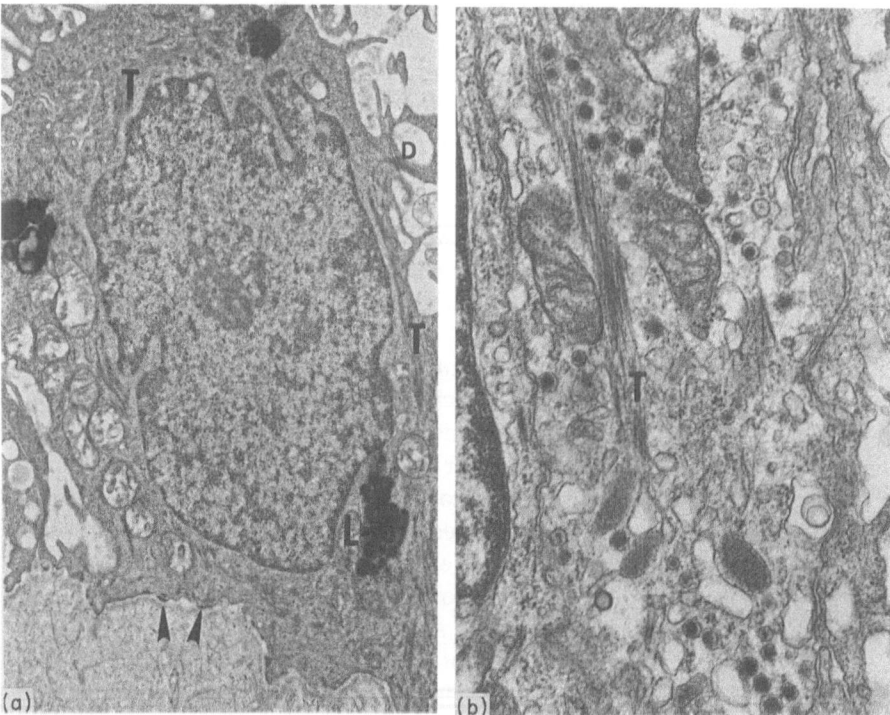

Fig. 3.8 (a) Basal cell. The cell is attached to the basal lamina by well-developed hemidesmosomes (arrowheads). The nuclear to cytoplasmic ratio is high because the cytoplasm is very scant. Tonofilament bundles (T) and lysosomes (L), filled with lipofuscin, lie in the cytoplasm. Desmosome (D). (Electron micrograph: × 9000.) (b) Dense-core granulated cell. The cytoplasm contains numerous dense-cored granules. Note tonofilament bundles (T), like those seen in basal cells. (Electron micrograph: × 22 000.)

because the cytoplasm is very scant. Polyribosomes are numerous but endoplasmic reticulum and Golgi apparatus are poorly developed. Tonofilament bundles, shown to be keratin by immunocytochemistry (Schlegel *et al.*, 1980; Mitchell and Gusterson, 1982), are often relatively abundant. A monoclonal antibody to keratin demonstrates determinants specific to basal cells (Blobel *et al.*, 1984).

Dense-core granulated (DCG) cells (Fig. 3.8b) (Synonyms: endocrine cells, Kultschitsky cells, K-cells, Feyrter cells, neuroendocrine cells, small-granule cells, neurosecretory cells, paracrine cells, APUD cells, etc.) are present in the surface epithelium and in the bronchial glands (Bensch *et al.*, 1965; Terzakis *et al.*, 1972; Tateishi, 1973; Hage, 1976; Hage *et al.*, 1977; Capella *et al.*, 1978). The cells are quite rare in the adult, although they are said to be more numerous in smaller than in larger bronchi (Tateishi, 1973).

They usually occur singly, but groups of cells are occasionally seen. Many cells are entirely basally located; that is, the apex of the cell does not reach the lumen, but some cells assume columnar form and reach to the airway lumen (Tateishi, 1973; McDowell et al., 1976; Sorokin et al., 1981). DCG cells possess long dendrite-like cytoplasmic processes that extend considerable distances within the intercellular spaces formed by neighboring epithelial cells.

Based on the ultrastructural characteristics of their dense-cored granules, at least three cell types have been described in the human fetus (Hage, 1973; Capella et al., 1978), but only one type has so far been identified in the adult. In the adult, the granules which are surrounded by a single membrane are small and round (100–140 nm diameter). They have a dense core surrounded by an electron-lucent halo. Bundles of filaments, which morphologically resemble the tonofilaments of basal cells, are commonly seen in the cytoplasm of normal DCG cells (Fig. 3.8b).

Although the cells are easily recognized ultrastructurally by their characteristic dense-cored granules, they are not readily distinguished from other cells at light microscopic level unless special stains are used. Sometimes they can be demonstrated using argyrophilic stains (Grimelius, 1968; Tateishi, 1973) or by their property of formaldehyde-induced fluorescence, although both techniques are notoriously unreliable. The latter reaction demonstrates biogenic amines and can be enhanced by prior incubation with 5-hydroxytryptophan or L-DOPA (Hage et al., 1977; Hage, 1980). Argyrophilia is a common cytochemical characteristic shared by a number of DCG cells that produce low molecular weight polypeptide hormones. Some of these cells can be demonstrated in paraffin sections using lead hematoxylin (Solcia et al., 1969) or basic dyes after acid hydrolysis (Solcia et al., 1968). The PAS-lead hematoxylin stain, used alone (Sorokin and Hoyt, 1978) or in conjunctive staining regimens (Sorokin et al., 1981), exquisitely demonstrates these cells by light microscopy in glycol-methacrylate-embedded sections.

Until recently no hormones or enzymes had been linked specifically with pulmonary DCG cells, but during the last decade, due largely to the application of immunocytochemical methods, serotonin (Lauweryns et al., 1972), bombesin (Wharton et al., 1978), calcitonin (Becker et al., 1980), leu-enkephalin (Cutz et al., 1981), and the enzyme neuron-specific enolase (Wharton et al., 1981; Sheppard et al., 1984) have been demonstrated, particularly in fetal and/or neonatal lungs. Immunostained serial sections indicated that neuron-specific enolase-positive cells also contained bombesin and/or serotonin-like reactivity. These observations point to heterogeneity between different types of DCG cells (Wharton et al., 1981).

The precise function of DCG cells is not known, but it has been postulated that they serve a chemoreceptor function in the regional control of vasodilation and vasoconstriction (Lauweryns and Cokelaere, 1973; Moosavi *et al.*, 1973). As described above, the biological characteristics of these cells suggest that they secrete bioactive humoral substances that react either within their immediate environment (paracrine action) or more distally (endocrine action).

A hypothesis was proposed that DCG cells of diverse types originated from the neural crest (Pearse, 1969). However, there is now strong evidence that these cells are of endodermal origin in the intestinal tract and lung (LeDouarin and Teillet, 1973; Andrew 1974, 1975, 1976; Pictet *et al.*, 1976; Fontaine and LeDouarin, 1977; Yesner, 1981; Sorokin *et al.*, 1982; Di Augustine and Sonstegard, 1984). However, neural crest cells do migrate into these regions to give rise to autonomic ganglia.

Reference is often made to so-called *intermediate cells*. The term is used loosely to describe several different cell types in normal and abnormal epithelia. For example, the term has been used to describe 'tall' basal cells, mature mucus-secreting cells with scant secretion product, and immature presecretory and preciliated cells. Confusion has arisen over many years by extrapolation of poorly defined functional concepts to poorly defined morphological criteria, and it is recommended that the term be dropped (McDowell *et al.*, 1983). Intermediate cells are perceived by some as undifferentiated cells with the capacity to differentiate directly into specialized cells and the term is often used to describe cells in the normal epithelium that lack obvious signs of specialization by light microscopy. These cells are spindle shaped and may extend from base to lumen. However, ultrastructural studies have demonstrated that the majority of cells deemed to be of 'intermediate' type based on light microscopic criteria are in fact specialized secretory cells with mucous granules in both normal (McDowell *et al.*, 1978) and abnormal (Trump *et al.*, 1978) epithelium. In metaplastic epithelium, pathologists have used the term in a spatial sense to describe cells that lie in a position 'intermediate' between basal and superficial layers. For further discussion the reader is referred to McDowell *et al.* (1983).

3.2.4 Bronchial glands

The submucosal glands are the major source of bronchial secretions. Glands occur throughout the bronchial tree in large, medium, and small bronchi, but they are absent from the bronchioles. They vary in number and size according to the size of the bronchus and are most highly developed in medium-sized bronchi. The glands are tubulo-acinar structures, each with a duct that opens into the airway lumen. They lie deep in the bronchial wall, usually external to the muscularis and internal to or between the cartilage plates (Fig. 3.3). It is estimated that there are 5000 glands in the human lung, and the area of the bronchial glandular epithelium far exceeds that of the bronchial surface epithelium. Studies suggest that the glands constitute some 40 times the volume of surface epithelial secretory cells (Reid, 1960; Tappan and Zalar, 1963).

Glandular reconstructions have been made from serial sections, and large glands are composed of four structural regions: the ciliated duct, the collecting duct, mucous tubules, and serous tubules (Meyrick et al., 1969). The ciliated duct, which is continuous with the surface epithelium, is lined by basal cells, columnar ciliated and mucous cells, similar to cells in the surface epithelium. This leads into the lower part of the duct, the collecting duct, which is lined by collecting duct cells (Fig. 3.9a). Collecting duct cells are tall columnar and contain numerous large densely-packed mitochondria which lie parallel to the lateral borders of the cell; the endoplasmic reticulum is poorly developed. These features cause the cells to stain intensely eosinophilic in sections stained with hematoxylin and eosin. The collecting duct cells have the appearance of oncocytes (Matsuba et al., 1972). They show high activity of oxidative enzymes, but they do not stain with periodic acid-Schiff (Azzopardi and Thurlbeck, 1968). It has been suggested that the collecting duct cells play a role in modulating the water and ionic content of the mucous secretions (Meyrick and Reid, 1970; Meyrick, 1977).

The secretory elements arise from the collecting duct. They are of two types, mucous or serous, depending upon the type of epithelial secretory cell. Mucous tubules, lined by mucous cells, branch from the collecting duct and end in clusters of blind-ended serous tubules. Some serous branches also arise from the sides of the mucous tubules (Fig. 3.9a). Thus, discrete regions within the gland are formed of either mucous cells or serous cells, in roughly equal proportions. Because of the structure of the glands, serous secretions (which are formed distally) flow through the proximal mucous tubules before they reach the airway.

Mucous cells and serous cells can be distinguished morphologically and histochemically (Meyrick and Reid, 1970; Meyrick, 1977; Bowes and Corrin, 1977). By light microscopy, mucous cells are characteristically distended with secretion product, while the cytoplasm of serous cells appears granular. The secretion granules of mucous glands stain blue or blue-purple with the AB-PAS stain, indicative of acidic glycoproteins (sulfo or sialomucins), whereas many of the serous cells stain magenta, indicative of neutral glycoproteins. Some serous cells show evidence of acidic secretions (Fig. 3.9b). Keratin is present in both serous cells and mucous cells (Gusterson et al., 1982; Blobel et al., 1984).

Mucous and serous cells are columnar and are characterized ultrastructurally by electron-dense cytoplasm and well-developed Golgi apparatus and rough endoplasmic reticulum. However, mucous cells contain

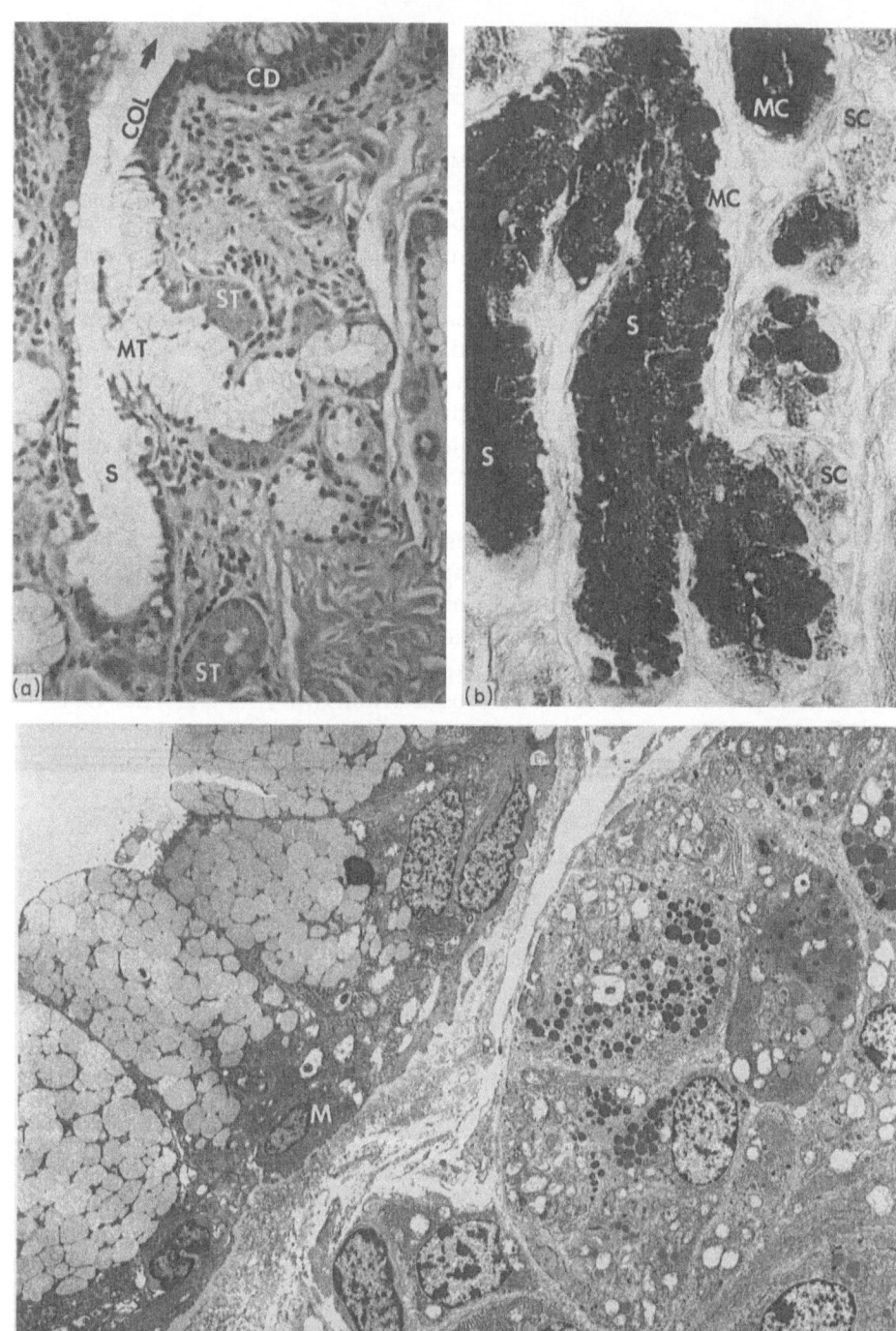

numerous large electron-lucent granules which often fuse one with another and distend the apical cytoplasm. On the other hand, serous cells contain electron-dense membrane-bounded granules which accumulate in the apical cytoplasm but which remain discrete and do not distend the apical portion of the cell (Fig 3.9c). The cells are joined laterally by small desmosomes and apically by tight junctions.

Bronchial changes in disease stimulate conversion of serous cells to mucous cells and in chronic bronchitis the majority of the glands are composed of distended mucous cells and granular serous cells are rare (Reid, 1960). Exposure to irritants such as tobacco smoke and sulfur dioxide also causes serous cells to transform into mucous cells and cells that contain both electron-dense (serous) and electron-lucent (mucous) granules (Jeffery et al., 1976; Jeffery and Reid, 1977b) are seen ultrastructurally.

Serous cells contain the enzyme muramidase (lysozyme) (Mason and Taylor, 1975; Klockars and Reitamo, 1975; Bowes and Corrin, 1977). Secretion of this enzyme, an important nonspecific antibacterial agent, appears to be a major function of serous cells, which are to be considered part of the bronchial defense system against infection. In chronic bronchitis, serous acini are rare, suggesting that muramidase secretions are reduced. This may have important implications with regard to bacterial infections frequently associated with chronic bronchitis (Bowes and Corrin, 1977).

Evidence is also increasing to support the view that serous cells are responsible for the transport of IgA across the glandular epithelium. Secretory component, a glycoprotein, is present in the cytoplasm and plasma membrane of the serous cells, including those of the bronchial glands (Poger and Lamm, 1974; Brandtzaeg, 1974; Harris and South, 1981). Interstitial plasma cells are the principal source of IgA in bronchial secretions and IgA-containing cells mostly cluster around the bronchial glands in the main and large bronchi (Soutar, 1976). It has been suggested that membrane-associated secretory component acts as a specific surface receptor for IgA produced in the lamina propria and that serous cells are

---

Fig. 3.9 (a) Bronchial gland. Ciliated duct (CD); collecting duct (COL); mucous tubule (MT) and serous tubules (ST). Secretions (S) lie within the glandular lumen. The arrow points in the direction of the airway. (Paraffin section stained with hematoxylin and eosin: × 220.) (b) Mucous and serous tubules of a bronchial gland stained with Alcian blue-PAS. The mucous cells (MC) are distended with acidic mucosubstances. Secretions (S) fill the glandular lumen. Serous cells (SC) are not distended with secretion; however, small discrete secretion granules are dispersed within them. (Paraffin section stained with Alcian blue-PAS: × 330.) (c) Mucous tubule (left); serous tubule (right). The mucous cells contain numerous electron-lucent granules which are coalescing and distend the apical cytoplasm. The serous cells contain discrete electron-dense granules. Myoepithelial cell (M). Reproduced with permission from Bowes and Corrin (1977). (Electron micrograph: × 2600.)

responsible for the molecular completion of secretory IgA and for selective external transfer of the antibody to the glandular lumen (Brandtzaeg, 1974).

Other cell types of the glandular epithelium include DCG cells (Bensch *et al.*, 1965) and myoepithelial cells. The latter, sometimes called basket cells, are located between the bases of the serous, mucous, and collecting duct cells and the basal lamina (Fig. 3.9c). It is likely that contraction of these cells aids in the passage of secretion from the gland into the airway lumen (Meyrick and Reid, 1970).

Human bronchial glands are innervated, and bundles of unmyelinated axons are found between the acini. Single terminal axons are seen above the basal lamina between serous, mucous, and collecting duct cells and between any of these cells and myoepithelial cells (Meyrick and Reid, 1970).

3.2.5   Epithelial cell kinetics

Surprisingly little is known about cell kinetics of the adult human tracheobronchial epithelium; although studied quite extensively in animals, the proliferative potentials of different cell types, the origins of nascent cells, and an appreciation of the full range of phenotypic expression remain to be clarified, and voids still exist in our understanding. One reason for this is that different investigators have varied perceptions of the nature and functions of the various epithelial cells.

In experimental animals the adult surface epithelium has a very low labeling index for tritiated thymidine and a low mitotic rate (reviewed in Boren and Paradise, 1978; Kauffman, 1980). This gives the undisturbed epithelium a proliferative profile of a stable cell population similar to that of kidney, liver, and pancreas. These epithelia normally demonstrate very low levels of replication, but the cells can undergo rapid division in response to a variety of stimuli and are capable of reconstituting the tissue of origin.

Although numerous studies in different species have demonstrated that basal cells and mucous cells can synthesize DNA and undergo mitosis, one body of opinion maintains that basal cells are the major progenitor cells from which all other cell types arise, including ciliated cells (reviewed by Breeze and Wheeldon, 1977). However, it has also been stated for over 100 years that mucous cells serve as transitional stages in the development of ciliated cells (Miller, 1932). Extensive kinetic analysis of undisturbed hamster trachea led Boren and Paradise (1978) to describe two kinetic compartments – a self-maintaining basal cell compartment which fed into a dividing mucous cell compartment. Nascent mucous and ciliated cells arose from division of mucous cells. The greatest amplification was ascribed to mucous cells since they far outnumbered basal cells and 80% of them divided. Moreover, the cell cycle time of mucous cells (97 hours) was much shorter than that of basal cells (159 hours). For additional comments on the genesis of different cell types in normal and abnormal states see Chapter 9.

We know of no kinetic analysis of the proliferative potentials of cells of the bronchial glands. Basal cells are absent from the glands and the secretory elements are composed of mucous cells and serous cells. During glandular development in the rat, mitotic figures were common in the secretory cells (Smolich et al., 1978). In the adult epithelium both mucous cells and serous cells are capable of division (Meyrick, 1977).

Available data suggest that DCG cells divide infrequently or not all in the normal adult epithelium (reviewed by Di Augustine and Sonstegard, 1984); it is generally agreed that ciliated cells of the respiratory tract are terminally differentiated and do not divide.

3.3 Conclusion to Part One

With this we conclude Part One of the book. The discussions of the choice of specimen which will likely provide the most relevant information at the least risk of morbidity to the patient, of the care necessary in processing specimens for examination, and a review of the normal structure of the airways and kinetics of the epithelial cells are intended to lay a foundation for the succeeding chapters which deal with specific abnormalities of the bronchi. The ability to correctly interpret biopsy material, particularly when the specimens are small, is very much dependent on the appropriate selection of specimens and their proper handling. We all too often discover that our difficulties in arriving at a useful diagnosis result from a lack of forethought. In more complex cases a joint discussion between the pathologist and the thoracic surgeon and/or pulmonary internist may prove invaluable. Although an understanding of normal structure and cell kinetics may not be considered essential for pathodiagnosis, such knowledge is important, for it allows rational interpretations which can guide the pathologist in a logical consideration of the lesion being examined, avoiding embarrassing pitfalls.

References

Andrew, A. (1974), Further evidence that enterochromaffin cells are not derived from the neural crest. *J. Embryol. Exp. Morph.*, **31**, 589–98.

Andrew, A. (1975), APUD cells in the endocrine pancreas and the intestine of chick embryos. *Gen. Comp. Endocrinology*, **26**, 485–95.

Andrew, A. (1976), An experimental investigation into the possible neural crest origin of pancreatic APUD (islet) cells. *J. Embryol. Exp. Morph.*, **35**, 577–93.

Azzopardi, A. and Thurlbeck, W.M. (1968), Oxidative enzyme pattern of the bronchial mucous glands. *Am. Rev. Resp. Dis.*, **97**, 1038–45.

Becker, K.L., Monaghan, K.G. and Silva, O.L. (1980), Immunocytochemical localization of calcitonin in Kulchitsky cells of human lung. *Arch. Pathol. Lab. Med.*, **104**, 196–8.

Bensch, K.G., Gordon, G.B. and Miller, L.R. (1965), Studies on the bronchial counterpart of the Kultschitzky (argentaffin) cell and innervation of bronchial glands. *J. Ultrastruct. Res.*, **12**, 668–86.

Blobel, G.A., Moll, R., Franke, W.W. and Vogt-Moykopf, L. (1984), Cytokeratins in normal lung and lung carcinomas. I. Adenocarcinomas, squamous cell carcinomas and cultured cell lines. *Virchows. Arch. (Cell Pathol.)*, **45**, 407–29.

Boren, H.G. and Paradise, L.J. (1978), Cytokinetics of lung. In *Pathogenesis and Therapy of Lung Cancer* (ed. C.C. Harris), Marcel Dekker, New York, pp. 369–418.

Bowes, D. and Corrin, B. (1977), Ultrastructural immunocytochemical localisation of lysozyme in human bronchial glands. *Thorax*, **32**, 163–70.

Boyden, E.A. (1955), *Segmental Anatomy of the Lungs. The Blackiston Division.* McGraw-Hill, New York.

Boyden, E.A. (1977), Development and growth of the airways. In *Development of the Lung* (ed. W.A. Hodson), Marcel Dekker, New York, pp. 3–35.

Brandtzaeg, P. (1974), Mucosal and glandular distribution of immunoglobulin components: differential localization of free and bound SC in secretory epithelial cells. *J. Immunol.*, **112**, 1553–9.

Breeze, R.G. and Wheeldon, E.B. (1977), State of the art. The cells of the pulmonary airways. *Am. Rev. Resp. Dis.*, **116**, 705–77.

Bucher, U. (1969), Development of cartilage. In *The Anatomy of the Developing Lung* (ed. J. Emery), Heinemann Medical Books, London, pp. 74–93.

Bucher, U. and Reid, L. (1961), Development of the mucus-secreting elements in human lung. *Thorax*, **16**, 219–25.

Campiche, M.A., Gautier, A., Hernandez, E.I. and Reymond, A. (1963), An electron microscope study of the fetal development of human lung. *Pediatrics*, **32**, 976–94.

Capella, C., Hage, E., Solcia, E. and Usellini, L. (1978), Ultrastructural similarity of endocrine-like cells of the human lung and some related cells of the gut. *Cell Tiss. Res.*, **186**, 25–37.

Conen, P.E. and Balis, J.U. (1969), Electron microscopy in study of lung development. In *The Anatomy of the Developing Lung* (ed. J. Emery), Heinemann Medical Books, London, pp. 18–48.

Cutz, E., Chan, W. and Track, N.S. (1981), Bombesin, calcitonin and leu-enkephalin immunoreactivity in endocrine cells of human lung. *Experientia*, **37**, 765–7.

Cutz, E., Chan, W., Wong, V. and Conen, P.E. (1975), Ultrastructure and fluorescence histochemistry of endocrine (APUD-type) cells in tracheal mucosa of human and various animal species. *Cell Tiss. Res.*, **158**, 425–37.

de Haller, R. (1969), Development of mucus-secreting elements. In *The Anatomy of the Developing Lung* (ed. J. Emery), Heinemann Medical Books, London, pp. 94–115.

Di Augustine, R.P. and Sonstegard, K.S. (1984), Neuroendocrine like (small granule) epithelial cells of the lung. *Environmental Health Perspectives*, **55**, 271–95.

Emery, J. (1969), Connective tissue and lymphatics. In *The Anatomy of the Developing Lung* (ed. J. Emery), Heinemann Medical Books, London, pp. 49–73.

Fontaine, J. and LeDouarin, N.M. (1977), Analysis of endoderm formation in the avian blastoderm by the use of quail-chick chimaeras. *J. Embryol. Exp. Morph.*, **41**, 209–22.

Grimelius, L. (1968), A silver nitrate stain for $\alpha_2$cells in human pancreatic islets. *Acta Soc. Med. Upsal.*, **73**, 243–70.

Gusterson, B., Mitchell, D., Warburton, M. and Sloane, J. (1982), Immunohistochemical localization of keratin in human lung tumors. *Virchows Arch. (Pathol. Anat.)*, **394**, 269–77.

Hage, E. (1973), Electron microscopic identification of several types of endocrine cells in the bronchial epithelium of human foetuses. *Z. Zellforsch. Mikrosk. Anat.*, **141**, 401–12.

Hage, E. (1976), Endocrine-like cells of the pulmonary epithelium. In *Chromaffin, Enterochromaffin and Related Cells* (eds R.E. Coupland and T. Fujita), Elsevier, New York, pp. 317–32.

Hage, E. (1980), Light and electron microscopic characteristics of the various lung endocrine cell types. *Invest. Cell Path.*, **3**, 345–51.

Hage, E., Hage, J. and Juel, G. (1977), Endocrine-like cells of the pulmonary epithelium of the human adult lung. *Cell Tiss. Res.*, **178**, 39–48.

Harris, J.P. and South, M.A. (1981), Secretory component. A glandular epithelial cell marker. *Am. J. Pathol.*, **105**, 47–53.

Jeffery, P.K. (1982), The innervation of bronchial mucosa. In *Cellular Biology of the Lung* (eds G. Cumming and G. Bonsignore), Plenum Press, New York, pp. 1–25.

Jeffery, P.K. and Reid, L.M. (1977a), Ultrastructure of airway epithelium and submucosal gland during development. In *Development of the Lung* (ed. W.A. Hodson), Marcel Dekker, New York, pp. 87–134.

Jeffery, P.K. and Reid, L.M. (1977b), The respiratory mucous membrane. In *Respiratory Defense Mechanisms. Part I.*, chapter 7 (eds J.D. Brain, D.F. Proctor and L.M. Reid), Marcel Dekker, New York, pp. 193–245.

Jeffery, P., Widdicombe, J.G. and Reid, L. (1976), Anatomical and physiological features of irritation of the bronchial tree. In *Air Pollution and the Lung* (eds E.F. Ahgrouson, A. Ben-David and M.A. Klinberg), Wiley, New York, pp. 253–67.

Kauffman, S.L. (1980), Cell proliferation in the mammalian lung. *Int. Rev. Exp. Pathol.*, **22**, 131–91.

Klockars, M. and Reitamo, S. (1975), Tissue distribution of lysozyme in man. *J. Histochem. Cytochem.*, **23**, 932–40.

Lamb, D. and Lumsden, A. (1982), Intra-epithelial mast cells in human airway epithelium: evidence for smoking-induced changes in their frequency. *Thorax*, **37**, 334–42.

Lauweryns, J.M. and Cokelaere, M. (1973), Hypoxia-sensitive neuro-epithelial bodies: intrapulmonary secretory neuroreceptors modulated by the CNS. *Z. Zellforsch.*, **145**, 521–40.

Lauweryns, J.M., Cokelaere, M. and Theunynck, P. (1972), Neuro-epithelial bodies in the respiratory mucosa of various mammals: a light optical, histochemical and ultrastructural investigation. *Z. Zellforsch.*, **135**, 569–92.

LeDouarin, N.M. and Teillet, M.A. (1973), The migration of neural crest cells to the wall of the digestive tract in avian embryo. *J. Embryol. Exp. Morph.*, **30**, 31–48.

Mason, D.Y. and Taylor, C.R. (1975), The distribution of muramidase (lysozyme) in human tissues. *J. Clin. Pathol.*, **28**, 124–32.

Masters, J.R.W. (1976), Epithelial-mesenchymal interaction during lung development: the effect of mesenchymal mass. *Developmental Biology*, **51**, 98–108.

Matsuba, K., Takizawa, T. and Thurlbeck, W.M. (1972), Oncocytes in human bronchial mucous glands. *Thorax*, **27**, 181–4.

McDermott, M.R., Befus, A.D. and Bienenstock, J. (1982), The structural basis for immunity in the respiratory tract. *Int. Rev. Exp. Pathol.*, **23**, 47–112.

McDowell, E.M., Barrett, L.A., Glavin, F., Harris, C.C. and Trump, B.F. (1978), The respiratory epithelium. I. Human bronchus. *J. Natl Cancer Inst.*, **61**, 539–49.

McDowell, E.M., Barrett, L.A. and Trump, B.F. (1976), Observations on small granule cells in adult human bronchial epithelium and in carcinoid and oat cell tumors. *Lab. Invest.*, **34**, 202–6.

McDowell, E.M., Combs, J.W. and Newkirk, C. (1983), A quantitative light and electron microscopic study of hamster tracheal epithelium with special attention to so-called 'intermediate cells'. *Exp. Lung Res.*, **4**, 205–26.

Meyrick, B. (1977), Mucus-producing cells of the tracheobronchial tree. In *Mucus in Health and Disease* (eds M. Elstein and D.V. Parke), Plenum Press, New York, pp. 61–76.

Meyrick, B. and Reid, L. (1970), Ultrastructure of cells in the human bronchial submucosal glands. *J. Anat.*, **107**, 281–99.

Meyrick, B., Sturgess, J.M. and Reid, L. (1969), A reconstruction of the duct system and secretory tubules of the human bronchial submucosal gland. *Thorax*, **24**, 729–36.

Miller, W.S. (1932), The epithelium of the lower respiratory tract. Section V. In *Special Cytology. The Form and Functions of the Cell in Health and Disease*, Vol. 1, 2nd edn, (ed. E.V. Dowdry), Paul B. Hoeber, New York, pp. 133–50.

Miller, W.S. (1947), The trachea and bronchi. In *The Lung*, 2nd edn, Charles C. Thomas, Springfield, Ill., pp. 12–21.

Mitchell, D.P. and Gusterson, B.A. (1982), Simultaneous demonstration of keratin and mucin. *J. Histochem. Cytochem.*, **30**, 707–9.

Monkhouse, W.S. and Whimster, W.F. (1976), An account of the longitudinal mucosal corrugations of the human tracheo-bronchial tree, with observations on those of some animals. *J. Anat.*, **122**, 681–95.

Moosavi, H., Smith, P. and Heath, D. (1973), The Feyrter cell in hypoxia. *Thorax*, **28**, 729–41.

Nagaishi, C. (1972), *Functional Anatomy and Histology of the Lung*, University Park Press, Baltimore.

Pearse, A.G.E. (1969), The cytochemistry and ultrastructure of polypeptide hormone-producing cells of the APUD series and the embryologic, physiologic and pathologic implications of the concept. *J. Histochem. Cytochem.*, **17**, 303–13.

Pictet, R.L., Rall, L.B., Phelps, P. and Rutter, W.J. (1976), The neural crest and the origin of the insulin-producing and other gastrointestinal hormone-producing cells. *Science*, **191**, 191–2.

Poger, M.E. and Lamm, M.E. (1974), Localization of free and bound secretory component in human intestinal epithelial cells. A model for the assembly of secretory IgA. *J. Exp. Med.*, **139**, 629–42.

Ramaekers, F., Huysmans, A., Noesker, O., Kant, A., Jap, P., Herman, C. and Vooijs, P. (1983), Monoclonal antibody to keratin filaments, specific for glandular epithelia and their tumors. Use in surgical pathology. *Lab. Invest.*, **49**, 353–61.

Reid, L. (1960), Measurement of the bronchial mucous gland layer. A diagnostic yardstick in chronic bronchitis. *Thorax*, **15**, 132–41.

Schlegel, R., Banks-Schlegel, S. and Pinkus, G.S. (1980), Immunohistochemical localization of keratin in normal human tissues. *Lab. Invest.*, **42**, 91–6.

Schneeberger, E.E., Walters, D.V. and Olver, R.E. (1978), Development of intercellular junctions in the pulmonary epithelium of the foetal lamb. *J. Cell Sci.*, **32**, 307–24.

Sheppard, M.N., Marangos, P.J., Bloom, S.R. and Polak, J.M. (1984), Neuron specific enolase: a marker for the early development of nerves and endocrine cells in the human lung. *Life Sci.*, **34**, 265–71.

Sleigh, M.A. (1981), Ciliary function in mucus transport. *Chest*, **80** (supplement), 791–5.

Smolich, J.J., Stratford, B.F., Maloney, J.E. and Ritchie, B.C. (1978), New features in the development of the submucosal gland of the respiratory tract. *J. Anat.*, **127**, 223–38.

Solcia, E., Capella, C. and Vassallo, G. (1969), Lead-hematoxylin as a stain for endocrine cells. Significance of staining and comparison with other selective methods. *Histochemie*, **20**, 116–26.

Solcia, E., Vassallo, G. and Capella, C. (1968), Selective staining of endocrine cells by basic dyes after acid hydrolysis. *Stain Technol.*, **43**, 257–63.

Sorokin, S. (1960), Histochemical events in developing human lungs. *Acta Anat.*, **40**, 105–10.

Sorokin, S. (1965), Recent work on developing lungs. In *Organogenesis* (eds R.L. DeHaan and H. Ursprung), Holt, Rinehart and Winston, New York, pp. 467–91.

Sorokin, S.P. (1968), Reconstruction of centriole formation and ciliogenesis in mammalian lungs. *J. Cell Sci.*, **3**, 207–30.

Sorokin, S.P. and Hoyt, R.F. (1978), PAS-lead hematoxylin as a stain for small-granule endocrine cell populations in the lungs, other pharyngeal derivatives and the gut. *Anat. Rec.*, **192**, 245–60.

Sorokin, S.P., Hoyt, R.F. and Grant, M.M. (1982), Development of neuroepithelial bodies in fetal rabbit lungs. I. Appearance and functional maturation as demonstrated by high-resolution light microscopy and formaldehyde-induced fluorescence. *Exp. Lung Res.*, **3**, 237–59.

Sorokin, S.P., Hoyt, R.F. and McDowell, E.M. (1981), An unusual bronchial carcinoid tumor analyzed by conjunctive staining. *Hum. Pathol.*, **12**, 302–13.

Soutar, C.A. (1976), Distribution of plasma cells and other cells containing immunoglobulin in the respiratory tract of normal man and class of immunoglobulin contained therein. *Thorax*, **31**, 158–66.

Sturgess, J.M. (1979), Mucous secretions in the respiratory tract. *Pediatric Clin. N. Am.*, **26**, 481–501.

Taderera, J.V. (1967), Control of lung differentiation *in vitro*. *Developmental Biology*, **16**, 489–512.

Tappan, V. and Zalar, V. (1963), The pathophysiology of bronchial mucus. *Ann. N.Y. Acad. Sci.*, **106**, 722–45.

Tateishi, R. (1973), Distribution of argyrophil cells in adult human lungs. *Arch. Pathol. Lab. Med.*, **96**, 198–202.

Terzakis, J.A., Sommers, S.C. and Andersson, B. (1972), Neurosecretory appearing cells of human segmental bronchi. *Lab. Invest.*, **26**, 127–32.

Tos, M. (1968), Development of the mucous glands in the human main bronchus. *Anat. Anz.*, **123**, 376–89.

Trump, B.F., McDowell, E.M., Glavin, F., Barrett, L.A., Becci, P.J., Schürch, W., Kaiser, H.E. and Harris, C.C. (1978), The respiratory epithelium. III. Histogenesis of epidermoid metaplasia and carcinoma *in situ* in the human. *J. Natl Cancer Inst.*, **61**, 563–75.

Valerio, M.G., Fineman, E.L., Bowman, R.L., Harris, C.C., Stoner, G.D., Autrup, H., Trump, B.F., McDowell, E.M. and Jones, R.T. (1981), Long-term survival of normal adult human tissues and xenografts in congenitally athymic nude mice. *J. Natl Cancer Inst.*, **66**, 849–58.

Van As, A. and Webster, I. (1972), The organization of ciliary activity and mucus transport on pulmonary airways. *S. Afr. Med. J.*, **46**, 347–50.

von Hayek, H. (1960), *The Human Lung*, Hafner, New York.

Wessells, N.K. (1970), Mammalian lung development: interactions in formation and morphogenesis of tracheal buds. *J. Exp. Zool.*, **175**, 455–66.

Wharton, J., Polak, J.M., Bloom, S.R., Ghatei, M.A., Solcia, E., Brown, M.R. and Pearse, A.G.E. (1978), Bombesin-like immunoreactivity in the lung. *Nature*, **273**, 769–70.

Wharton, J., Polak, J.M., Cole, G.A., Marangos, P.J. and Pearse, A.G.E. (1981), Neuron-specific enolase as an immunocytochemical marker for the diffuse neuroendocrine system in human fetal lung. *J. Histochem. Cytochem.*, **29**, 1359–64.

Yesner, R. (1981), The dynamic histopathologic spectrum of lung cancer. *Yale J. Biol. Med.*, **54**, 447–56.

Part two:
Diseases of the bronchi

4 Micro-organisms

In this chapter our attention will be centered on the various micro-organisms which cause pulmonary disease. Clearly any attempt to be thorough in this coverage would be beyond the scope of the book; rather we will discuss only those micro-organisms which cause lesions that can be diagnosed from bronchial biopsy and in particular those with morphological features which allow recognition in specimens. The histological reactions to these organisms are in themselves often distinctive and will be discussed with more detail in Chapters 5 and 8.

4.1 Viruses

There are more than 200 serologically distinct viruses which cause respiratory disease (Douglas, 1979). They are commonly referred to as the respiratory viruses. Most cause diseases which, although significant in terms of morbidity, rarely lead to hospitalization or the need to establish a specific etiologic diagnosis. Detection by culture takes between 3 days and 1 week. Although nearly instantaneous diagnosis is technically possible using negatively-stained specimens examined in the transmission electron microscope (Doane et al., 1967; Bishop et al., 1974; Chernesky, 1979), high titers of virus particles are necessary, and few electron microscope laboratories have had experience with these techniques. It is more common to have surgical pathologists diagnose viral infections on the basis of changes in appearance of infected cells and specifically on the presence of inclusion bodies which can result from several different phenomena. Inclusion bodies may be collections of the virions themselves, often closely packed so as to form geometrically regular arrays, or they may be accumulations of viral precursor materials clustered in a portion of the host cell as part of the replication process. They may also be accumulations of nonviral material, or at least material not directly involved in assembly of new virus, within the cell. The inclusions may be located within the nucleus or in the cytoplasm. Although these inclusions become conspicuous/distinctive only when they become fairly large, they represent a stage of interaction between the infecting virus and the host cell and smaller forms must exist. These inclusions are more easily seen in poorly-fixed specimens since they tend to be more resistant to fixation abuse than the surrounding cellular material; often an artefactual space surrounding the inclusion makes it more easily detected.

Considerable knowledge of the viruses themselves, their processes of replication and their effects on the host cell are available with tissue culture models. Much less is available on the same processes as they occur in the respiratory system of man. One problem with reports from clinical material is that positive identification of the causative virus is not always available. 'Diagnosis' is often made by the recognition of 'characteristic' features, which are then described as being specific for that virus.

There are three commonly visible morphological effects of viral infection on the host cell: necrosis, often (but not always) necessary for release of the replicated virus particles; multinucleation; and cytomegaly. Unfortunately, the diagnostically important respiratory viruses are each capable of causing any or all of these cellular reactions. In the following discussions we will try to deliniate those microscopic features which will help in the identification of the infections by adenovirus, cytomegalovirus, Herpes simplex, influenza and measles. Table 4.1 gives some of the principal diagnostic features of these viruses.

4.1.1   Adenovirus

This virus is less frequently detected than the others discussed below, but it does cause a bronchitis and pneumonia in adults (most frequently reported in military recruits), children (Pinkerton and Carroll, 1971) and patients with various predisposing problems. In the last group Zahradnik *et al.* (1980) included bone marrow and renal transplant recipients; patients with drug-induced pancytopenia, asthma and chronic obstructive pulmonary disease, Hodgkin's disease, and breast cancer; and prematurely born infants. The disease is usually self-limiting but may rarely be a significant cause of death.

This DNA virus replicates within the nucleus of the infected cell and the virions form into a compact array of particles as they accumulate (Pinkerton and Carroll, 1971; Myerowitz *et al.*, 1975). The crystalline accumulation of virions gives the characteristic basophilic intranuclear inclusions seen in the H&E-stained sections. There may be a thin rim of residual heterochromatin demarking the nuclear margin or the inclusions may appear to spread out into the surrounding cytoplasm (the smudge cells). The uniform density of the particles within the crystalline arrays gives a ground-glass appearance or homogeneity to the stained inclusions. The basophilia of the inclusions and the minimal or absent cleared zone (halo) surrounding them helps in differentiation from the inclusions of

Table 4.1 Some characteristics of the respiratory viruses potentially detected in bronchial specimens

Name	Form	Site of replication	Inclusions	Effect on host cell	Principal host cell in lung
Adenovirus	DNA, icosahedral	Nucleus	Intranuclear (smudge cells)	Enlargement	Bronchial epithelium
Cytomegalovirus	DNA, icosahedral, envelope	Nucleus	Intranuclear (variable cytoplasm)	Cytomegaly	Pneumocyte
Herpes simplex	DNA, icosahedral, envelope	Nucleus	Intranuclear	Multinucleation (moulding)	Squamous cell, bronchial epithelium
Influenza	RNA, helical, envelope	Nucleus cytoplasm	None reliably	Ciliocytophoria	Bronchial
Measles	RNA, helical, envelope	Nucleus	Intranuclear and cytoplasmic	Cytomegaly, (syncytial) multinucleation	Bronchial epithelium, pneumocytes

herpes and cytomegalovirus. Most observers have not seen cytomegaly and/or multinucleation with adenovirus bronchitis, although some increase in the size of the host cell is reported (Craighead, 1970; Pinkerton and Carroll, 1971). Ciliated cells are common targets of infection and frequently retain their cilia (Craighead, 1970), but alveolar cells have also been seen with inclusions in a necrotizing interstitial pneumonitis (Myerowitz *et al.*, 1975). Adenovirus-infected epithelial cells with intranuclear inclusions have been detected in cytology specimens (Frable *et al.*, 1977).

4.1.2 *Cytomegalovirus*

Clinically this virus may be the most important of the group being considered here. This DNA virus belongs in the same group as Herpes simplex but has a different presentation. Cytomegalic inclusion disease is a rare cause of disseminated disease in infants (Stagno *et al.*, 1981) but in

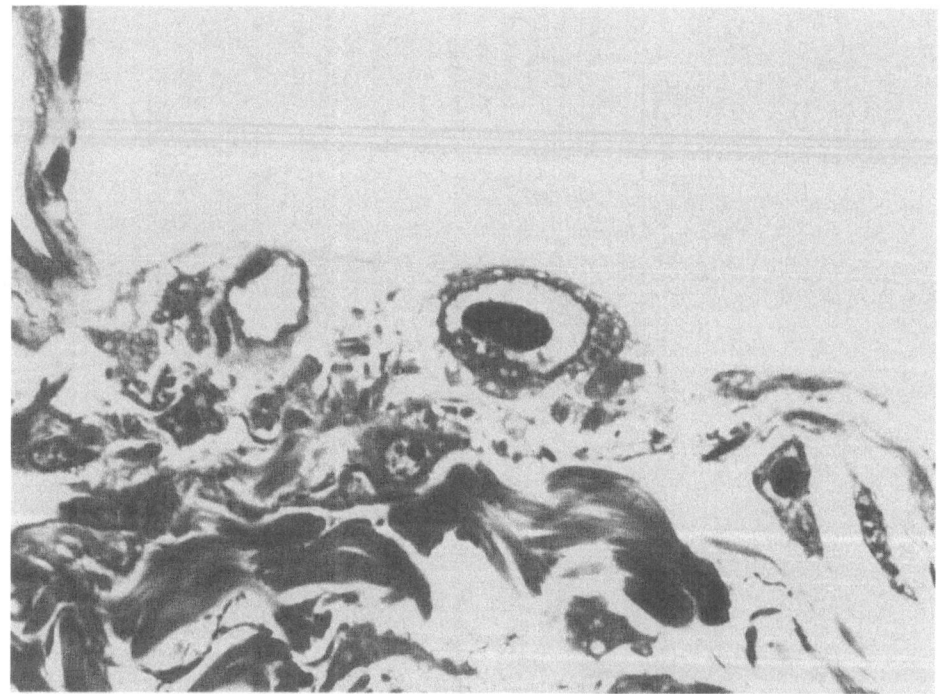

Fig. 4.1 Very enlarged pneumocyte with characteristic large intranuclear inclusion body of cytomegalovirus infection. There is a wide area of clearing between the inclusion and the nuclear membrane. (Epon/Araldite section stained with toluidine blue: × 800.)

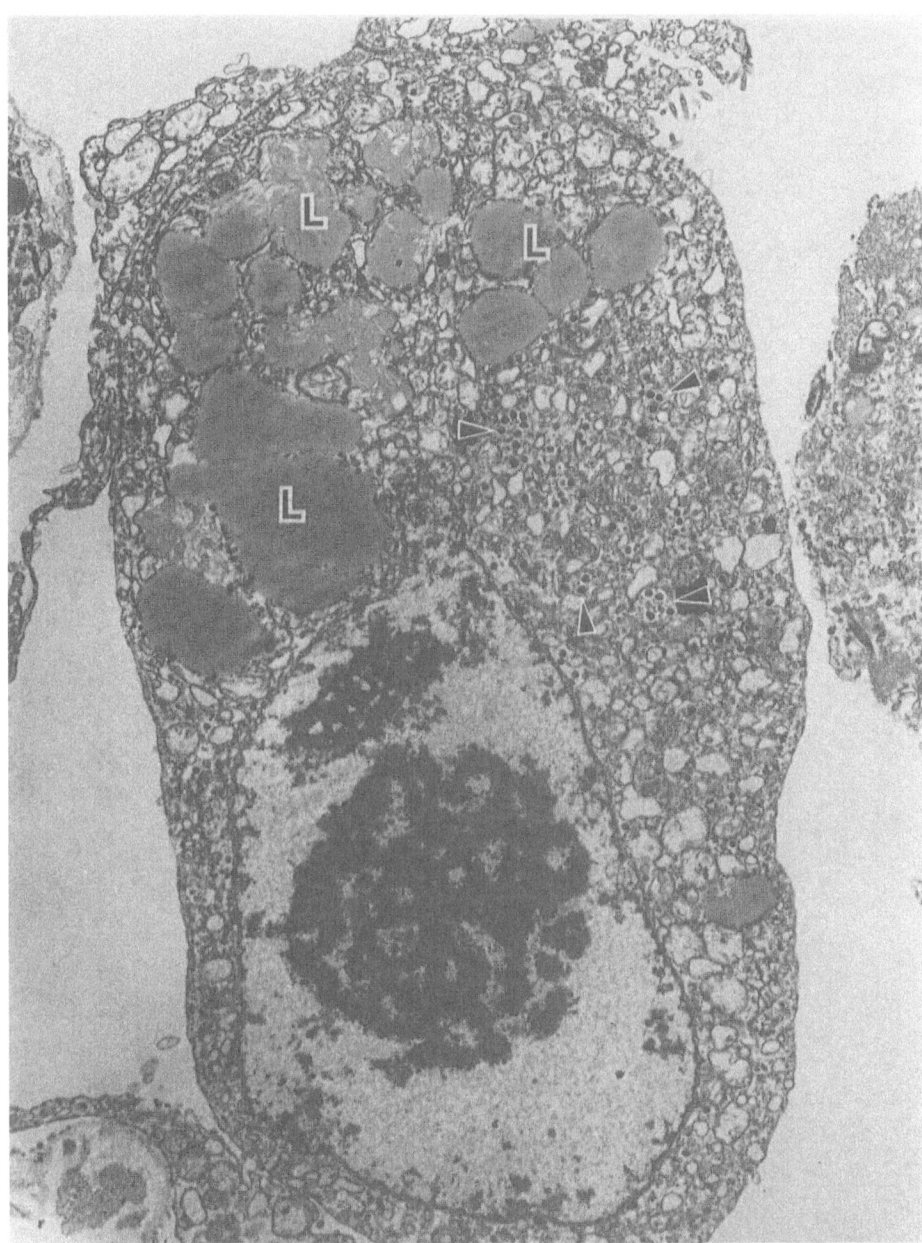

Fig. 4.2 Figs 4.2 and 4.3 are transmission electron micrographs of a cytomegalo-virus-infected pneumocyte with central large and adjacent smaller intranuclear inclusion bodies. Although these inclusions look remarkably like macronucleoli, they are viral precursor material and assembled viral particles. Fig. 4.2 is low magnification of whole cell. The clustered, irregular homogeneous bodies in the cytoplasm are lipidic droplets (L). Very small uniformly round particles surrounded by a cleared halo in the cytoplasm are virus (arrows) which have migrated through the nuclear membrane. The large electron-dense intranuclear inclusions have a somewhat reticulated appearance. (× 7 900)

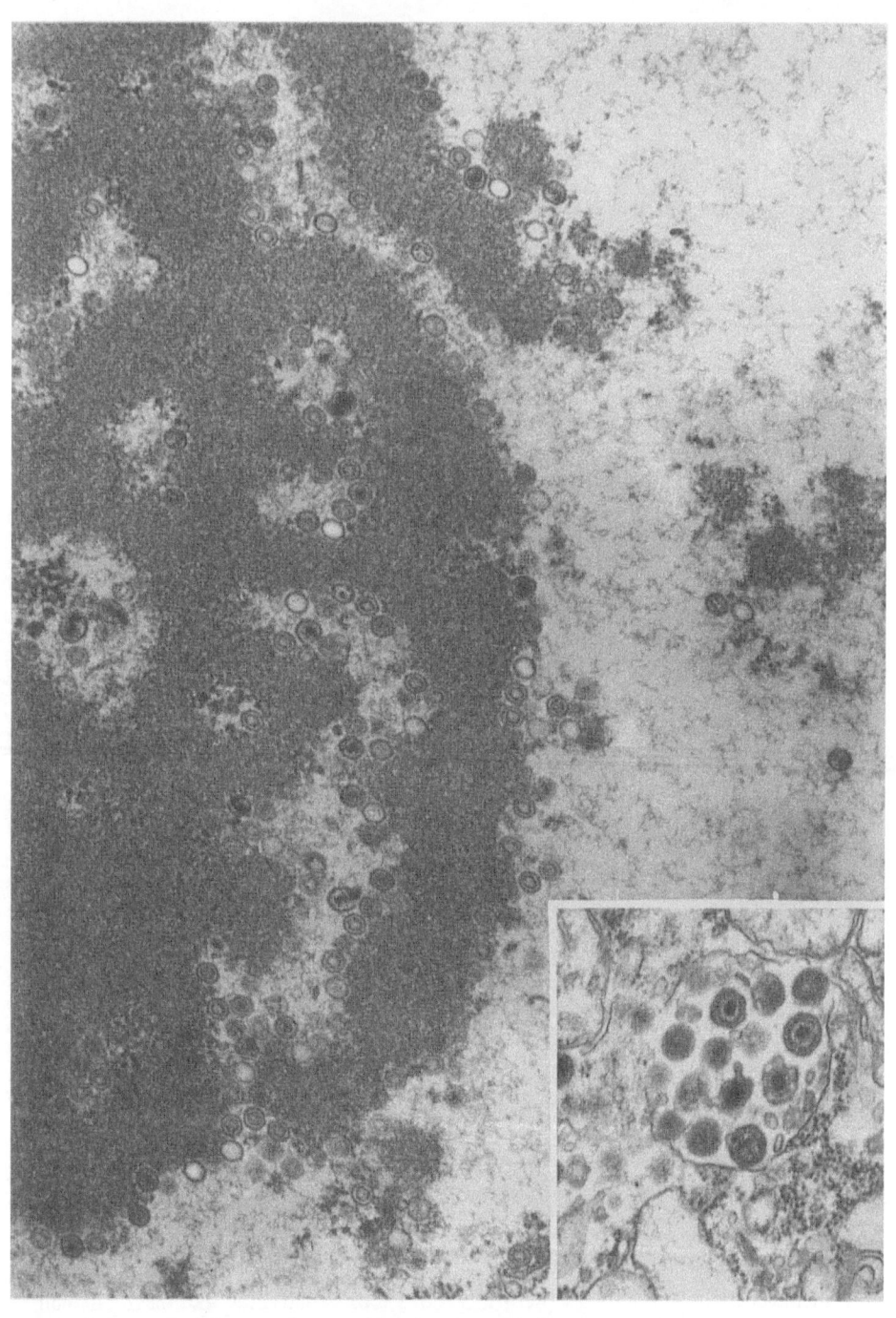

our current practice most cases are in immunocompromised patients. The virus is apparently ubiquitous and latent infections are common. Disseminated disease is probably hematogenously spread. Renal transplant recipients are at high risk. Fiala *et al.* (1975) were able to detect active cytomegalovirus infections in 96% of their renal transplant recipients. Some of these patients had clinical evidence of pneumonitis. Bone marrow recipients are also at high risk (Neiman *et al.*, 1977). The diagnosis is frequently made only after death but bronchoscopic diagnosis is possible (Behrens and Quick, 1974). Culture is more sensitive than the detection of cytomegalic inclusion cells (Craighead, 1971; Smith *et al.*, 1975; Abdallah *et al.*, 1976). The pneumonitis may be an incidental finding at autopsy (Craighead, 1971), and concurrent infection with other pathogens is common (Abdallah *et al.*, 1976). The most frequent copathogen is *Pneumocystis carinii* (see Section 4.5).

Recent attention has been drawn to a new clinical setting for cytomegalovirus infection. The homosexual male and the Haitian immigrant to the USA have been found to be at significant risk for several infections, including cytomegalovirus and Kaposi's sarcoma (Urmacher *et al.*, 1982; see Section 4.5 for a more detailed account). There is some suspicion that the cytomegalovirus plays a key role in the acquired immune deficiency syndrome.

In the lung, pneumocytes are the principal sites of morphologically detectable infection and they can be seen in transbronchial biopsies. The cells become greatly enlarged, and a centrally located, dense intranuclear inclusion with a definite cleared zone between the inclusion and the nuclear border is distinctive (Fig. 4.1). The intranuclear inclusions are usually described as basophilic but they may be eosinophilic (Macasaet *et al.*, 1975). Intracytoplasmic inclusions are also described but are less reliable markers of this infection. The large central intranuclear inclusion is seen ultrastructurally to be precursor material from which assembled virions emerge (Figs 4.2, 4.3). The virions acquire an envelope as they pass through the nuclear envelope into the cytoplasm. Cytomegalovirus-infected cells are rarely seen in sputa but are seen in bronchoscopic material submitted for cytological examination (Jain *et al.*, 1973; Frable *et al.*, 1977).

Fig. 4.3 At higher magnification of the same cell as in Fig. 4.2 the inclusion body is composed of finely granular material and numerous viral capsids, which can be seen in various stages of assembly within cleared areas of the inclusion body. The cytomegalovirus migrates through the nuclear envelope and acquires a surrounding membrane called an envelope. (× 36 000) *Inset*: The enveloped virus are clustered within a cytoplasmic vacuole. (× 36 000)

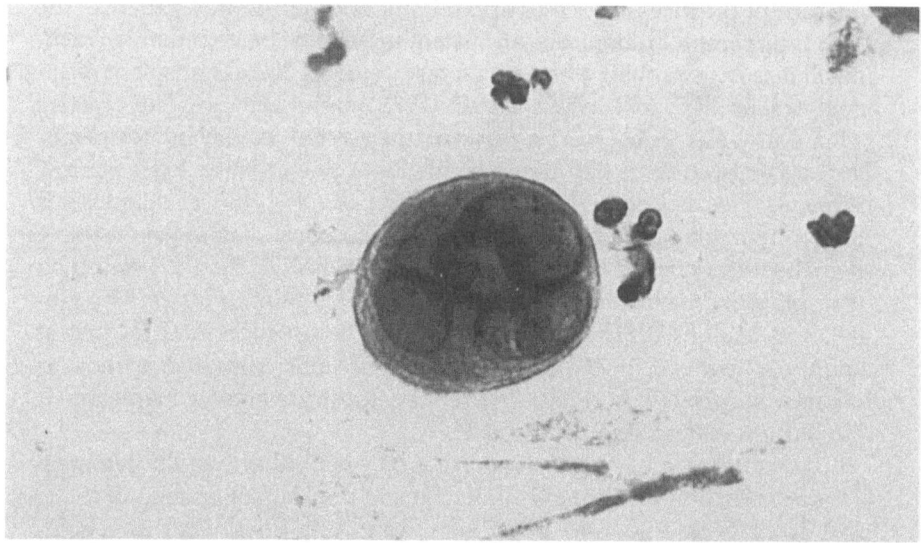

Fig. 4.4 Epithelial cell infected with Herpes simplex virus. The cell is somewhat enlarged and contains seven or more nuclei crowded together in the center. These nuclei do not have discernible inclusions. (Papanicolaou sputum smear: × 600.)

4.1.3   Herpes simplex

Herpetic tracheobronchitis is a necrotizing infection seen primarily in patients with severe underlying disease and not uncommonly as a part of the terminal illness. Patients hospitalized with severe burns are at significant risk (Nash, 1972). It is uncommon for the pulmonary infection to be clinically recognized. The agent is a DNA virus which replicates in the nucleus and migrates to the cytoplasm of the host cell, acquiring an envelope as it traverses the nuclear membrane. Like its close relative cytomegalovirus it is probably ubiquitous, and reactivation of latent herpes (that is, persistent infection of cells without recognizable cellular effect or

Fig. 4.5 Cells infected with herpes simplex. (a) Herpes-simplex-infected multinucleated epithelial cell with the ground-glass type of intranuclear inclusion. The heterochromatin is marginated and a hyaline material fills the nuclei. The nuclei mold each other in the crowded arrangement and there is scant cytoplasm. (Papanicolaou sputum smear: × 1000.) (b) Metaplastic cell in sputum specimen. The dense type of herpetic intranuclear inclusions is present in the four closely-packed nuclei. This form of inclusion is eosinophilic in H&E-stained sections. Their size and the cleared zones which surround them distinguish them from nucleoli. (Epon/Araldite section stained with toluidine blue: × 650.)

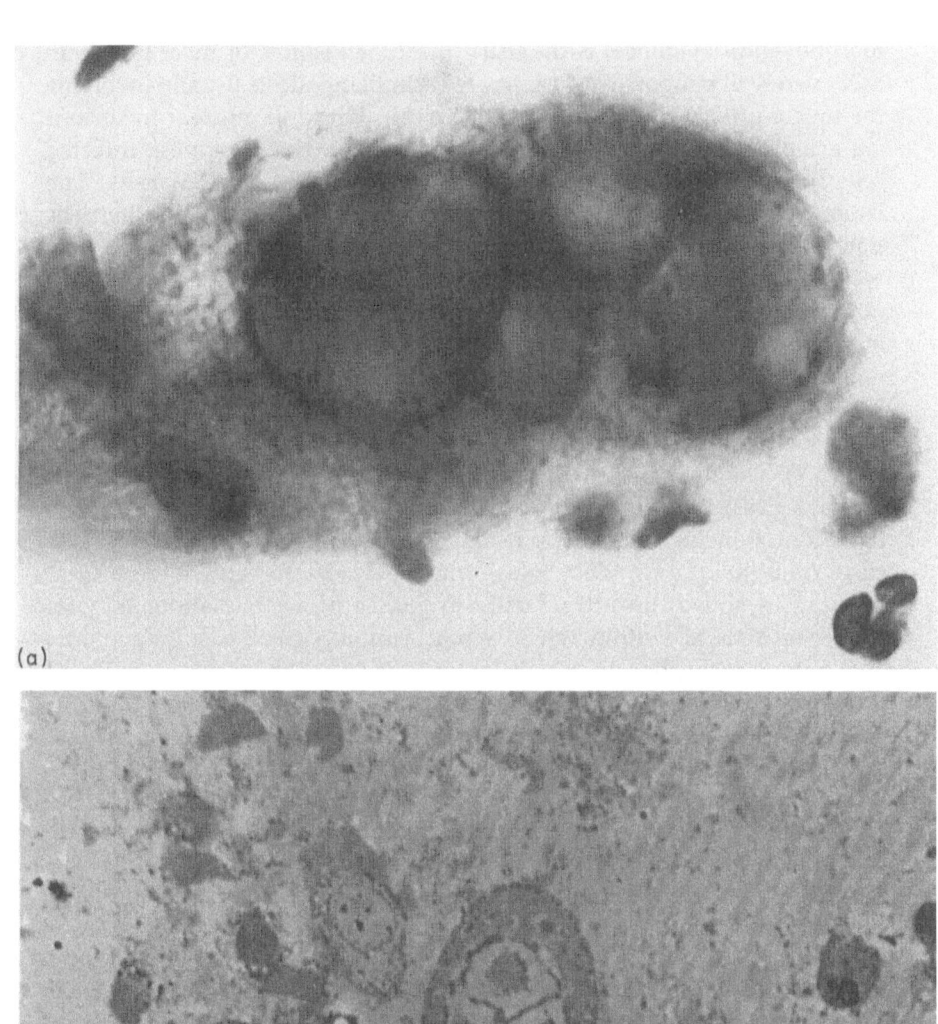

morphological evidence) is the usual presumed source of most lesions in the severely ill patient. The lesions are necrotizing ulcers usually involving the mucosa of the respiratory tree. The cells with intranuclear inclusions are usually seen along the advancing margins of the ulceration. Infected cells include columnar and squamous metaplastic epithelial cells. The latter are more frequently infected. Many patients who develop herpetic tracheobronchitis had antecedent irritation of the respiratory mucosa; epidermoid (squamous) metaplasia may precede the infection in these cases. Nash (1972) suggests that the more rare disseminated herpes infection, which causes a necrotizing pneumonitis, may be hematogenously spread rather than by extension from upper airway infections, as is postulated in the more common herpes bronchitis. The infected cells do not usually enlarge appreciably but multinucleation is frequently seen (Fig. 4.4). The intranuclear inclusions are of two types – a homogeneous (ground-glass) type (Fig. 4.5a) which involves the entire nucleus and a large central inclusion which is usually eosinophilic and surrounded by a clear zone (halo) (Fig. 4.5b) (Nash and Foley, 1970). This large central inclusion is shown ultrastructurally to consist of accumulations of viral precursor material within which virion assembly proceeds. Adenovirus and herpes inclusions have similar ground-glass appearances by light microscopy but they differ ultrastructurally. The herpes inclusion is composed of large numbers of scattered virions (Fig. 4.6) (Frable and Jay, 1977), whereas adenovirus inclusions are virions in a compact crystalline array. The multinucleation in herpes infection results in a cluster of nuclei which mold tightly together (Figs 4.4, 4.5) and are usually surrounded by only a modest amount of cytoplasm (Vernon, 1982). Jordan et al. (1975) found less tendency to multinucleation in infected columnar epithelial cells than in epidermoid (squamous) metaplastic cells.

Herpes-infected exfoliative cells (referred to in general as virocytes by the cytopathologists) are more frequently seen in sputa and bronchial cytology specimens than are the other viruses discussed (Frable et al., 1977). The herpetic lesions are superficial and tend to involve more proximal airways; therefore the infected cells are more likely to exfoliate into the cytology specimens. The frequency with which herpes is seen in cytology specimens is consequently disproportionately greater than their relative incidence as pulmonary pathogens.

4.1.4 Influenza

Influenza causes significant respiratory illness but is rarely detected by bronchoscopic examination. This RNA virus replicates as long helically symmetrical virions within infected respiratory epithelial cells, exits through the cell membrane, acquiring an envelope in the process, and

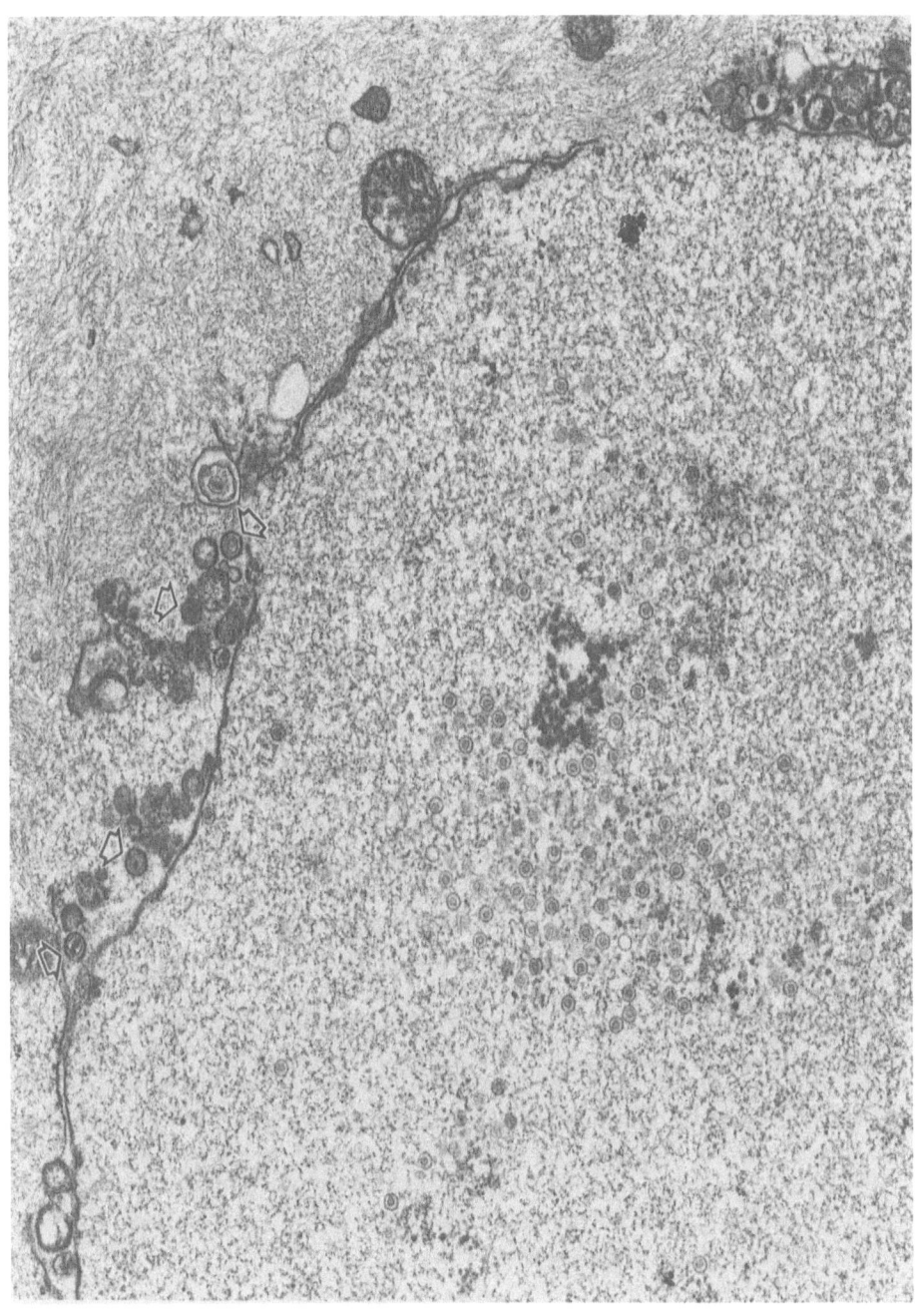

Fig. 4.6 The ultrastructural appearance of a nucleus with the ground-glass herpes simplex inclusion like that shown in Fig. 4.5a. The individual herpes virions are scattered through the nucleus which is otherwise featureless. The nuclear membrane is fragmented and a few cytoplasmic virus particles can be seen along the nuclear membrane with their additional envelope (arrows). (Sputum specimen, transmission electron micrograph: × 21 500.)

rarely results in identifiable inclusion bodies. There is a striking epithelial hyperplasia in the bronchial mucosa with a pseudoneoplastic appearance (Hers *et al.*, 1958). Cytological evidence of influenza pneumonia was proposed by Papanicolaou with the observation of apical decapitation of ciliated epithelial cells (termed ciliocytophthoria). Ciliocytophthoria was felt to be a significant feature of viral respiratory infection by Kim *et al.* (1964). It is probably not a specific finding, however, and although frequently seen in viral pneumonias it may be due to many different factors (Koss, 1979a).

4.1.5   Measles

Measles pneumonia may be an extension of the disseminated disease most commonly seen in infants and can be fatal. A form of pneumonia identified as giant cell pneumonia which is not accompanied by a skin rash has been shown to be due to the measles virus as well (Weller, 1952; Enders *et al.*, 1959). Mitus *et al.* (1959) describe identical diseases in patients who had preceding measles and died with pneumonia, all of whom were leukemics. The virus is RNA with helically formed virions which may accumulate in the nucleus or cytoplasm and result in detectable inclusion bodies (Archibald *et al.*, 1971). Both ciliated cells and pneumocytes may be infected and evolve into the characteristic syncytial giant cells with both intranuclear and less common intracytoplasmic inclusions (Weller, 1952; Archibald *et al.*, 1971; Becroft and Osborne, 1980). Becroft and Osborne (1980) report a pseudoneoplastic epithelial hyperplasia which accompanies the infection in the respiratory mucosa and alveoli. The giant cells in measles pneumonia are easily accepted as syncytial because of their appearance (Fig. 4.7) and have abundant cytoplasm and small- to moderate-sized nuclei which frequently are clustered, but do not form a compact group with molding as is seen in herpes (Sherman and Ruckle, 1958). The intranuclear inclusions may be visible in a few or most of the clustered nuclei (Fig. 4.8) and large numbers of intranuclear and cytoplasmic inclusions can be very dramatic in tissue sections (Fig. 4.9). Little *et al.* (1981) report a case of giant cell pneumonia caused by parainfluenza and cautioned against presuming a measles etiology when giant cells are seen without intranuclear inclusions. Frable *et al.* (1977) describe measles giant cells in bronchial cytology specimens.

4.2   Mycoplasma and chlamydia

Mycoplasma pneumoniae [originally called the Eaton agent and subsequently referred to as pleuropneumonia-like organisms (PPLO)] are reported to cause pneumonia in 1 out of 1000 persons each year. The

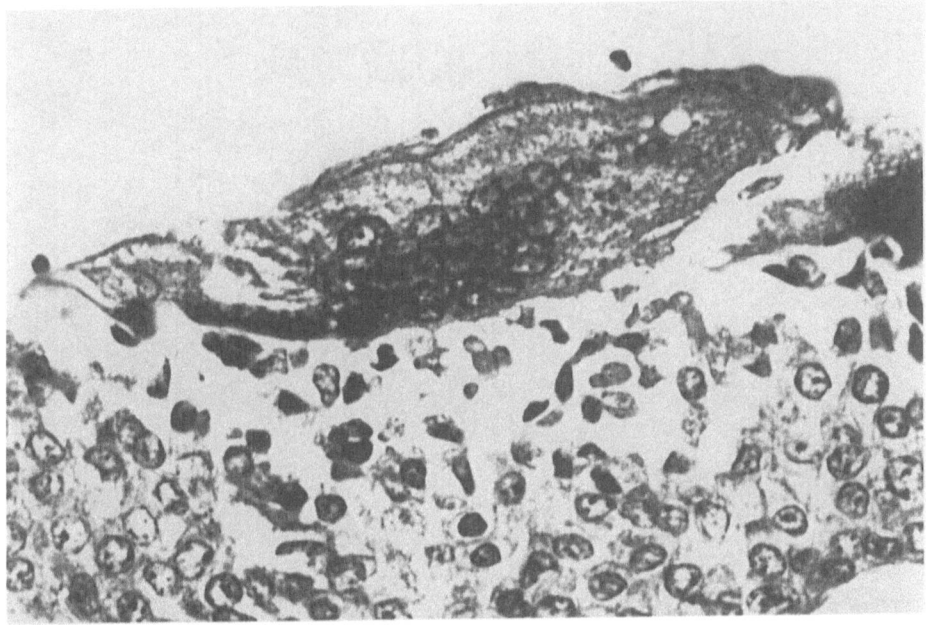

Fig. 4.7 Bronchial epithelium infected with measles virus. In the superficial layers a very large multinucleated giant cell has developed (syncytium). Remnants of the cilia can be seen on its upper surface. (Paraffin-embedded section stained with H&E: × 450. Courtesy of Dr A. Flint, University of Michigan).

diagnosis is made by sputum culture and bronchoscopic material. Biopsies are extremely rarely obtained. About 10–20% of all pneumonias are due to this very small organism which lacks a cell wall but is capable of growth on cell-free media (Cherry and Welliver, 1976). Most 'atypical pneumonias' were probably caused by this organism. The histological changes are totally nonspecific; however, bronchial epithelial cells may contain the organism which can be specifically stained with immunofluorescent techniques (Liu, 1957).

Chlamydia are intracellular obligate parasites which cause a limited number of human infections including ornithosis (psittacosis), caused by *Chlamydia psittaci*, and inclusion conjunctivitis, neonatal pneumonia, lymphogranuloma venereum and genital tract infections, caused by *Chlamydia tracheomatis* (Guze *et al.*, 1982). The uterine cervical infection at the time of birth has now been shown to transmit the organism to the newborn, who may develop pneumonia within the first few months of life (Arth *et al.*, 1978; Frommell *et al.*, 1979). Chlamydial pneumonitis has also been seen in an immunocompromised adult (Ito *et al.*, 1982). The organism is detected by inoculation of infected material from the patient in tissue

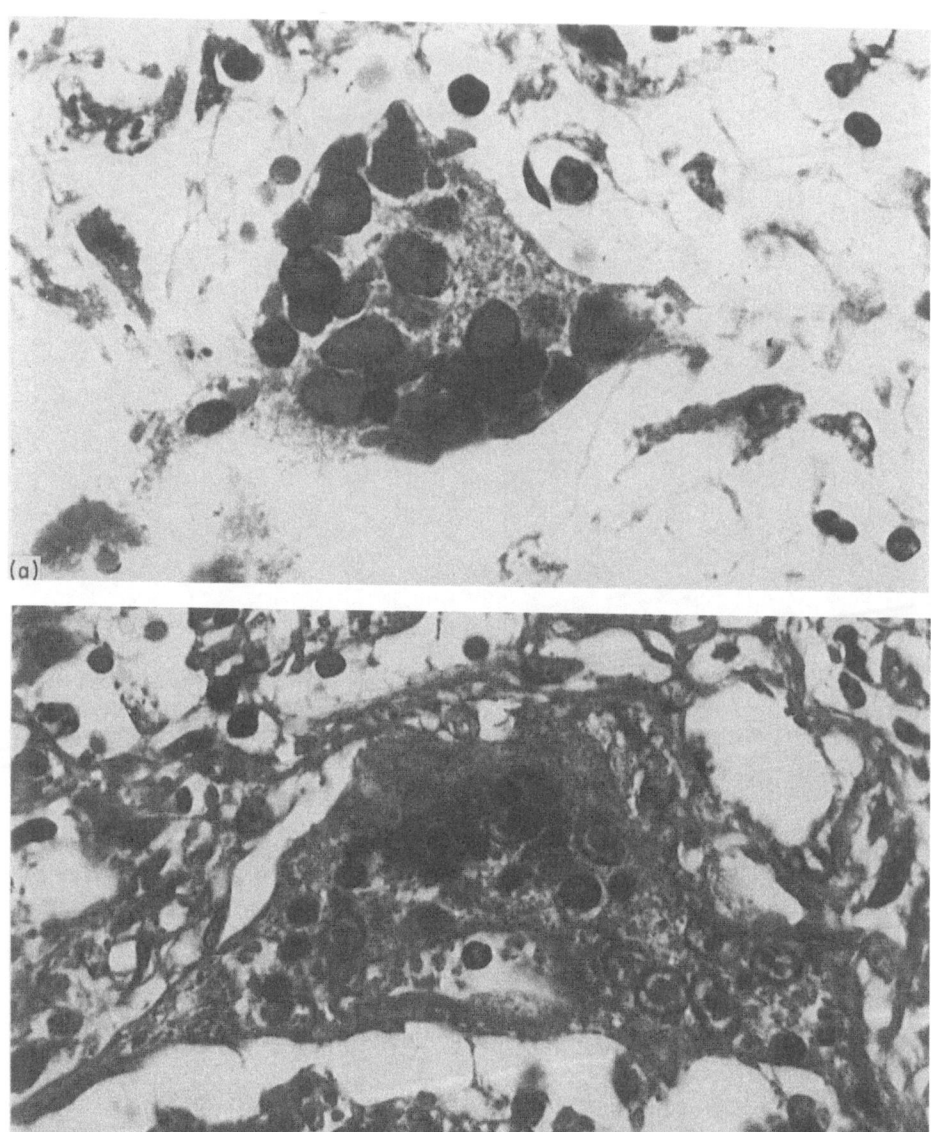

Fig. 4.8 Alveolar giant cells in measles pneumonia. Large numbers of nuclei are surrounded by abundant cytoplasm. (a) Cell with predominantly ground-glass type of intranuclear inclusions. (b) Giant cell with several compact intranuclear inclusions with surrounding cleared zone. (Paraffin embedded sections stained with H&E: × 600. Courtesy of Dr A. Flint, University of Michigan.)

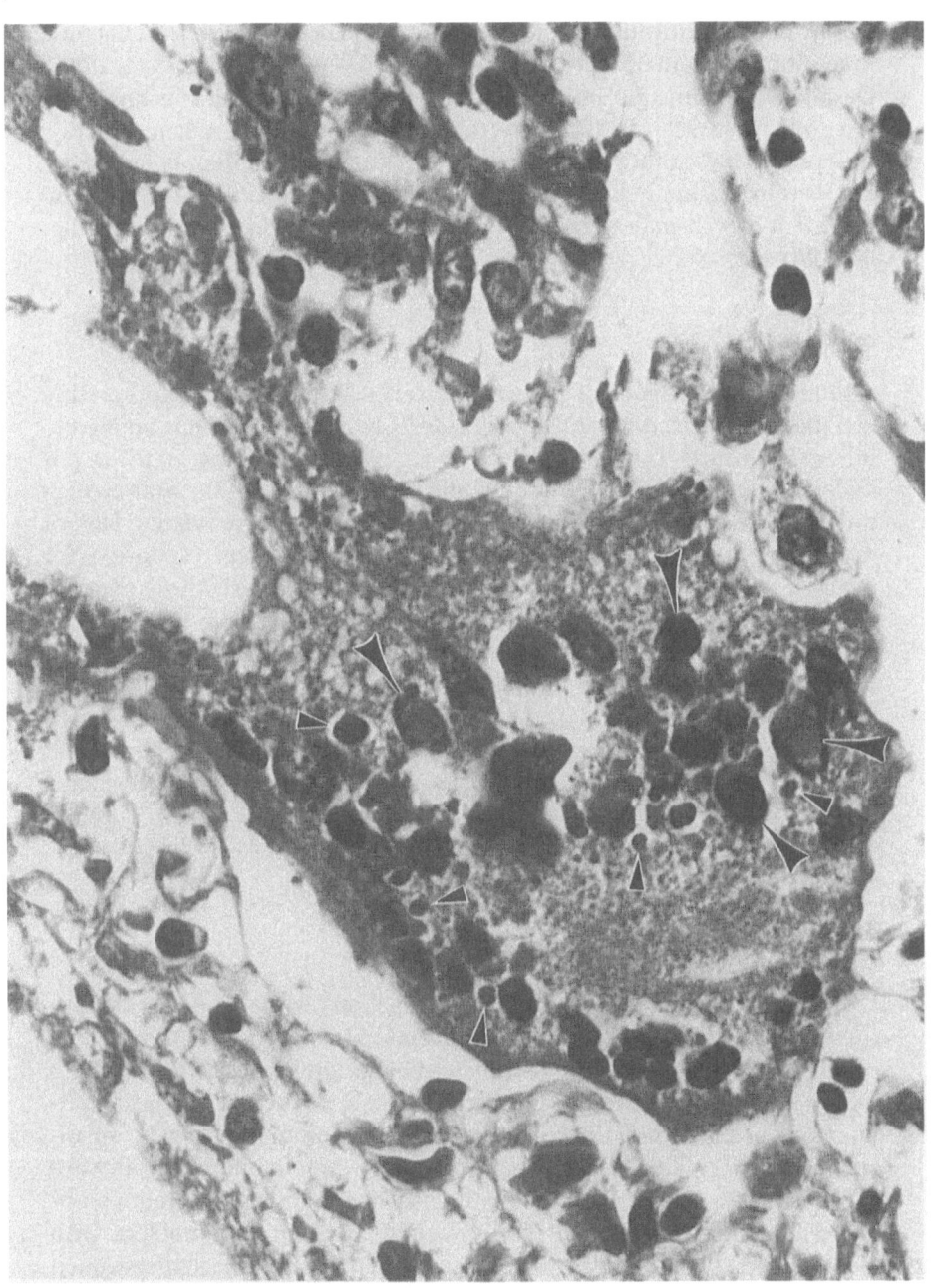

Fig. 4.9 Very large alveolar giant cell with measles virus intranuclear inclusion bodies (large arrows) and numerous cytoplasmic inclusions (smaller arrows). (Paraffin-embedded sections stained with H&E: × 700. Courtesy of Dr A. Flint, University of Michigan.)

culture and identification of the cytoplasmic inclusion bodies with Giemsa, immunofluorescent or other stains (Johnson, 1975; Woodland *et al.*, 1982). Despite the distinctive morphology of the cytoplasmic inclusions, they have not been seen in biopsies from pneumonias even when infection was proven by culture of the same material. The cytoplasmic inclusions are seen in the epithelial cells of conjunctival and genital infections and persistent search may eventually demonstrate them in bronchial epithelium as well.

4.3   Bacteria

Although the incidence of pneumonia caused by bacteria is appreciably less than that caused by viruses, considerably more attention is applied to these organisms. This is undoubtedly a reflection of the state of our understanding of culture techniques and the availability of therapies which can alter the course of the bacterial pneumonias and the relative lack of the same for viral infections. Acute bacterial pneumonia is responsible for much of the terminal illness of our population, particularly those who are hospitalized at the time of death. Most of the bacteria which cause pulmonary infections are widespread in our environment, and the list of known factors which allows them to become established pathogens within the lungs is growing. Damage to the normal mucociliary clearance mechanisms, altered immunological status and concurrent viral infection are all known to predispose to bacterial pneumonia. Because of the frequency with which the bronchial biopsy is used to establish the cause of pneumonia in the immunocompromised individual, this will be considered specifically at the end of this chapter (Section 4.6).

4.3.1   Pyogenic bacteria

The diagnosis of most acute bacterial infections is made without bronchoscopy or biopsy. Sputum smears examined with the Gram stain and cultures are usually adequate to initiate specific antibiotic therapy in those patients with clinical evidence of acute infection. When the clinical characteristics suggest bacterial infection but the sputum yields only microorganisms which are frequent colonizers of the mouth and upper airways or organisms inconsistent with the course of the disease, secretions obtained bronchoscopically can be selectively cultured. The problem with bronchoscopic material remains contamination of the collected specimen by organisms from the upper airways during introduction of the bronchoscope. *In vitro* and clinical trials of several available catheters have shown that uncontaminated specimens can be obtained with a bronchial brush carried through the bronchoscope channel within a plastic tube which is itself protected by an outer plastic tube and sealed distally with a plug (Wimberley et al., 1979). The entire assembly is advanced to the site of suspected infection, the plug is pushed out of the outer sheath by advancing the inner sheath several additional centimeters and then the brush is advanced several more centimeters into the bronchus and rotated to collect secretions. The brush is withdrawn into the inner sheath and the whole cannula is removed from the bronchoscope.

Although the various common acute bacterial infections have characteristic inflammatory cellular responses and the tissue reactions may help in their identification, the pathologist rarely has the opportunity to use this information in biopsy specimens unless it is incidental to other findings such as a neoplasm. Large colonies of bacteria are occasionally seen in necrotic debris adjacent to malignancy and can be easily appreciated with the Brown and Brenn Gram stain (Luna, 1968). The finding of occasional bacteria in the inflammatory exudate in bronchial biopsies is not generally acceptable as a diagnostic finding since contamination or colonization is so common.

4.3.2   Actinomyces and nocardia

These organisms are usually associated with chronic pneumonia and may occur as primary infections or as infections superimposed on tuberculosis or other underlying pulmonary disease. Actinomyces israelii is an anaerobic branching filamentous organism which forms distinctive colonies in tissue (Fig. 4.10). They are not readily seen in H&E-stained sections but are found within necrotic debris as groups of radiating thin (0.5 μm) Gram-positive filaments with outer club-shaped projections. These structures, called sulfur granules, may be large enough to be visible to the unaided eye. The filaments of actinomyces characteristically do not stain with the acid-fast stain (Robboy and Vickery, 1970), but are easily appreciated with silver stains (Fig. 4.11). The distinctive clubs are seen with high magnification as sheaths surrounding the filaments. Multinucleated giant cells and histiocytes are occasionally seen adjacent to the sulfur granules.

Actinomyces granules have been detected in sputum samples submitted for cytologic examination (Lazzari et al., 1981). In sputa the colonies of actinomyces were surrounded by leukocytes and necrotic debris. For a thorough discussion of the morphology and staining reactions of actinomyces granules see the work of Gupta (1982).

Nocardia asteroides is also a Gram-positive branching, filamentous organism. It does not form sulfur granules in pulmonary infections (Palmer et al., 1974). Nocardia are irregularly acid fast and can be more easily seen in the modified Ziehl-Neelsen stain using a weaker acidic rinse (Robboy and Vickery, 1970). They cause a necrotizing tissue reaction. Culture is

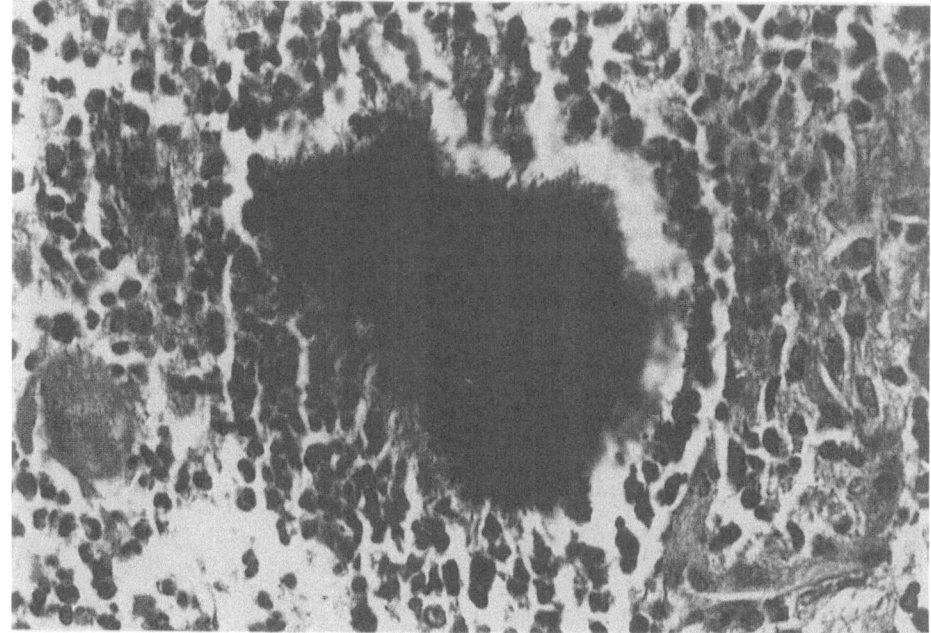

Fig. 4.10   Actinomyces colony forming a 'sulfur granule' surrounded by a dense infiltrate of leukocytes in lung parenchyma. (Paraffin-embedded section stained with PAS: × 700.)

difficult and biopsy may be required to identify the organism. The filaments of both Actinomyces and Nocardia are best seen with oil immersion objectives.

Pollock *et al.* (1978) describe the use of fluorescent-labeled antibodies to distinguish Actinomyces from Nocardia in cases in which the other staining reactions are equivocal. Actinomyces and Nocardia may be present in the immunocompromised person (see Section 4.6).

4.3.3   *Legionella*

The intense search for the cause of Legionnaires' disease in 1976 has led to the recognition of a new bacterial genus, Legionella. Certainly the incidence of the pneumonias caused by the several species now known in this group is not as great as many other uncommon pneumonias but the diagnosis can be established by identifying the characteristic bacillary forms, which are seen in both intracellular and extracellular locations in transbronchial biopsy. The Dieterle stain (Van Orden and Greer, 1977) is the most reliable method. This stain, originally developed as a means of detecting spirocetes (Dieterle, 1927), also stains *Calymmatobacteria*

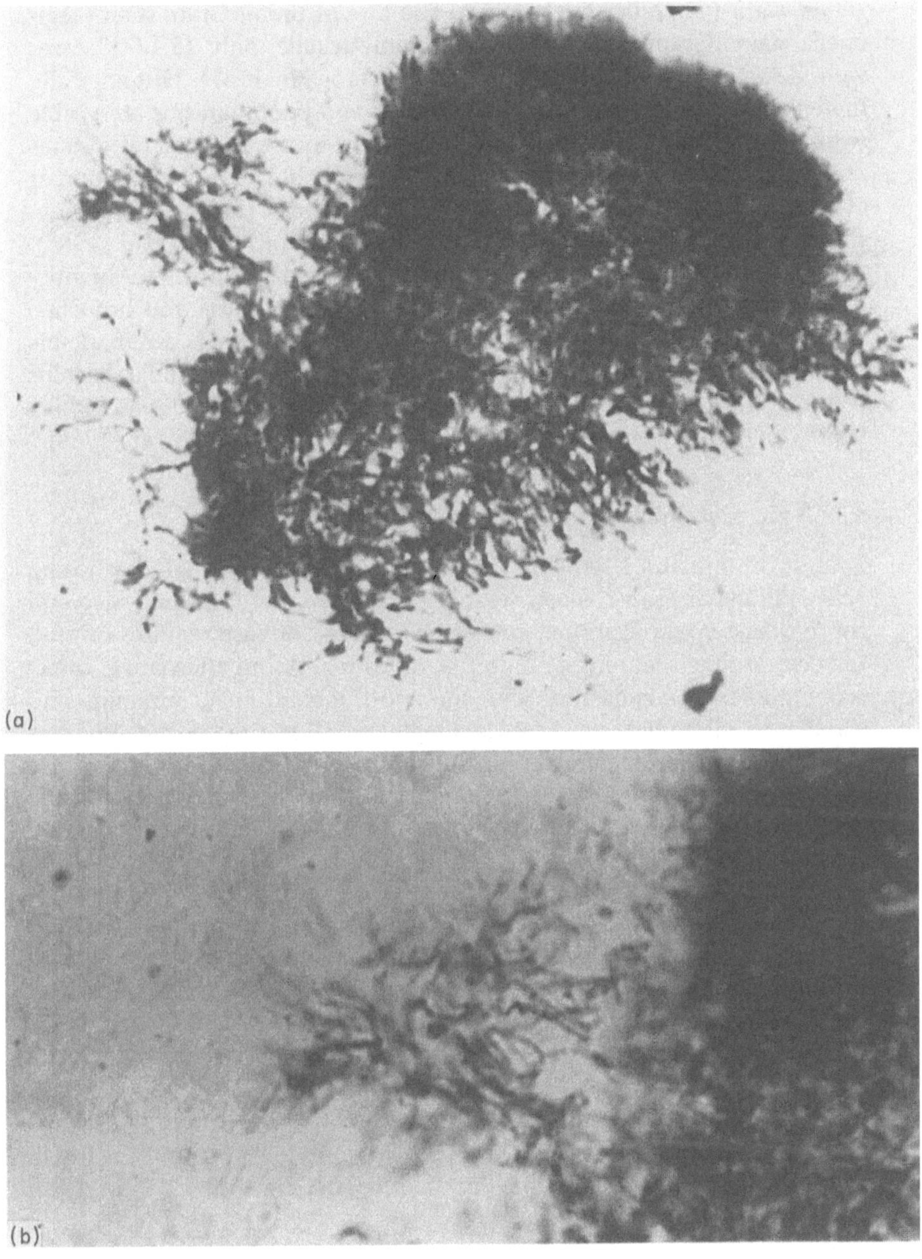

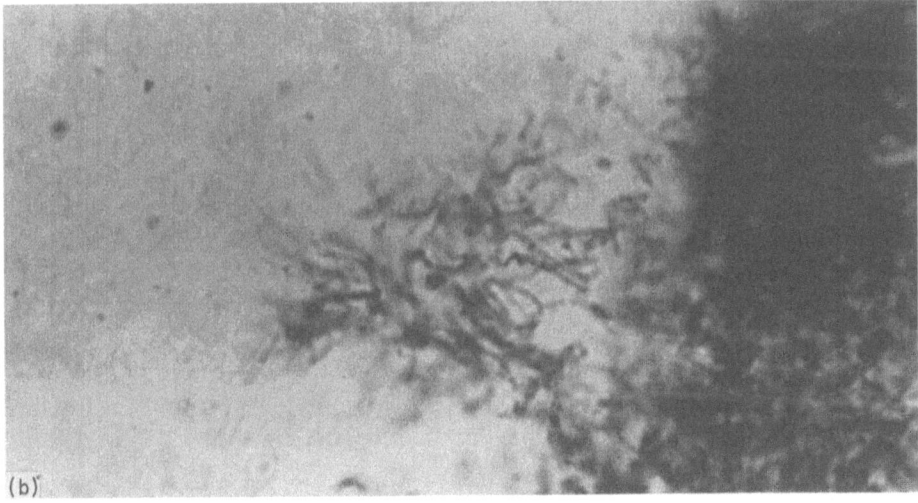

Fig. 4.11 Colony of Actinomyces. The individual filamentous forms are easily seen with a silver stain. (a) Whole colony (× 800) (b) Edge of colony with branching filaments (× 900). (Paraffin-embedded sections stained with Gomori's silver methenamine.)

granulomatis (Chandler *et al.*, 1977). The Brown-Brenn Gram stain (Legionella stains Gram negative) gives variable results; only 12 of 28 cases were detected in one series (Winn and Myerowitz, 1981). Histologically there is an acute bronchiolitis and alveolitis and the organisms are visible within the inflammatory exudate. Diagnosis by serological techniques remains the most common method used clinically but a significant number of cases have relied on morphological identification of the bacilli in biopsy, sputa, endobronchial aspirates and bronchial washings (Kirby *et al.*, 1980).

Direct immunofluorescent techniques can be used to confirm the identity of suspected bacilli on tissue sections as well as in sputa and bronchial washings (Broome *et al.*, 1979; Kirby *et al.*, 1980). There is a remarkable similarity in the ultrastructural appearance of this intracellular bacillus (Winn and Myerowitz, 1981) and the bacillus of Whipple's disease which is extremely rarely seen as a pneumonic infection (Winberg *et al.*, 1978).

4.3.4 *Mycobacteria*

Sputum examination remains the most common means of diagnosing active pulmonary tuberculosis. The Ziehl-Neelsen staining of digested and concentrated sputa from patients with suspected disease requires careful, time consuming scanning at high magnification. As an alternative, direct staining of the mycobacillus with the two fluorochromes, auramine and rhodamine, first introduced by Hageman (1938), is a rapid screening test that can be performed at lower magnification (Truant *et al.*, 1962). Because of the 'oversensitivity' of the fluorochrome staining, restaining with the Ziehl-Neelsen stain is necessary to confirm the diagnosis (Joseph and Houk, 1968).

Although some have suggested that transbronchial biopsy is the preferred method of diagnosis in rapidly progressing tuberculosis (Geppert and Leff, 1979), most concluded that bronchoscopic specimens should be obtained only when sputa are negative microscopically for the acid-fast bacilli (Sahn and Levin, 1975; Banner, 1979; Danek and Bower, 1979; Wallace *et al.*, 1981; Jett *et al.*, 1981). Cultures obtained through bronchoscopy are less often successful than from sputa (Wallace *et al.*, 1981), which could be due to inhibition of growth by the local anesthetic agents used. Conte and Laforet (1962) have shown inhibition of growth of fungi, *M. tuberculosis* and nontuberculous bacteria by several of the common anesthetics.

The histological pattern of tuberculosis seen in bronchial biopsy is variable, as might be expected, due to the variety of types of tuberculous reaction as well as the minimal amount of tissue sampled. In proven cases of tuberculosis, Wallace *et al.* (1981) found transbronchial specimens to be mostly nonspecific chronic inflammatory reactions (48%); 13% had noncaseous granulomas and there were an equal number of caseous granulomas. Nine per cent of their transbronchial biopsies were normal. Forty-eight per cent of the specimens obtained at bronchoscopy in this series had acid-fast bacilli (Fig. 4.12), and 17% of the granulomas had acid-fast bacilli. In their series, 20% of the sputum-negative cases yielded positive bronchoscopic cultures (brushings and washings). Jett *et al.* (1981) found that although only 47% of their tuberculous cases had positive cultures from bronchoscopy, 95% of their atypical mycobacterial cases yielded positive cultures. In miliary tuberculosis, sputum cultures are less successful and the course of the disease often prompts bronchoscopic examination (Sahn and Levin, 1975; Geppert and Leff, 1979).

The sputum cytology findings of patients with tuberculosis are not specific. However, the presence of numerous histiocytes and multinucleated giant cells (of either Langhans' or foreign body types) are suggestive (Nasiell *et al.*, 1972; Roger *et al.*, 1972). Calcospherites in sputum cytology

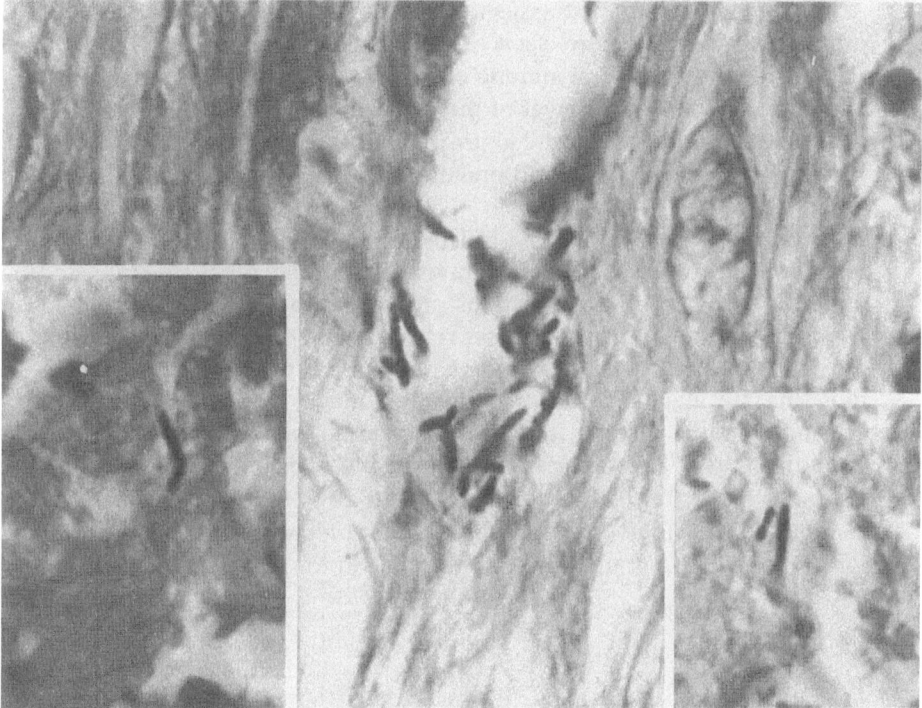

Fig. 4.12 The acid-fast bacilli of tuberculosis in necrotic tissue stained with the Ziehl-Neelsen stain. Insets are bacilli from other areas, since they tend to be widely scattered. Some of the apparent differences in shape are due to the optical plane of the photomicrographs. The beaded appearance is real and helps to identify this mycobacterium. (Paraffin-embedded sections with Ziehl-Neelsen stain: × 1000.)

specimens can be seen in tuberculosis but are also seen as a nonspecific finding in chronic pulmonary disease (Koss, 1979b). Calcospherites in sputum are characteristic of pulmonary alveolar microlithiasis, an extremely rare disease of the lung (Saputo *et al.*, 1979).

Further discussion of mycobacterial pneumonia will be found in Chapter 8 within the context of the differential diagnosis of granulomatous disease. Both *M. tuberculosis* and the atypical mycobacteria can be found in immunocompromised persons (Section 4.6).

4.4 Fungi

Biopsy specimens with mycotic infections of the lungs are usually from immunocompromised patients. The specific approach to the evaluations of these biopsies will be discussed in Section 4.6. In this section each of the more frequently encountered fungi will be described with emphasis on diagnostic features.

All of the fungi are distinguished by the presence of a cell wall. This usually refractile structure, seen in H&E-stained sections, surrounds the cell outside the plasma membrane and the microscopic appearance of the membrane and the outer layer of the cell wall are traditionally referred to as double contoured. Table 4.2 gives an outline of the diagnostically useful characteristics of the fungi and pneumocystis (which will be discussed in Section 4.5).

Aspergillus, Candida and the Mucorales are ubiquitous in our environment, frequently colonize the respiratory tract, rarely cause true infections under predisposing host conditions and are capable of systemic spread which can be fatal. Their diagnoses rely heavily on histologic evidence of infection. In contrast Blastomyces, Coccidioides, Cryptococcus and Histoplasma are generally soil-inhabiting organisms which are capable of causing sporadic disease in otherwise normal persons exposed to the airborne spores. They are capable of causing subclinical infections. The disease which they cause tends to occur in recognizable geographic distribution. Blastomyces, Coccidioides, Cryptococcus and Histoplasma sometimes evoke a granulomatous response in the lung (Chapter 8).

4.4.1 *Aspergillus*

Aspergillus may colonize the tracheobronchial tree without significant effect except for the uncommon occurrence of allergic bronchopulmonary aspergillosis (see Chapter 6). Alternatively the fungus may grow as a mass, usually within a pre-existing cavity as an aspergilloma or as invasive aspergillosis in the immunocompromised patient. Infections with Aspergillus have been reported in patients who have no evidence of immuno-

Table 4.2 Diagnostic characteristics of some of the micro-organisms which cause respiratory infections

Organism	Size/diameter	Morphology	Silver stain	Where to look
Aspergillus	3–5 μm	Hyphae, septate, branching at 45°		Extracellular, in necrosis, vessel walls
Candida	3–7 μm	Yeast, multiple buds with narrow attachments, pseudohyphae		Extracellular, inflammatory exudates
Mucorales	10–35 μm	Large irregular hyphae, nonseptate, branching at 90°		Extracellular, in necrosis, vessel walls
Blastomyces	8–15 μm	Yeast, single bud with broad attachment, multiple nuclei		Necrotic debris, within histiocytes and multinucleated giant cells
Coccidioides	10–80 μm	Spherules		Extracellular, within multinucleated giant cells
	2–5 μm	Endospores		
Cryptococcus	5–20 μm	Yeast, single bud with narrow attachment, gelatinous capsule		Extracellular, intracellular within multinucleated giant cells
Histoplasma	1.5–3.5 μm	Ovoid yeast		Extracellular in necrosis or intracellular in histiocytes
Pneumocystis	5–8 μm	Cysts		Extracellular within alveolar
	2–12 μm	Trophozoites		

compromise (Brown *et al.*, 1980). The case shown in Fig. 4.17 happens to be from a patient with no known immunological problem, although both this patient and that reported by Brown *et al.* were cirrhotics, which could be a factor.

The airborne spores of this fungus are universally found in our environment. They grow as hyphae which are septate and characteristically branch at an acute angle. These characteristics can be seen in H&E-stained sections but scattered hyphae are more easily detected with the silver methenamine stain (Fig. 4.13a). The hyphae are 3–5 μm in diameter and have a fairly uniform contour at the septa and branches (Figs 4.13, 4.14, 4.15). The silver stains localize within the cell wall material (including the septae which are the same material). When these organisms die their cell walls and septae survive for some time; therefore hyphal structures visible with the silver stains are not necessarily viable.

When invasive, the hyphae have a predilection for the walls of blood vessels, and necrosis which frequently accompanies the fungal infection may be in part due to vascular occlusion and infarction. A necrotic background with sparse acute inflammatory cellular infiltrate and branching hyphae can be seen in bronchial and transbronchial biopsies as well as in bronchial brushings and washings. The vascular invasion, however, is rarely seen in these specimens because it tends to occur in the large blood vessels. In cytological material the hyphae are easily visualized with the Papanicolaou stain (Johnston *et al.*, 1969).

Aspergillomas are mycelia (masses of hyphae) of the fungus usually growing within a pre-existing pulmonary cavity such as from tuberculosis, bronchiectasis, bullous emphysema or an area of necrosis caused by invasive aspergillosis. The classic radiologic image of a fungus ball is an air-filled space with discrete wall within which a central mass moves about with various positions of the patient. Biopsy of the aspergilloma itself consists almost entirely of the characteristic hyphae. In addition the asexual fruiting body of the fungus (which must have free air to develop) may be seen with its chains of small conidiospores.

Most of the human pulmonary infections are with the species *fumigatus*; however, one of the other species, *niger*, may be accompanied by a distinctive accumulation of crystals of calcium oxalate in the surrounding tissue (Kurrein *et al.*, 1975; Severo *et al.*, 1981). In one reported case, death was due to oxalosis with renal failure and calcium oxalate crystals

---

Fig. 4.13 Aspergillus infection. (a) Mass of hyphae (mycelium) in a transbronchial biopsy. The septate uniform hyphae with occasional branches traverse in and out of the section resulting in ovoid cut 'ends'. (Paraffin-embedded section stained with Gomori's methenamine silver: × 500.) (b) Mycelium in transbronchial biopsy. (Scanning electron micrograph: horizontal width of field = 270 μm.)

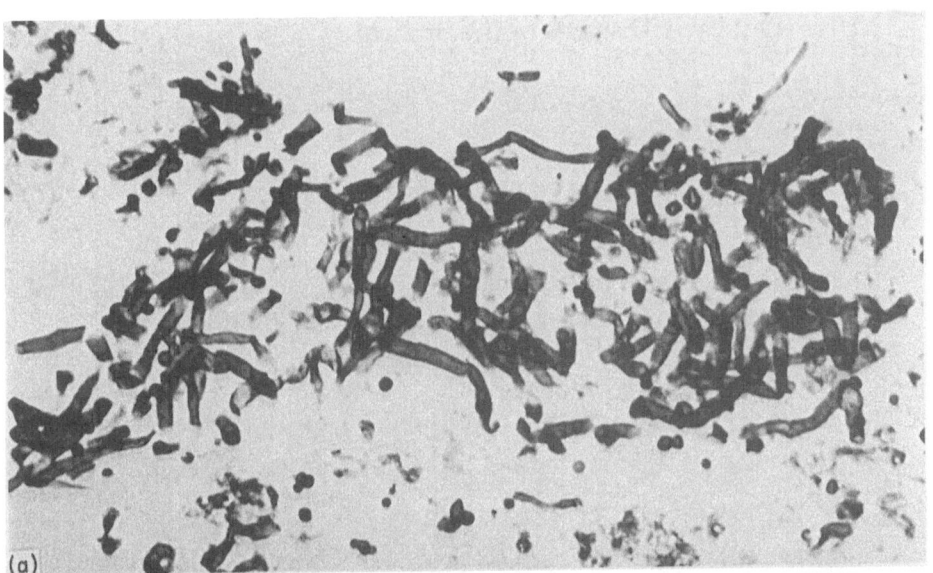

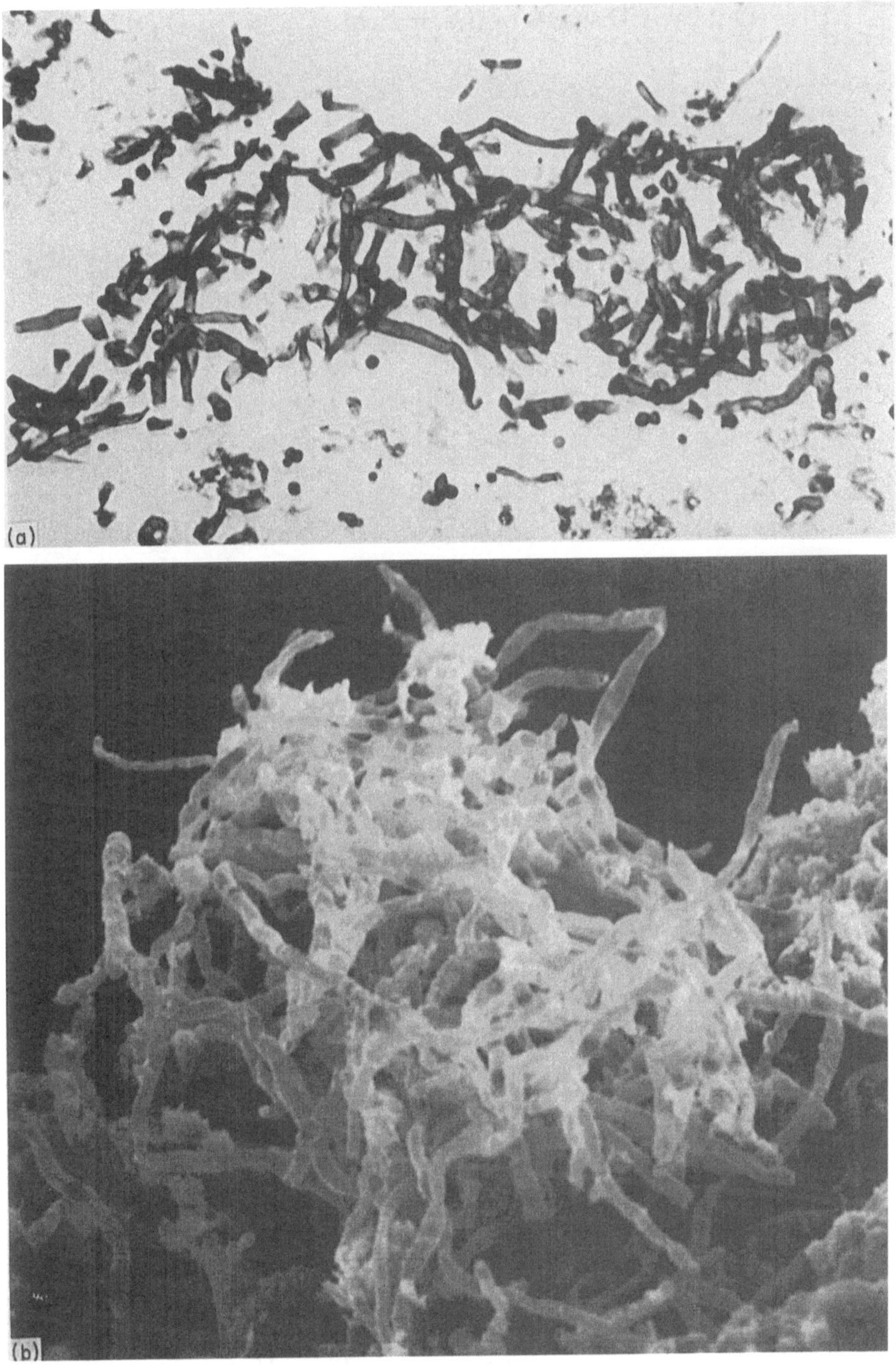

(a)

(b)

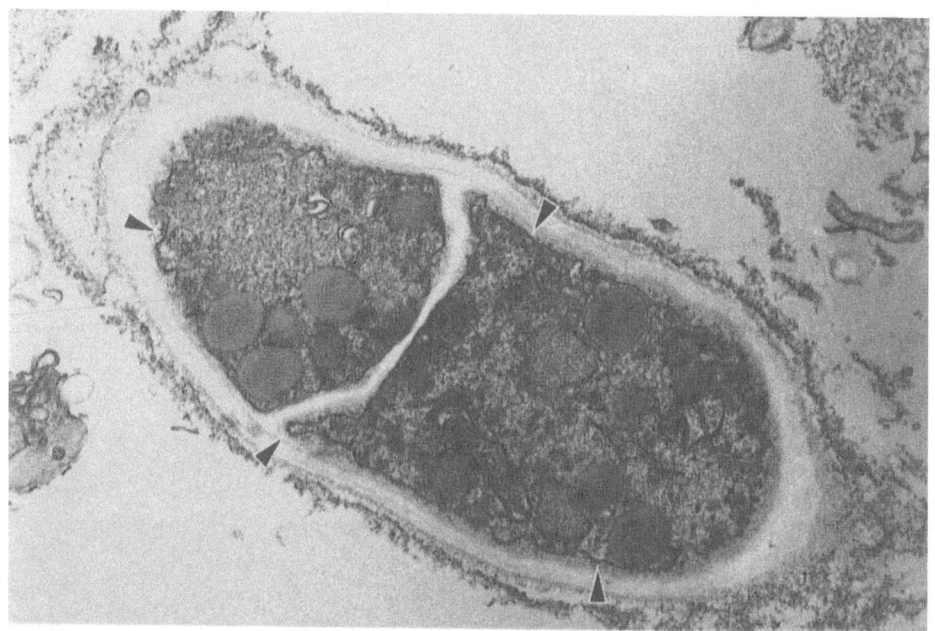

Fig. 4.14 Transmission electron micrograph of Aspergillus hyphae from a biopsy specimen of a lung abscess. The cytoplasm contains the usual organelles. The plasma membrane (arrows) is covered with a cell wall which has a layered appearance of variable electron density. The section cuts through the fungus at a septum dividing two adjacent cells. (× 17 500)

were found in the tissues from 11 of 68 cases of aspergillosis (Nime and Hutchins, 1973). The crystals have been seen in sputa, pleural effusions, bronchial washings and bronchial biopsies in one patient who had *Aspergillus niger* cultured from each of these sources (Reyes *et al.*, 1979). The phenomenon results from the reaction of oxalic acid, a fermentation product of *Aspergillus niger* (Müller, 1975; Müller and Frosch, 1975; Raper and Fennel, 1977) with calcium and the formation of the birefringent crystals (Figs 4.16, 4.17) in the vicinity of the infections.

4.4.2 *Candida*

This yeast is the most frequently seen fungus in pulmonary specimens, but invasive candidiasis is exceedingly uncommon. When it does occur nearly all of the patients have malignancies and the infection with candida is part of the terminal illness (Masur *et al.*, 1977). Hematogenous spread in severely ill patients is more likely than aspiration pneumonia (Rose and

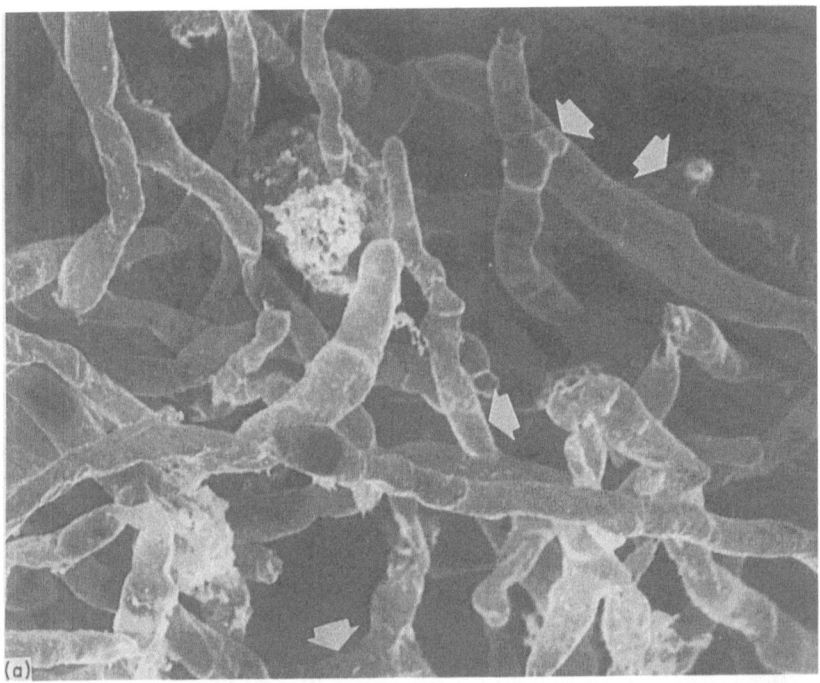

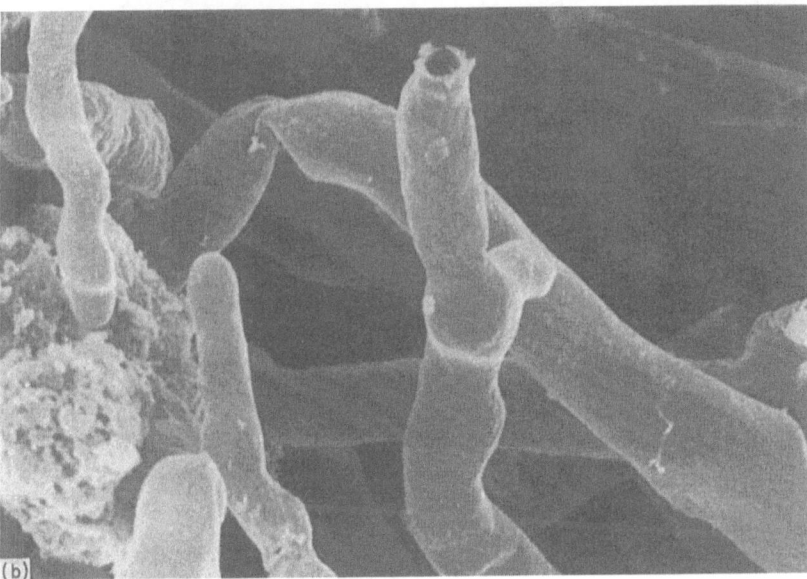

Fig. 4.15 Aspergillus hyphae. By SEM only the outer surface is visible so the septae cannot be seen, but the branching is shown. (a) Uniform surface contours with branches (arrows). (Scanning electron micrograph: horizontal width of field = 100 μm.) (b) Higher magnification of the above with cut end of one hypha. The 'kink' in the adjacent hypha is probably an artefact. (Horizontal width of field = 50 μm.)

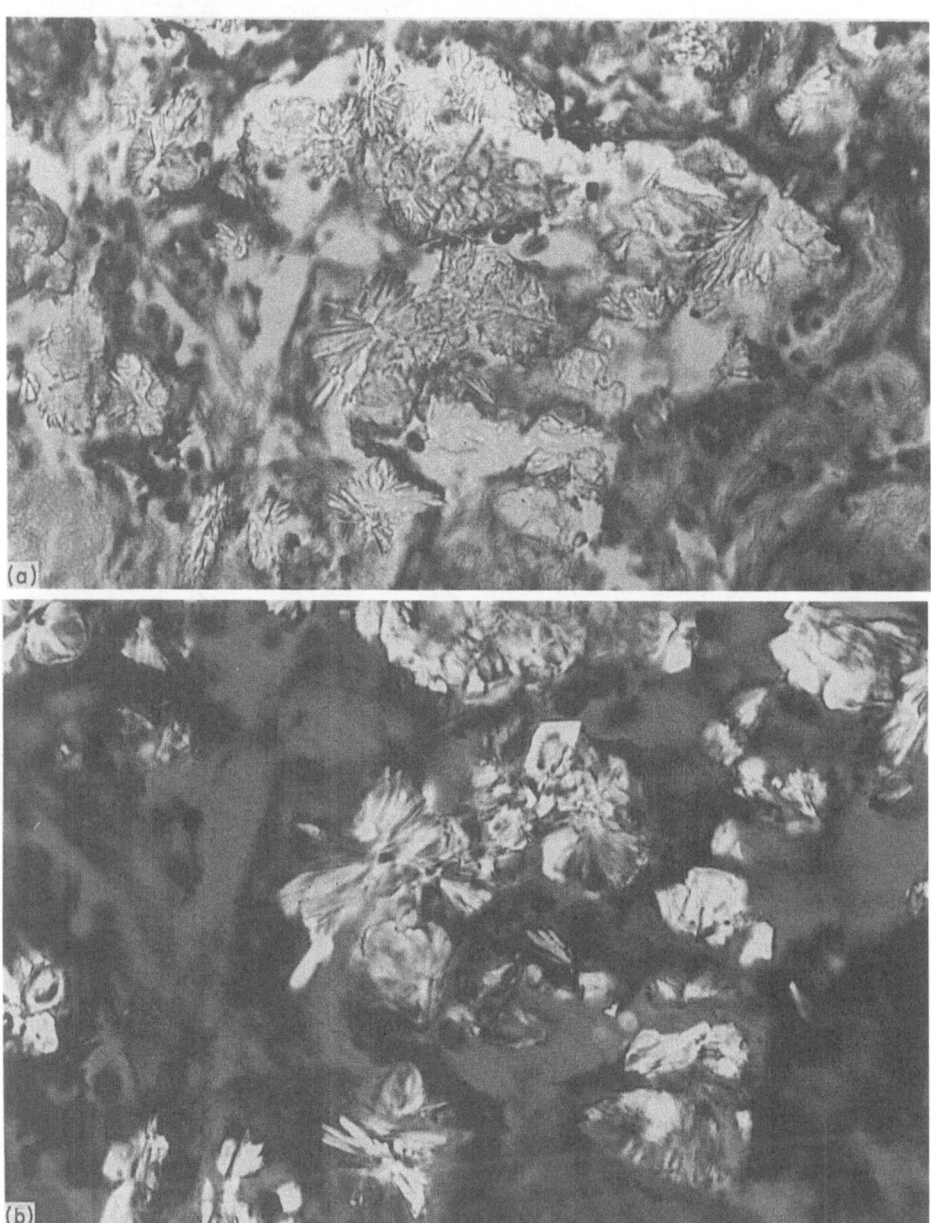

Fig. 4.16 Crystals of calcium oxalate in transbronchial biopsy of *Aspergillus niger* mycetoma (fungus ball). (a) Regular illumination of the section. The crystals can be discerned among the inflammatory cells. (b) Same field but with polarized light to demonstrate the birefringent property of the crystals. (Paraffin-embedded section stained with H&E: × 300.)

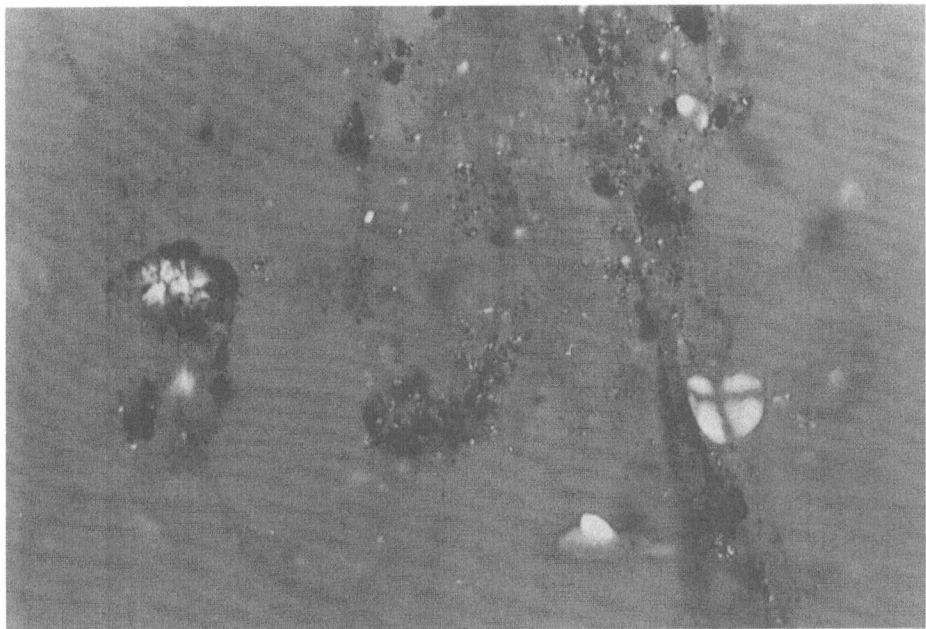

Fig. 4.17 Calcium oxalate crystals in bronchial brushing from a patient with aspergilloma formed by the species *niger*. By polarizing the light the numerous small oxalate fragments are brightly illuminated. One cluster of calcium oxalate crystals is present in some of the exudate on the left and the 'Maltese cross' pattern is seen on the right from a starch grain from the bronchoscopist's gloves. (Papanicolaou preparation of bronchial brushing: × 100.)

Sheth, 1978). The yeast is ovoid, 3–7 μm long, with a tendency to taper more at one end (Fig. 4.18). Pseudohyphae, formed by linear budding without detachment, are common in tissue sections (Figs 4.19, 4.20). This appearance could be confused with Aspergillus, which has hyphae of the same general diameter; however, the pseudohyphae of candida have a constricted appearance between the individual cells, whereas the hyphae of Aspergillus have a smooth contour without constriction at the septae. Cross-sections of Aspergillus hyphae can appear oval but do not have buds and often appear hollow. With invasive candidiases there is usually a necrotizing reaction. The finding of candida in sputa, bronchial washings and brushings, as well as the culture of this organism from these sources, is nearly always of no clinical significance since they are usually oral contaminants or colonization rather than true invasive infection. Although visible in H&E-stained sections the silver methenamine stains make the organisms more easily seen.

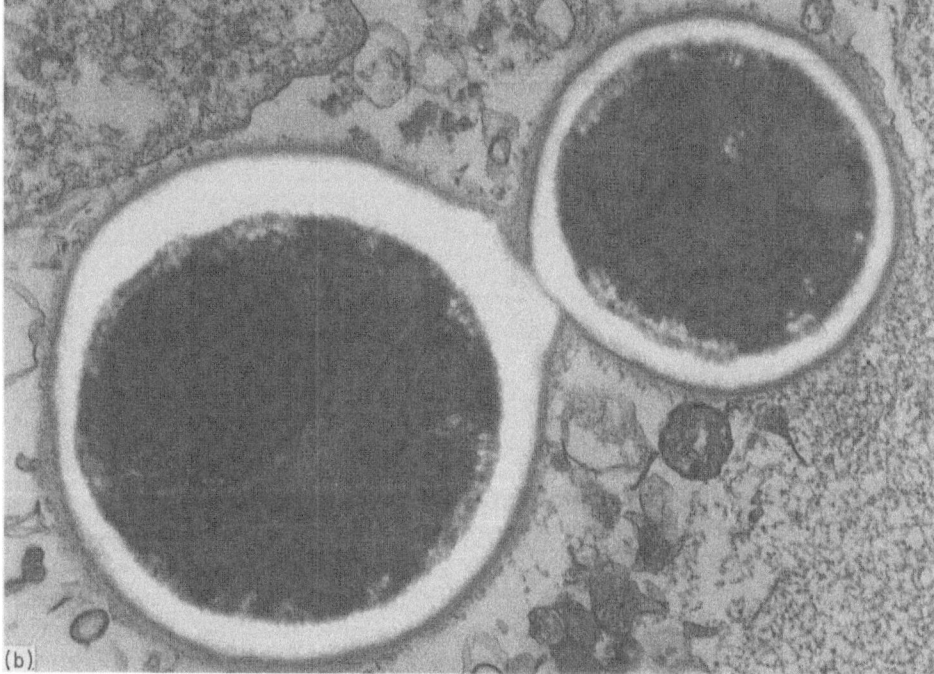

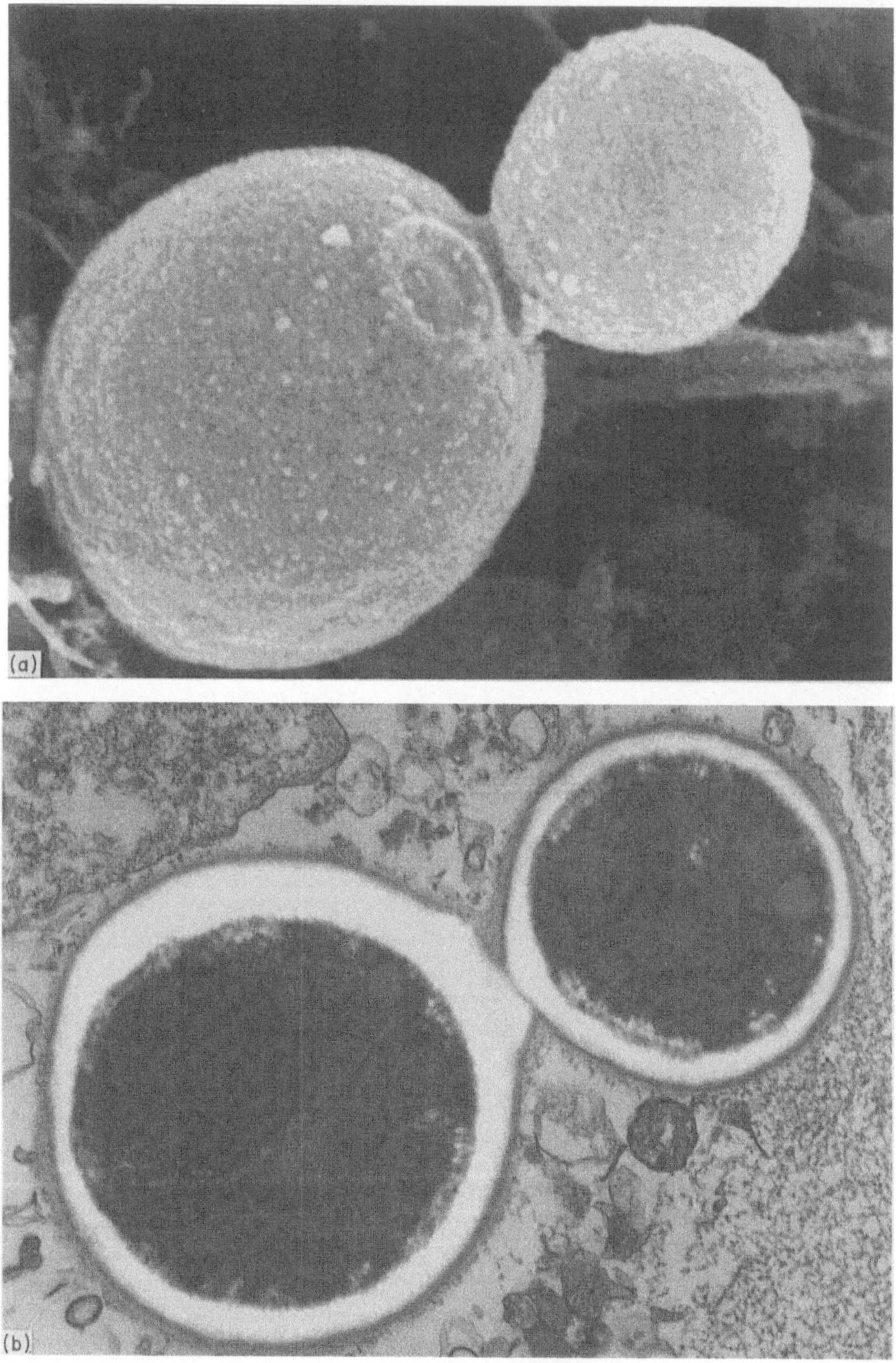

4.4.3 Mucorales

Because the taxonomic system is primarily derived from differences in the morphology of the sexual fruiting structures, and since the human pathogens rarely form these structures, there is some confusion on the correct name to apply to individual cases of infection with these fungi. Phycomycosis and mucormycosis are probably the most commonly used terms. At one time mucormycosis was a rare disease of patients with diabetes mellitus, leukemia or lymphoma (Baker, 1956; Straatsma et al., 1962). It is now more commonly seen and has earned the status of an opportunistic fungus which causes invasive pulmonary disease in a variety of patients under medical care (Agger and Maki, 1978; Lehrer et al., 1980). Unfortunately, many infections remain undiagnosed until autopsy, but some have been diagnosed by bronchial biopsy and successfully treated (Medoff and Kobayashi, 1972).

The two most common pulmonary pathogens are Rhizopus and Mucor. All of the fungi in this group have nonseptate hyphae which branch at right angles and are somewhat larger than those of Aspergillus. The hyphae are more variable in contour with a diameter of 15–35 μm (Fig. 4.21). In sections, the hyphae are often fragmented and present with an odd assortment of ovoid profiles, bulbous short hyphae and irregular fragments. The fragmentation, which can make morphological identification difficult, results from sectioning since the hyphae are larger in diameter than the thickness of our routine paraffin sections. If these irregular hyphae are cut in cross-section they can be mistaken for round yeast forms (Fig. 4.21). These problems in recognition are most troublesome in the smaller biopsies from bronchoscopy. Although the hyphae stain well with hematoxylin, it is easier to identify the broken and sectioned profiles of this fungus with a more contrasting stain such as methenamine silver.

Ultrastructurally the cell walls are electron dense (Fig. 4.22) and have a textured surface (Fig. 4.23). Hyphae are well demonstrated in Papanicolaou-stained cytology smears. In these preparations they tend to be less fragmented and the branching is more easily appreciated (Johnston et al., 1969).

Fig. 4.18 Bronchial biopsy with budding yeast of *Candida sp.* with one attached bud and separation wound of another. The cells are slightly elongated and there is a narrow neck at the attachment. (a) Scanning electron micrograph: horizontal width of field = 9.2 μm. (b) Transmission electron micrograph: × 8000.

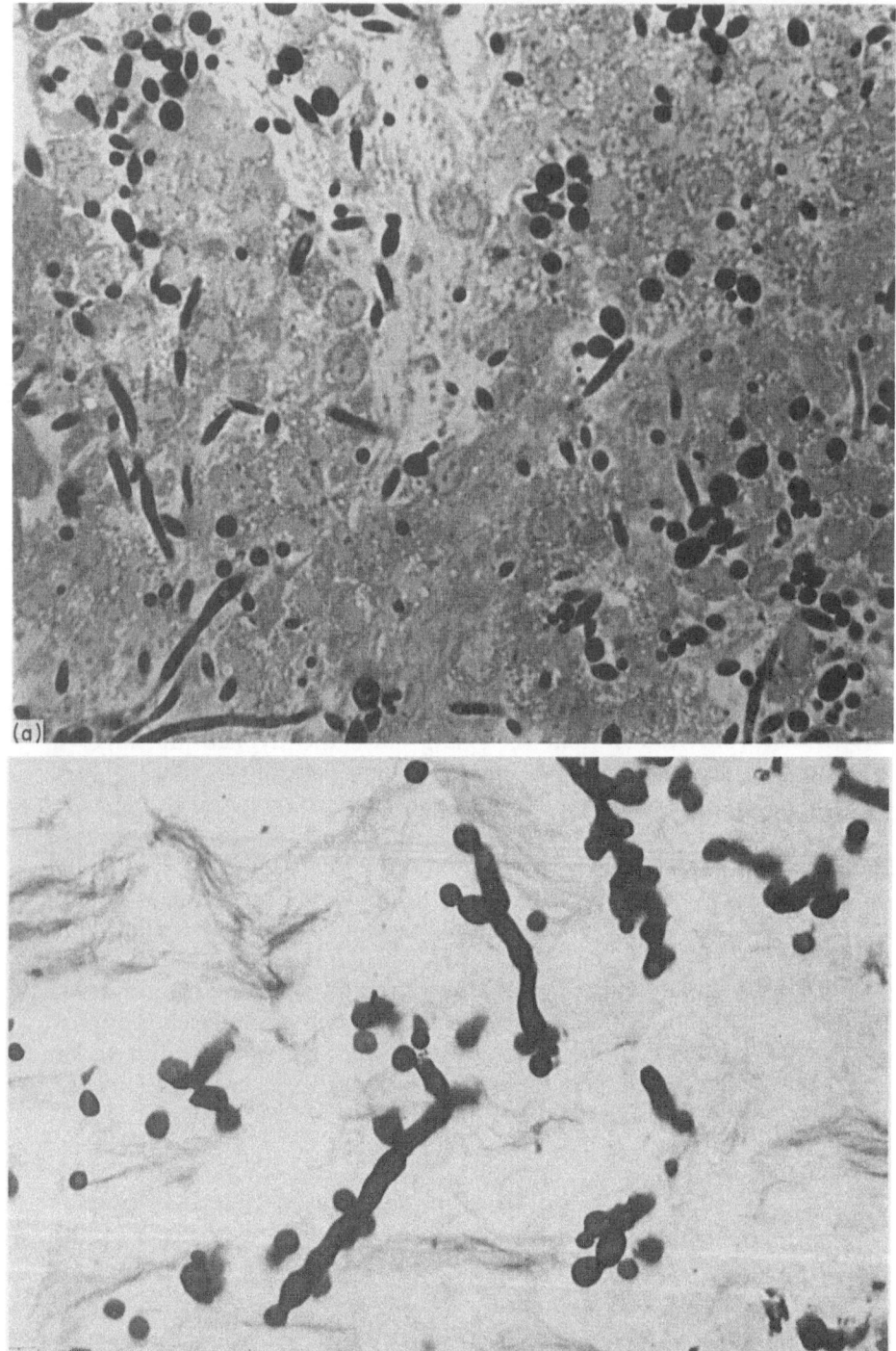

(a)

(b)

4.4.4 Blastomyces

Pulmonary infections with *Blastomyces dermatitidis* can be an acute, usually self-limiting pneumonia which can be asymptomatic. Progression to a disseminated form is uncommon. It can also present in chronic form some time after the initial acute infection. The fungus grows with a hyphal morphology in the soil (which tends to have temperatures below 37°C) and presumably infects as airborne spores. At 37°C the blastomyces grows as an 8–15 μm yeast with single occurring buds which attach over a broad surface of the parent cell (Fig. 4.24). The cell wall is thick and stains darkly with the silver methenamine stains. The cell has multiple nuclei, which distinguish it from the other pathogenic fungi with yeast forms (Schwarz and Salfelder, 1977). The silver stains obscure this internal feature and some prefer the PAS stain which gives a dark pink color to the thick wall but does not obscure the nuclei.

The tissue reaction is extremely variable and the organism may be difficult to identify in biopsy material. Multinucleated giant cells of both Langhans' and foreign body types are frequently seen. Granulomas, often with central necrosis or suppuration, are seen. There may be only a few yeast or masses of them with little or no leukocytic response (Sarosi and Davies, 1979). In their review of 37 cases of pulmonary blastomycosis, Schwarz and Salfelder (1977) found 7 with necrosis and the remaining 30 with hard sarcoid-like granulomas. One third of their cases had an ulcerative bronchitis, many with granulomas in the bronchi, and they suggest that these lesions should be easily detected in bronchial biopsy material.

Sputum cytology smears are excellent sources for detecting the yeast but the observer must be alert to objects other than abnormal cells (Johnston *et al.*, 1969). Sanders *et al.* (1977) found 4 cases in a routine cytology service but retrospectively were able to find 3 additional cases from patients with culture-proven infections which had been overlooked initially.

4.4.5 Coccidioides

Coccidioides immitis is predominantly a pulmonary pathogen. Like blastomycosis, coccidioidomycosis usually presents as an acute pneumonia which is often asymptomatic and self-limiting. In 5% of cases, the pneumonia will persist as a symptomatic pneumonia involving one or a few

---

Fig. 4.19 Candida with a mixture of budding yeast forms and pseudohyphae. (a) Sputum colonized with *Candida albicans*. (Epon/Araldite section stained with toluidine blue: × 240.) (b) Transbronchial biopsy of invasive *Candida albicans*. (Paraffin-embedded section stained with Gomori's silver methenamine: × 480.)

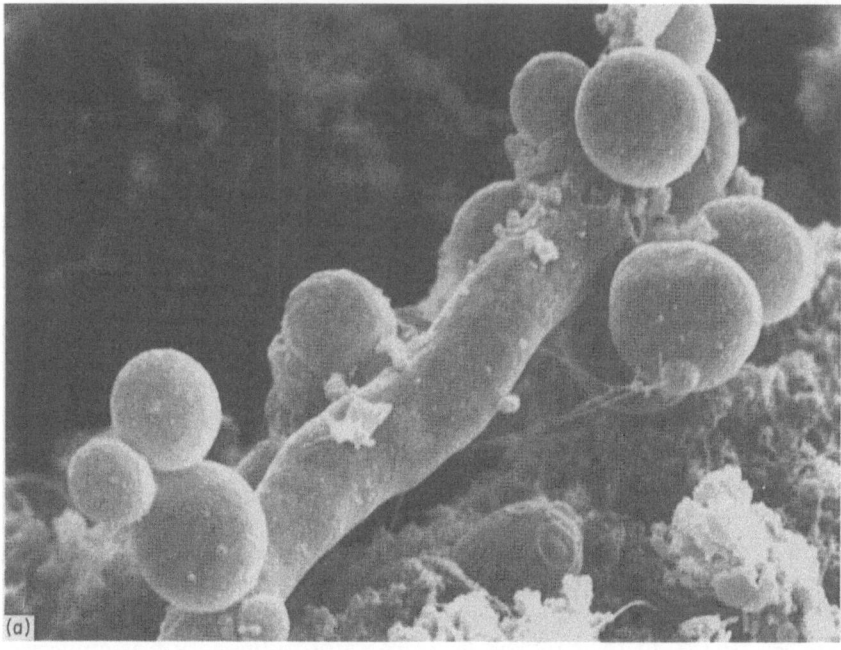

Fig. 4.20   Candida pseudohyphae with multiple budding. Even in the pseudo-hyphae there is a slight tapering of the cell toward the attachment sites. Trans-bronchial biopsy. Scanning electron micrographs: (a) Horizontal width of field = 15.9 μm. (b) and (c) Horizontal width of field = 8.5 μm.

areas of lung (Deppisch and Donowho, 1972). Most of the persistent lesions are peripherally located and often in a subpleural site. Persistent infection with a miliary pattern is only rarely seen. Disseminated coccidi-oidomycosis is uncommon. Pulmonary infection occurs from airborne spores which usually are lifted up by the wind from dry sandy soil. The soils of southwestern USA are the most frequent source, and the epide-miology has some remarkable tales of infections traveling over long distances in dust storms as well as infections acquired during archeological digs.

In tissue the fungus grows as nonbudding spherules. These are variable in size with diameters of 10–80 μm. As the fungus matures they form endospores (Fig. 4.25) which are 2–5 μm in diameter within the larger spherules (Drutz and Catanzaro, 1978). Spherules are frequently found within multinucleated giant cells of either Langhans' or foreign body types. The spherules are often seen within necrotic areas and leukocytes can be abundant. The silver methenamine stain helps to see the smaller spherules, but the stain tends to obscure the endospores. The large

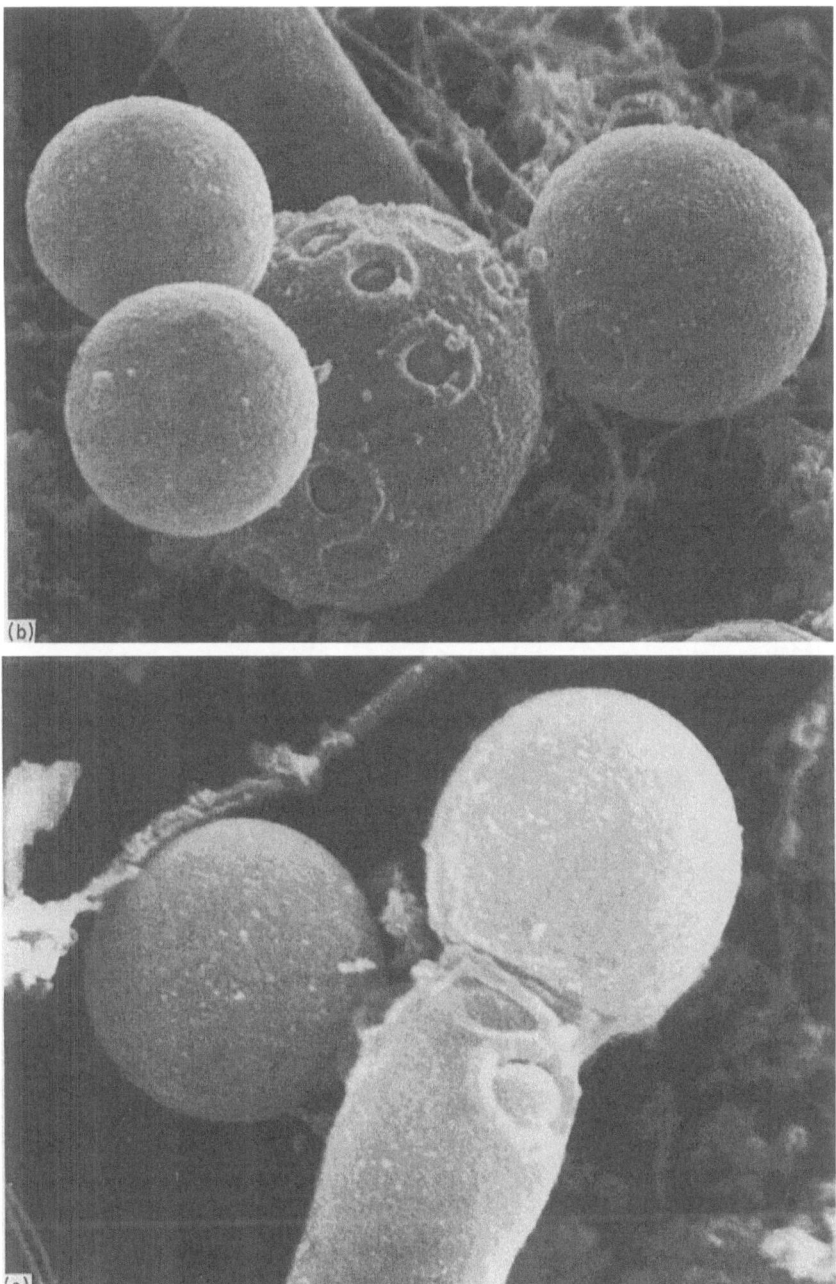

(b)

(c)

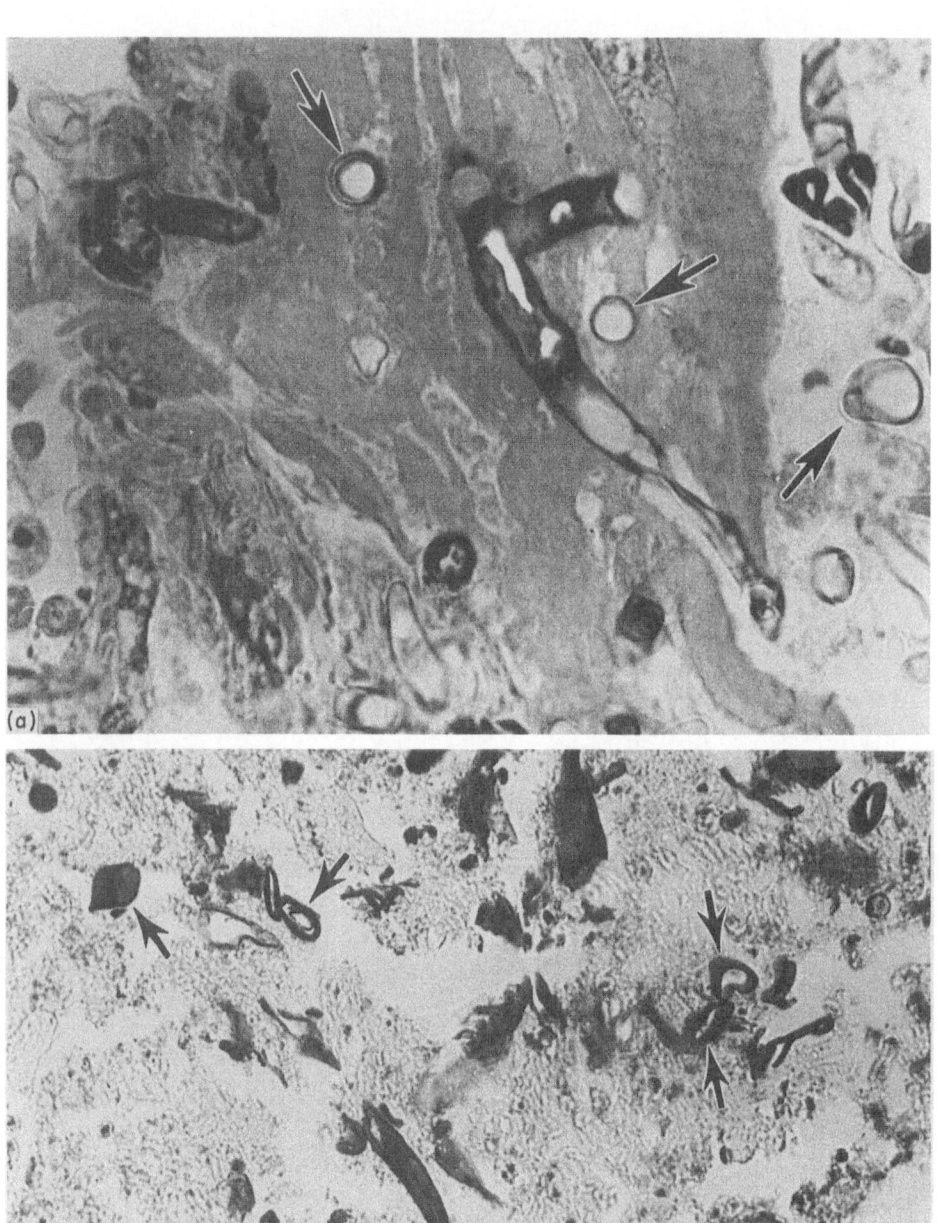

(a)

(b)

spherules are hard to miss with H&E or PAS stains. The Papanicolaou stain demonstrates the spherules and endospores extremely well (Guglietti and Reingold, 1968). Because of their large size they can be mistaken for pollen grains.

The spherules and endospores are not infectious to humans; however, in culture arthrospores are produced which present a serious biohazard in the microbiology laboratory (Drutz and Catanzaro, 1978). Subsequently, extraordinary procedures must be utilized to prevent the spread of these airborne spores and infection of laboratory personnel. Because of the hazard which accompanies culturing, the histological diagnosis becomes more important in this disease.

4.4.6 Cryptococcus

Cryptococcus, like the other fungi in this group, infects lung to produce an asymptomatic self-limiting disease in most of the individuals who are exposed. A chronic persistent form of pulmonary infection may become clinically recognized. *Cryptococcus neoformans* is more likely to present as a disseminated disease, with meningitis a very frequent initial diagnosis (Kerkering *et al.*, 1981). Taylor (1970) and Hatcher *et al.* (1971) both report that only 10% of the diagnosed cases were primary pneumonias. Of the 24 cases of pulmonary cryptococcosis in the Hatcher series, 5 were diagnosed from sputum cultures. Most cases (16) were diagnosed by lung biopsy, 2 by fine needle aspirates and 1 by scalene lymph node biopsy. Sixty-seven per cent of their cases required thoracotomy for diagnosis. Taylor reported an even greater percentage of necessary diagnostic thoracotomies. It is not uncommon to see this organism in tissue biopsies which are negative on culture.

The fungus has a yeast form with nearly spherical shape, 5–20 μm in diameter, with the formation of single buds which are attached by a narrow neck to the parent cell (Fig. 4.26). They have a gelatinous capsule which does not stain with H&E or the silver stains but can be seen with PAS or mucicarmine stains (Luna, 1968). Both the frequency of budding

---

Fig. 4.21 Mucorales infection. (a) One of the Mucorales (genus undetermined) in lung tissue. The characteristic 90° branching and nonseptate hyphae can be seen. The yeast-like structures (arrows) are cross-sections of the hyphae passing vertically through the block. (Epon/Araldite-embedded section stained with toluidine blue: × 560.) (b) Considerable fragmentation and obliquely sectioned profiles make the Mucorales difficult to distinguish from necrotic debris. The silver stains give enhanced contrast and make identification more easy. Ovoid and cross-sectioned hyphae are indicated with arrows. Transbronchial biopsy. (Paraffin-embedded section stained with Gomori's silver methenamine: × 400.)

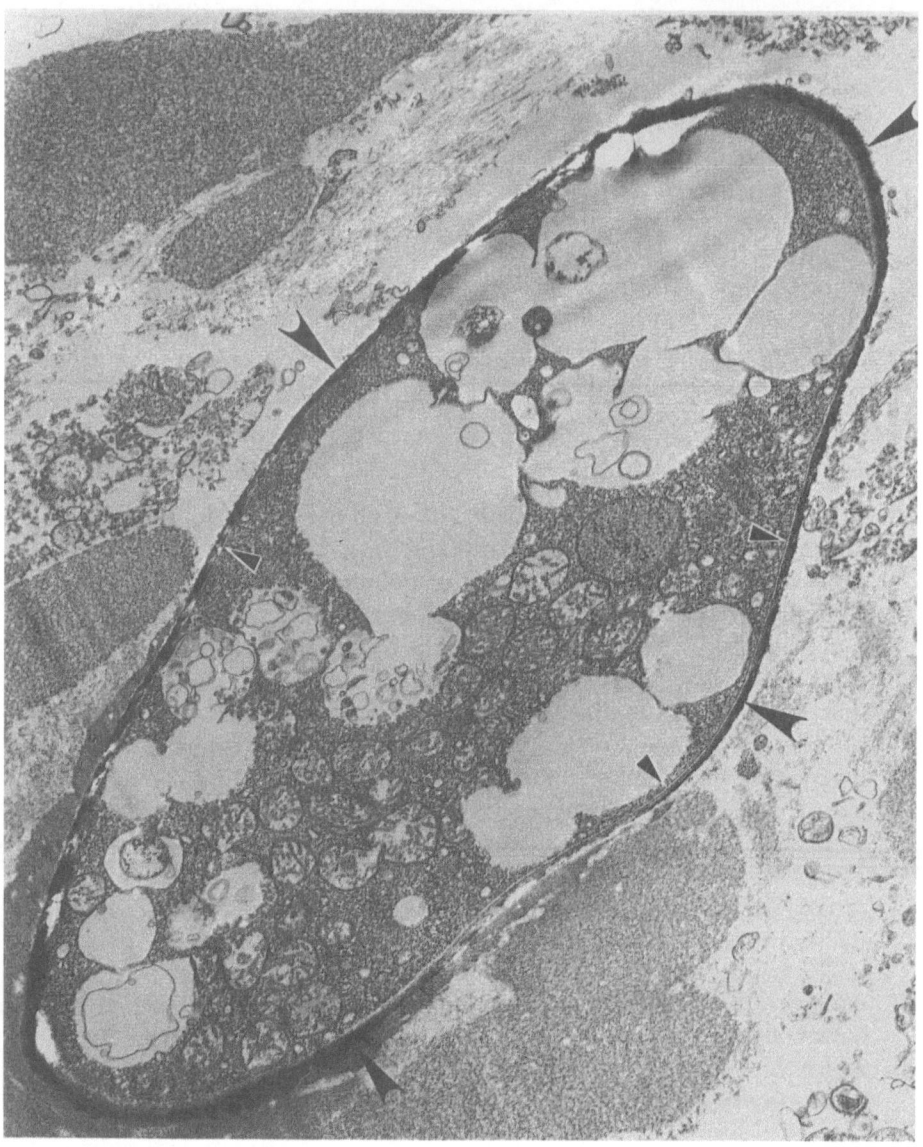

Fig. 4.22 Invasive mucormycosis in lung. The fungal cell contains an assortment of organelles and vacuoles. The plasma membrane (small arrows) can be seen just inside the thicker, electron-dense cell wall (larger arrows). (Transmission electron micrograph: × 7000.)

Fig. 4.23 The Mucorales cell wall is very electron dense and composed of irregular layers. (a) In this transmission electron micrograph of a bronchial biopsy an empty hyphal wall is surrounded and apparently invaded by neutrophilic leukocytes. (× 8000) (b) The surface of the hyphae are textured in the scanning electron micrograph, unlike those of Aspergillus (compare with Fig. 4.15). Transbronchial biopsy. (Scanning electron micrograph: horizontal width of field = 108 μm.)

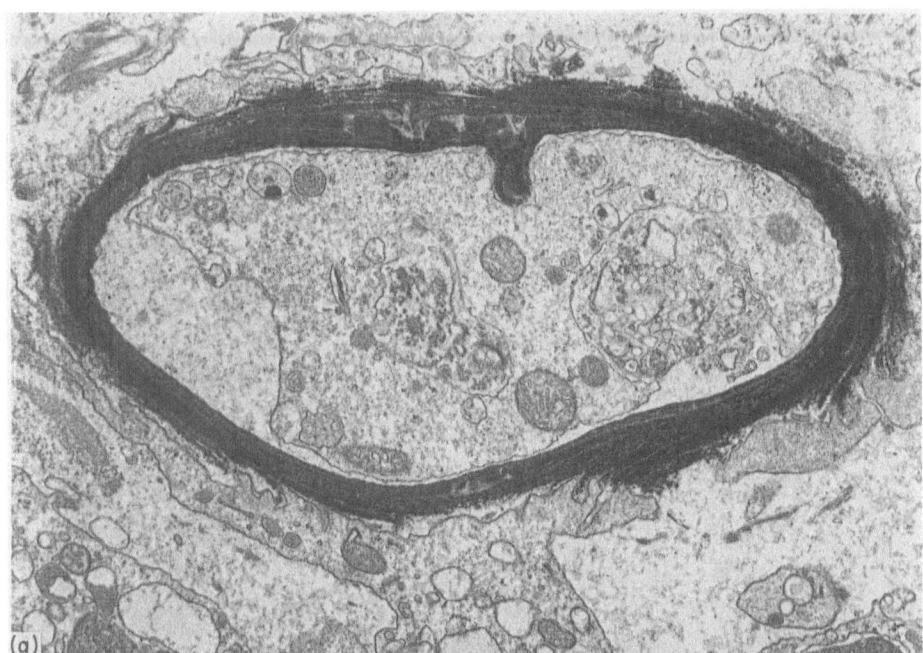

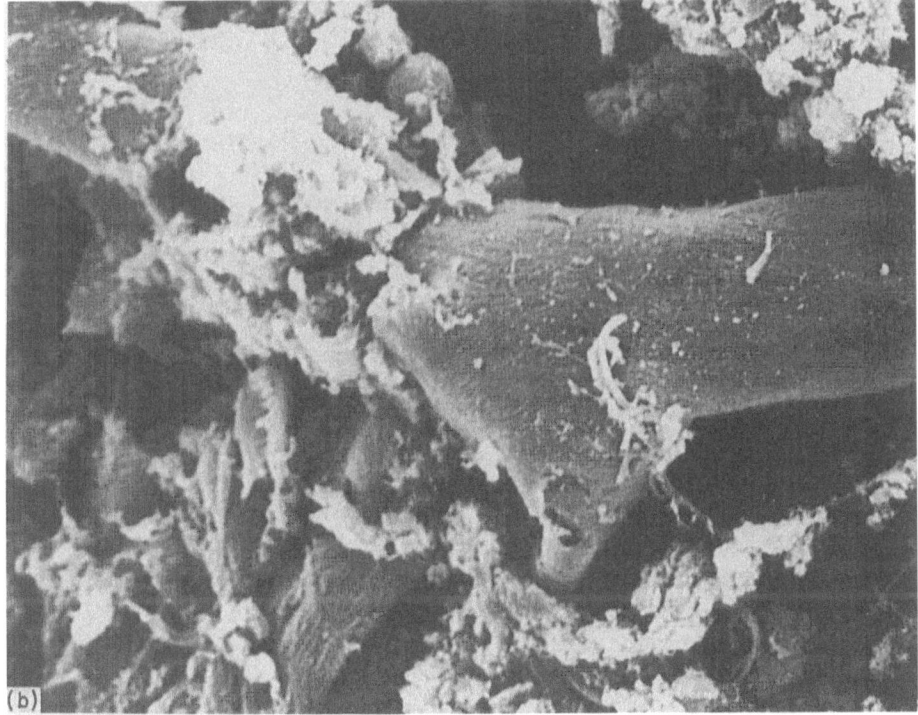

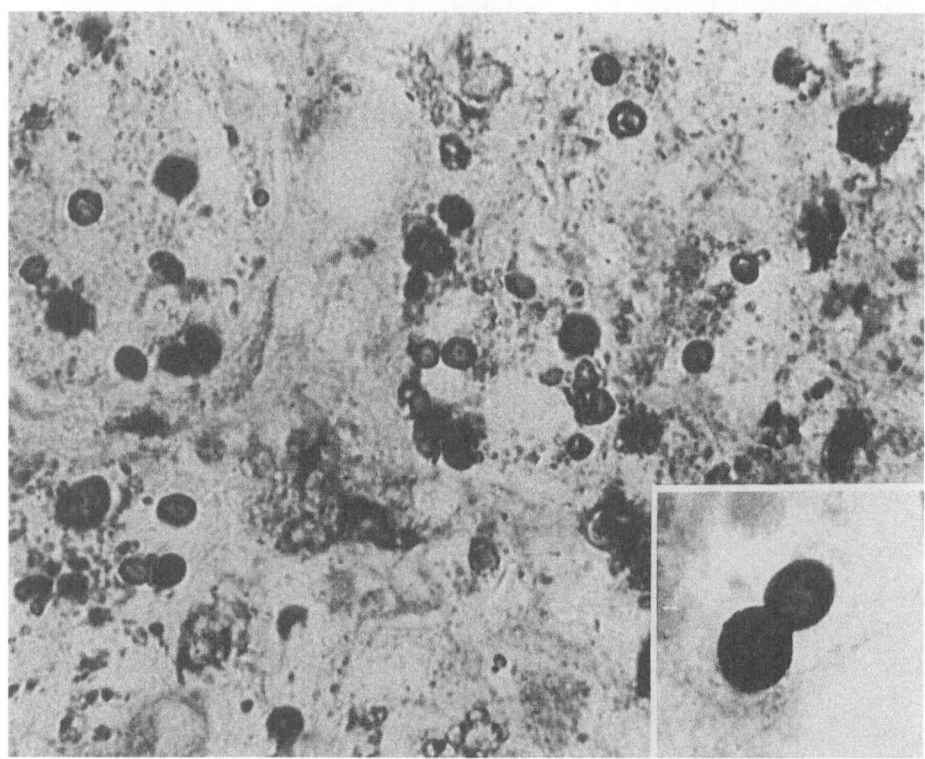

Fig. 4.24 Pulmonary blastomycosis. Numerous nearly spherical, thick walled yeast are present among the necrotic debris. (× 400) *Inset*: Higher magnification of one of the uncommon budding yeast showing the broad attachment between the bud and the parent cells. (× 900) (Paraffin-embedded section stained with Gomori's silver methenamine).

and the thickness of the capsule are variable, which sometimes makes difficult a definite judgement based on these characteristics. In the chronic and disseminated forms of cryptococcosis the tissue reaction is granulomatous with small or large nodules, some of which may have central necrosis. The yeast may be seen in the cytoplasm of multinucleated giant cells (Fig. 4.27), but more frequently lying within the necrotic debris or simply scattered in the tissue adjacent to the granuloma. Baker (1976), after diligent search, has been able to demonstrate rare lymph node extension similar to that which is seen in tuberculosis, histoplasmosis and coccidioidomycosis.

If watched for carefully, cryptococcus can be spotted in cytology smears from sputa (Fig. 4.28), bronchial washings and brushings (Prolla *et al.*, 1970; Gleason *et al.*, 1980; Rosen and Koprowska, 1982). In the reported

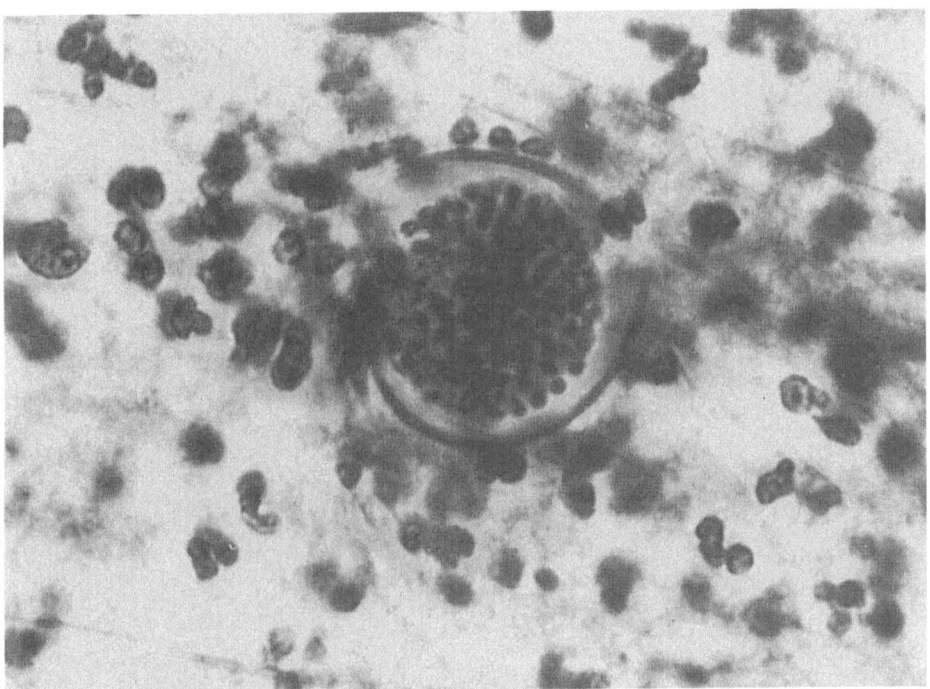

Fig. 4.25 *Coccidioides immitis.* Large spherule (60 μm in diameter) containing large numbers of developing endospores. The spherule, which is surrounded by neutrophils, is broken open. Although the endospores are released from the spherules by rupture of the wall, the breakage is more likely in this situation due to the pressure of the coverslip on this very large object. (Papanicolaou smear: × 630.)

cases, fresh material or the initial smears were subsequently stained with PAS or mucicarmine to make a more confident diagnosis.

4.4.7   Histoplasma

Histoplasmosis is endemic in the midwestern states of the USA but is seen in other parts of the world where the conditions are correct for growth of this fungus in soil (usually enriched with bird droppings). There is a spectrum of disease resulting from airborne infection similar to those described for Blastomyces, Coccidioides and Cryptococcus, as well as caused by *Mycobacteria tuberculosis.* Straub and Schwarz (1962), in an extensive study which makes use of experimental and clinical material, give a clear account of these similarities in both pathobiology of the infections and morphology of their tissue reactions. *Histoplasma*

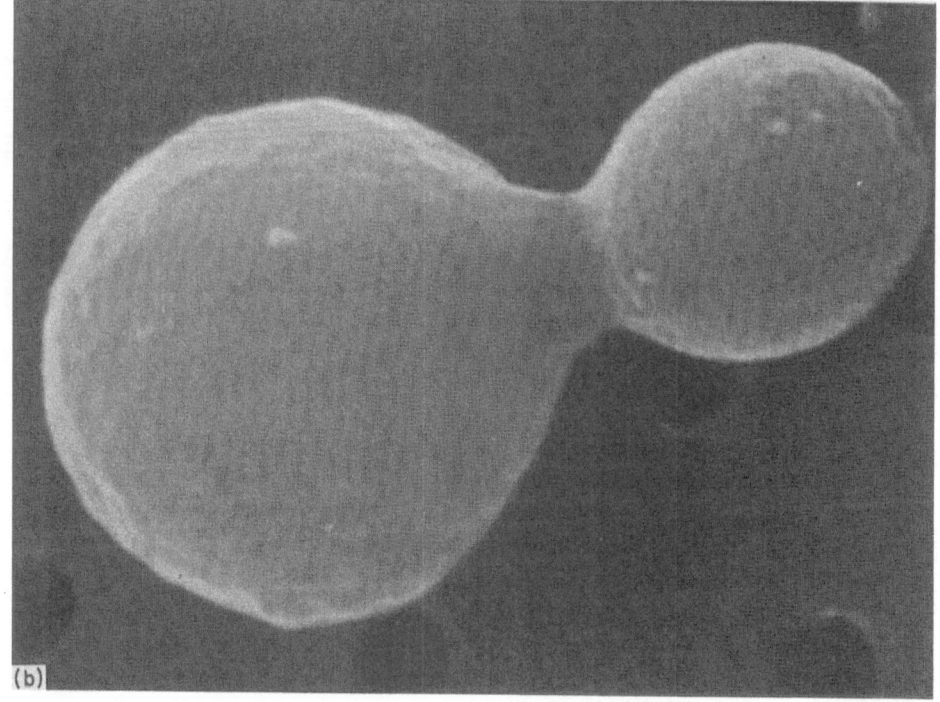

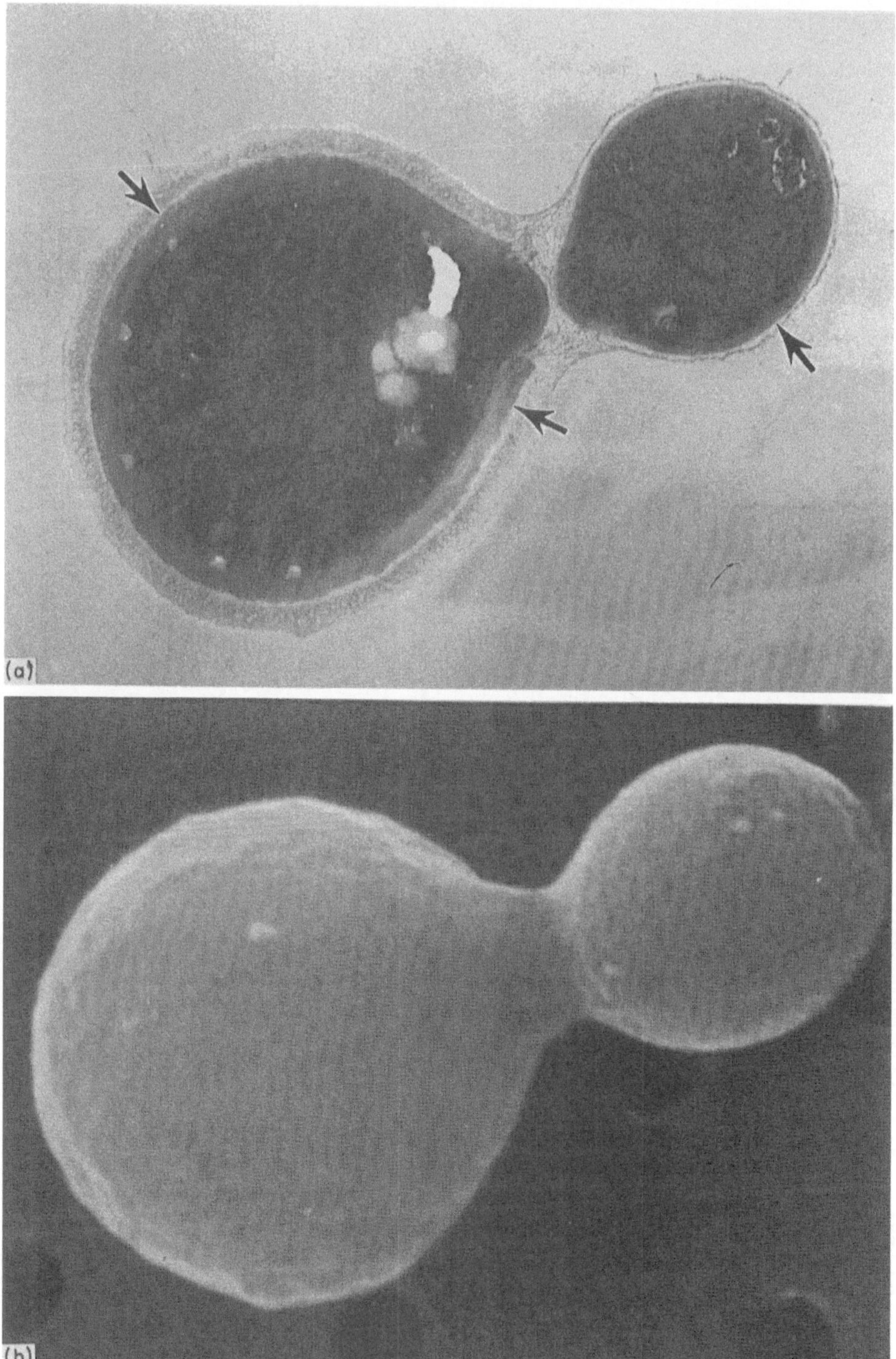

capsulatum (the most common species) is a highly infectious fungus but has low pathogenicity. The chronic form of histoplasmosis which usually overlays other pre-existing chronic pulmonary disease is the form which provides most of the biopsy specimens. With unusually heavy exposure an acute pulmonary histoplasmosis develops which is different from the usually subclinical incidental infection in the endemic areas, only because of a more diffuse pulmonary infection (Goodwin and Des Prez, 1978). Histoplasmosis is most frequently diagnosed by serology.

This fungus, like Blastomyces and Coccidioides, grows as hyphae in the soil environment, but as yeast forms at body temperature. The airborne spores enter the airways and are phagocytized by histiocytes. They apparently parasitize the phagocyte and multiply intracellularly. The intracellular form is ovoid, 1.5–3.5 μm. Small buds can be seen occasionally attached to the smaller pole of the parent cell (Fig. 4.29, arrows). Extracellular yeast are likewise ovoid but tend to be somewhat larger and consequently somewhat more easily seen (Goodwin *et al.*, 1981). The extracellular yeast are most commonly scattered in the necrotic centers of granulomas (Fig. 4.29). All of the forms of this yeast are nearly undetectable in routine H&E-stained sections but are well stained with silver methenamine. The silver-stained cell walls can frequently be seen in old granulomas and may not indicate clinically active disease. The granulomas tend to be larger than those in tuberculosis and calcify readily. In fulminant cases of disseminated histoplasmosis, macrophages are seen with distended cytoplasm filled with the small yeast forms (Goodwin *et al.*, 1980). Calcospherites can be seen in sputa from individuals with calcified histoplasmosis granulomas.

4.5 Pneumocystis

The controversy which surrounds determining whether *Pneumocystis carinii* belongs with the protozoa or the yeast is essentially irrelevant when discussing the diseases this organism produces. There is a pneumocystis pneumonia in young otherwise healthy neonates and infants between the ages of 2 and 12 weeks, which in one study accounted for 14% of hospitalized pneumonias in this age group (Stagno *et al.*, 1980). In some-

Fig. 4.26 Budding yeast of *Cryptococcus neoformans*. (a) The cytplasm is very electron dense and is surrounded by a thick, laminated, moderately electron-dense cell wall (arrows). The characteristic gelatinous capsule is continuous over both the parent cell and the bud and appears somewhat fibrillary, although this may be an artefact of fixation. (Transmission electron micrograph: × 15 000.) (b) Narrow attachment zone between bud and parent cell of *Cryptococcus neoformans*. The gelatinous capsule has condensed around the yeast during processing. (Scanning electron micrograph: horizontal field width = 5.5 μm.)

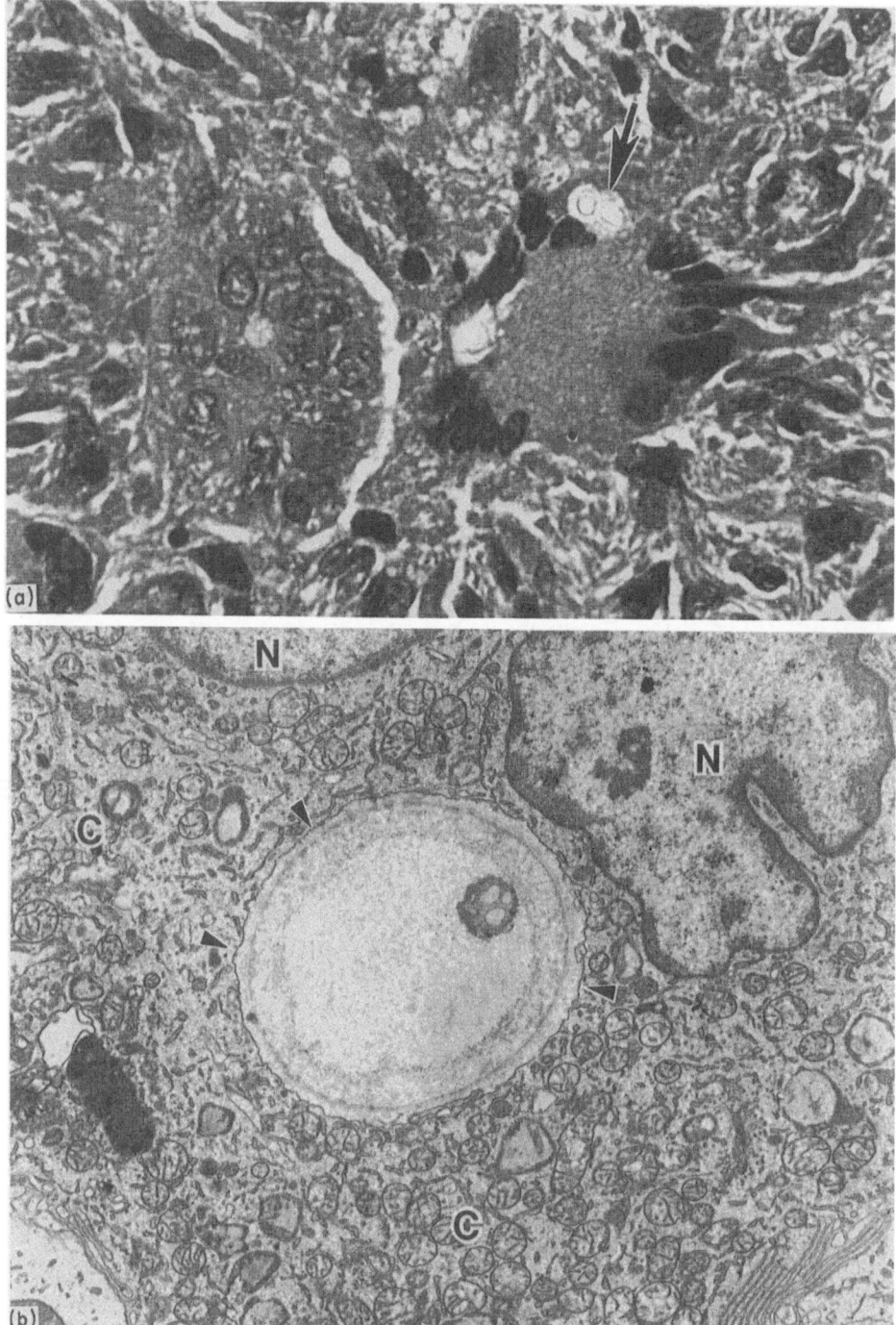

(a)

(b)

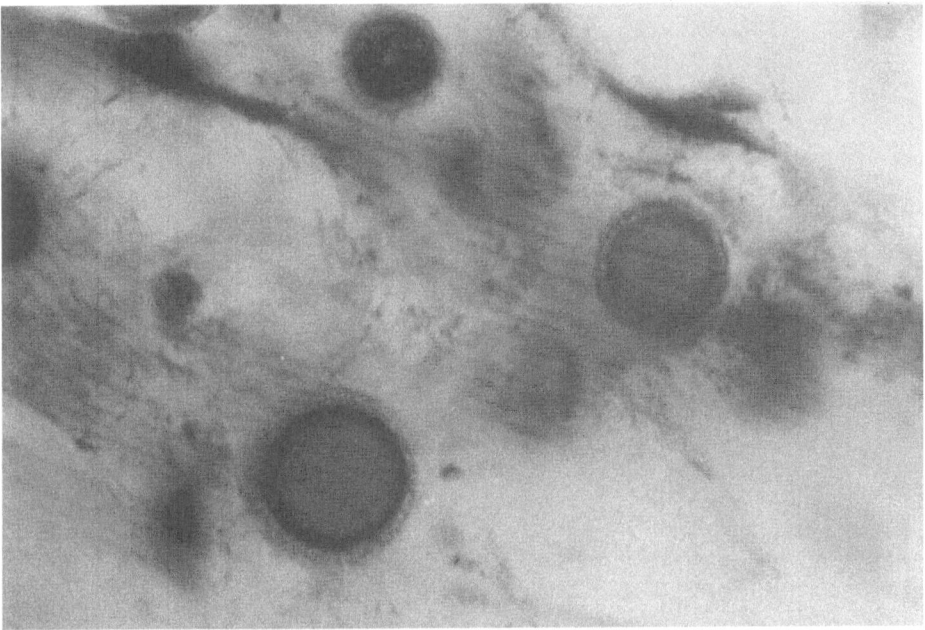

Fig. 4.28 Several yeast of *Cryptococcus neoformans* in sputum specimen. The patient, who was being treated for leukemia, had pulmonary and meningeal infections. All sputa from this patient contained masses of the fungus which were well stained with the Papanicolaou stain. Notice that the capsule is also slightly stained (pink). (Papanicolaou sputum smear: × 1800.)

what older children pneumocystis pneumonia is a complication in 1% of patients with acute leukemia (Walzer *et al.*, 1974). Infections are also a serious risk in patients with renal or bone marrow transplants (Neiman *et al.*, 1977) as well as the other causes of immunocompromise (Weber *et al.*, 1977) and in a patient with Cushing's syndrome (Anthony and Greco, 1981). Nearly all of the infections diagnosed by biopsy are in immuno-compromised individuals and in this setting it is a dramatic rapidly progressive disease which until recently was invariably fatal.

The organism is ubiquitous in humans and grows principally in the

Fig. 4.27 Cryptococcosis. (a) Multinucleated giant cells, one of which contains a budding yeast (arrow). The halo surrounding the double-layered cell wall of the parent and bud is caused by the presence of the gelatinous capsule. Bronchial biopsy. (Paraffin-embedded section stained with H&E: × 560.) (b) Multinucleated giant cell with Cryptococcus within a cytoplasmic phagosome. Nucleus (N), cytoplasm (C) of the giant cell. The phagosomal membrane (arrows) can be seen surrounding the yeast. Bronchoscopic biopsy. (Transmission electron micrograph: × 8900.)

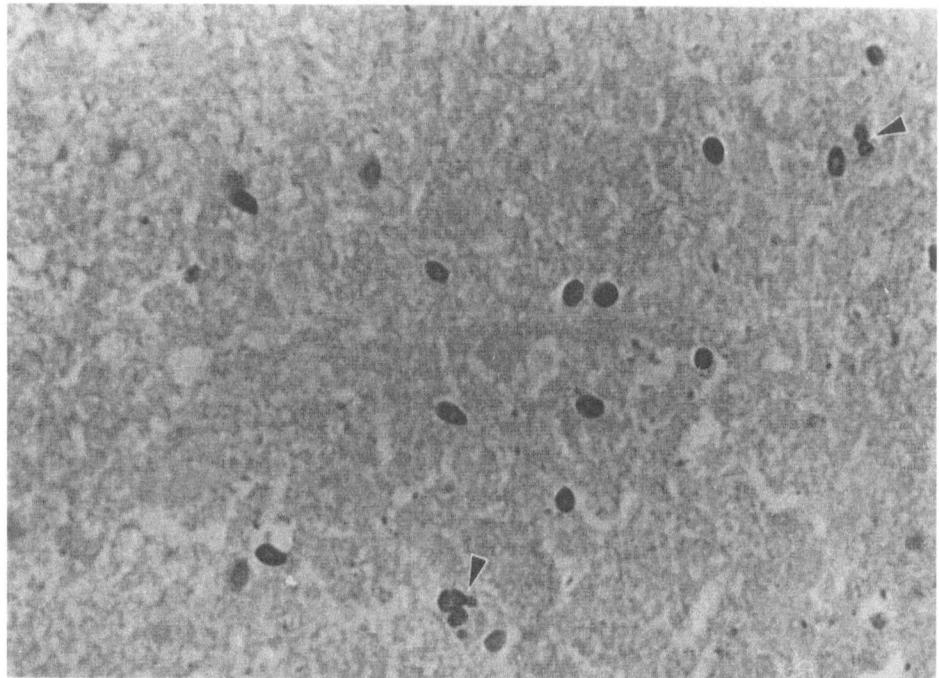

Fig. 4.29 Pulmonary histoplasmosis. Within the nearly amorphous necrotic debris within a large granuloma, the ovoid rarely budding (arrows) yeast are distinguishable with the silver methenamine stain. They are about 2 μm in width but somewhat longer. (Paraffin-embedded section stained with Gomori's silver methenamine: × 1000.)

alveolar spaces. There is an indistinguishable organism found in rodents which is probably epidemiologically unrelated to the disease in humans. The pneumonia in newborns is characterized by a lymphocytic interstitial infiltrate with conspicuous plasma cells, leading to its frequent designation as interstitial plasma cell pneumonia. In immunocompromised patients the reaction is influenced by the patient's impairment (frequently a leukopenia) and the histological changes may be minimal. The diagnostic foamy intra-alveolar eosinophilic material (occasionally incorrectly called an exudate) is a mass of the organisms, frequently with no inflammatory cellular or proteinaceous exudate. The distinctive feature which allows differentiation from the numerous exudative materials in alveoli is the presence of numerous 'holes' within the eosinophilic material which can be appreciated in H&E-stained sections (Fig. 4.30). Ultrastructural examination of the eosinophilic material shows it to be masses of cystic (3–4 μm) and trophozoic (2–12 μm) forms (Fig. 4.31) (Campbell, 1972; Hasleton *et al.*, 1981; Yoneda *et al.*, 1982). An ultrastructural study of all stages of the life cycle was made by Vavra and Kücera (1970). The cysts account for the 'holes' seen in paraffin sections stained with H&E. Intracystic forms develop (Fig. 4.32) which are released as trophozoites (Fig. 4.33). The trophozoites have numerous tubular expansions of their cell walls (Figs 4.32, 4.33, 4.34) which make up most of the eosinophilic material seen by light microscopy. Silver stains make the cysts very conspicuous (Fig. 4.35) and a variety of modifications are available, particularly aimed at reducing the time necessary to complete the staining and allow more rapid definitive diagnoses (Chalvardjian and Grawe, 1963; Churukian, 1977; Musto *et al.*, 1982). A characteristic dot can be seen in a few of the cysts. This is occasionally labeled as a nucleus in the older literature, but is actually a focal thickening of the cyst wall (Fig. 4.36). The trophozoites stain with cresyl violet (Bowling *et al.*, 1973) and toluidine blue (Pritchett *et al.*, 1977). Demicco *et al.* (1979) recommend using tissue with pneumocystis as positive control for these stains because of some difficulty in staining reactions not appreciated if the usual control tissue with fungi are used. Red blood cells, partially stained with the silver stains, are sometimes difficult to distinguish from the cysts, which are similar in size and shape, but the focal thickening in the wall of the cysts allows differentiation.

The pathologist is usually alerted to the need to search for the intra-alveolar foam by the clinical history or a specific notation that the specimen was obtained because of the clinical suspicion of pneumocystis pneumonia. Recently, however, there have been reports of clusters of pneumocystis infections in patients who were recognized as being immunodeficient only when they were discovered to have various infections and/or Kaposi's sarcoma. The outbreaks of acquired immune deficiency syndrome have attracted scientific and lay interest. At risk are homosexual males (Follansbee *et al.*, 1982; Gottlieb *et al.*, 1981; Laurens *et al.*, 1982), but also Haitian emigrants to the USA (Hawkins and Smith, 1982) and intravenous drug users as well as others with no apparent epidemiological pattern (Haverkos and Curran, 1982).

A task force on the acquired immune deficiency syndrome coordinated by Curran (1982) has reported more than 200 cases, most of which had pneumocystis pneumonia. In a review later in the same year the total had nearly reached 700 (Haverkos and Curran, 1982). Pneumocystis was identified in these cases by morphological detection in a variety of specimen sources including open lung biopsy, transthoracic fine needle aspiration, bronchial washings and lavage, as well as transbronchial biopsy. The organism is rarely detected in sputa but special stains allow rapid detection in the cytology specimens from bronchoscopy and fine needle aspirations (see Section 2.4.3). In their population of immunosuppressed

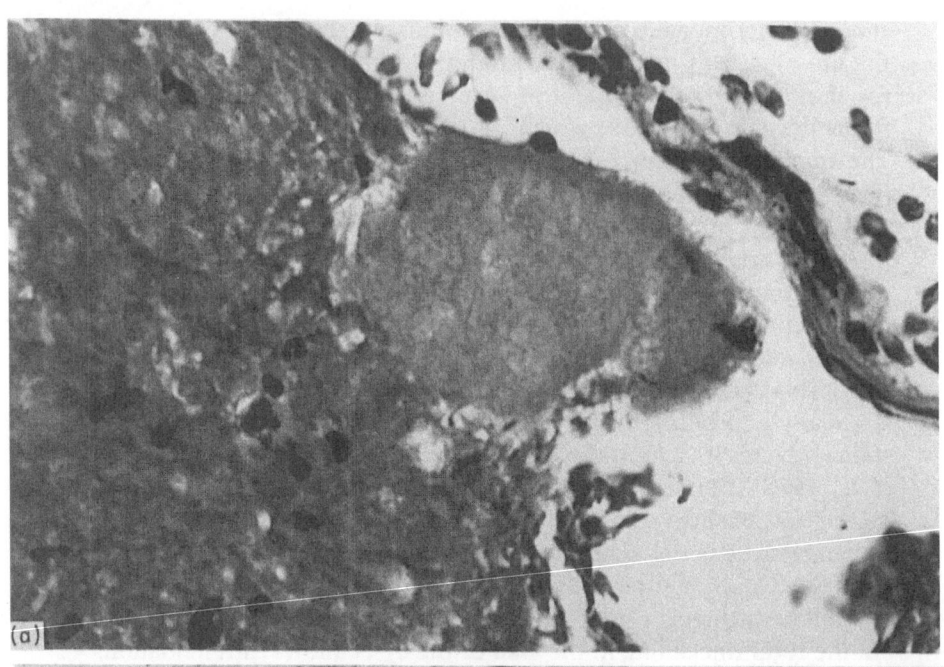

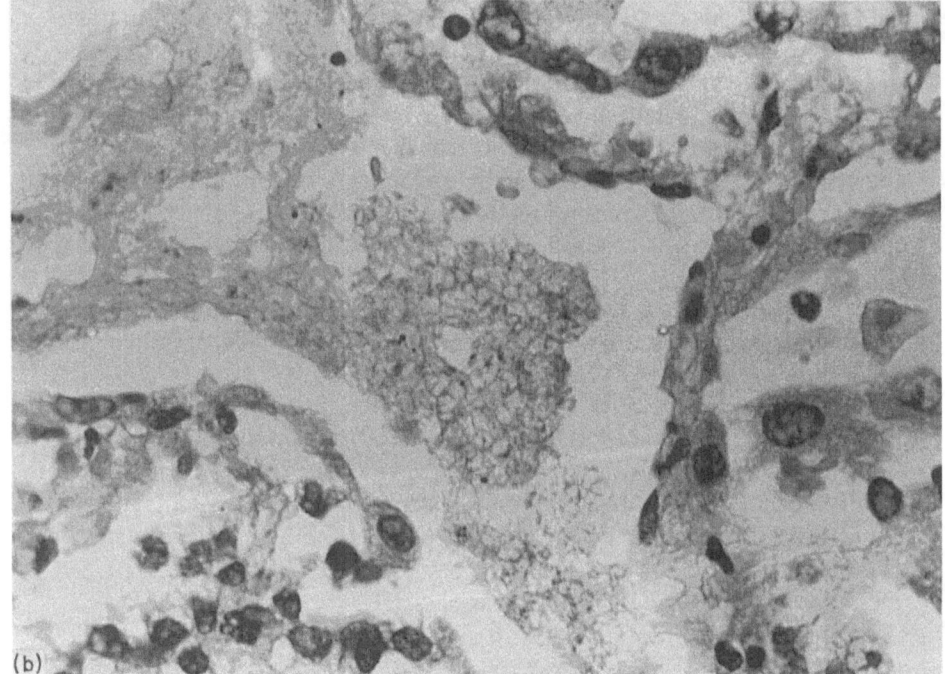

patients with proven pneumocystis pneumonia, Walzer *et al.* (1974) had diagnostic yields of 64% in the open lung biopsies, 62% in the bronchial biopsies and 55% in the lung needle aspirates. The high percentage of false negative specimens may be due to sampling, but it is interesting that the usually reliable open biopsy is only slightly more sensitive than bronchoscopic material. In the large number of cases now accumulating with acquired immune deficiency syndrome, most of the diagnoses are made by bronchoscopy, either in transbronchial biopsies or bronchial washings/lavage.

Pneumocystis pneumonia can be treated, but even with the current therapy nearly one half of the cases are fatal. Although the current drug is less toxic than that used in the recent past, a full course of treatment is usually dependent on morphological identification of the organism. As mentioned in Section 4.1.2, cytomegalovirus is a common copathogen with *Pneumocystis carinii.*

4.6   The immunocompromised individual

The etiological diagnosis of airway infection by micro-organisms is important for prompt appropriate treatment in these individuals. The full spectrum of common pathogens is expanded to include many not-so-common pathogens as well as a number of opportunistic micro-organisms (not ordinarily considered pathogens) in these patients. In many cases the diagnosis relies wholly or in part on the morphologic detection and identification of the organisms themselves. Many of the culprits have been discussed under separate sections in this chapter.

As commented above, most of these patients have clinically recognized immunocompromise and the specimens are obtained with that in mind. Open lung biopsy through a thoracotomy remains the most accurate and sensitive means of histologically identifying the etiology of their disease (which of course is not always infectious). Bronchoscopic specimens are nearly as adequate and there is less risk to the patient. Culture both from

Fig. 4.30 Exudative materials in alveoli. (a) An eosinophilic fibrinous intra-alveolar exudate which does not contain any internal structure. Transbronchial biopsy from a patient *without* pneumocystis. (b) In sharp distinction to the exudate above, this foamy eosinophilic material from another patient has the characteristics of *Pneumocystis carinii.* The adjacent pneumocytes are not very reactive and there are no inflammatory cells in the alveolar space. (Paraffin-embedded sections stained with H&E: × 300.)

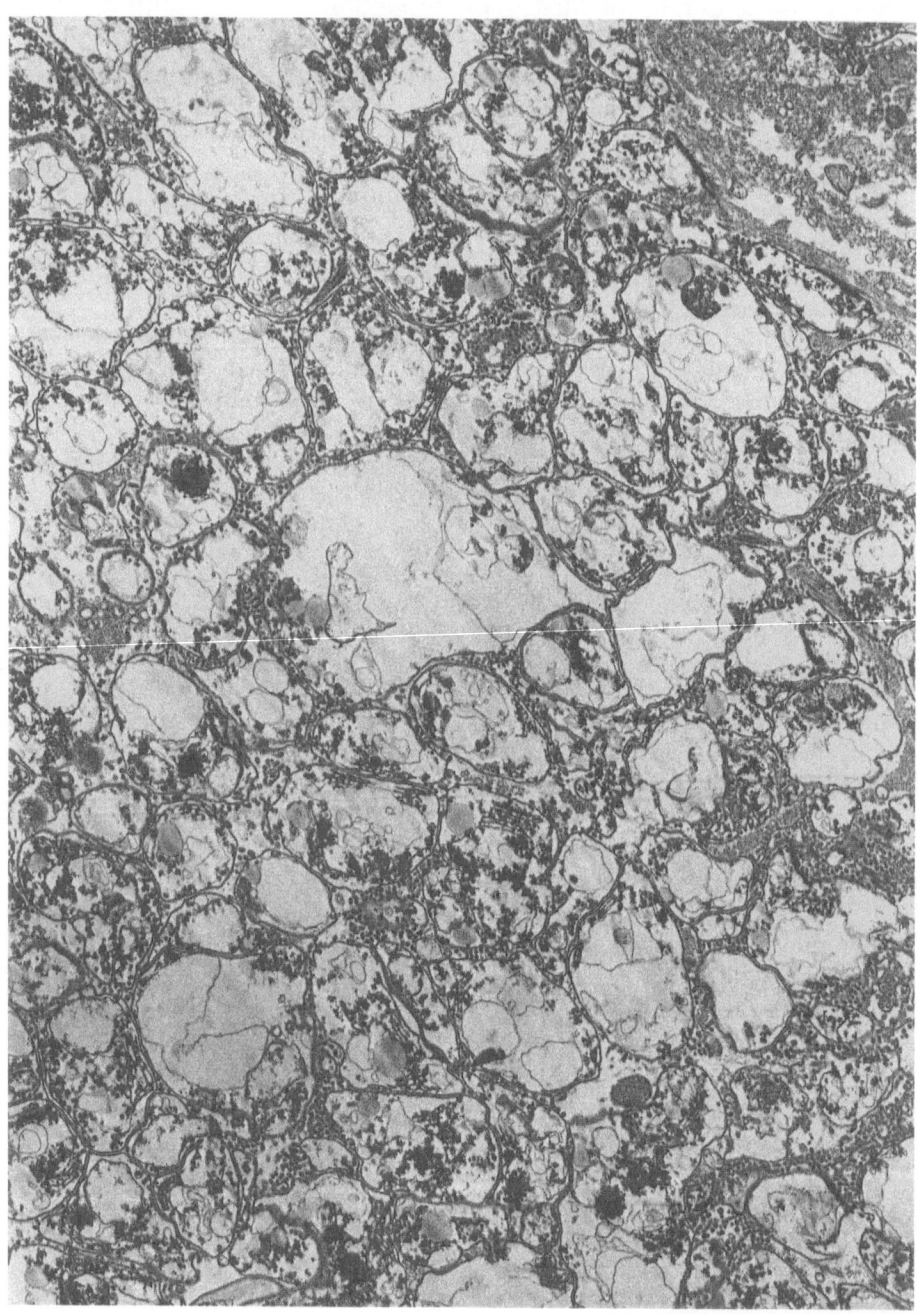

Fig. 4.31 Low magnification of the intra-alveolar foam (as in Fig. 4.30b) in a case of pneumocystis pneumonia. The foam is a mass of the organisms with very little other material. Most of the forms here are trophozoites. (Transmission electron micrograph: × 7700.)

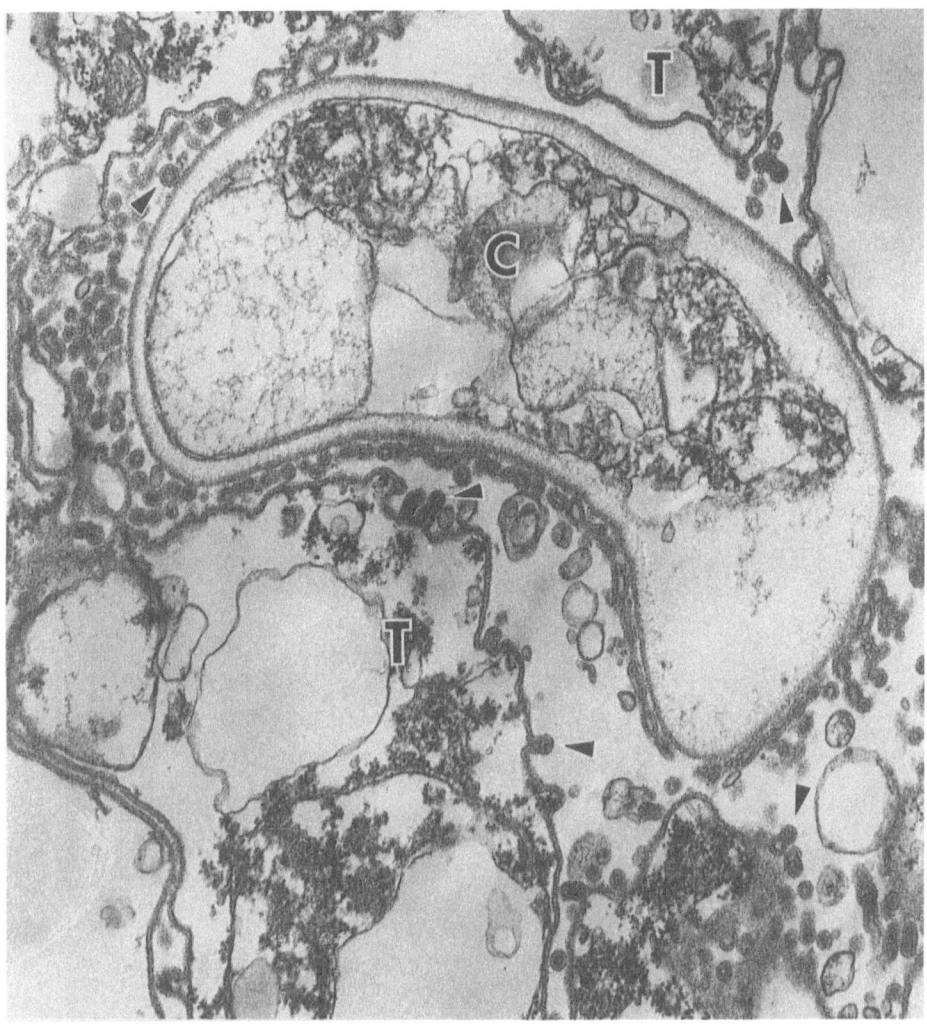

Fig. 4.32 Cysts (C) of *Pneumocystis carinii* with newly developing intracystic forms. The tubular expansions are well shown here (arrows) mostly associated with the walls of trophozoites (T). (Transmission electron micrograph: × 31 500.)

washings and the tissue itself should always be obtained, but we will be concerned here only with the microscopic detection. If pneumocystis is suspected, a rapid diagnosis is important and direct tissue imprints (air dried) and frozen sections of tissue are stained with one of the rapid stains

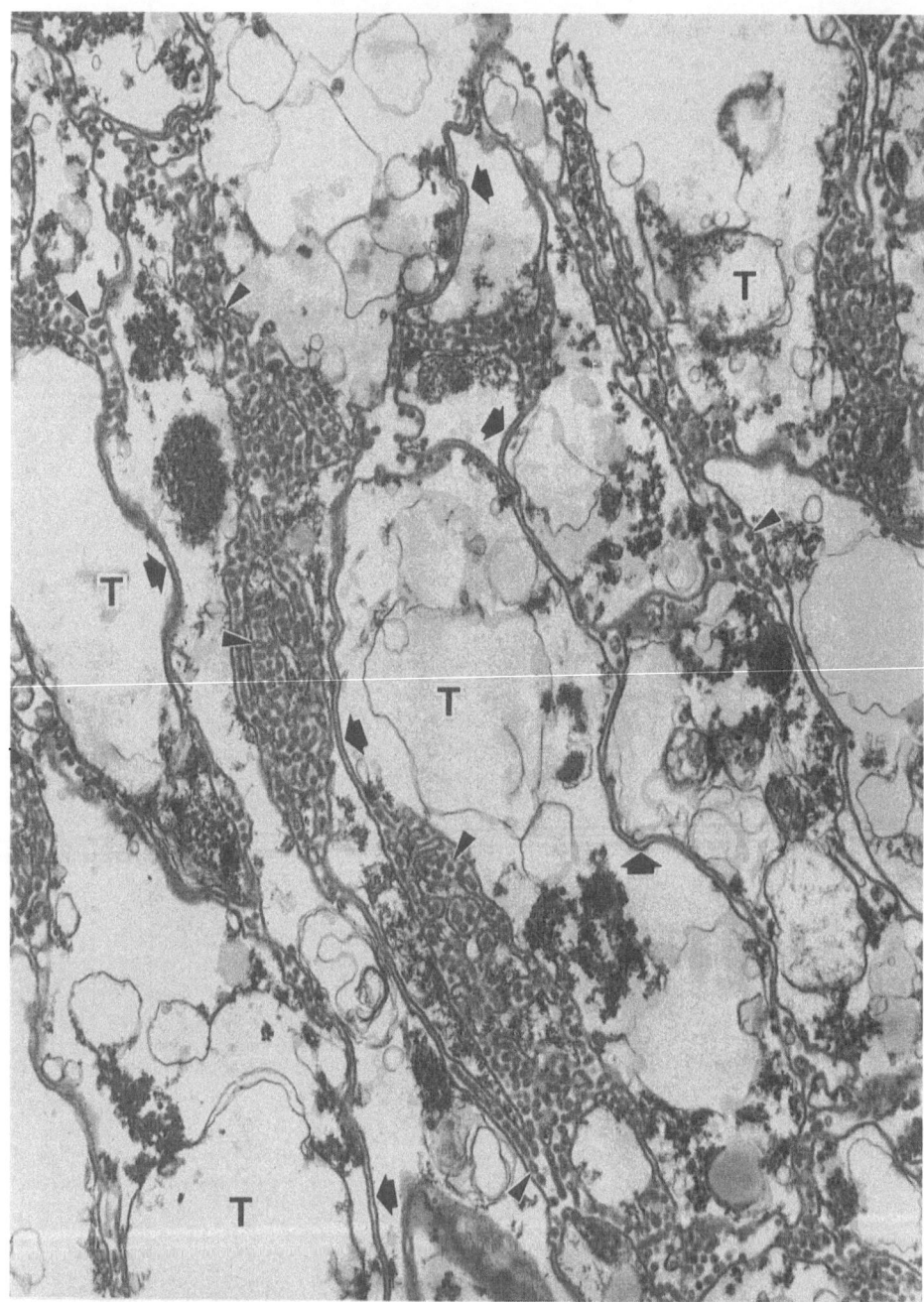

Fig. 4.33 Trophozoites (T) of *Pneumocystis carinii* with very irregular shapes outlined by their cell walls which have a double-layered appearance (broad arrows) and crowded together to form the intra-alveolar material seen in H&E sections. There are extensive profiles of the tubular extensions (thin arrowheads) which become compressed between adjacent organisms. (Transmission electron micrograph: × 16 300.)

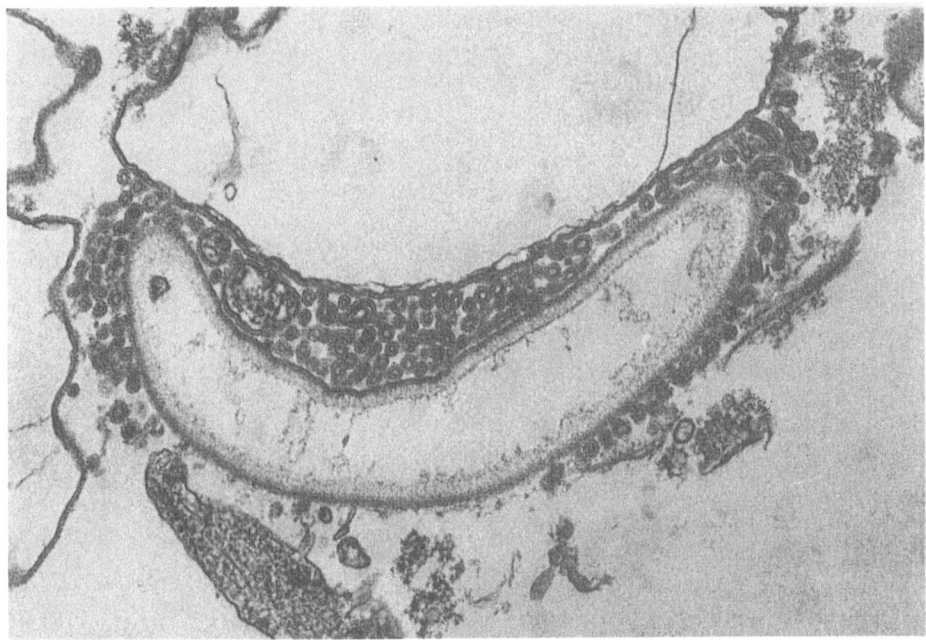

Fig. 4.34 Banana-shaped pneumocystis with thickened cell wall. The numerous tubular extensions, mostly cut in cross section here, are not arising from the cell wall of this organism but are from neighboring trophozoites. This form would stain with the silver stains (see Fig. 4.35). (Transmission electron micrograph: × 30 000.)

discussed in Section 4.5. For the other organisms the usual specimen turn around times are generally acceptable.

Routinely we recommend methenamine silver, Ziehl-Neelsen, Brown and Brenn and PAS stains on all tissue biopsies from these patients. Step sections through the small endobronchial and transbronchial biopsies, with intervening paraffin sections saved on slides for additional examinations if necessary, should be cut. If done at the time of original sectioning this can save much technician time, minimize delays in determining as accurate and specific a diagnosis as is possible from the specimen and increase the diagnostic yield. Cytology specimens can also be examined with special stains if necessary (see Section 2.4.3). If the specimen is inadequate (for transbronchial biopsies there must be tissue which includes alveoli) or if the findings are nonspecific, this information must be immediately communicated to the physician caring for the patient. If culture results are also noncontributory, additional specimens may be required.

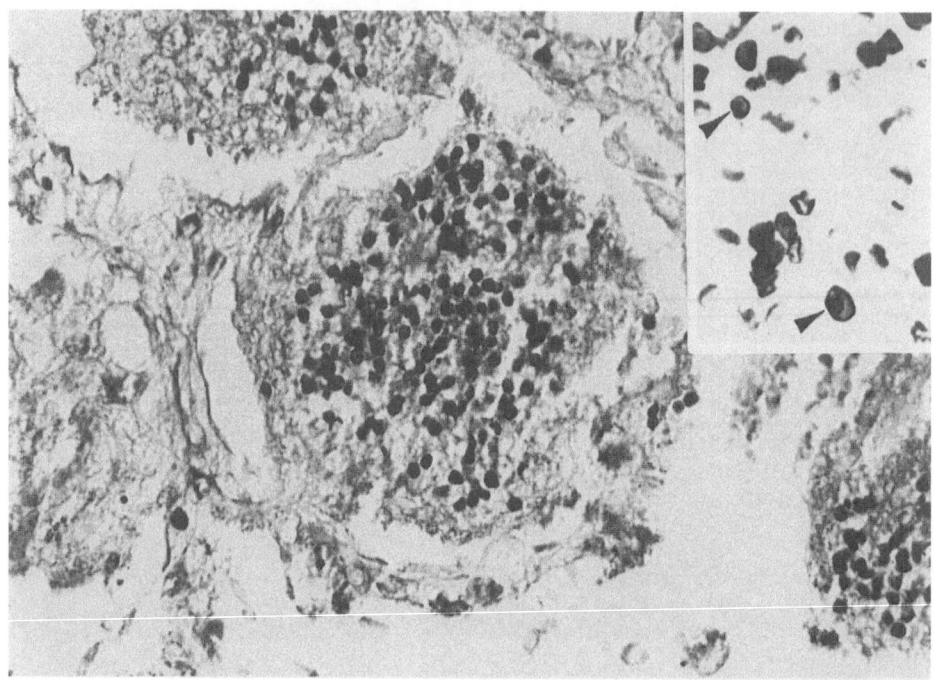

Fig. 4.35 Pneumocystis pneumonia with cystic forms well shown with silver staining. The remaining portions of the foam are trophozoites which are not stained by this technique. Biopsy of the lung. (× 200) *Inset*: Dark dot 'within' cyst which helps to differentiate pneumocystis from red blood cells; the latter are occasionally stained with the silver reactions but lack this feature. This dot is actually a thickened region of the cell wall of the cyst (see Fig. 4.36). (× 530) (Paraffin-embedded section stained with Gomori's methenamine silver.)

All of the organisms described in this chapter can be overlooked in specimens sent for examination but there is no reason, when one is alerted to the possibility of their presence, that they should be missed. Constant vigilance for even the smallest hint (a group of active histiocytes, a multinucleated giant cell, necrosis, hyperplastic epithelial cells in an inflammatory background or alveolar hyaline membranes) should lead to special stains and a diligent search for an identifiable etiologic agent. When dealing with these organisms, the old adage 'you won't find them if you don't look for them' is particularly pertinent. Nash (1982) has a very thorough review of diagnosis of infection in the immunocompromised host.

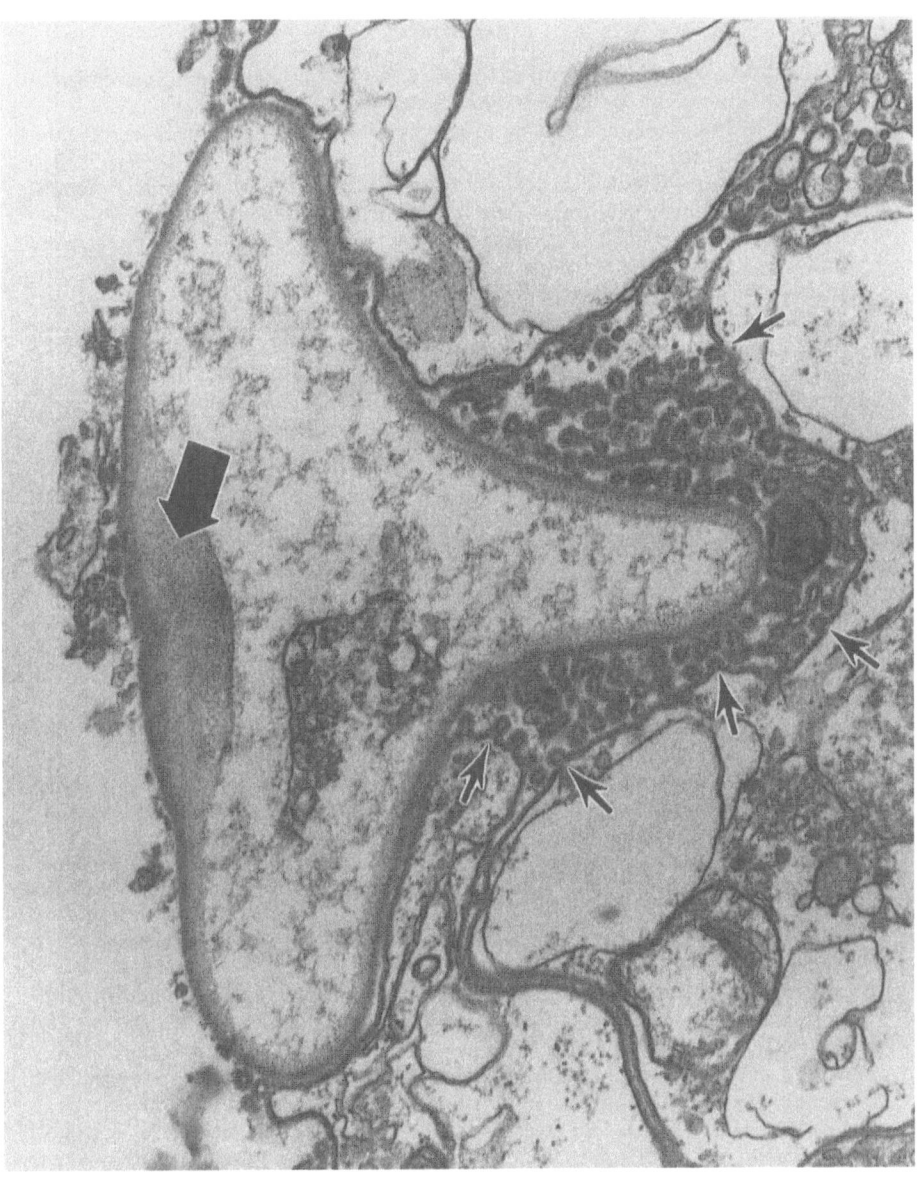

Fig. 4.36 Cystic form of *Pneumocystis carinii* which has been sectioned in a way which shows the characteristic thickened region (broad arrow) of its cell wall. Notice also the numerous tubular extensions, some of which can be seen arising from the thinner cell wall of a neighboring trophozoite (thinner arrows). (Transmission electron micrograph: × 34 000.)

References

Abdallah, P.S., Mark, J.B.D. and Merigan, T.C. (1976), Diagnosis of cytomegalovirus pneumonia in compromised hosts. *Am. J. Med.*, **61**, 326–32.

Agger, W.A. and Maki, D.G. (1978), Mucormycosis. A complication of critical care. *Arch. Intern. Med.*, **138**, 925–7.

Anthony, L.B. and Greco, F.A. (1981), *Pneumocystis carinii* pneumonia: a complication of Cushing's syndrome. *Ann. Intern. Med.*, **94**, 488–9.

Archibald, R.W.R., Weller, R.O. and Meadow, S.R. (1971), Measles pneumonia and the nature of the inclusion-bearing giant cells. A light- and electron-microscope study. *J. Pathol.*, **103**, 27–34.

Arth, C., von Schmidt, B., Grossman, M. and Schachter, J. (1978), Chlamydial pneumonitis. *J. Pediatr.*, **93**, 447–9.

Baker, R.D. (1956), Pulmonary mucormycosis. *Am. J. Pathol.*, **32**, 287–313.

Baker, R.D. (1976), The primary pulmonary lymph node complex of cryptococcosis. *Am. J. Clin. Pathol.*, **65**, 83–92.

Banner, A.S. (1979), Tuberculosis. Clinical aspects and diagnosis. *Arch. Inter. Med.*, **139**, 1387–90.

Becroft, D.M.O. and Osborne, D.R.S. (1980), The lungs in fatal measles infection in childhood: pathological, radiological and immunological correlations. *Histopathol.*, **4**, 401–12.

Behrens, H.W. and Quick, C.A. (1974), Bronchoscopic diagnosis of cytomegalovirus infection. *J. Infect. Dis.*, **130**, 174–6.

Bishop, R.F., Davidson, G.P., Holmes, I.H. and Ruck, B.J. (1974), Detection of a new virus by electron microscopy of fecal extracts from children with acute gastroenteritis. *Lancet*, **i**, 149–51.

Bowling, M.C., Smith, I.M. and Wescott, S.L. (1973), A rapid staining procedure for *Pneumocystis carinii*. *Am. J. Med. Tech.*, **39**, 267–8.

Broome, C.V., Cherry, W.B., Winn, W.C., Jr. and MacPherson, B.R. (1979), Rapid diagnosis of Legionnaires' disease by direct immunofluorescent staining. *Ann. Intern. Med.*, **90**, 1–4.

Brown, E., Freedman, S., Arbeit, R. and Come, S. (1980), Invasive pulmonary aspergillosis in an apparently nonimmunocompromised host. *Am. J. Med.*, **69**, 624–7.

Campbell, W.G., Jr. (1972), Ultrastructure of *Pneumocystis* in human lung. *Arch. Pathol.*, **93**, 312–24.

Chalvardjian, A.M. and Grawe, L.A. (1963), A new procedure for the identification of *Pneumocystis carinii* cysts in tissue sections and smears. *J. Clin. Pathol.*, **16**, 383–4.

Chandler, F.W., Hicklin, M.D. and Blackmon, J.A. (1977), Demonstration of the agent of Legionnaires' disease in tissue. *New Engl. J. Med.*, **297**, 1218–20.

Chernesky, M.A. (1979), The role of electron microscopy in diagnostic virology. In *Diagnosis of Viral Infections. The Role of the Clinical Laboratory* (eds D.A. Lennette, S. Specter and K.D. Thompson), University Park Press, Baltimore, pp. 125–42.

Cherry, J.D. and Welliver, R.C. (1976), Mycoplasma pneumoniae infections of adults and children. *West. J. Med.*, **125**, 47–55.

Churukian, C.J. (1977), Rapid Grocott's methenamine-silver nitrate method for fungi and *Pneumocystis carinii*. *Am. J. Clin. Pathol.*, **68**, 427–8.

Conte, B.A. and Laforet, E.G. (1962), The role of the topical anesthetic agent in modifying bacteriologic data obtained by bronchoscopy. *New Engl. J. Med.*, **267**, 957–60.

Craighead, J.E. (1970), Cytopathology of adenoviruses type 7 and 12 in human respiratory epithelium. *Lab. Invest.*, **22**, 553–7.

Craighead, J.E. (1971), Pulmonary cytomegalovirus infection in the adult. *Am. J. Pathol.*, **63**, 487–504.

Curran, J.W. (1982), Epidemiologic aspects of the current outbreak of Kaposi's sarcoma and opportunistic infections. *New Engl. J. Med.*, **306**, 248–52.

Danek, S.J. and Bower, J.S. (1979), Diagnosis of pulmonary tuberculosis by flexible fiberoptic bronchoscopy. *Am. Rev. Resp. Dis.*, **119**, 677–9.

Demicco, W.A., Stein, A., Urbanetti, J.S. and Fanbury, B.L. (1979), False negative biopsy in *Pneumocystis carinii* pneumonia. *Chest*, **75**, 389–90.

Deppisch, L.M. and Donowho, E.M. (1972), Pulmonary coccidioidomycosis. *Am. J. Clin. Pathol.*, **58**, 489–500.

Dieterle, R.R. (1927), Method for demonstration of *Spirochaeta pallida* in single microscopic sections. *Arch. Neurol. Psychiatry*, **18**, 73–80.

Doane, F.W., Anderson, N., Chatiyanonda, K., Bannatyne, R.M., McLean, D.M. and Rhodes, A.J. (1967), Rapid laboratory diagnosis of paramyxovirus infection by electron microscopy. *Lancet*, **ii**, 751–3.

Douglas, R.G. (1979), Viral respiratory illness: the role of diagnostic virology. In *Diagnosis of Viral Infections. The Role of the Clinical Laboratory* (eds D.A. Lennette, S. Specter and K.D. Thompson), University Park Press, Baltimore, pp. 215–27.

Drutz, D.J. and Catanzaro, A. (1978), Coccidioidomycosis. Part I. *Am. Rev. Resp. Dis.*, **117**, 559–85.

Enders, J.F., McCarthy, K., Mitus, A. and Cheatam, W.J. (1959), Isolation of measles virus at autopsy in cases of giant-cell pneumonia without rash. *New Engl. J. Med.*, **261**, 875–81.

Fiala, M., Payne, J.E., Berne, T.V., Moore, T.C., Henle, W., Montgomerie, J.Z., Chatterjee, S.N. and Guze, L.B. (1975), Epidemiology of cytomegalovirus infection after transplantation and immunosuppression. *J. Infect. Dis.*, **132**, 421–33.

Follansbee, S.E., Busch, D.F., Wofsay, C.B., Coleman, D.L., Bullet, J., Aurigemma, G.P., Ross, T., Hadley, W.K. and Drew, W.L. (1982), An outbreak of *Pneumocystis carinii* pneumonia in homosexual men. *Ann. Int. Med.*, **96**, 705–13.

Frable, W.J., Frable, M.A. and Seney, F.D., Jr. (1977), Virus infections of the respiratory tract. Cytopathologic and clinical analysis. *Acta Cytol.*, **21**, 32–6.

Frable, W.J. and Jay, S. (1977), Herpes virus infection of the respiratory tract. Electron-microscopic observation of the virus in cells obtained from a sputum cytology. *Acta Cytol.*, **21**, 391–3.

Frommell, G.T., Rothenberg, R., Wang, S., McIntosh, K., Wintersgill, C., Allaman, J. and Orr, I. (1979), Chlamydial infection of mothers and their infants. *J. Pediatr.*, **95**, 28–32.

Geppert, E.F. and Leff, A. (1979), The pathogenesis of pulmonary and miliary tuberculosis. *Arch. Intern. Med.*, **139**, 1381–3.

Gleason, T.H., Hammar, S.P., Barthas, M., Kasprisin, M. and Bockus, D. (1980), Cytological diagnosis of pulmonary cryptococcosis. *Arch. Pathol. Lab. Med.*, **104**, 384–7.

Goodwin, R.A., Jr. and Des Prez, R.M. (1978), Histoplasmosis. *Am. Rev. Resp. Dis.*, **117**, 929–56.

Goodwin, R.A., Loyd, J.E. and Des Prez, R.M. (1981), Histoplasmosis in normal hosts. *Medicine*, **60**, 231–66.

Goodwin, R.A., Jr., Shapiro, J.L., Thurman, G.H., Thurman, S.S. and Des Prez, R.M. (1980), Disseminated histoplasmosis: clinical and pathologic correlations. *Medicine*, **59**, 1–33.

Gottlieb, M.S., Schroff, R., Schanker, H.M., Weisman, J.D., Fann, P.P., Wolf, R.A. and Saxon, A. (1981), *Pneumocystis carinii* pneumonia and mucosal candidiasis in previously healthy homosexual men. Evidence of a new acquired cellular immunodeficiency. *New Engl. J. Med.*, **305**, 1425–31.

Guglietti, L.C. and Reingold, I.M. (1968), The detection of *Coccidioides immitis* in pulmonary cytology. *Acta Cytol.*, **12**, 332–4.

Gupta, P.K. (1982), Intrauterine contraceptive devices. Vaginal cytology, pathologic changes and clinical implications. *Acta Cytol.*, **26**, 571–613.

Guze, P.A., Bayer, A.S., Anthony, B.F., Tillman, D.B. and Bills, R. (1982), Spectrum of human chlamydial infections. *West. J. Med.*, **135**, 208–25.

Hageman, von P.K.H. (1938), Fluoreszenfarbung von tuberkelbakterien mit auramin. *München. Med. Wschr.*, **85**, 1066–8.

Hasleton, P.S., Curry, A. and Rankin, E.M. (1981), *Pneumocystis carinii* pneumonia: a light microscopical and ultrastructural study. *J. Clin. Pathol.*, **34**, 1138–46.

Hatcher, C.R., Jr., Sehdeva, J., Waters, W.C., III, Schulze, V., Logan, W.D., Jr., Symbas, P. and Abbott, O.A. (1971), Primary pulmonary cryptococcosis. *J. Thorac. Cardiovasc. Surg.*, **61**, 39–49.

Haverkos, H.W. and Curran, J.W. (1982), The current outbreak of Kaposi's sarcoma and opportunistic infections. *Cancer*, **32**, 330–9.

Hawkins, J.N. and Smith, J.G., Jr. (1982), Loss of immunocompetency in homosexuals: a new problem. *So. Med. J.*, **75**, 516–18.

Hers, J.F., Masurel, N. and Mulder, J. (1958), Bacteriology and histopathology of the respiratory tract and lungs in fatal Asian influenza. *Lancet*, **ii**, 1141–3.

Ito, J.I., Jr., Comess, K.A., Alexander, E.R., Harrison, H.R., Ray, C.G., Kiviat, J. and Sobonya, R.E. (1982), Pneumonia due to *Chlamydia trachomatis* in an immunocompromised adult. *New Engl. J. Med.*, **307**, 95–8.

Jain, U., Mani, K. and Frable, W.J. (1973), Cytomegalic inclusion disease: cytologic diagnosis from bronchial brushing material. *Acta Cytol.*, **17**, 467–8.

Jett, J.P., Cortese, D.A. and Dines, D.E. (1981), The value of bronchoscopy in the diagnosis of mycobacterial disease. A five year experience. *Chest*, **80**, 575–8.

Johnson, F.W.A. (1975), A comparison of staining techniques for demonstrating group A chlamydia in tissue culture. *Med. Lab. Technol.*, **32**, 233–8.

Johnston, W.W., Schlein, B. and Amatulli, J. (1969), Cytopathologic diagnosis of fungus infections. I. A method for the preparation of simulated cytopathologic material for the teaching of fungus morphology in cytology specimens. II. The presence of fungus in clinical material. *Acta Cytol.*, **13**, 488–95.

Jordan, S.W., McLaren, L.C. and Crosby, J.H. (1975), Herpetic tracheobronchitis. *Arch. Intern. Med.*, **135**, 784–8.

Joseph, S.W. and Houk, V.N. (1968), Evaluation and application of the fluorochrome stain for microscopic detection of Mycobacteria in clinical specimens. *Am. Rev. Resp. Dis.*, **98**, 1044–7.

Kerkering, T.M., Duma, R.J. and Shadomy, S. (1981), The evolution of pulmonary cryptococcosis. Clinical implications from a study of 41 patients with and without compromising host factors. *Ann. Intern. Med.*, **94**, 611–16.

Kim, C.J., Ko, I. and Bukantz, S.C. (1964), Ciliocytophthoria (CCP) in asthmatic children with references to viral respiratory infection and exacerbation of asthma. *J. Allergy*, **35**, 159–68.

Kirby, B.D., Snyder, K.M., Meyer, R.D. and Finegold, S.M. (1980), Legionnaires' disease: report of sixty-five nosocomially acquired cases and review of the literature. *Medicine*, **59**, 188–205.

Koss, L.G. (1979a), In *Diagnostic Cytology and Its Histopathologic Bases*, 3rd edn, J.B. Lippincott, Philadelphia, pp. 554–5.

Koss, L.G. (1979b), Histology and cytology of the normal respiratory tract. In *Diagnostic Cytology and Its Histopathologic Bases*, 3rd edn, J.B. Lippincott, Philadelphia, p. 547.

Kurrein, F., Green, G.H. and Rowles, S.L. (1975), Localized deposition of calcium oxalate around a pulmonary *Aspergillus niger* fungus ball. *Am. J. Clin. Pathol.*, **64**, 556–63.

Laurens, R.G., Jr., Pine, J.R. and Schwarzmann, S.W. (1982), *Pneumocystis carinii* pneumonia in a male homosexual. *So. Med. J.*, **75**, 638–9.

Lazzari, G., Vineis, C. and Cugini, A. (1981), Cytologic diagnosis of primary pulmonary actinomycosis. Report of two cases. *Acta Cytol.*, **25**, 299–301.

Lehrer, R.I., Howard, D.H., Sypherd, P.S., Edwards, J.E., Segal, G.P. and Winston, D.J. (1980), Mucormycosis. *Ann. Intern. Med.*, **93**, 93–108.

Little, B.W., Tihen, W.S., Dickerman, J.D. and Craighead, J.E. (1981), Giant cell pneumonia associated with parainfluenza virus type 3 infection. *Human Pathol.*, **12**, 478–81.

Liu, C. (1957), Studies on primary atypical pneumonia. *J. Exp. Med.*, **106**, 455–66.

Luna, L.G. (ed.) (1968), In *Manual of Histologic Staining Methods of the Armed Forces Institute of Pathology*, 3rd edn, McGraw-Hill, New York, pp. 222–5.

Macasaet, F.F., Holley, K.E., Smith, T.F. and Keys, T.F. (1975), Cytomegalovirus studies of autopsy tissue. II. Incidence of inclusion bodies and related pathologic data. *Am. J. Clin. Pathol.*, **63**, 859–65.

Masur, H., Rosen, P.P. and Armstrong, D. (1977), Pulmonary disease caused by Candida species. *Am. J. Med.*, **63**, 914–25.

Medoff, G. and Kobayashi, G.S. (1972), Pulmonary mucormycosis. *New Engl. J. Med.*, **286**, 86–7.

Mitus, A., Enders, J.F., Craig, J.M. and Holloway, A. (1959), Persistence of measles virus and depression of antibody formation in patients with giant-cell pneumonia after measles. *New Engl. J. Med.*, **261**, 882–9.

Müller, H.M. (1975), Oxalate accumulations from citrate by *Aspergillus niger*. I. Biosynthesis of oxalate from its ultimate precursor. *Archiv. Microbiol.*, **103**, 185–9.

Müller, H.M. and Frosch, F. (1975), Oxalate accumulation from citrate by *Aspergillus niger*. II. Involvement of tricarboxylic acid cycle. *Archiv. Microbiol.*, **104**, 159–62.

Musto, L., Flanigan, M. and Elbadawi, A. (1982), Ten-minute silver stain for *Pneumocystis carinii* and fungi in tissue sections. *Arch. Pathol. Lab. Med.*, **106**, 292–4.

Myerowitz, R.L., Stalder, H., Oxman, M.N., Levin, M.J., Moore, M., Leith, J.D., Gantz, N.M. and Pellegrini, J. (1975), Fatal disseminated adenovirus infection in a renal transplant recipient. *Am. J. Med.*, **59**, 591–8.

Nash, G. (1972), Necrotizing tracheobronchitis and bronchopneumonia consistent with herpetic infection. *Human Pathol.*, **3**, 283–91.

Nash, G. (1982), Pathologic features of the lung in the immunocompromised host. *Human Pathol.*, **13**, 841–58.

Nash, G. and Foley, F.D. (1970), Herpetic infection of the middle and lower respiratory tract. *Am. J. Clin. Pathol.*, **54**, 857–63.

Nasiell, M., Roger, V., Nasiell, K., Ernstad, I., Vogel, B. and Bisther, A. (1972), Cytologic findings indicating pulmonary tuberculosis. I. The diagnostic significance of epithelioid cells and Langhan's giant cells found in sputum or bronchial secretions. *Acta Cytol.*, **16**, 146–51.

Neiman, P.E., Reeves, W., Ray, G., Flournoy, N., Lerner, K.G., Sale, G.E. and Thomas, E.D. (1977), A prospective analysis of interstitial pneumonia and opportunistic viral infection among recipients of allogeneic bone marrow grafts. *J. Infect. Dis.*, **136**, 754–67.

Nime, F. and Hutchins, G. (1973), Oxalosis caused by *Aspergillus* infection. *Johns Hopkins Med. J.*, **133**, 183–94.

Palmer, D.L., Harvey, R.L. and Wheeler, J.K. (1974), Diagnostic and therapeutic considerations in *Nocardia asteroides* infection. *Medicine*, **53**, 391–401.

Pinkerton, H. and Carroll, S. (1971), Fatal adenovirus pneumonia in infants. Correlation of histologic and electron microscopic observations. *Am. J. Pathol.*, **65**, 543–8.

Pollock, P.G., Valicenti, J.F., Jr., Meyers, D.S., Frable, W.J. and Durham, J.B. (1978), The use of fluorescent and special staining techniques in the aspiration of nocardiosis and actinomycosis. *Acta Cytol.*, **22**, 575–9.

Pritchett, P.S., Murad, T.M. and Webster, M.J. (1977), Identification of *Pneumocystis carinii* infection in cytology specimens. *Acta Cytol.*, **21**, 784–5.

Prolla, J.C., Rosa, U.W. and Xavier, R.G. (1970), The detection of *Cryptococcus neoformans* in sputum cytology. Report of one case. *Acta Cytol.*, **14**, 87–91.

Raper, K.B. and Fennel, D.I. (1977), *The Genus Aspergillus*, R.E. Krieger, New York.

Reyes, C.V., Kathuria, S. and MacGlashan, A. (1979), Diagnostic value of calcium oxalate crystals in respiratory and pleural fluid cytology. A case report. *Acta Cytol.*, **23**, 65–8.

Robboy, S.J. and Vickery, A.L., Jr. (1970), Tinctorial and morphologic properties distinguishing actinomycosis and nocardiosis. *New Engl. J. Med.*, **282**, 593–6.

Roger, V., Nasiell, M., Nasiell, K., Hjerge, A., Enstad, I. and Bisther, A. (1972), Cytologic findings indicating pulmonary tuberculosis. II. The occurrence in sputum of epithelioid cells and multinucleated giant cells in pulmonary tuberculosis, chronic non-tuberculosis inflammatory lung disease and bronchogenic carcinoma. *Acta Cytol.*, **16**, 538–42.

Rose, H.D. and Sheth, N.K. (1978), Pulmonary candidiasis. A clinical and pathological correlation. *Arch. Intern. Med.*, **138**, 964–5.

Rosen, S.E. and Koprowska, I. (1982), Cytologic diagnosis of a case of pulmonary cryptococcosis. *Acta Ctyol.*, **26**, 499–502.

Sahn, S.A. and Levin, D.C. (1975), Diagnosis of miliary tuberculosis by transbronchial lung biopsy. *Brit. Med. J.*, **ii**, 667–8.

Sanders, J.S., Sarosi, G.A., Nollet, D.J. and Thompson, J.I. (1977), Exfoliative cytology in the rapid diagnosis of pulmonary blastomycosis. *Chest*, **72**, 193–6.

Saputo, V., Zocchi, M., Mancosu, M., Bonaldi, U. and Croce, P. (1979), Pulmonary alveolar microlithiasis. A case report with a discussion of differential diagnosis. *Helv. Paediat. Acta*, **34**, 245–55.

Sarosi, G.A. and Davies, S.F. (1979), Blastomycosis. *Am. Rev. Resp. Dis.*, **120**, 911–38.

Schwarz, J. and Salfelder, K. (1977), Blastomycosis. A review of 152 cases. In *Current Topics in Pathology* (eds E. Grandman and W.H. Kristen), Springer-Verlag, Berlin, no. 65, pp. 165–200.

Severo, L.C., Londero, A.T., Geyer, G.R. and Picon, P.D. (1981), Oxalosis associated with an *Aspergillus niger* fungus ball. Report of a case. *Mycopathol.*, **73**, 29–31.

Sherman, F.E. and Ruckle, G. (1958), *In vivo* and *in vitro* cellular changes specific for measles. *Arch. Pathol.*, **65**, 587–99.

Smith, T.F., Holley, K.E., Keys, T.F. and Macasaet, F.F. (1975), Cytomegalovirus studies of autopsy tissue. I. Virus isolation. *Am. J. Clin. Pathol.*, **63**, 854–8.

Stagno, S., Brasfield, D.M., Brown, M.B., Cassell, G.H., Pifer, L.L., Whitley, R.J. and Tiller, R.E. (1981), Infant pneumonitis associated with cytomegalovirus,

Chlamydia, Pneumocystis and *Ureaplasma*: a prospective study. *Pediatr.*, **68**, 322–9.

Stagno, S., Pifer, L.L., Hughes, W.T., Brasfield, D.M. and Tiller, R.E. (1980), *Pneumocystis carinii* pneumonitis in young immunocompetent infants. *Pediatr.*, **66**, 56–62.

Straatsma, B.R., Zimmerman, L.E. and Gass, J.D.M. (1962), Phycomycosis: a clinicopathologic study of fifty-one cases. *Lab. Invest.*, **11**, 963–85.

Straub, M. and Schwarz, J. (1962), Histoplasmosis, coccidioidomycosis and tuberculosis: a comparative pathological study. *Pathol. Microbiol.*, **25**, 421–77.

Taylor, E.R. (1970), Pulmonary cryptococcosis. Analysis of 15 cases from the Columbian area. *Ann. Thorac. Surg.*, **10**, 309–16.

Truant, J.P., Brett, W.A. and Thomas, W., Jr. (1962), Fluorescence microscopy of tubercle bacilli stained with auramine and rhodamine. *Henry Ford Hosp. Med. Bull.*, **10**, 287–96.

Urmacher, C., Myskowski, P., Ochoa, M., Jr., Kris, M. and Safai, B. (1982), Outbreak of Kaposi's sarcoma with cytomegalovirus infection in young homosexual men. *Am. J. Med.*, **72**, 569–75.

Van Orden, A. and Greer, P. (1977), Modification of the Dieterle spirochete stain. *J. Histotechnol.*, **1**, 51.

Vavra, J. and Kücera, K. (1970), *Pneumocystis carinii* Delanoë: its ultrastructure and ultrastructural affinities. *J. Protozool.*, **17**, 463–83.

Vernon, S.E. (1982), Cytologic features of nonfatal herpes virus tracheobronchitis. *Acta Cytol.*, **26**, 237–42.

Wallace, J.M., Deutsch, A.L., Harrell, J.H. and Moser, K.M. (1981), Bronchoscopy and transbronchial biopsy in evaluation of patients with suspected active tuberculosis. *Am. J. Med.*, **70**, 1189–94.

Walzer, P.D., Perl, D.P., Krogstad, D.J., Rawson, P.G. and Schultz, M.G. (1974), *Pneumocystis carinii* pneumonia in the United States. Epidemiologic, diagnostic, and clinical features. *Ann. Intern. Med.*, **80**, 83–93.

Weber, W.R., Askin, F.B. and Dehner, L.P. (1977), Lung biopsy in *Pneumocystis carinii* pneumonia. A histopathologic study of typical and atypical features. *Am. J. Clin. Pathol.*, **67**, 11–19.

Weller, R.W. (1952), Giant cell pneumonia with inclusions. *Pediatr.*, **10**, 681–6.

Wimberley, N., Faling, L.J. and Bartlett, J.G. (1979), A fiberoptic bronchoscopy technique to obtain uncontaminated lower airway secretions for bacterial culture. *Am. Rev. Resp. Dis.*, **119**, 337–43.

Winberg, C.D., Rose, M.E. and Rappaport, H. (1978), Whipple's disease of the lung. *Am. J. Med.*, **65**, 873–80.

Winn, W.C., Jr. and Myerowitz, R.L. (1981), The pathology of the Legionella pneumonias. A review of 74 cases and the literature. *Human Pathol.*, **12**, 401–22.

Woodland, R.M., Malam, J. and Darougar, S. (1982), A rapid method for staining inclusions of *Chlamydia psittaci* and *Chlamydia trachomatis*. *J. Clin. Pathol.*, **35**, 642–4.

Yoneda, K., Walzer, P.D., Richey, C.S. and Birk, M.G. (1982), *Pneumocystis carinii*: freeze-fracture study of stages of the organism. *Exp. Parasitol.*, **53**, 68–76.

Zahradnik, J.M., Spencer, M.J. and Porter, D.D. (1980), Adenovirus infection in the immunocompromised patient. *Am. J. Med.*, **68**, 725–32.

5 Bronchial inflammatory reactions

5.1 Acute bronchitis

Acute bronchitis, characterized by leucocytes (predominantly neutrophils) over the surface of the mucosa and in the adjacent lamina propria, capillaries made conspicuous by swelling with increased numbers of erythrocytes, and interstitial edema, is undoubtedly the most frequent lesion of the bronchial tree. Infectious acute bronchitis is caused by either bacteria, the pleuropneumonia-like organisms (PPLO), or virus and is usually treated empirically with antibiotics. Microbiological cultures are rarely obtained in general medical practice. When cultures are requested it is with the intention of altering the therapy should an unexpected agent be discovered. Nearly all cases are treated without hospitalization and the surgical pathologist has little involvement.

Acute inflammation of the bronchial mucosa is a frequent ancillary finding in endobronchial biopsies taken for other purposes, such as for identifying a tumor. Occasionally, specific micro-organisms can be seen in biopsies taken to diagnose neoplasia, e.g. *Candida sp.*, bacteria, herpes virus and *Aspergillus* (Chapter 4). The relevance of the presence of such organisms when accompanying malignant bronchial tumors is not known since most are capable of colonizing the bronchi under conditions which alter the normal bronchial clearance mechanism. They should not be considered pathogens in the absence of clinical evidence of infection. Even the bronchoscopy itself with local physical trauma from the tip, suctioning and introduction of forceps and/or brushes will elicit an acute inflammatory reaction within minutes (Fig. 5.1).

Hospitalized patients who develop bronchitis should be more vigorously examined to identify specific etiologic agents. This is particularly true if the patient is immunocompromised, either from the patient's primary disease (leukemia, lymphoma, lupus erythematosis, or carcinomatosis) or from therapeutic procedures, particularly cytotoxic drugs. In this setting it is essential, and frequently life saving, to determine if the pulmonary condition is a result of direct involvement by the primary disease process, a reaction to therapy (Sections 5.9, 5.10) or due to an infectious agent. Bronchoscopic biopsy, particularly transbronchial biopsy, may be a rapid, minimally invasive, initial approach to the clarification of this differential

140

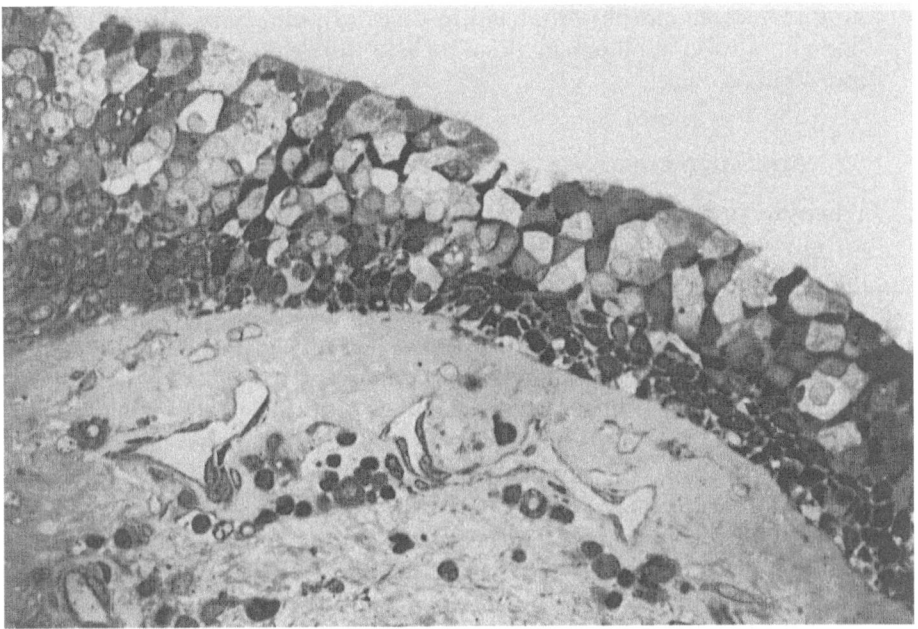

Fig. 5.1 Biopsy of normal bronchial mucosa. There are a few neutrophils in the superficial lamina propria elicited by the 'trauma' of the bronchoscope during examination prior to the biopsy. (Plastic specimen, stained with toluidine blue: × 470.)

diagnosis (Lauver *et al.*, 1979; Katzenstein and Askin, 1980; Hedemark *et al.*, 1982). To maximize the specimen yield, special stains and a diligent search for the etiologic agent(s) are required and it is suggested that a protocol for handling these specimens be prepared, such as that suggested in Section 4.6. Specific infectious agents are discussed in detail in Chapter 4. Nash (1982) has an excellent recent review of the differential diagnosis in these cases.

Acquired immune deficiency syndrome (AIDS) is a special case of host compromise because the patient may not be considered to be immunocompromised until after the diagnosis of acute infection. The extensive coverage of this syndrome in the lay and medical press has caused a heightened sensitivity and most specimens are sent with the comment of clinical suspicion for AIDS. As more patients are evaluated, additional infectious agents are being found, including some heretofore not generally considered to be opportunistic (Cohen *et al.*, 1983; Croxson *et al.*, 1983) (Section 4.5).

If bronchoscopically obtained material is inadequate for a specific diagnosis or if the findings are inconsistent with the clinical setting, open lung biopsy should be considered in cases of pulmonary disease in the immunocompromised patient (Rossiter *et al.*, 1979; Gaensler and Carrington, 1980).

5.2   Aspiration bronchitis

When the bronchi are contaminated with foreign liquids or when solids are introduced from the oropharynx, the process is referred to as aspiration. The severity and nature of the tissue reaction is variable depending on the offending material. Solid objects such as safety pins, gold crowns from teeth, coins, etc. are usually simply a problem of retrieval. Other materials such as gastric contents may contain infectious agents, chemical irritants and foreign organic material and often cause a necrotizing bronchitis. A necrotizing bronchitis occurs in alcoholics who, in their impaired state, may aspirate the vomitus which they inadequately clear from their mouths. The same may also occur in patients with inadequate control of the clearing mechanisms of the oropharynx and airways, or epiglottic closure, in patients with esophageal obstruction and in patients with gastric feeding tubes. In newborns, tracheoesophageal fistula is a rare cause of aspiration bronchitis.

The bronchitis and pneumonia which often follow aspiration tend to be necrotizing (Fig. 5.2) and abscess development is a common complication. Infections are usually due to anaerobic bacteria. The bronchi of these patients are rarely biopsied for diagnostic purposes, unless the pattern of infection is patchy and mistaken for neoplasm.

5.3   'Chronic bronchitis' and chronic obstructive lung disease

Chronic bronchitis as used in the general medical literature is a clinical entity and not a morphological description of chronic inflammatory infiltrates within the bronchial mucosa. The clinical disorder is defined by excessive mucus secretion in the bronchial tree. This is manifested by chronic or recurrent productive cough. Arbitrarily the symptoms should be present on most days for a minimum of 3 months in the year and for not less than 2 successive years. Other specific diseases which may have these symptoms are excluded to make the entity more clinically meaningful (Harris *et al.*, 1962). This is not only a clinical definition but is exclusionary as well. Chronic obstructive pulmonary disease (COPD) is likewise a clinically defined entity, the abnormality being functional: a decrease in the forced expiratory volume and flow. The principal symptom is dyspnea. Emphysema is defined anatomically as permanent enlargement of distal air spaces accompanied by destruction of alveolar septal tissue. Although chronic bronchitis, COPD and emphysema are often clinically associated,

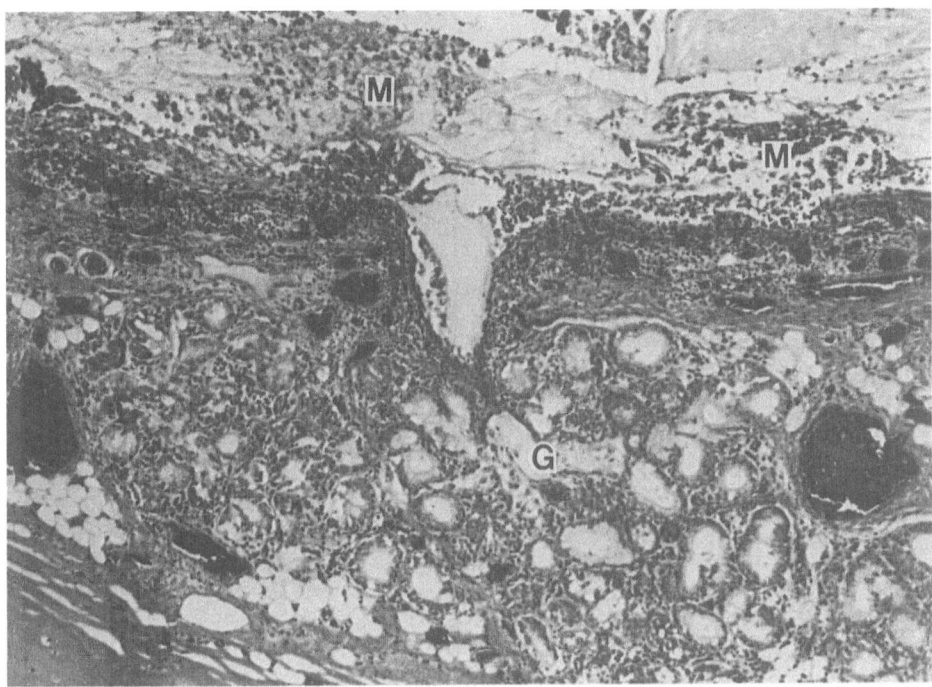

Fig. 5.2 Necrotizing bronchitis resulting from aspiration of gastric material. The epithelium is replaced with layers of mucus, containing numerous neutrophils (M). Beneath this, lymphocytes surround congested vessels and the adjacent bronchial glands (G). (Paraffin section, H&E stain: × 108.)

considerable confusion has resulted from the indiscriminate usage of these terms. Cigarette smoking is the single most significant cause of COPD (Thurlbeck *et al.*, 1970; Surgeon General of The United States, 1982).

Since Reid (1954) demonstrated quantitative changes in the volume of mucous cells in the bronchial mucosa, there have been many attempts to clarify the relationship between chronic bronchitis and histopathological changes in the airways (Reid, 1960; Glynn and Michaels, 1960; Thurlbeck *et al.*, 1970; Takizawa and Thurlbeck, 1971; Heard *et al.*, 1979; Douglas, 1980; Snider, 1981). Increased numbers of mucous 'goblet' cells in the surface epithelium and in the submucosal glands can be seen (Fig. 5.3). There may also be chronic inflammatory cell infiltrates and focal epidermoid (squamous) metaplasia, although this is not consistent. There is an increase in the bronchial glandular volume in cigarette smokers (Douglas *et al.*, 1982). Much of the apparent inconsistencies and even arguments between investigators can be explained by returning to the definition which is clinical and not histopathological. More recently there has been

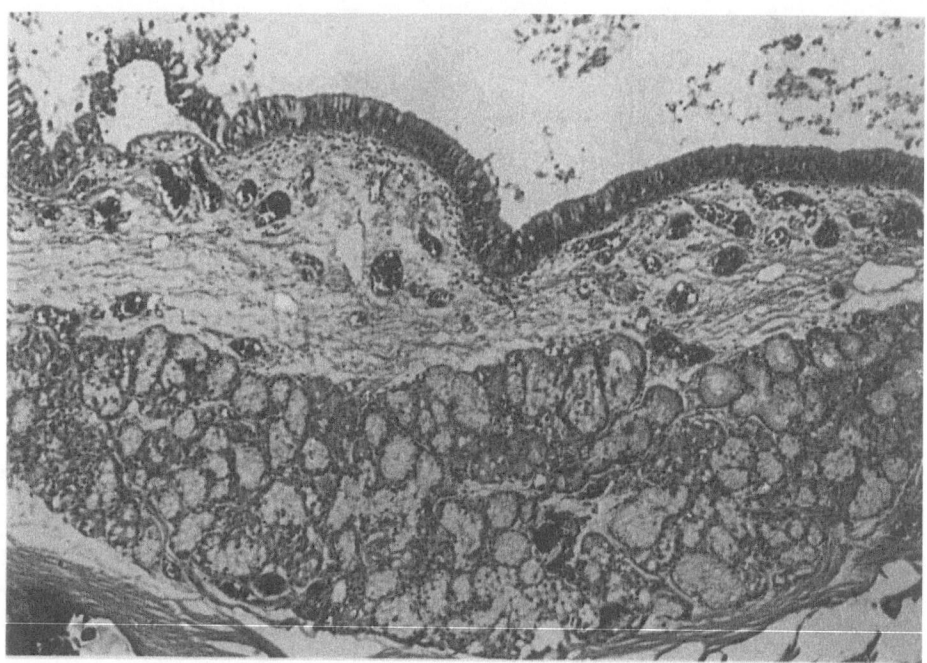

Fig. 5.3 Bronchial wall of a male smoker with chronic bronchitis. There is some increase in the number of mucous cells in the surface epithelium and an increase in the number of bronchial mucous glands. Lymphocytes are scattered in the upper lamina propria. (Paraffin section, H&E stain: × 108.)

a general acceptance of this definitional problem and there have been fewer attempts to establish quantitative changes seen in biopsy specimens with severity of chronic bronchitis. In any event bronchial biopsy is not currently used to diagnose, grade or follow chronic bronchitis clinically.

The abundant sputum produced by patients with chronic bronchitis contains mixed inflammatory cells and may contain Curschmann's spirals. These spirals, first reported by Curschmann (1885), are best appreciated in whole mount preparations of sputa (Fig. 5.4). They are inspissated mucus formed into coiled strands of variable size, from 20 μm long to some which are visible with the unaided eye. They are generally reported

Fig. 5.4 Curschmann's spirals. (a) The irregular loose coiling is visible in this spiral contained in the sputum of a patient with chronic bronchitis. (Papanicolaou stained smear: × 100.) (b) At higher magnification of two other spirals the structure can be seen to consist of a central core of dense mucus, formed into an irregular coil. (Papanicolaou stained smear: × 710.) (c) The fuzzy appearance, likened to a pipe-cleaner, is due to loosened filamentous mucus spreading away from the central core. (Papanicolaou stained smear: × 800.)

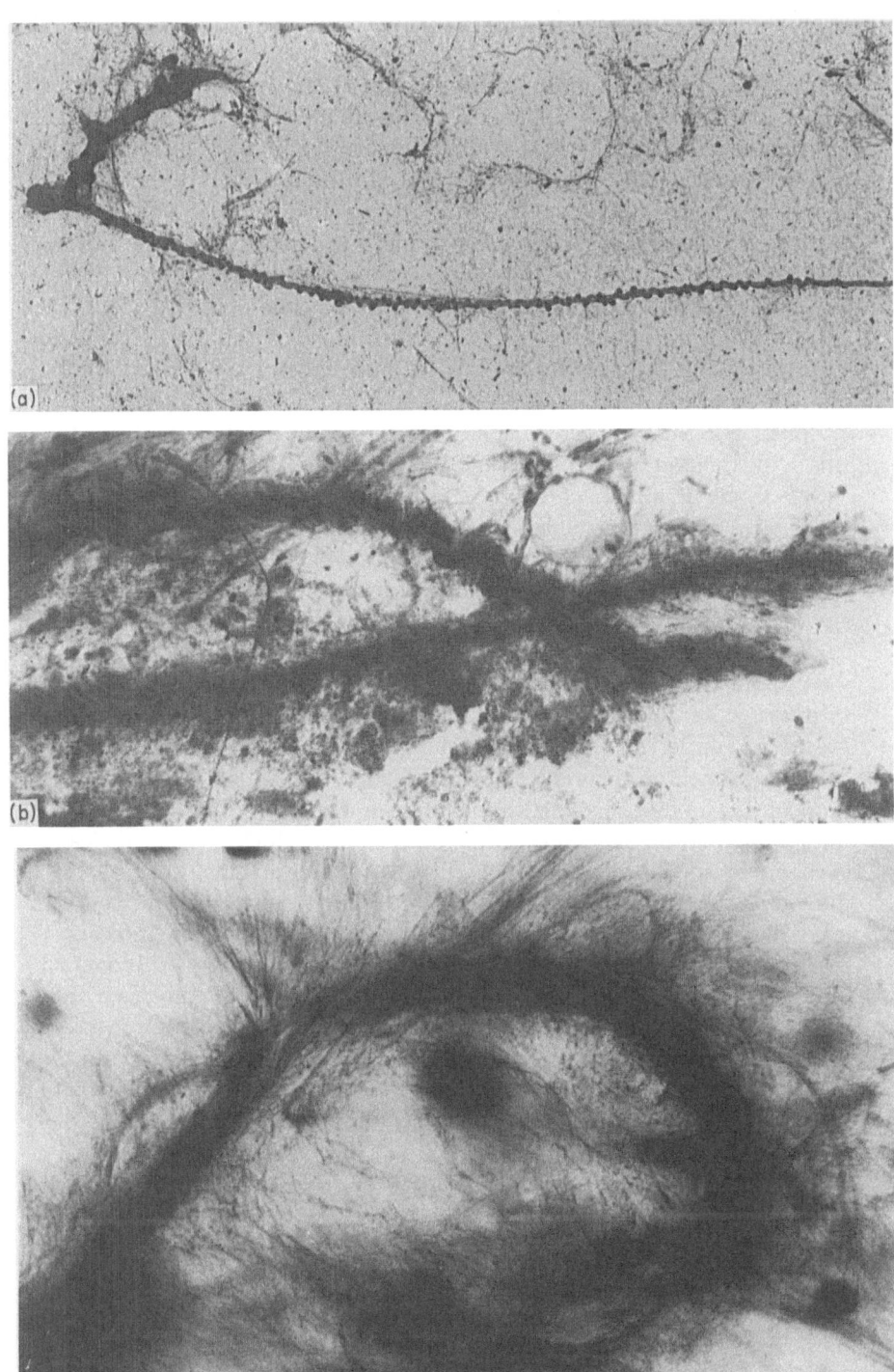

as being 'casts' of small bronchi. The smaller spirals, however, are considerably smaller than any of the bronchi which contain mucous cells. Alternatively they may be the extruded mucus from hyperactive bronchial glands, twisting slightly as they emerge into the bronchial lumen. Their appearance has been likened to that of a pipe-cleaner because the central portion of the spiral is more compact, and radiating filamentous mucus extends outward giving it a fuzzy appearance. In the Papanicolaou stain, the spirals stain variably bluish, purple or orange. Although characteristically seen in the sputum of chronic bronchitics and asthmatics (Section 5.8), they have been found by Walker and Fullmer (1970) in 94% of cigarette smokers. They found from 1 to 916 spirals in individual aliquots of sputa, but the number of spirals could not be related to either the length of smoking or the amount of cigarettes smoked daily.

Deficiency of alpha$_1$-antitrypsin is a specific genetic defect causing progressive airway obstruction in a small number of cases (Cutz and Cox, 1979; Snider, 1981). The histopathological changes are seen in the distal air spaces and there are no diagnostic features observed in bronchial specimens from these individuals which would distinguish them from the variety of other causes of COPD.

Accumulations of chronic inflammatory cells in the bronchial wall with mixtures of lymphocytes, plasma cells and in some cases eosinophils are present in a variety of bronchial infections (Fig. 5.5). This histopathological 'chronic bronchitis' may be superimposed on existing clinical chronic bronchitis. The mycobacterial infections are discussed in Chapter 6 with the granulomatous reactions. Fungal infections, which characteristically elicit a chronic inflammatory response in the bronchial mucosa, are individually discussed in Section 4.4. Although culture of the specific agent remains the most widely used method of diagnosing these infections, the finding of appreciable chronic inflammatory reaction in a bronchial biopsy specimen should cause a diligent search for micro-organisms within the tissue using special stains (Sections 2.3.3 and 4.6). Radiation (Section 5.10) and reactions to drugs (Section 5.9) may also evoke a chronic inflammatory reaction. Although the usual hallmark of viral infection is lymphocytic infiltrates, specific viral infections with adenovirus and herpes are recognized in the bronchus because of intranuclear inclusion bodies (Section 4.1). Herpetic bronchitis is usually ulcerative with surrounding acute inflammation (Nash, 1972).

5.4 Bronchiectasis

Bronchiectasis is the permanent, abnormal dilation of bronchi, often associated with infections (Thurlbeck *et al.*, 1970; Heard *et al.*, 1979). A careful study of surgical specimens by Whitwell (1952) did much to elucidate the spectrum of morphological types and their pathogenesis. The

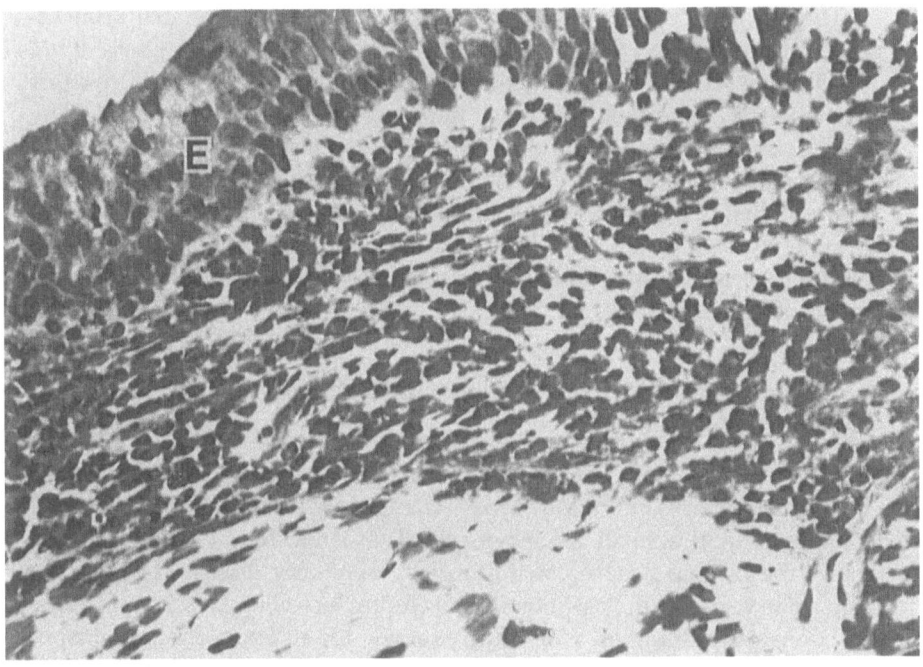

Fig. 5.5 Bronchial mucosa with accumulations of chronic inflammatory cells (predominantly lymphocytes) in the lamina propria. The overlying epithelium (E) is intact. This reaction was present in a biopsy immediately adjacent to an infiltrative bronchial carcinoma. (Paraffin section, H&E stain: × 470.)

incidence of bronchiectasis has decreased with the general use of antibiotics for the treatment of pulmonary infections (Ellis *et al.*, 1981; Davis *et al.*, 1983). The diagnosis is suspected clinically by the intermittent production of copious amounts of putrid smelling sputum, which may result from changes in position of the patient. It is confirmed by radiological examination and bronchoscopic visualization of the abnormal bronchi. There are no specific findings, or any differences in the various types of bronchiectasis, in biopsy specimens.

Bronchiectasis has an increased association with situs inversus, first reported by Kartagener (1933) and subsequently by others (Olsen, 1942; Torgersen, 1949). This is attributed to a genetic abnormality of the axoneme of cilia (Afzelius, 1976). The bronchiectasis is undoubtedly an acquired abnormality in these syndromes, secondary to the inadequate mucociliary clearance and consequent recurring infections (Section 7.3).

Bronchiectasis may be seen as a complication of alpha$_1$-antitrypsin deficiency (Cutz and Cox, 1979). About one half of the patients with cystic fibrosis (Section 8.2) develop bronchiectasis (Davis *et al.*, 1983).

There is a very rare form of congenital and perhaps familial bronchiectasis (Mitchell and Bury, 1975; Wayne and Taussig, 1976; Davis *et al.*, 1983). This bronchiectasis is generalized throughout the lungs in contrast to the focal nature of the much more common acquired forms. The underlying abnormality is a deficiency of bronchial cartilage, particularly in the more distal airways (Williams and Campbell, 1960). The cartilage in the Williams-Campbell syndrome is histologically normal but is diminished in amount and occurs as thin plates (Mitchell and Bury, 1975). The review by Davis *et al.* (1983) gives a very good discussion of the familial forms of bronchiectasis.

5.5 Pulmonary fibrosis and chronic inflammatory infiltrates

There are a large number of histopathological reactions in the lung which are characterized by fibrosis, generalized or specific accumulations of inflammatory cells of various types, changes in alveolar lining cells and alterations in the small blood vessels. These reactions can be grouped under the general heading of infiltrative pulmonary disease. They represent some very specific pathobiological entities as well as loosely associated reactions still waiting for a unifying etiology. Many represent the nonspecific end stages of a variety of inflammatory diseases. Crystal *et al.* (1981) recently reviewed this subject. At least some of the specific forms are undoubtedly immunological diseases, and the more recent techniques of inflammatory cell identification, localization of immunological markers and cellular enzyme analysis may help to clarify the sometimes overwhelming differential diagnoses. As the use of bronchial lavage became more widespread, particularly in analyzing the diffuse diseases (Hunninghake *et al.*, 1979; Haslan *et al.*, 1980), it was hoped that this less invasive technique would be available to diagnose this group of reactions. However, at this time, the open lung biopsy remains the single most reliable specimen for accurate and meaningful analysis (Carrington and Gaensler, 1978; Rossiter *et al.*, 1979; Gaensler and Carrington, 1980; Wall *et al.*, 1981). Since these pulmonary lesions are best understood by open lung biopsy, their discussion will be found in another volume in this series (Hayes, 1986) which discusses pulmonary parenchymal pathology.

5.6 Asthma

The Committee on Diagnostic Standards for Nontuberculous Respiratory Disease defines asthma as 'disease characterized by increased responsiveness of the trachea and bronchi to various stimuli and manifested by a respiratory function. Respiratory dysfunction when present consists primarily of an increased resistance to airflow' (Harris *et al.*, 1962). Others stress the reversibility and episodic character of the airway obstruction (Karr, 1980; Middleton *et al.*, 1981; Mathews, 1982). Asthma afflicts as much as 5% of the world's population. About 3000 patients die from asthma each year in the United States and about 1500 in the United Kingdom (Middleton *et al.*, 1981; Stellman *et al.*, 1982). Asthma is a significant clinical syndrome and can be subclassified into two major pathophysiological groups: (1) those which are immunologic responses to antigenically active agents (IgE mediated) and (2) those without evidence of immune mechanism involvement (intrinsic) (Middleton *et al.*, 1981; Sly, 1982). Approximately half of the patients with asthma are in each group. The immunologic mechanisms in IgE-mediated asthma are becoming well documented. However, the pathophysiological mechanism(s) in the second group are, at the present state of knowledge, generally attributed to an increased sensitivity of the bronchi. In this group the eliciting factors include exercise, changes in air temperature and emotional stress as well as air pollutants. Occupational asthma is a socially and legally important subclassification which separates those incitors which are related to work environment (Dosman *et al.*, 1981; Patterson and Goldstein, 1982; Pepys, 1982; Fish, 1982). In his review, Taylor (1980) reports that more than 200 agents had been identified in this category. Belin (1980) has a good review with extensive references to the agents which are implicated. A detailed history from the patient is the key to diagnosis in these cases (Chan-Yeung, 1982).

As stated above, asthma is a clinical entity and like chronic bronchitis (Section 5.3) is difficult to characterize histologically. The key features are bronchospasm and changes in the character of mucus, resulting in mucous plugging. At least in the early stages, the bronchospasm is a function of smooth muscle tone and there may be no morphological changes. Mucous plugs are more frequently a finding at autopsy (Leff, 1982; Hogg, 1982). It is not surprising, therefore, that the histopathological characteristics of asthma are confusing, controversial and inconsistent. Classical dogma equates asthma with mucous plugs, bronchial smooth muscle hyperplasia, mucous gland hyperplasia and thickening of the epithelial basement membrane (Fig. 5.6). However, these characteristics are those seen at autopsy of chronic asthmatics who died in status asthmaticus and do not reflect the changes in early disease; nor can they be related to severity of the disease attacks (Dunnill *et al.*, 1969; Thurlbeck *et al.*, 1970). Cutz *et al.* (1978) studied open lung biopsies of asthmatic children at times between attacks, as well as autopsy specimens from children who died in status asthmaticus, and reported mucous (goblet) cell hyperplasia, peribronchial smooth muscle hypertrophy, an eosinophilic leukocytic infiltrate, basement membrane thickening and mucous plugs which contained exfoliated epithelial cells. They commented that the thickened basement

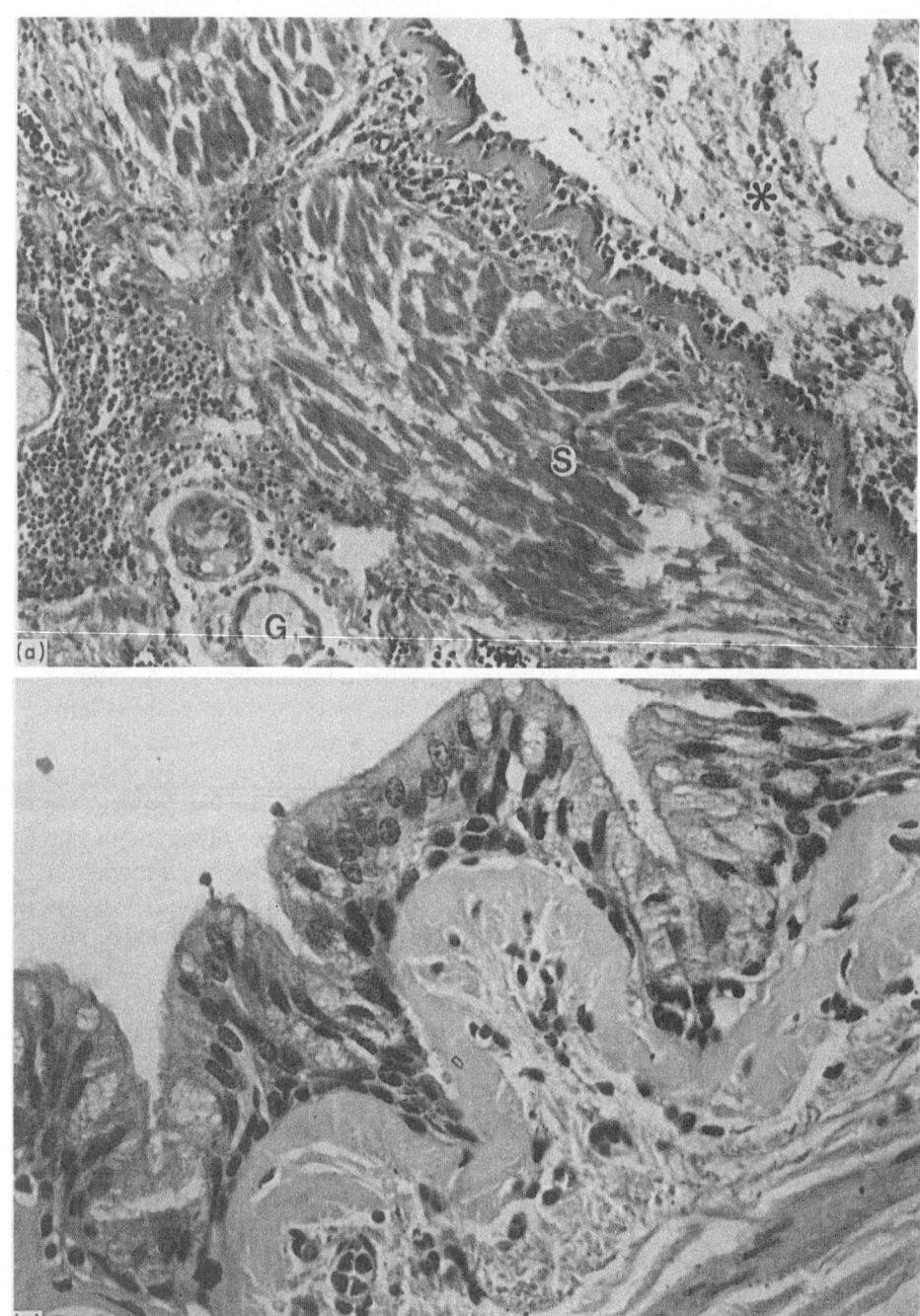

membrane seen by light microscopy was actually collagen adjacent to the basal lamina and not a true thickening of the basement membrane. They also reported numerous mast cells, some of which were intraepithelial.

Comparisons of bronchial changes in asthmatics and chronic bronchitics show some differences in basement membrane thickness (thicker in some asthmatics), variable changes in volume/number of mucous cells and smooth muscle and focal epidermoid 'squamous' metaplasia in both; because of overlap of these features and variability between patients, no clear histological characteristics can distinguish these two clinical entities (Glynn and Michaels, 1960; Thurlbeck *et al.*, 1970; Takizawa and Thurlbeck, 1971; Callerame *et al.*, 1971a, 1971b). Fortunately, surgical pathologists are rarely asked to diagnose either chronic bronchitis or acute asthma. In fact it is very uncommon to see biopsy material from asthmatics unless incidental to the diagnosis of bronchial masses.

Jelihovsky (1983) compared light microscopic sections of mucous plugs from asthmatics and patients with mucoid impaction (Section 5.7). Plugs from asthmatics were distinguished by the concentric layering and exfoliated sheets of bronchial epithelial cells.

Sputum from asthmatics frequently contains eosinophils and an occasional Charcot-Leyden crystal (Fig. 5.7); however, these may also be seen in allergic bronchopulmonary aspergillosis (Section 5.7), in chronic eosinophilic pneumonia, and in some drug reactions and parasitic infestations (Schatz *et al.*, 1981). Charcot-Leyden crystals were described by Charcot and Robin in 1853 in a patient with leukemia and by Leyden in 1872 in asthmatics. The crystals are seen in whole mounts as slender eosinophilic rods, tapered at each end (Fig. 5.7a, b), and are hexagonal in cross-section (Fig. 5.7c, d). They may be present whenever large numbers of eosinophils accumulate, particularly if degranulation is occurring. Interestingly, the protein which aggregates in orderly arrangements to form these crystals is not the same as the principal component of the eosinophilic granules called major basic protein (Gleich *et al.*, 1976).

Fig. 5.6 Asthma. Bronchi from patients with chronic asthma. (a) Mucus with a mixture of inflammatory cells and some exfoliated bronchial epithelium (*). Only the basal cells remain in the epithelium. The 'basement membrane' is very prominent. Conspicuous bundles of smooth muscle (S) are surrounded by chronic inflammatory cells including eosinophils. A few bronchial glands (G) are present in the section. (Paraffin section, H&E stain: × 108.) (b) Another specimen with intact mucosa. The dense hyaline layer (basement membrane) contains a few fibrocytes. The hyaline layer is dense collagen deposited beneath the true basement membrane. The distinctive undulated appearance of the mucosa is an inconsistent finding in asthmatics' bronchi and may be a reflection of bronchospasm or hyperplastic smooth muscle bundles in the wall. (Paraffin section, H&E stain: × 470.)

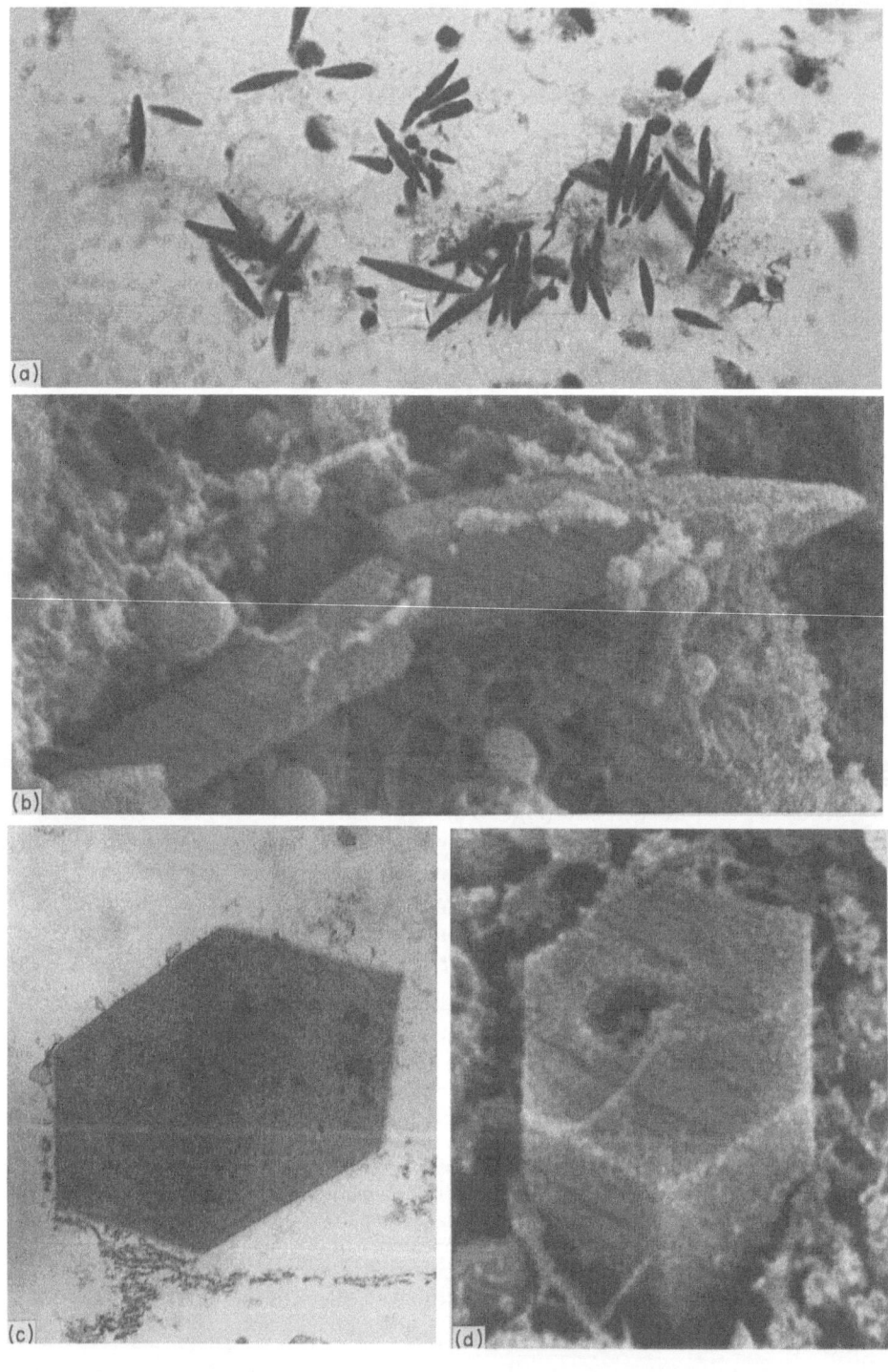

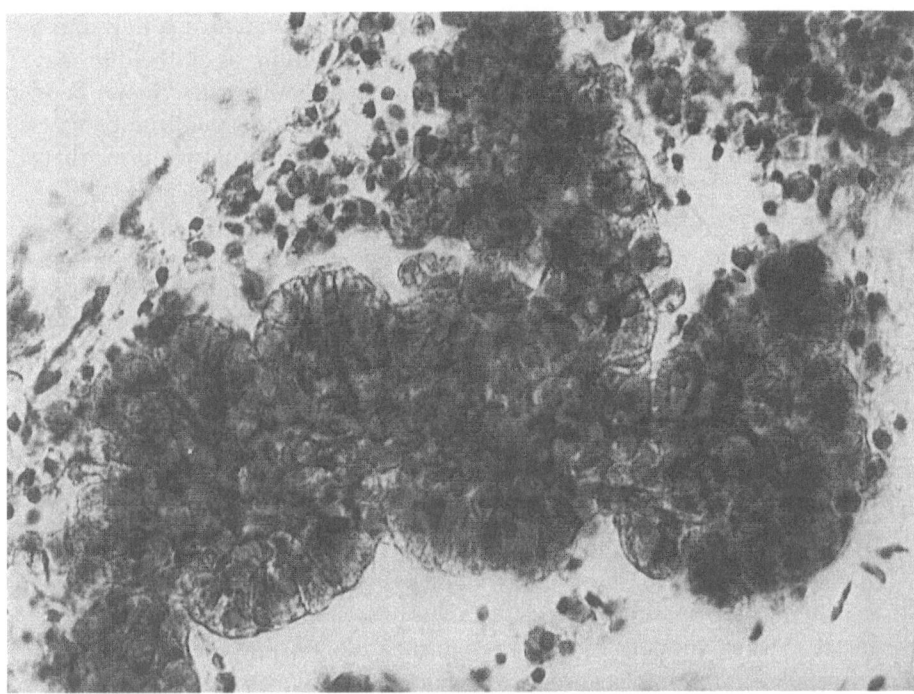

Fig. 5.8 Creola body. Exfoliated bronchial epithelial cells have been shed as a large clump and condensed to form a solid mass which mimicks the appearance of adenocarcinoma. The uniformity of the nuclei and the low nuclear/cytoplasmic ratio distinguishes this as benign. Although these clumps are seen characteristically in the sputa of active asthmatics they can also be seen in chronic bronchitics. (Papanicolaou stained smear: × 180.)

Curschmann's spirals (Fig. 5.4) and exfoliated epithelial cells are found in sputa of asthmatics (Naylor and Railey, 1964; Sanerkin and Evans, 1965), but they are not specific for this disease (Mathews, 1982). The tendency of the bronchial epithelium to exfoliate during acute asthmatic attacks was studied by Naylor (1962), who introduced the term Creola body to describe large sheets of exfoliated epithelium which condense to form spherical or elongated masses in the overlying mucous layer (Fig. 5.8). Nearly half of the sputa from asthmatics studied in his cytopathology

Fig. 5.7 Charcot-Leyden crystals. (a) Unusually large number of crystals in a sputum smear from a patient during acute asthmatic attack. Smear courtesy of Dr B. Naylor, University of Michigan. (Papanicolaou stained smear: × 710.) (b) Whole crystals. (Scanning electron micrograph: horizontal width of field = 8 μm.) (c) Crystal cut obliquely but almost in cross-section. (Transmission electron micrograph: × 17 700.) (d) Freeze-fracture preparation with fractured crystal protruding from the background debris. (Scanning electron micrograph: horizontal width of field = 3.6 μm.)

laboratory had Creola bodies, half contained Curschmann's spirals and a few contained Charcot-Leyden crystals. The shedding of epithelium may be related to a protein derived from eosinophil granules called major basic protein. This protein was found in the sputa of most hospitalized patients with asthma and causes bronchial epithelial cells in culture to exfoliate (Frigas et al., 1981).

There is a well-recognized triad of aspirin intolerance, asthma and nasal polyposis (Samter and Beers, 1968; Delaney, 1975; Stenius and Lemola, 1976; Lewis et al., 1983). Individuals usually have the non-IgE-mediated type of asthma and may also have intolerance to tartrazine (a food coloring agent) and indomethacin. The polyposis in this triad does not extend to the lower respiratory tree.

5.7 Hypersensitivity reactions in lung

Hypersensitivity pneumonitis generally refers to diffuse infiltrative lung disease which is initiated by antigens (usually inhaled) after a prior sensitizing exposure. Unlike asthma, these reactions develop in the more distal airways, produce dyspnea not bronchospasm, and are characterized by cellular immunological reactions. Some pathologists classify hypersensitivity pneumonitis as extrinsic allergic alveolitis. The reactions are initially characterized by increased numbers of macrophages and lymphocytes with the development of interstitial granulomas; eosinophils may also accumulate. Several recent reviews summarize the present understanding of the pathophysiology and the ever expanding list of identified antigens (Ward et al., 1978; Reed and deShazo, 1982; Schlueter, 1982). Bronchial biopsy is rarely obtained and the histopathological changes are not specific for this group of reactions and certainly not for the various diseases associated with specific antigen exposure. The granulomas tend to be poorly formed and are surrounded by infiltrates of lymphocytes, two features which may suggest hypersensitivity pneumonitis rather than sarcoidosis (see Chapters 6 and 8). Eventually, with repeated exposure, diffuse pulmonary fibrosis results. Cellular and chemical analysis of bronchoalveolar lavage may be helpful in distinguishing these reactions and may eventually play a role in their specific diagnosis (Reynolds et al., 1977; Ward et al., 1978; Hunninghake et al., 1979; Fink, 1982; Epstein et al., 1982).

Farmer's lung, bird breeder's disease, bagassosis, cheese-washer's lung, maple bark stripper's lung, isocyanate disease and suberosis (from moldy cork) are but a few examples of the colorful names which show both the diversity and sometimes remarkable specificity of the diseases which have been associated with antigen inhalation. Berylliosis, usually considered a pneumoconiosis, may more properly belong with these reactions (Karkinen-Jääskeläinen *et al.*, 1982; Epstein *et al.*, 1982).

Mucoid impaction, occasionally with the coughing up of mucoid casts of the bronchial tree, is frequently associated with a hypersensitivity reaction to aspergillus. This condition, best referred to as allergic bronchopulmonary aspergillosis, is a noninvasive form of pulmonary aspergillosis (see Section 4.4.1). It can clinically present as asthma (see Section 5.6), but is best considered a specific form of hypersensitivity pneumonitis (Riley *et al.*, 1975; Khan *et al.*, 1976; Rosenberg *et al.*, 1977; Ein *et al.*, 1979). Some also include allergic bronchopulmonary aspergillosis in the group of eosinophilic pneumonias (Schatz *et al.*, 1981; Reed and deShazo, 1982). Unlike most hypersensitivity reactions in lung, these patients are asthmatics and the tissue reaction includes an infiltrate with numerous eosinophils.

Clinically these patients have asthma and positive skin reactions to aspergillus antigens. Frequently, but not always, Aspergillus is cultured from their sputa. The species *fumigatus* is most frequently implicated but others have been isolated (Khan *et al.*, 1976). There is some suggestion that other fungi could be the cause of an identical disease, but none has been confirmed with skin tests. There are increased numbers of eosinophils in the walls of the bronchi and rare granulomas are located in a peribronchial pattern. The most distinctive histological findings are in the mucoid impactions (plugs) themselves. The plugs may be removed by bronchoscopy (lifted out intact by grasping the plug and withdrawing the bronchoscope) to relieve obstruction and reduce the complications in the more distal parenchyma. Histologically there is a geometric arrangement of the eosinophils and laminated layers of mucin in the mucoid plugs from both the more common asthmatics and those with bronchopulmonary aspergillosis (Jelihovsky, 1983). In the latter, the mucus forms in the pattern of a wheel with a central hub and spokes. Eosinophils cluster in pyramidal-shaped wedges (in the outline of a fir tree) with apex pointing toward the hub of the wheel. Hyphae of aspergillus are frequently found in sections of these plugs. They are particularly noticeable when silver methenamine stains are used (Section 4.4.1). The patient can be given a specimen jar containing formalin fixative and instructed to collect plugs which are coughed up, by placing them into the jar. They should be oriented in the paraffin blocks so as to provide cross-sections and both H&E and silver methenamine stains should be routinely prepared. In contrast to this specialized pattern, the mucoid plugs from the more common forms of asthma have a whorled pattern in the mucus laminations and the eosinophils tend to be layered in the same swirled fashion. There are often clumps of exfoliated bronchial epithelial cells entrapped in the mucus, which is not seen in the plugs from bronchopulmonary aspergillosis.

5.8 Inhaled mineral dusts

A variety of mineral dusts evoke pulmonary tissue reactions (Wagner, 1980). The vast majority of patients with lung disease attributable to such dusts are exposed during work-related activities. The general term used to encompass all of these lung disorders is pneumoconiosis, and those which are work related are categorized as occupational pneumoconioses (Dosman *et al.*, 1981). Many agents encountered in the work environment may cause asthma (Patterson and Goldstein, 1982) (Section 5.6). Because of the complexities of our current work environment, mixtures of various dusts may combine to give a unique pneumoconiosis, such as the case of a metal and mold worker who was exposed for 6 years to silica, asbestos, talc and beryllium in a particular work situation. He developed diffuse pulmonary infiltrates and subsequently died (Mark *et al.*, 1979). Rarely the offensive mineral dust is inhaled deliberately. A tragic case was reported by Gong and Tashkin (1979) in which a 10-year-old child inhaled cleaning powder (which contained abundant silica) daily for about 2 months. She developed clinically apparent silicosis by age 21 and died from progressive silicosis at 35. In most situations, because of extensive historical medical experience, the particular mineral which causes disease is known, work practices which lead to significant exposure are documented and the risks are known to the employer and employees.

Definite diagnosis of the pneumoconioses usually requires open lung biopsy. Pathologists examining bronchial specimens can make three types of contributions. By the identification of specific pneumoconioses we can alert the clinicians to unrecognized exposure (which would lead to a more intense review of the patient's environment) and clarify which particular mineral is present when pneumoconiosis is suspected yet the patient's exposure contains several dusts. Moreover, the presence of mineral particles in specimens obtained for other diagnostic purposes such as tumor or infection can be determined which may be of immediate and long term value in establishing relevant associations of mineral inhalation and other disease processes (Abraham, 1978; Mark, 1981).

The pulmonary reaction to inhaled particles can be of the immunologic hypersensitivity type (Section 5.7), granulomatous (Chapter 6), or fibrotic. Large amounts of coal dust may accumulate in the lung parenchyma with little apparent reaction. The remarkable ability of the lung to rid itself of foreign inhaled material can be appreciated from the observation that although coal workers may have inhaled 6 kg of coal dust during their years working, less than 80 g may be present in their lungs at death (Gross, 1971). In the following sections several of the readily recognized pneumoconioses will be discussed in more detail, followed by descriptions of techniques for the identification of mineral dusts in tissue specimens and diseases associated with exposure of mineral dusts. The first four sections illustrate four different tissue reactions to inhaled mineral dusts: *asbestosis*, in which the filamentous mineral asbestos is associated with widespread, irregular pulmonary fibrosis; *silicosis*, in which crystalline silica evokes discrete spherical nodules of fibrosis with contained silica particles; *coal dust*, which may accumulate in large quantities in lung tissue with very little reaction; and the formation of granuloma in *berylliosis*.

5.8.1   Asbestos

Asbestos is a mined mineral fiber of several crystalline configurations, used extensively in a multitude of commercial processes and products, and which has become nearly ubiquitous in our modern environment (Becklake, 1976; Churg and Warnock, 1981). The fibers are most often inhaled but are also present in water and probably in food. Within the lungs, parenchymal fibrosis is the usual reaction. Because of legal questions raised in recent years, the diagnosis, clinical significance and dose/disease relationships have become very controversial. There are documented associations with mesothelioma and relationships with other malignancies (Section 5.8.7). Diagnostic criteria and grading schema were presented by a Commission on Pneumoconiosis of the College of American Pathologists to the National Institute of Occupational Safety and Health (Craighead *et al.*, 1982). This group describes asbestosis as pulmonary fibrosis consequent to the accumulation of airborne asbestos in the lung. They concluded that radiological and clinical history were usually adequate for diagnosis and recognized that transbronchial biopsy or transthoracic biopsies were not adequate to establish the diagnosis and were certainly not reliable in excluding the diagnosis.

The exact pathogenesis of asbestosis is still subject to question (Heppleston, 1979; Gee, 1980; Becklake, 1982; Craighead *et al.*, 1982; deShazo, 1982). Although there may be acute pulmonary reactions in heavily exposed workers, most of the symptomatic disease becomes clinically significant years after exposure.

In the lungs one of the reactions to asbestos results in the distinctive coating of the fibers with an iron-containing material (Fig. 5.9). The fibers apparently acquire this material while phagocytized by macrophages and are then freed into the extracellular space (Becklake, 1976). The deposition may continue with build-up around the fibers, resulting in some very large structures. Typically, the encrustation forms in a beaded pattern (Fig. 5.10a, c), which may be the result of flexion of the fiber during the initial phases of coating. While the coating is very thin, bending of the fiber causes discontinuities in the coating material along the fiber's length. As

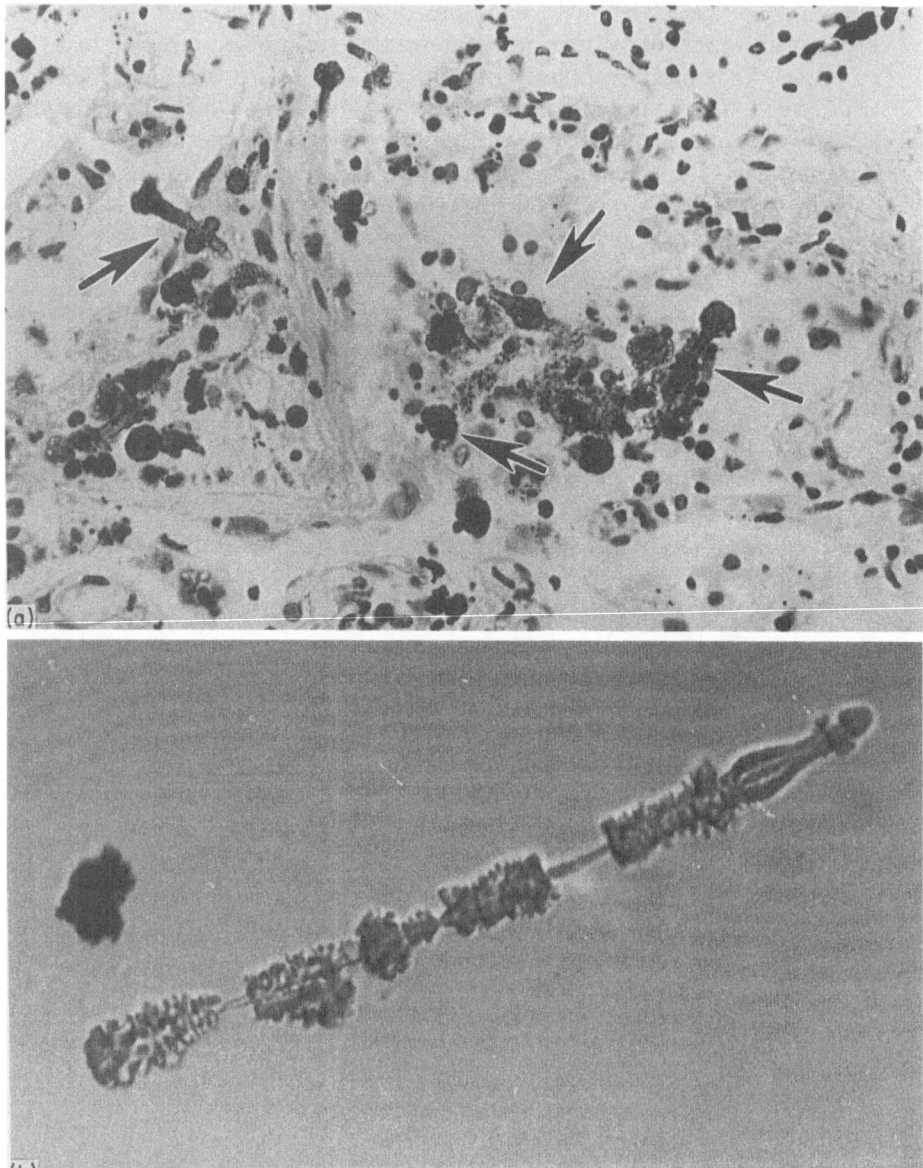

Fig. 5.9 Asbestos bodies. (a) Tissue section containing asbestos bodies (arrows). During sectioning the bodies are often fragmented and can be displaced by the knife. (Paraffin section, H&E stain: × 470.) (b) Asbestos body in a digested sputum specimen from a patient with a heavy exposure to asbestos in his work environment. (Unstained digestion concentrate: × 710.)

the deposition proceeds, the build-up occurs at the portions previously coated, and the gaps are perpetuated by continuation of the flexion at those gaps. The ends of fibers tend to accumulate more of the encrustation and the result is a dumb-bell shape (Figs 5.9a, 5.10b, c). The coating, which is retained during the digestive processes used to concentrate the bodies from tissue specimens (Section 2.4.3), is yellow or gold-brown colored which allows their identification in unstained preparations.

These bodies were originally called asbestos bodies. When it was recognized that similar encrustation occurred around nonasbestos fibers or particles, the term ferruginous bodies was coined. Currently there is a general acceptance that if a slender, transparent, fiber core is seen the term asbestos body is acceptable, since the vast majority of these bodies found in the general population have been shown to be asbestos (Warnock and Churg, 1980). A recent analysis of asbestos-exposed workers has revealed asbestos fibers encrusted with calcium oxalate rather than the typical iron-protein complex (deVuyst et al., 1982b). The 'oxalate bodies' were initially detected as birefringent fibers in a bronchoalveolar lavage from one asbestos worker.

Analysis of lungs from the general population demonstrates that asbestos bodies are nearly universal today (Rosen et al., 1972; Bhagavan and Koss, 1976; Churg and Warnock, 1979; Churg and Warnock, 1981; Modin et al., 1982; Churg, 1982). There are large numbers of asbestos bodies in the lungs of asbestos miners (Roggli et al., 1980a; Roggli et al., 1980b) and others who develop asbestosis (Whitwell et al., 1977; Churg and Warnock, 1981). They can be collected by bronchoalveolar lavage (Gaudichet et al., 1978; deVuyst et al., 1982a). Most of these analyses have been performed on concentrated, digested lung specimens or on tissue sections from bulk specimens, but not on bronchial specimens.

Ashcroft and Heppleston (1973) determined that phase contrast light microscopy increases the counts of visible fibers. However, their electron microscopic counts show that only 12% to 30% of the actual fibers are counted, even with this enhanced optical system. Their work indicated that the distribution of fiber sizes was more or less constant, so that light microscopic counts can be used as relative numbers, but should not be cited as actual numbers. Scanning electron microscopy demonstrates the encrusted bodies very well (Fig. 5.10) and uncoated fibers are visible (Fig. 5.10b). Although most asbestos bodies have the beaded appearance, rare ones have a continuous smooth coating (Fig. 5.10b). In one case report of pulmonary fibrosis analyzed by electron microscopy, numerous chrysotile asbestos fibers were documented, well below the size which could be detected in the light microscope, raising the possibility that some asbestos pulmonary reactions may go undetected without examination at higher resolution (Miller et al., 1975).

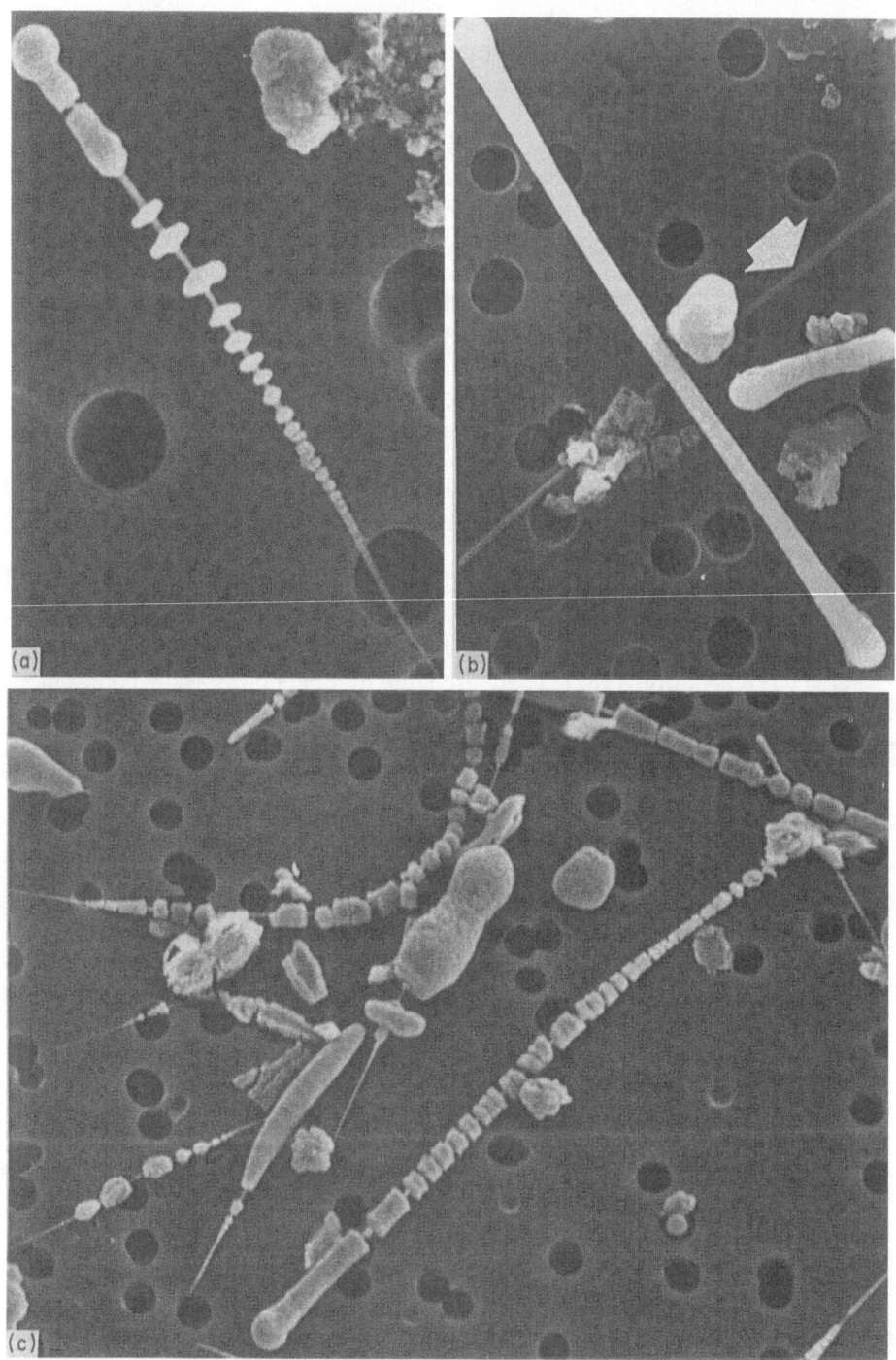

Asbestos bodies are occasionally identified in sputum specimens and studies have shown a strong correlation of their presence with significant pulmonary disease (Whitaker, 1978; Modin et al., 1982) or exposure (Naylor, 1977; Roggli et al., 1980b; McLarty et al., 1980; Craighead et al., 1982). In a cytology study of asbestos workers' sputa (McLarty et al., 1980) it was also found that those workers who smoked cigarettes yielded increased numbers of asbestos bodies in their routine smears. When asbestos bodies are found in sputa they should prompt a clinical review (if the patient had not been known to have significant exposure to asbestos) but are not adequate in themselves to establish the diagnosis of asbestosis.

Becklake (1982) has an extensive review if the reader wishes a more inclusive coverage of asbestosis. A thorough review of the epidemiologic aspects of asbestos-related diseases were published as a monograph from the International Agency for Research on Cancer (IARC) (Rall, 1977).

5.8.2 Silica

Most silicosis results from prolonged, extensive exposure of workers to the free crystalline silica. Silica itself may be the mined material, such as quartz, or it may occur as a contaminant in the mining of other minerals, such as gold. Heating of diatomaceous earth (diatoms are micro-organisms with abundant silica in their bivalved walls) produces high concentrations of forms of silica which are more reactive in tissue than quartz particles. Silica is used in abrasives and in pottery but is not present in our urban environment as widely as asbestos (Ziskind et al., 1976).

More is understood about the pathogenesis of the pulmonary reaction to silica than to asbestos. Silica particles of 1–3 μm length are phagocytized by macrophages in the distal airways and alveoli. There is a direct cytotoxic effect on the macrophages, causing release of substances including lysosomal enzymes, free radicals, fibrogenic factors and chemotactic factors for neutrophils. The phagocytized silica is also released and may continue its cytotoxicity with subsequent phagocytosis by additional macrophages (Gee, 1980; deShazo, 1982). This nidus of activity produces an expanding spherical nodule of fibrosis with a distinctive histological pattern

---

Fig. 5.10 Scanning electron microscopy of asbestos bodies from digested specimens. The smooth background with holes is the filter onto which the material was collected for examination. (a) Typical appearance. In this particular body one end of the fiber is encrusted with abundant material while the other end tapers to a point. (Horizontal width of field = 3 μm.) (b) One body with a continuous coating. There is also an uncoated fiber in the field (white arrow). (Horizontal width of field = 6 μm.) (c) Variability in length of fibers and thickness of coating gives a wide range of sizes. The smaller bodies would not be visible in the light microscope. The flexibility of the bodies can be seen as they drape across each other in their deposition on the filter. (Horizontal width of field = 19 μm.)

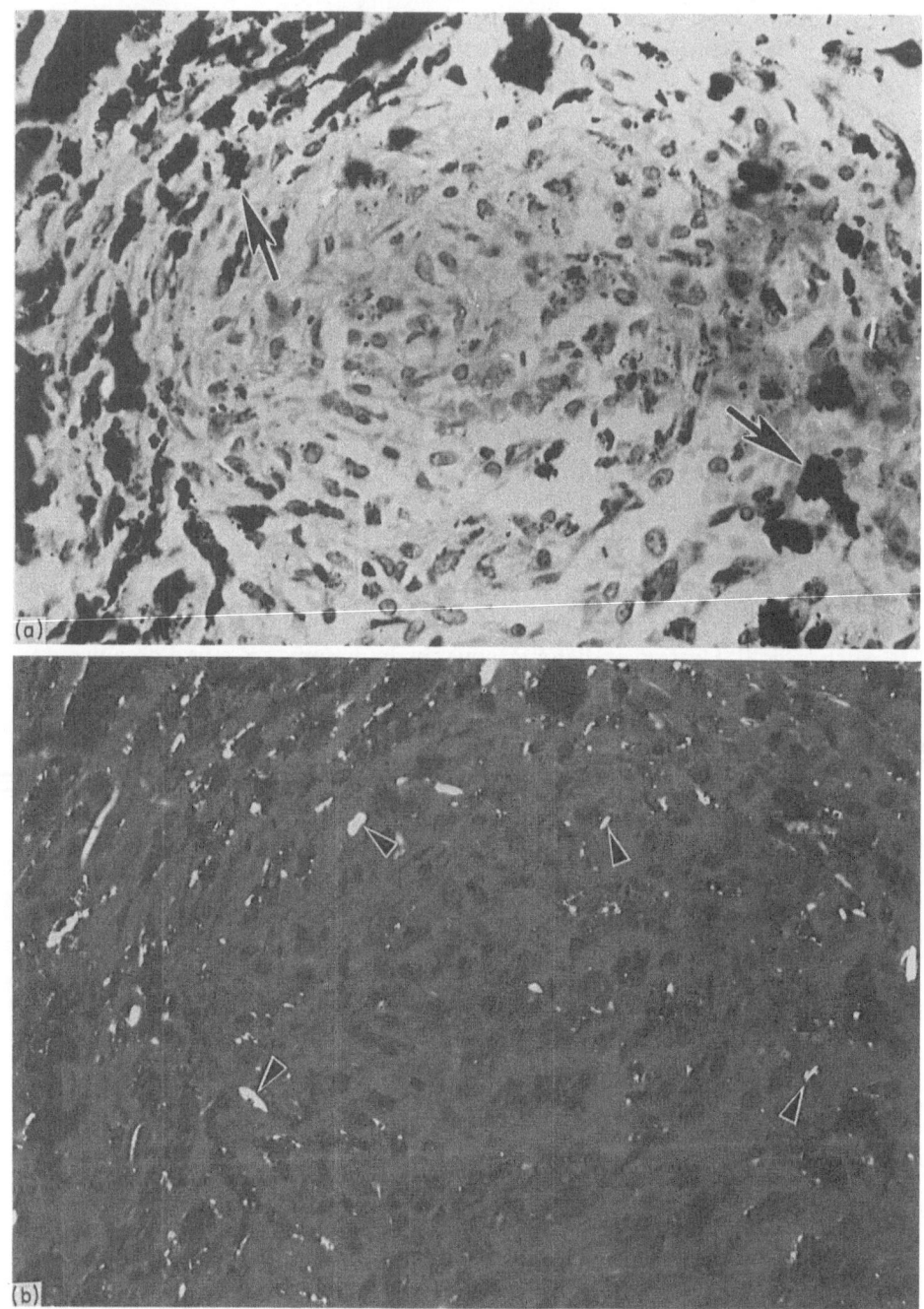
(a)

(b)

(Fig. 5.11). There is a central nidus of hyalinized collagen in a whorled pattern surrounded by concentric layers of collagen fibers and inactive fibrocytes (which form the bulk of the silicotic nodule) and an outer mantle of less orderly fibrous tissue. These nodules are well circumscribed, tend to originate near terminal airways and may continue to expand (Heppleston, 1979). Silica can be seen scattered throughout the mature nodule as birefringent triangular spicules (Section 5.8.6) (Fig. 5.11b). In a postmortem study of granite workers, Craighead and Vallyathan (1980) found histological lesions in 15 workers who did not have radiological evidence of pneumoconiosis. Of particular interest was their finding, using scanning electron microscopy and x-ray spectrometry, that silica crystals were present within the lesions. The crystals were smaller than could be detected by a polarizing light microscope. They suggest that the active silica in lesions may be 'submicroscopic' and that the usual criteria for attributing fibrotic nodules to silica by demonstration of birefringent particles may be inadequate. It is generally accepted that particles greater than 3 μm do not reach the terminal airways, but the lower size limit for active silica crystals is unknown.

The associations of silicosis with rheumatoid arthritis and tuberculosis are discussed in Section 5.8.7.

5.8.3 Coal dust

Coal dust is a mixture of particulate material and not simple carbon. Anthracotic pigment, a very nonspecific term used by most pathologists to refer to any intrinsically black-colored material in tissue, should not be used as a synonym for coal dust. In our urban population anthracotic pigment is a common finding in alveolar macrophages and tissues of the lung, in lymph nodes and even in sites distant from the lungs.

Coal worker's pneumoconiosis is accepted as the pulmonary response following heavy exposure to coal dust, and pathological standards have been proposed (Kleinerman et al., 1979). Using these standards it is necessary to have at least 50 g of wet fresh lung for inspection to determine

---

Fig. 5.11 Silicotic nodule in peribronchial tissue. (a) Characteristic end-stage fibrotic reaction to inhaled silica particles. Collagen and fibrocytes form a solid spherical nodule (shown here as a round cross-section). There is a suggestion of refractile material in the tissue. Surrounding the nodule there are extensive accumulations of anthracotic material (large arrows). (b) In the same field illuminated with nearly crossed polarizing filters, the spicules of birefringent silica (arrowheads) are easily seen in the nodule and adjacent connective tissue. (Paraffin section, H&E stain: × 470.)

if pneumoconiosis exists. The National Coal Workers' Autopsy Study in the United States has been accumulating data to clarify some of the unresolved issues in this form of pneumoconiosis (Cassidy, 1972), but the current status of this program is in some question.

The increased risk of granulomatous infections in coal workers is discussed in Section 5.8.7. Particulate black pigment may be found free in sputum and often in alveolar macrophages, particularly in cigarette smokers, but this observation has no known diagnostic value.

5.8.4 Beryllium

The pulmonary reaction to beryllium is fibrosis with fibrotic granuloma. It is indistinguishable from the histopathology of sarcoidosis (Williams, 1958; Freiman and Hardy, 1970) (for a discussion of the differential diagnosis of granuloma in bronchial specimens see Chapter 6). Prior to 1948 many fluorescent light bulbs had beryllium in the internal coating of the tubes and this was the major source of exposure. Since then most risk is to workers using beryllium compounds in metal alloys, window material for x-ray machines, cathode-ray tubes, ceramics, atomic power plants and aircraft brakes and to workers extracting the metal from ores (Nelsen, 1980). Because of the sporadic occurrence, beryllium has become one of the classic examples of long term sequelae from 'incidental' exposure to a pulmonary reactant. Karkinen-Jääskeläinen et al. (1982) describe a case of fatal beryllium granulomatous lung disease in a man who became exposed during the replacement of 1000 old fluorescent light bulbs (most were broken to reduce their bulk for transporting them away). The worker became symptomatic from this heavy, single dose within 3 months and died 2 years later. The key to diagnosis is careful history-taking and tissue analysis (Section 5.8.6). It has been suggested that the pulmonary reaction to beryllium is a form of hypersensitivity (Section 5.7) (Epstein et al., 1982; Karkinen-Jääskeläinen et al., 1982).

5.8.5 Talc

Talc is a granular or flat crystal of magnesium silicate. It evokes a foreign body type granulomatous reaction. Pulmonary disease follows very extensive exposure to the dust which often contains various other potentially active minerals such as asbestos and silica. In one well-documented case a soapstone polisher for 38 years became clinically recognized as a pneumoconiosis patient 32 years after initial exposure (Berner et al., 1981). This individual died and there was a diffuse pulmonary fibrosis with scattered 2–3 mm nodules with macrophages and multinucleated giant cells containing birefringent crystals. Analytical techniques (Section 5.8.6) confirmed that the massive amounts of crystalline material in these nodules, as well as within alveoli, were talc. Three dimensional techniques demonstrate that although the crystals of talc often look needle-like (particularly in crossed polarized microscopy), they are actually flat plates which are nearly invisible when viewed in their flat orientation, but distinctive when viewed on end (Fig. 5.12).

Talc is rarely used on surgical gloves now that its reactivity is appreciated. The birefringent objects seen in biopsy specimens which originate from glove powder are more commonly starch. Unlike the plate-like talc, starch is ovoid in shape and gives a characteristic Maltese cross image in crossed polarized microscopy and should not be confused with any talc which might be within the specimen itself (Fig. 4.17). Starch is not reactive in tissue.

The surgical pathologist is most likely to see talc reactions in the patient with diffuse pulmonary disease who has introduced talc intravenously as an unanticipated complication of drug abuse (Tomashefski and Hirsch, 1980; Sieniewicz and Nidecker, 1980). The reaction in these cases tends to be associated with small blood vessels. For a more detailed account of the histopathology of intravenous foreign particulate reaction see Chapter 6.

5.8.6 Identification of dust particles in biopsy material

The key to the pathological diagnosis of pulmonary reactions to particulate material is the detection and subsequent analysis for identification of the specific mineral or foreign matter. In the past this has required significant volumes of lung tissue, usually from autopsy or open biopsy of the lung, and involved either direct analysis or analysis of digested (Section 2.4.3) or ashed tissues (Whitwell et al., 1977). Clearly this type of quantitative and/or qualitative analysis requires a greater volume of tissue than would be available in bronchial biopsies, and so bronchoscopy was seldom considered as a diagnostic approach. However, with more recent advances in technology there is a definite role for the bronchoscopic specimen (Roggli and Shelburne, 1982).

The size of particles is of interest for an understanding of pathophysiology (Leineweber, 1981) but rarely is essential for identification. With the use of electron microscopy, it is becoming evident that the light microscope underappreciates the full range of particulate size (Ashcroft and Heppleston, 1973; Miller et al., 1975). Measurements of size and size distribution require the higher resolution of the electron microscope. Specific localization of identified particles is critical to our understanding of the relationship of the tissue reactions to the dust. These relationships are obliterated by digestion or ashing procedures, but can be appreciated

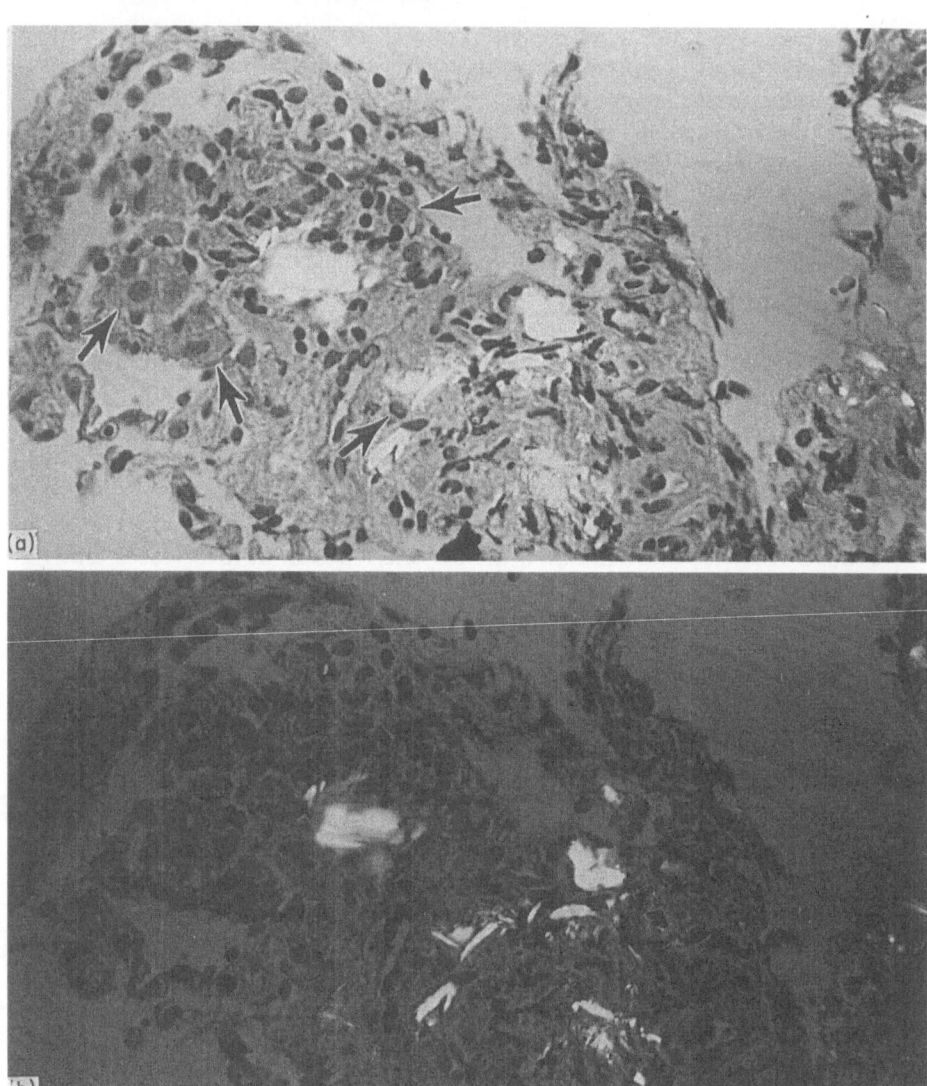

Fig. 5.12 Talc inclusions in transbronchial biopsy. (a) Macrophages (arrows), lymphocytes and fibrous tissue in lung parenchyma from intravenously introduced particles of talc. (b) With nearly crossed polarizing filters the birefringent plates of talc are easily seen, viewed on edge as well as occasional larger aggregates. (Paraffin section, H&E stain: × 470.)

in biopsy tissue sections (Johnson, 1972; Roggli and Shelburne, 1982). Unfortunately, the more sophisticated new techniques may simply give us a detailed analysis of accumulated material in the diseased tissues, without defining which are important etiologically and which are incidental (Lapenas *et al.*, 1982).

With the exception of black-colored material, which is so frequently seen as to invite dismissal, most mineral particles will not be seen in the light microscope without inserting polarizers (Mason *et al.*, 1982). Johnson (1972) has a very good review of the use of polarizing light microscopy to identify mineral particles. Silica, talc, asbestos, calcium oxalate, graphite, barium sulfate and other contrast media used for radiology are all detectable with crossed polarized optics. Johnson also gives histochemical techniques for identifying calcium, carbonates, calcium oxalate, iron and thorium dioxide in tissue sections. Kleinerman *et al.* (1979) caution about interpretation of all birefringent needle-like crystals as silica, since they find that most particles with this shape are silicates. Silica has a roughly triangular shape and is not needle-shaped.

Initially the transmission electron microscope (TEM) (Henderson *et al.*, 1970; Churg and Warnock, 1977; Lee and Fisher, 1979; Cook, 1979) and currently the scanning electron microscope (SEM) (Berry *et al.*, 1976; Abraham, 1978; Crocker *et al.*, 1980; Craighead and Vallyathan, 1980; Pickett *et al.*, 1980; Berner *et al.*, 1981; Lapenas *et al.*, 1982; Shelburne *et al.*, 1983) have been used to successfully identify particulate material in tissue specimens. The TEM allows direct imaging of the particles for size, shape and counting as well as electron diffraction for crystallographic identification, but the analysis is tedious.

SEM techniques include backscatter electron imaging and x-ray energy spectrometry. Analysis can be performed on formalin-fixed tissues from paraffin blocks, or even from previously mounted sections if that is the only available material (Pickett *et al.*, 1980). By mounting sections on clear plastic substrates it is possible to do light microscopy and SEM/x-ray energy spectrometry on the same section, without transferring the tissue (Kupke *et al.*, 1983). Although the equipment is becoming widely available for such analysis (much of it in the industrial sector), trained persons experienced with biological tissues, particularly specimens of pathological interest, are still hard to find. Additional experience with biopsy material may help to clarify some pathological problems and increase the practical applications of these extremely sensitive and precise techniques. It is now possible to visualize single submicroscopic particles within cells and make precise chemical and crystallographic analysis. We all need to be reminded, however, that unless we are alert to the possible involvement of foreign material (both inorganic and organic compounds) in the histologic sections we examine, we will never detect their presence or their importance (Berry *et al.*, 1976; Abraham, 1978; Mark, 1981). The finding of specific foreign material should prompt a thorough interview with the patient concerning occupational or other environmental sources for the dust. As our environment becomes more cluttered with increased amounts and types of substances, the lungs will certainly be a major source for discovery of the untoward reactions which must surely be our fate as we breathe. The bronchial biopsy may be the first opportunity to make the relevant associations of disease with environmental contaminants. With the current state of the art in TEM and SEM analysis we have the tools to do this and we need only watch carefully.

5.8.7   *Increased risk of secondary disease*

As if the pneumoconioses were not enough, there are several classical disease associations which arise from increased risk, either to the dust or to the reactions they evoke. It has been appreciated for decades that coal workers have a higher risk for tuberculosis than the general population (Kleinerman *et al.*, 1979; Sluis-Cremer, 1980). There is a significant risk for tuberculosis in workers exposed to silica dusts (Bailey *et al.*, 1974; Snider, 1978). Careful study seems to indicate that the increased risk in coal workers is related to their exposure to silica in the coal dust and not specifically associated with the carbon dust (Sluis-Cremer, 1980). Abraham (1978) suggests that much of the fibrosis in coal worker's pneumoconiosis may also be a reaction to the trace amounts of silica and silicates they have found mixed with the carbon. Many workers who have silicosis (Snider, 1978) and coal worker's pneumoconiosis die from tuberculosis (Sluis-Cremer, 1980). It is easy to speculate that the increased risk is related to the particular macrophage cytotoxicity of silica (Snider, 1978). Individuals with silicosis also have an increased incidence of the other granulomatous infections including atypical mycobacteria and histoplasmosis.

Caplan (1953) described massive fibrotic nodules in coal miners who had rheumatoid arthritis. Caplan's lesion may also be found in silicosis when coexistent with rheumatoid arthritis. Silica is frequently found in these large nodules. The size of the lesion results from coalescence of somewhat large (1 cm) nodules. The lesions may cavitate (Gough *et al.*, 1955) and be mistaken for pulmonary malignancy. Tuberculosis is even

---

Fig. 5.13 Chemotherapy effects on epithelial cells. The two most frequent morphological changes seen are giantism of cells and multinucleation. All micrographs are at the same magnification. (a) Nearly normal epithelial cells for comparison. Neutrophils (arrows) help reference for size in both (a) and (b). (b) Enlarged but normally shaped ciliated cell. (c) Enlarged epithelial cell with a flat apical surface but no visible cilia. This cell is definitely abnormal. (d) Slightly enlarged columnar cell with multinucleation and an adjacent normal ciliated cell. (e) Enlarged multinucleated cell with flat apical surface surrounded by more normal ciliated cells. (f) Multinucleated epithelial cell. (g) Giant epithelial cell which retains the overall shape of a ciliated cell but cilia are absent. Notice that both the nuclear and cytoplasmic volumes are increased. (Papanicolaou-stained bronchial washing: × 710.)

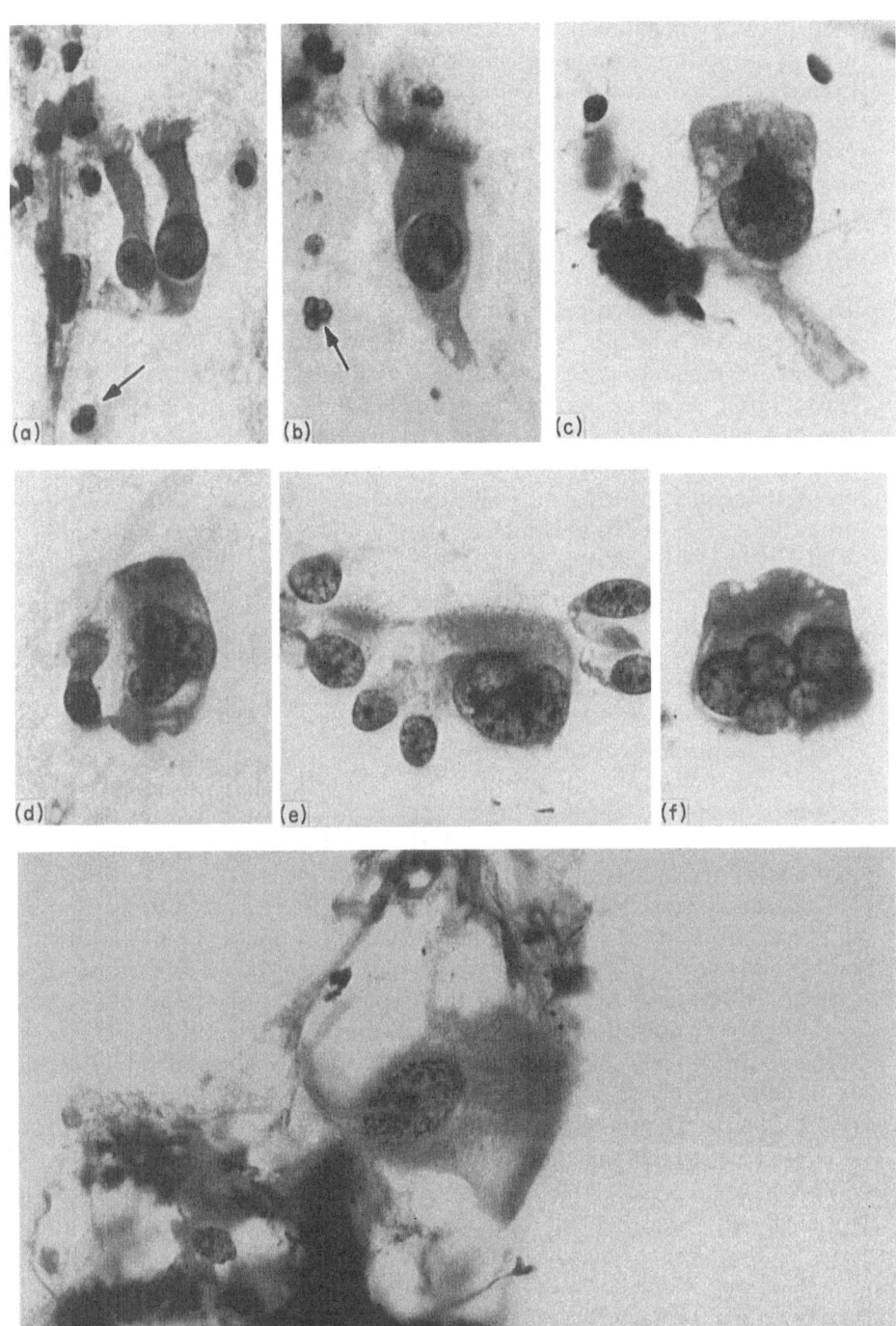

more prevalent in patients with Caplan's lesion, and acid-fast stains should always be performed if these lesions are biopsied. Central liquifaction necrosis and unusually prominent pallisading macrophages are a clue that the fibrotic nodule is not simply silicotic.

For an extensive review of the risk of cancer from mineral exposure see the IARC monograph on this subject (Wagner, 1980).

5.9 Reactions to drugs

The list of drugs which cause pulmonary lesions is long and continually expanding. The reader is referred to several reviews for a more extensive coverage (Whitcomb, 1973; Sostman et al., 1977; Weiss and Muggia, 1980; Nash, 1982). Most of the reactions involve the pulmonary interstitium and alveolae. In most cases the patients have received a variety of cytotoxic drugs, radiation (Section 5.10) and oxygen, which makes it difficult to precisely identify the offending agent(s). Both radiation and oxygen may produce additive effects in combination with some of the agents (Einhorn et al., 1976; Weiss and Muggia, 1980; Tryka et al., 1982). The most convincing evidence implicating specific agents is the lack of progression, or in some cases regression, of the pulmonary changes after discontinuation of the drug. Although the interstitial and alveolar changes which result from these drugs may be seen in transbronchial biopsy (Orwoll et al., 1978; McCrea et al., 1981; Michael and Rudin, 1981; Perlow et al., 1981), these reactions can be nonspecific histologically and because of the extent and clinical importance of the differential diagnosis, open lung biopsy is generally preferred if tissue specimens are required. The discussion here will focus on those agents which cause histopathological changes in the bronchial tissues.

Epidermoid (squamous) metaplasia (Section 9.1.4) was seen in reaction to Mitomycin (Orwoll et al., 1978) and Bleomycin (Jones, 1978) and the metaplasia was often atypical (Section 9.6.1) (Luna et al., 1972; Krous and Hamlin, 1973; Orwoll et al., 1978). Atypical metaplasia may also be associated with Busulfan therapy (Podall and Winkler, 1974). Nuclear atypia associated with Bleomycin and with Busulfan was reported by Koss et al. (1965), Luna et al. (1972), Whitcomb (1973), and Sostman et al. (1977). Koss et al. (1965) comments that the nuclear atypia is similar to that seen with radiation and was present in uterine cervix as well as bronchial and alveolar cells. The severe atypia caused Koss (1979) to speculate that bronchogenic carcinoma might develop in patients who received Busulfan and survived from their treated malignancy a sufficient length of time. Giant epithelial cells and/or multinucleation are characteristic reactions, particularly to Busulfan (Fig. 5.13) (Koss, 1979; Nash, 1982). The atypical cells can be seen in sputa and can be mistaken for malignant

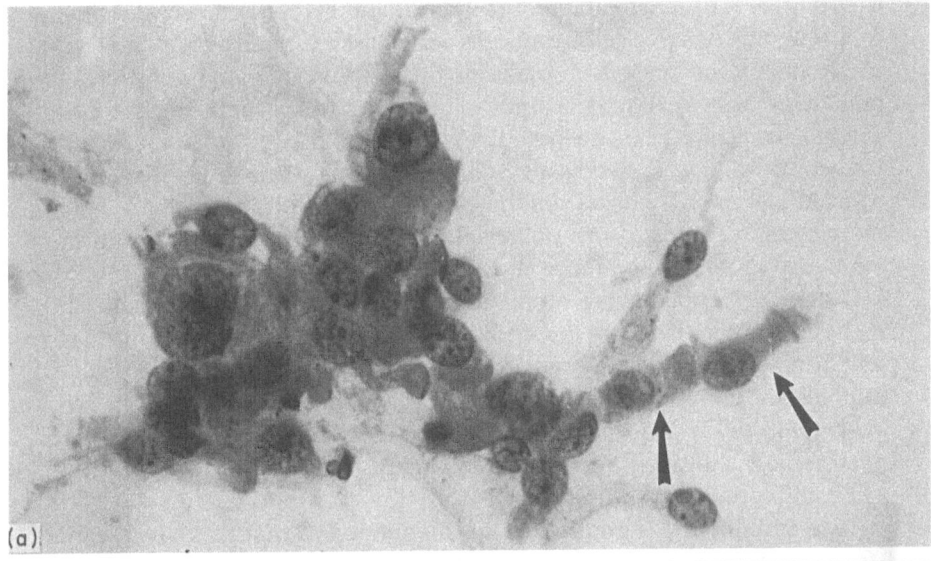

(a)

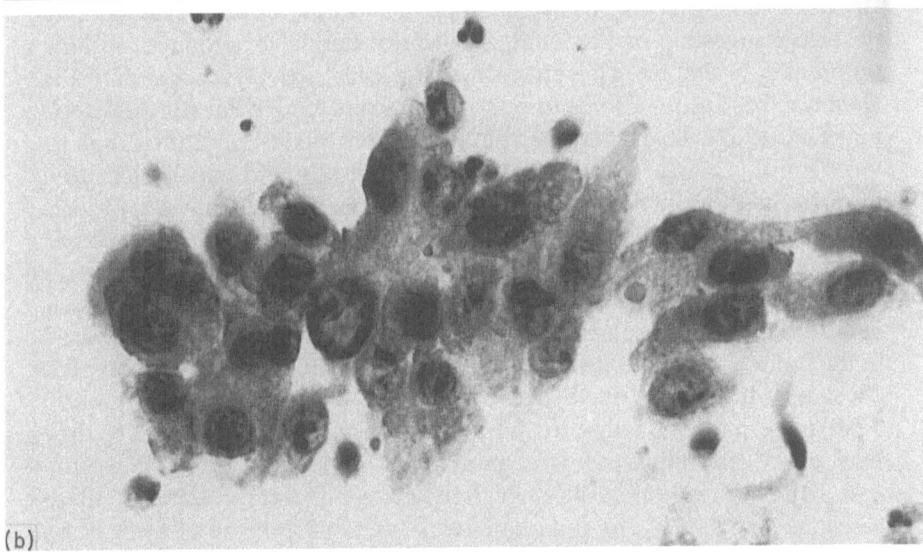

(b)

Fig. 5.14 Effect of chemotherapeutic agent on bronchial epithelial cells. Although the multinucleation and giantism shown in Fig. 5.13 would not be mistaken for neoplasia because the epithelial cells retain their characteristic shape or have cilia, some atypia is difficult if not impossible to distinguish from malignant cells as seen in these two different clusters of cells. Some more normal ciliated cells are present. (a) Sputum. There are some recognizable ciliated cells (arrows). (b) Bronchial brushing. (Papanicolaou stained smears: × 710.)

cells (Fig. 5.14). Concomitant large nuclear and cytoplasmic volumes help to distinguish reactive cells from cells which are exfoliative from bronchial malignancy. The presence of cilia or their basal bodies on questionably malignant cells is a reliable indication that the cells are benign since ciliated bronchial cells do not divide (Section 3.2.5) and there are no ciliated bronchogenic neoplasms. Clinical information is the best deterrent to overdiagnosis. Bronchial epithelial reactions to these drugs are much more common (and may be universal) than the more clinically significant interstitial lesions of the lung.

Roeckel (1973) describes a papilloma of atypical cells in a patient who received antineoplastic treatment with cobalt radiation, nitrogen mustard, vinblastine, vincristine, prednisone and several antibiotics. Reports of noncaseous granuloma in patients receiving Methotrexate are cited by Whitcomb (1973) and Sostman et al. (1977). The latter group also described dystrophic calcification and ossification in lung as a long term complication of Busulfan therapy.

Two additional situations will be mentioned, although they are not strictly speaking reactions to 'therapeutic' drugs. Both accidental and deliberate ingestion of Paraquat, a powerful herbicide, produces striking pulmonary reactions. The alveolar lining cells actively accumulate the chemical, producing a focal toxicity which leads to alveolar fibrosis (Keeling et al., 1981). There may be a severe necrotizing lesion of the oropharynx (Thurlbeck and Thurlbeck, 1976). Periodically and usually localized in major metropolitan centers, intravenous drug abusers may adopt local fads which evoke pulmonary reactions. This reaction is not to the drugs' direct effect, such as in overdose, but is secondary to the injection of foreign particulate material into the venous system. The reaction takes years to develop. The particulate material is most frequently the filler used in the fabrication of tablets intended by the manufacturer for oral use, but chosen by the abuser for a particular 'effect' (Tomashefski and Hirsch, 1980). The particles lodge in the pulmonary capillary beds where they may evoke thrombosis and/or granulomas depending on their nature. Talc is the most common filler which results in pulmonary lesions in these cases (Szwed, 1970). The granulomatous reactions in some of these cases is more fully discussed in Chapter 6. Even without a granulomatous reaction it is easy to detect talc particles in small blood vessels in suspected cases using polarizing filters, since the particles are birefringent (Fig. 5.12) (Johnson, 1972).

5.10   Radiation effects

There are a variety of effects from therapeutic radiation of the lung (Roswit and White, 1977; Gross, 1977; Fajardo and Berthrong, 1978; Nash, 1982).

There is some damage to lung parenchyma within the field of radiation in all patients receiving radiotherapy. The severe complications, however, are usually insidious, commencing weeks after completion of treatment, involve the exposed lung parenchyma, and may become irreversible with progressive interstitial fibrosis. Both acute and chronic radiation pneumonitis are less common in current practice, but still remain significant complications in as much as 10% of patients whose radiation field includes the lungs (Gross, 1977). Risk factors include total radiation dose, fractionation schedule, exposed lung volume, and individual sensitivity (Roswit and White, 1977).

Cellular atypia (Section 9.6.1) is a common sequela to radiation. The changes are similar to those previously described as reactions to cytotoxic drugs (Section 5.9) and are undoubtedly more common than the serious complications of radiation-induced pneumonitis. The surgical pathologist or cytopathologist may be confronted with specimens from patients with known bronchial carcinoma who have received radiation and asked if there is evidence of residual or recurrent malignancy. Aside from the question of determining if truly malignant cells which might be present are biologically active or irreparably damaged by the radiation, the atypia resulting from radiation in non-neoplastic cells is sometimes difficult, if not impossible, to distinguish from malignancy (Fig. 5.15). Cell enlargement, often with proportional nuclear enlargement (Fig. 5.16), is the most common visible alteration in epithelial and mesenchymal cells following radiation. Focal epidermoid (squamous) metaplasia (Section 9.1.4) may result from radiotherapy and persist for months after completion of therapy. Atypical changes in these metaplastic foci may be difficult to distinguish from malignancy (Fig. 5.15) in both biopsy and cytology specimens. For these reasons Koss (1979) advocates a conservative approach to the diagnosis of bronchial carcinoma with a history of recent radiation to the lung.

Features which are helpful in distinguishing radiation-induced atypia include very large cells with abundant cytoplasm and one or more large nuclei, a generalized reaction in which epithelial cells as well as adjacent fibrocytes and endothelial cells are abnormal, and normal appearing cells intermixed with bizarre cells. There are no studies to indicate how long the radiation-induced changes can be expected to persist in human bronchial epithelium but in our personal experience changes may be present at least one year following termination of radiation exposure.

5.11 Pulmonary alveolar proteinosis

This relatively uncommon pulmonary reaction is characterized by accumulations of proteinaceous, lipid rich material within alveoli and was first

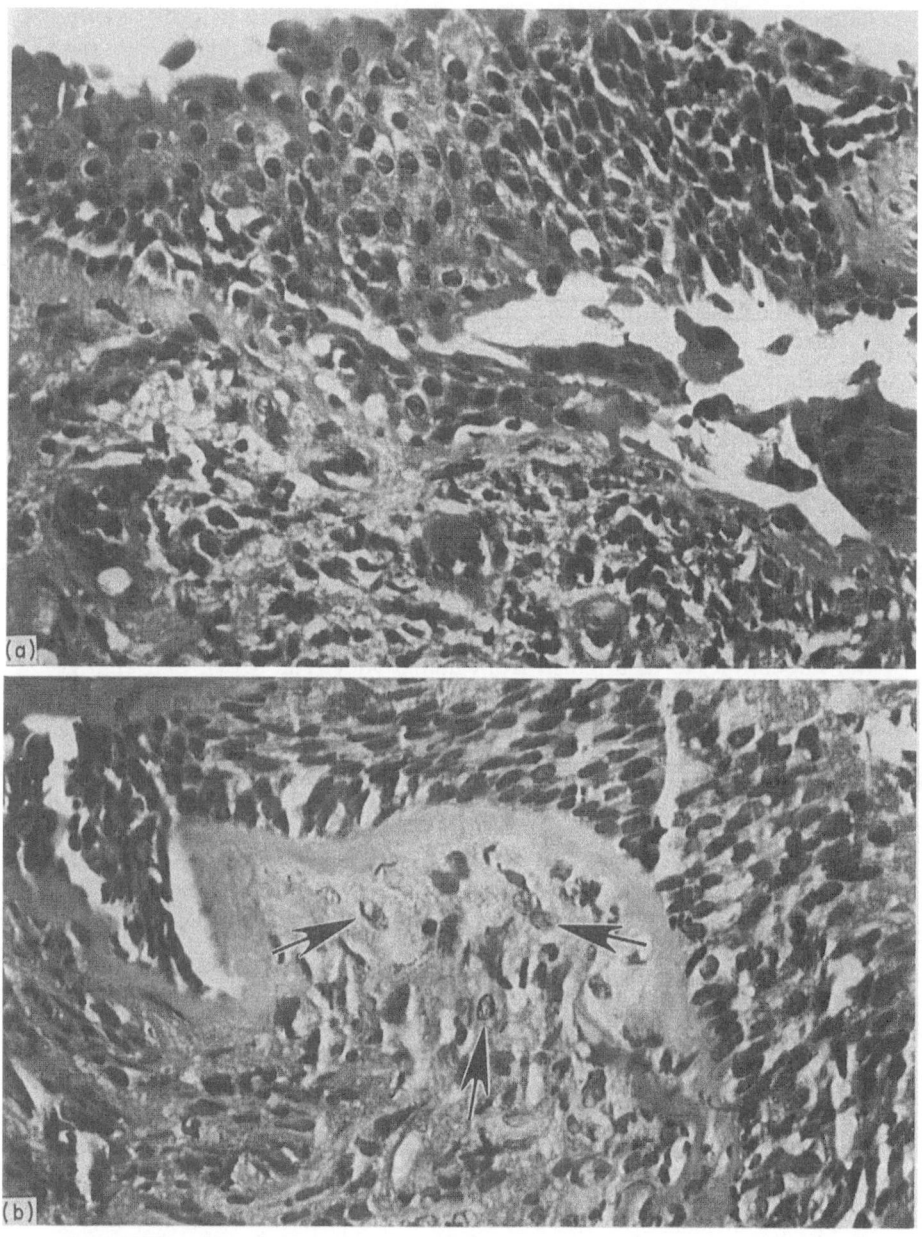

Fig. 5.15 Radiation effects on bronchial epithelium. (a) Marked atypical changes mimicking carcinoma are present in the metaplastic epithelium. (b) However, reactive enlarged endothelial cells and fibrocytes (arrows) can also be seen in the underlying connective tissue demonstrating the universal effect and suggesting the diagnosis of radiation changes. (Paraffin section, H&E stain: × 470.)

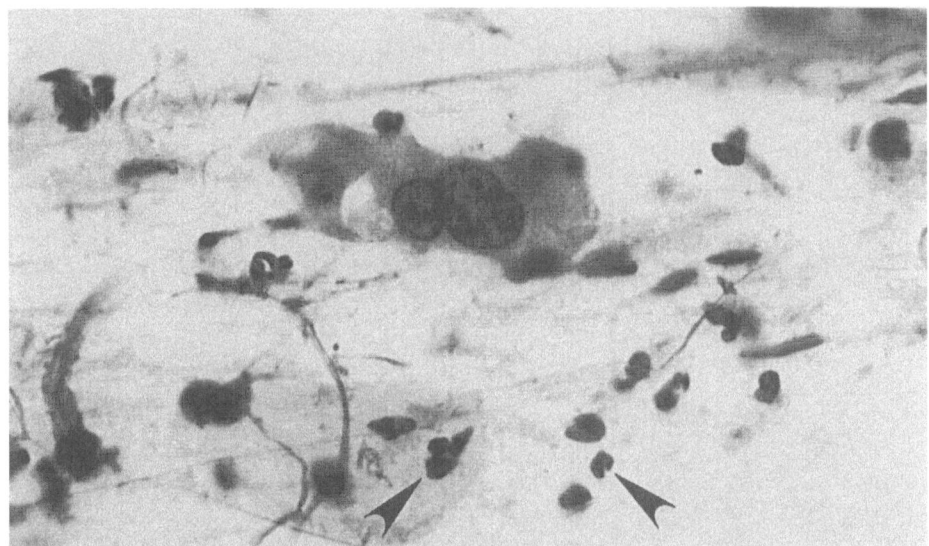

Fig. 5.16 Atypical epithelial cell in sputum from a patient who had received therapeutic radiation several months previously. Both the cytoplasmic and nuclear volumes are greatly increased and the two nuclei are probably in one cell. Adjacent neutrophils (arrows) give a size reference. Cells like this could easily be mistaken for malignancy if the history of prior radiation treatment was not known to the pathologist. (Papanicolaou stained sputum smear: × 710.)

recognized by Rosen *et al.* (1958). Histologically the material is granular, floccular and acidophilic. It is PAS positive, and although the alveoli are filled (sometimes distended) there is minimal visible alteration of the alveolar lining cells or adjacent interstitum. Currently it is suspected that this is a particular form of reaction and can be associated with a variety of initiating events including heavy silica dust exposure and various infections (Costello *et al.*, 1975; Green *et al.*, 1980; Rubin *et al.*, 1980). The lesion can be produced in experimental animals by exposure to silica. Although more common in adults, the condition has been diagnosed in children (Colon *et al.*, 1971; McCook *et al.*, 1981) and even in four siblings (Teja *et al.*, 1981).

Treatment is extensive bronchoalveolar lavage (to remove the alveolar material) and it may be necessary to repeat this procedure. Despite this treatment, cases are frequently fatal. Originally, open lung biopsy was used to make the diagnosis. However, bronchoalveolar lavage is capable of distinguishing this reaction (Hunninghake *et al.*, 1979; Martin *et al.*, 1980; Smith, 1981; Fulmer, 1982) by the presence of large acellular eosinophilic bodies in a background of granular eosinophilic material with very few macrophages.

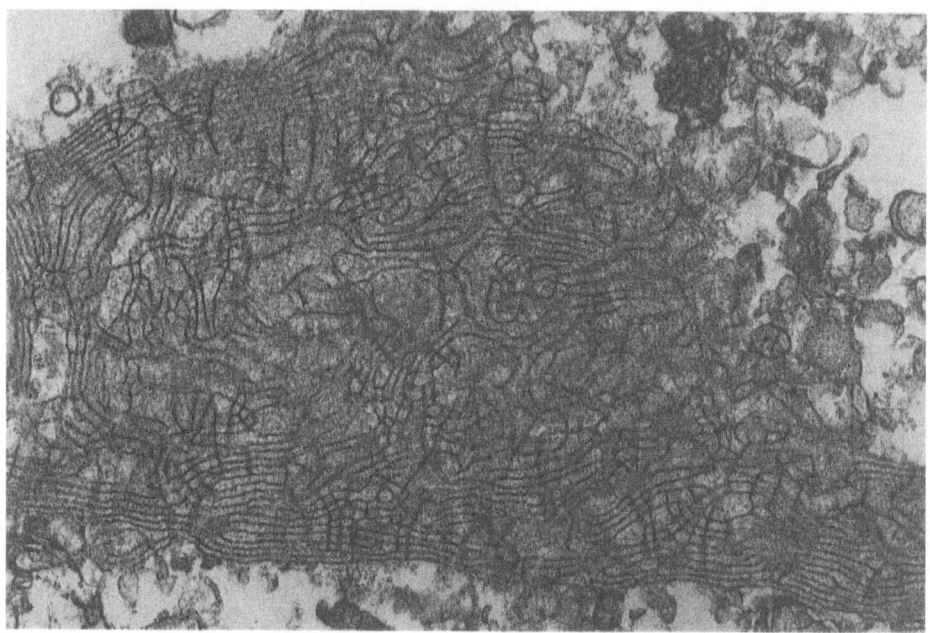

Fig. 5.17 Electron microscopic appearance of characteristic material contained in sputa and bronchoalveolar lavages from patients with alveolar proteinosis. Identical materials seen in bronchoalveolar lavages from patients with many different chronic respiratory diseases. (Electron micrograph: × 34 700.)

Analysis of the material obtained by therapeutic bronchoalveolar lavage shows abundant phospholipids (mostly lecithin), cholesterol, free fatty acids and elevated amounts of IgG (Ito *et al.*, 1978). Ultrastructural examination shows the material to contain distinctive lamellar structures (Costello *et al.*, 1975; Hook *et al.*, 1978; Shelburne *et al.*, 1983). Some of these structures are similar in appearance to the whorls seen in the cytoplasm of the type 2 alveolar lining cells, while others (Fig. 5.17) are distinctly different. The same structures can be seen in the sputa produced by these patients (Costello *et al.*, 1975; Shelburne *et al.*, 1983). However, indistinguishable structures have been seen in patients with chronic bronchitis and pneumocystis infections without the clinical features of pulmonary alveolar proteinosis.

5.12 Tracheobronchopathia osteoplastica

This rare pathological curiosity has been known for more than 100 years but still is capable of eliciting some controversy about the nature of the lesion. The abnormality is recognizable to the unaided eye as an irregular

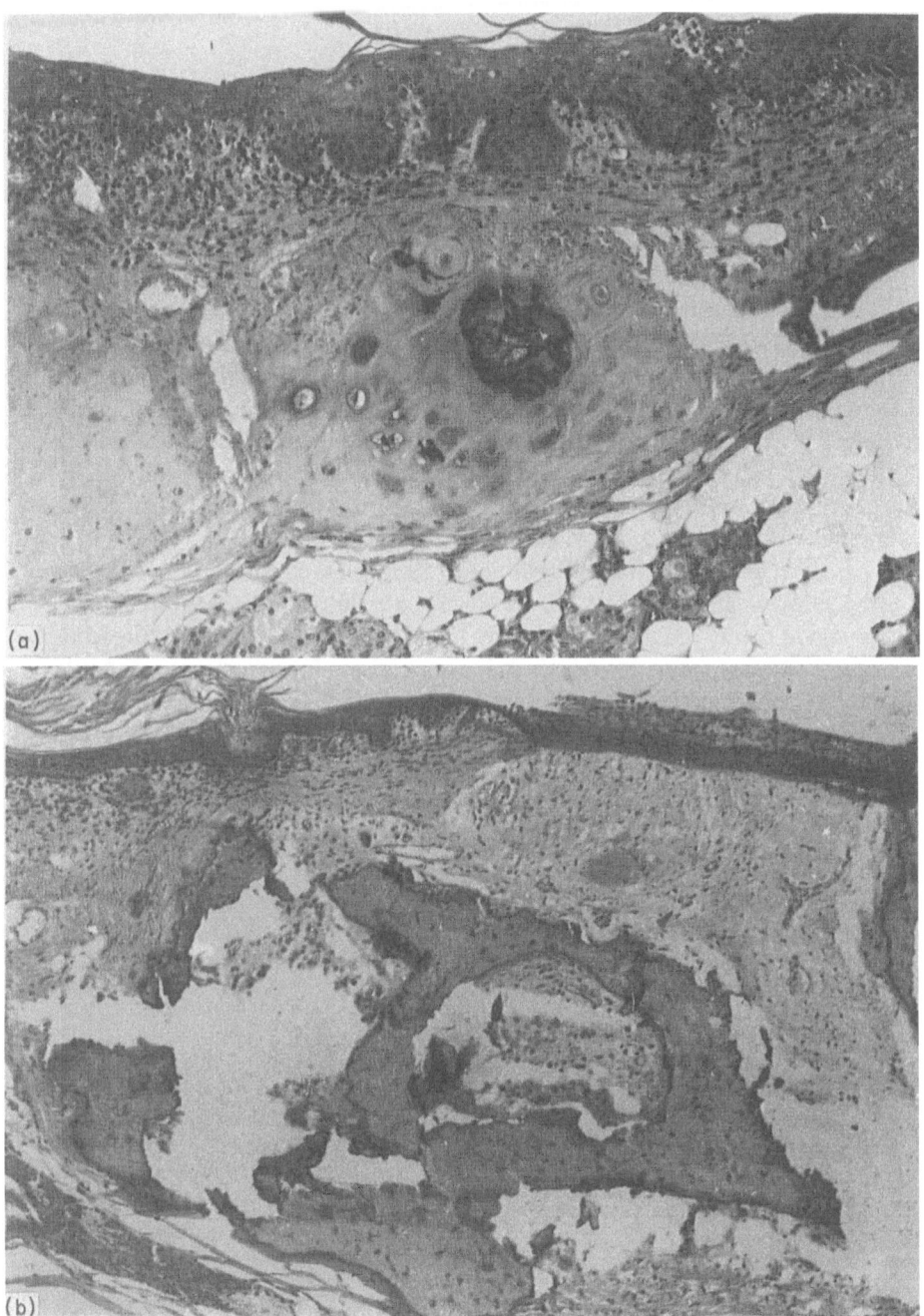

Fig. 5.18 Tracheobronchopathia osteoplastica. (a) Bronchus with keratinizing epidermoid metaplasia and nodules of cartilage, portions of which are becoming calcified. Beneath the cartilage are fat and bronchial glands. (Paraffin section, H&E stain: × 180.) (b) Adjacent area contains mature bone. This process extended bilaterally in the major bronchi and into the distal trachea. (Paraffin section, H&E stain: × 108.)

knobby appearance of the wall of the airways. The lower two thirds of the trachea are most commonly involved but the major bronchi are also abnormal in one quarter of the cases (Pounder and Pieterse, 1982). In the bronchoscope the irregularities appear papillary and submucosal. They are yellow-white and hard. The overlying mucosa is usually normal in appearance. The lesion is usually not distinguishable on x-rays. The papillary (knobby) appearance is the result of development of nodules of cartilage and normal lamellar bone between the cartilaginous rings and the mucosa (Fig. 5.18). The bone rarely forms over the membranous portions of the trachea. Serial sections have demonstrated continuity with the perichondrium of the underlying tracheal (bronchial) rings (Pounder and Pieterse, 1982). There may also be mature (ectopic) cartilage and the lamellar bone frequently contains normal bone marrow. Serum calcium and phosphorus concentrations are normal and this lesion is not associated with abnormal calcification at other locations.

In a review of the world literature in 1968, Sakula found only 125 cases reported, including his own. In the recent literature it has arisen with renewed vigor. This is undoubtedly the by-product of the widespread use of the bronchoscope. Its incidence is not precisely known; however, Ashley (1970) found 0.4% in an autopsy series and Lundgren and Stjernberg (1981) found the same percentage in their bronchoscopy series. However, in a much larger series of bronchoscopies, Van Nierop et al. (1983) found only 0.02% had the abnormality. Although in one large series Härmä and Suurkari (1977) had one case in an 11 year old, it is discovered more

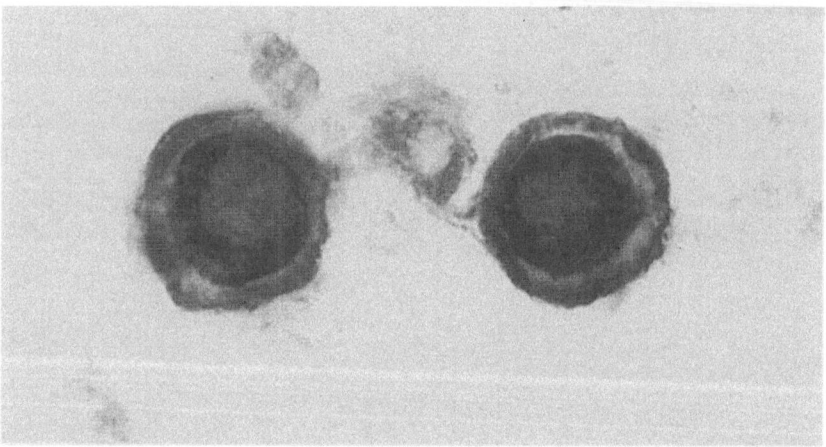

Fig. 5.19   Microliths (calcospherites) in sputum from a patient with chronic bronchitis. These are nonspecific calcific concretions in the mucus of patients with a variety of chronic inflammatory lesions and not just in pulmonary microlithiasis, which is a very rare abnormality. (Papanicolaou stained smear: × 710.)

frequently in older persons and appears to have no unfavorable consequences. Van Nierop *et al.* (1983) followed one case for 25 years with no evidence of symptoms. There have been a number of suggested etiologies but none has been present in all of the cases reported (Primer, 1979; Young *et al.*, 1980).

The principal importance of this lesion is in distinguishing it from neoplasm. In biopsy material it is difficult to distinguish from degenerative changes with foci of osseous metaplasia, but if the bronchoscopist describes a knobby appearance, suspects neoplasm and bone is found in the submucosa, tracheobronchia osteoplastica should be suspected.

5.13   Pulmonary microlithiasis

This is an equally rare abnormality of lung, diagnosed almost always by its distinctive radiological changes. Unlike tracheobronchopathia

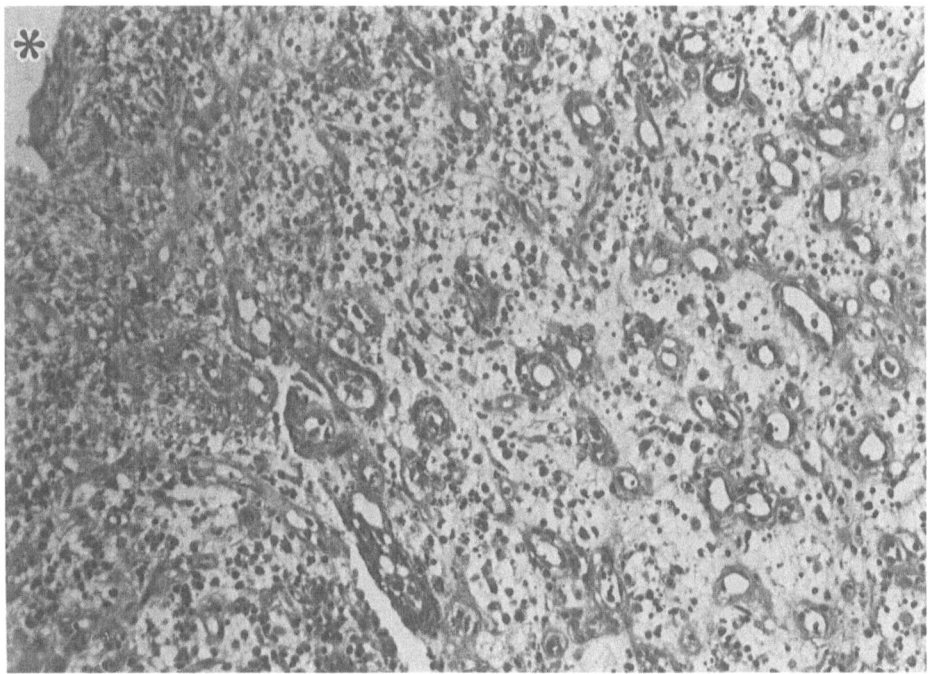

Fig. 5.20   Granulation tissue nodule in bronchus at the site of previous biopsy. The bronchoscopist saw an irregular mucosal nodule and considered it potentially neoplastic. Sections show proliferation of capillaries, spindle-shaped cells with a mixture of lymphocytes and neutrophils, with edema. This was the site of a biopsy taken 8 days previously and is a reparative reaction. The asterisk is at the luminal surface. (Paraffin section, H&E stain: × 180.)

osteoplastica, the progression of this lesion may result in airflow restrictions. The microliths (calcospherites) are apparently formed within alveoli as roughly spherical amorphous material which, in tissue sections, is concentrically laminated, basophilic and PAS positive (Miro *et al.*, 1982; Prakash *et al.*, 1983). Chemical analysis shows calcium and phosphorus, but no iron or silica. Transbronchial biopsy can retrieve specimens which contain the alveolar microliths, but the diagnosis is primarily made by the radiological findings of very fine sand-like micronodularity involving lower portions of both lungs.

Microliths can be found in the sputa from these patients. They are spherical and stain dark purple or brown with the Papanicolaou stain (Fig. 5.19). Tao (1978) has shown that about one out of four patients with chronic obstructive pulmonary disease have microliths in their sputa. One of the cases in this series also had tuberculosis, and Koss (1979) comments that they can be seen in sputa with any of the calcific granulomatous pulmonary diseases. The findings of calcified concretions in sputum, therefore, should not be interpreted as alveolar microlithiasis.

5.14   Bronchial inflammatory lesions mimicking neoplasia

A number of endobronchial lesions mimic neoplasia to either the bronchoscopist or the surgical pathologist. Perhaps the most embarrassing for the bronchoscopist is the new polypoid nodule which forms at the site of recent bronchial biopsy. This looks histologically like a pyogenic granuloma (Fig. 5.20) and may be covered with regenerating metaplastic epithelium (Chapter 9). The formation of these polypoid lesions following mechanical injury has been studied in the hamster trachea. The excrescences are covered with keratinizing metaplastic regenerating epithelium and develop within 48 hours in this model (Keenan *et al.*, 1983). Tracheobronchopathia osteoplastica (Section 5.12) can suggest neoplasm to the unwary bronchoscopist, resembling extensive submucosal spread. Wright *et al.* (1983) reported a case of pulmonary actinomycosis which simulated a bronchial neoplasm at bronchoscopy. Liebow and Carrington (1969) reported two cases of eosinophilic pneumonia with endobronchial polypoid masses which looked histologically like nasal polyps. Similar endobronchial polyps can also be seen as incidental findings not associated with any specific pulmonary disease. Histologically they appear reparative and not neoplastic (Fig. 5.21), as are the more common nasal polyps.

Fig. 5.21 Endobronchial polyp. (a) Papillary lesion with both columnar and stratified epidermoid (squamous) epithelium with a core of connective tissue. (Plastic section, toluidine stain: × 110.) (b) Same lesion seen by the scanning electron microscope. (Scanning electron micrograph: horizontal width of field = 1.3 mm.)

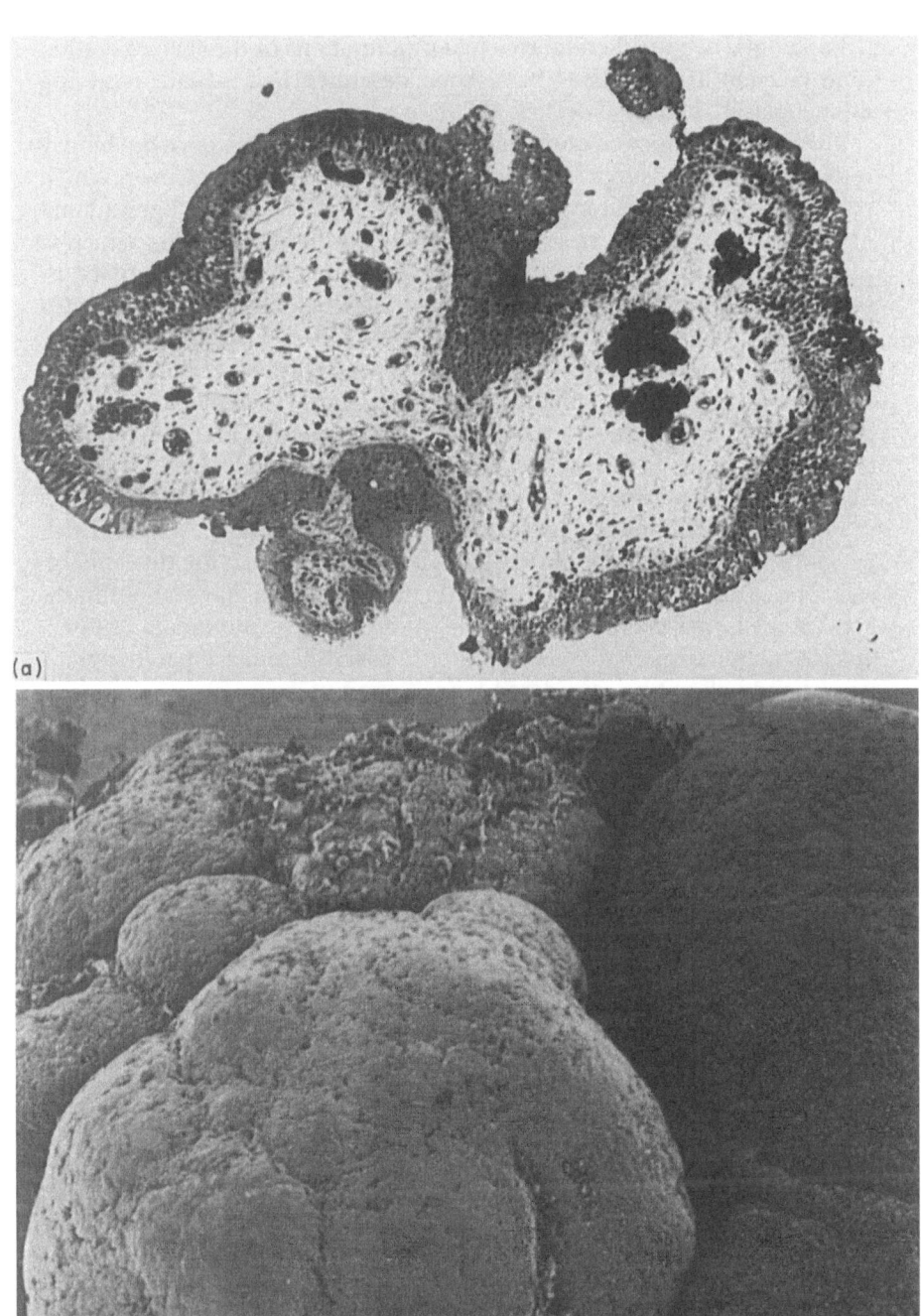

Papillomas are small endobronchial proliferations of the surface epithelium (Section 10.5.1). They have been described in a patient receiving antineoplastic therapy (Roeckel, 1973).

The lesions mentioned above should cause no difficulty once the biopsy is examined by the surgical pathologist. There are some, however, which require some judgement on the basis of histology. Plasma cell granuloma of the lung can present as a pedunculated endobronchial lesion which is histologically identical to its more common parenchymal counterpart. In sections there is a mixture of whorled spindle-shaped cells admixed with numerous plasma cells. Lymphocytes, eosinophils and macrophages are a variable component. Foamy macrophages can occasionally be abundant. Electron microscopic examination has not helped to understand or distinguish this lesion, probably because of the limited cases and the diversity of the tissue patterns (Buell *et al.*, 1976; Alvarez-Fernandez and Escalona-Zapata, 1983). Two things are important about these lesions. They are the most common pulmonary 'tumor' in young people, and they should not be confused with true plasma cell neoplasms (which lack the diversity of cell types seen in plasma cell granuloma and which have abnormally appearing plasma cells). The two other interesting pseudotumors of lung, 'sclerosing hemangioma' and lymphocytic pseudotumor are parenchymal lesions and will not be considered here.

There has been a suggestion that many of the benign mesenchymal endobronchial tumors are in fact hamartomatous growths (Tomashefski, 1982). They will be discussed in Chapter 11 along with the other nonepithelial neoplasms.

References

Abraham, J.L. (1978), Recent advances in pneumoconiosis: the pathologist's role in etiologic diagnosis. In *The Lung Structure, Function and Disease* (eds W.M. Thurlbeck and M.R. Abell), Williams and Wilkins, Baltimore, pp. 96–137.

Afzelius, B.A. (1976), A human syndrome caused by immotile cilia. *Science*, **193**, 317–19.

Alvarez-Fernandez, E. and Escalona-Zapata, J. (1983), Pulmonary plasma cell granuloma – an electron microscopic and tissue culture study. *Histopathol.*, **7**, 279–86.

Ashcroft, T. and Heppelston, A.G. (1973), The optical and electron microscopic determination of pulmonary asbestos fibre concentration and its relation to the human pathological reaction. *J. Clin. Pathol.*, **26**, 224–34.

Ashley, D.J.B. (1970), Bony metaplasia in trachea and bronchi. *J. Pathol.*, **102**, 186–8.

Bailey, W.C., Brown, M., Buechner, H.A., Weill, H., Ichinose, H. and Ziskind, M. (1974), Silico-mycobacterial diseases in sandblasters. *Am. Rev. Resp. Dis.*, **110**, 115–25.

Becklake, M.R. (1976), Asbestos-related diseases of the lung and other organs:

their epidemiology and implications for clinical practice. *Am. Rev. Resp. Dis.*, **114**, 187–227.

Becklake, M.R. (1982), Asbestos-related disease of the lungs and pleura. Current clinical issues. *Am. Rev. Resp. Dis.*, **126**, 187–94.

Belin, L. (1980), Occupational asthma and allergic alveolitis. *Europ. J. Resp. Dis.*, **61** (suppl. no. 107), 133–83.

Berner, A., Gylseth, B. and Levy, F. (1981), Talc dust pneumoconiosis. A case report. *Acta Pathol. Microbiol. Scand. Sect. A*, **89**, 17–21.

Berry, J.P., Henoc, P., Galle, P. and Pariente, R. (1976), Pulmonary mineral dust. A study of ninety patients by electron microscopy, electron microanalysis and electron microdiffraction. *Am. J. Pathol.*, **83**, 427–56.

Bhagavan, B.S. and Koss, L.G. (1976), Secular trends in prevalence and concentration of pulmonary asbestos bodies--1940-1972. A necropsy study. *Arch. Pathol. Lab. Med.*, **100**, 539–41.

Buell, R., Wang, N.-S., Seemayer, T.A. and Ahmed, M.N. (1976), Endobronchial plasma cell granuloma (xanthomatous pseudotumor). *Human Pathol.*, **7**, 411–26.

Callerame, M.L., Condemi, J.J., Bohrod, M.G. and Vaughan, J.H. (1971a), Immunologic reactions of bronchial tissues in asthma. *New Engl. J. Med.*, **284**, 459–64.

Callerame, M.L., Condemi, J.J., Ishizaka, K., Johansson, S.G.O. and Vaughan, J.H. (1971b), Immunoglobulins in bronchial tissues from patients with asthma with special reference to immunoglobulin E. *J. Allergy*, **47**, 187–97.

Caplan, A. (1953), Certain unusual radiological appearances in the chests of coalminers suffering from rheumatoid arthritis. *Thorax*, **8**, 29–37.

Carrington, C.B. and Gaensler, E.A. (1978), Clinical-pathologic approaches to diffuse infiltrative lung disease. In *The Lung Structure, Function and Disease* (eds W.M. Thurlbeck and M.R. Abell), Williams and Wilkins, Baltimore, pp. 58–87.

Cassidy, E.P. (1972), The National Coal Workers' Autopsy Study. The development and implementation of an occupational necropsy study. *Arch. Pathol.*, **94**, 133–6.

Chan-Yeung, M. (1982), Occupational assessment of asthma. In *Advances in Assessment and Therapy of Asthma* (eds S.W. Epstein and E.W. Middleton), *Chest*, **82** (suppl.), 24s–27s.

Charcot, J.M. and Robin, C. (1853), Observations de leucocythemie. *Comptes Rendus Séances Mem. Soc. Biol.*, **5**, 44–50.

Churg, A. (1982), Fiber counting and analysis in the diagnosis of asbestos-related disease. *Human Pathol.*, **13**, 381–92.

Churg, A. and Warnock, M.L. (1977), Analysis of the cores of ferruginous (asbestos) bodies from the general population. *Lab. Invest.*, **37**, 280–6.

Churg, A.M. and Warnock, M.L. (1979), Numbers of asbestos bodies in urban patients with lung cancer and gastrointestinal cancer and in matched controls. *Chest*, **76**, 143–9.

Churg, A.M. and Warnock, M.L. (1981), Asbestos and other ferruginous bodies. Their formation and clinical significance. *Am. J. Pathol.*, **102**, 447–56.

Cohen, R.J., Samoszuk, M.K., Busch, D. and Lagios, M. (1983), Occult infections with *M. intracellulare* in bone-marrow biopsy specimens from patients with AIDS. *New Engl. J. Med.*, **308**, 1475–6.

Colon, A.R., Jr., Lawrence, R.D., Mills, S.D. and O'Connell, E.J. (1971), Childhood pulmonary alveolar proteinosis (PAP). Report of a case and review of the literature. *Am. J. Dis. Child.*, **121**, 481–5.

Cook, P.M. (1979), Preparation of extrapulmonary tissues and body fluids for quantitative transmission electron microscope analysis of asbestos and other mineral particle concentrations. *Ann. N. Y. Acad. Sci.*, **330**, 717–24.

Costello, J.F., Moriarty, D.C., Branthwaite, M.A., Turner-Warwick, M. and Corrin, B. (1975), Diagnosis and management of alveolar proteinosis: the role of electron microscopy. *Thorax*, **30**, 121–32.

Craighead, J.E., Abraham, J.L., Churg, A., Green, F.H.Y., Kleinerman, J., Pratt, P.C., Seemayer, T.A., Vallyathan, V. and Weill, H. (1982), The pathology of asbestos-associated diseases of the lungs and pleural cavities: diagnostic criteria and proposed grading schema. *Arch. Pathol. Lab. Med.*, **106**, 544–97.

Craighead, J.E. and Vallyathan, N.V. (1980), Cryptic pulmonary lesions in workers occupationally exposed to dust containing silica. *J. Am. Med. Assoc.*, **244**, 1939–41.

Crocker, P.R., Doyle, D.V. and Levison, D.A. (1980), A practical method for identification of particulate and crystalline material in paraffin-embedded tissue specimens. *J. Pathol.*, **131**, 165–73.

Croxson, T.S., Ebanks, D. and Mildvan, D. (1983), Atypical mycobacteria and Kaposi's sarcoma in the same biopsy specimens. *New Engl. J. Med.*, **308**, 1476.

Crystal, R.G., Gadek, J.E., Ferrans, V.J., Fulmer, J.D., Line, B.R. and Hunninghake, G.W. (1981), Interstitial lung disease: current concepts of pathogenesis, staging and therapy. *Am. J. Med.*, **70**, 542–68.

Curschmann, H. (1885), Einege Bemerkungen über die im Bronchialsecret vorkommenden Spiralen. *Deutsches Arch. f. Kin. Med.*, **36**, 578–85.

Cutz, E. and Cox, D.W. (1979), Alpha$_1$-antitrypsin deficiency: the spectrum of pathology and pathophysiology. In *Perspectives in Pediatric Pathology*, Vol. 5 (eds H.S. Rosenberg and R.P. Bolande), Masson, New York, pp. 1–39.

Cutz, E., Levison, H. and Cooper, D.M. (1978), Ultrastructure of airways in children with asthma. *Histopathol.*, **2**, 407–21.

Davis, P.B., Hubbard, V.S., McCoy, K. and Taussig, L.M. (1983), Familial bronchiectasis. *J. Pediat.*, **102**, 177–85.

Delaney, J.C. (1975), Asthma, nasal polyposis, and aspirin idiosyncrasy. *Clin. Allergy*, **5**, 234–5.

deShazo, R.D. (1982), Current concepts about the pathogenesis of silicosis and asbestosis. *J. Allergy Clin. Immunol.*, **70**, 41–9.

deVuyst, P., Jedwab, J., Dumortier, P., Vandermoten, G., Van de Weyer, R. and Yernault, J.C. (1982a), Asbestos bodies in bronchoalveolar lavage. *Am. Rev. Resp. Dis.*, **126**, 972–6.

deVuyst, P., Jedwab, J., Robience, Y. and Yernault, J.-C. (1982b), 'Oxalate bodies', another reaction of the human lung to asbestos inhalation? *Europ. J. Resp. Dis.*, **63**, 543–9.

Dosman, J.A., Cockcroft, D.W. and Hoeppner, V.H. (1981), Airways obstruction in occupational pulmonary diseae. *Med. Clin. No. Am.*, **65**, 691–706.

Douglas, A.N. (1980), Quantitative study of bronchial mucous gland enlargement. *Thorax*, **35**, 198–201.

Douglas, A.N., Lamb, D. and Ruckley, V.A. (1982), Bronchial gland dimensions in coalminers: influence of smoking and dust exposure. *Thorax*, **37**, 760–4.

Dunnill, M.S., Massarella, G.R. and Anderson, J.A. (1969), A comparison of the quantitative anatomy of the bronchi in normal subjects, in status asthmaticus, in chronic bronchitis, and in emphysema. *Thorax*, **24**, 176–9.

Ein, M.E., Wallace, R.J., Jr. and Williams, T.W., Jr. (1979), Allergic bronchopulmonary aspergillosis-like syndrome consequent to aspergilloma. *Am. Rev. Resp. Dis.*, **119**, 811–20.

Einhorn, L., Krause, M., Hornback, N. and Furnas, B. (1976), Enhanced pulmonary toxicity with Bleomycin and radiotherapy in oat cell lung cancer. *Cancer*, **37**, 2414–16.

Ellis, D.A., Thornley, P.E., Wightman, A.J., Walker, M., Chalmers, J. and Crofton, J.W. (1981), Present outlook in bronchiectasis: clinical and social study and review of factors influencing prognosis. *Thorax*, **36**, 659–64.

Epstein, P.E., Dauber, J.H., Rossman, M.D. and Daniele, R.P. (1982), Bronchoalveolar lavage in a patient with chronic berylliosis: evidence for hypersensitivity pneumonitis. *Ann Intern. Med.*, **97**, 213–16.

Fajardo, L.F. and Berthrong, M. (1978), Radiation injury in surgical pathology. Part 1. *Am. J. Surg. Pathol.*, **2**, 159–94.

Fink, J.N. (1982), Evaluation of the patient for occupational immunologic lung disease. *J. Allergy Clin. Immunol.*, **70**, 11–14.

Fish, J.E. (1982), Occupational asthma: a spectrum of acute respiratory disorders. *J. Occup. Med.*, **24**, 379–86.

Freiman, D.G. and Hardy, H.L. (1970), Beryllium disease. The relation of pulmonary pathology to clinical course and prognosis based on a study of 130 cases from the U.S. Beryllium Case Registry. *Human Pathol.*, **1**, 25–44.

Frigas, E., Loegering, D.A., Solley, G.O., Farrow, G.M. and Gleich, G.J. (1981), Elevated levels of eosinophil granule major basic protein in the sputum of patients with bronchial asthma. *Proc. Mayo Clin.*, **56**, 345–53.

Fulmer, J.D. (1982), Bronchoalveolar lavage. *Am. Rev. Resp. Dis.*, **126**, 961–3.

Gaensler, E.A. and Carrington, C.B. (1980), Open biopsy for chronic diffuse infiltrative lung disease: clinical, roentgenographic and physiological correlations in 502 patients. *Ann. Thorac. Surg.*, **30**, 411–26.

Gaudichet, A., Sebastien, P., Bientz, M., Jaurand, M.C., Atassi, R., Bonnaud, J. and Bignon, J. (1978), Metrologic des fibres d'amiante recueillies par lavage bronchoalveolaire. *Rev. Fr. Mal. Resp.*, **6**, 345–51.

Gee, J.B.L. (1980), Cellular mechanisms in occupational lung disease. *Chest*, **78** (suppl.), 384–7.

Gleich, G.J., Leogering, D.A., Mann, K.G. and Maldonado, J.E. (1976), Comparative properties of the Charcot-Leyden crystal protein and the major basic protein from human eosinophils. *J. Clin. Invest.*, **57**, 633–40.

Glynn, A.A. and Michaels, L. (1960), Bronchial biopsy in chronic bronchitis and asthma. *Thorax*, **15**, 142–53.

Gong, H., Jr. and Tashkin, D.P. (1979), Silicosis due to intentional inhalation of abrasive scouring powder. Case report with long-term survival and vasculitic sequelae. *Am. J. Med.*, **67**, 358–62.

Gough, J., Rivers, D. and Seal, R.M.E. (1955), Pathological studies of modified pneumoconiosis in coal-miners with rheumatoid arthritis (Caplan's syndrome). *Thorax*, **10**, 9–18.

Green, D., Dighe, P., Ali, N.O. and Katele, G.V. (1980), Pulmonary alveolar proteinosis complicating chronic myelogenous leukemia. *Cancer*, **46**, 1763–6.

Gross, N.J. (1977), Pulmonary effects of radiation therapy. *Ann. Intern. Med.*, **86**, 81–92

Gross, P. (1971), Some aspects of pneumoconiosis. In *Pathology Annual 1971* (ed. S.C. Sommers), Appleton-Century-Crofts, New York, pp. 61–79.

Härmä, R.A. and Suurkari, S. (1977), Tracheopathia chondro-osteoplastica. A clinical study of thirty cases. *Acta Otolaryngol.*, **84**, 118–23.

Harris, H.W. (chairman), Meneely, G.R., Renzetti, A., Jr., Steele, J.D. and Wyatt, J.P. (1962), Chronic bronchitis, asthma, and pulmonary emphysema. A statement by the Committee on Diagnostic Standards for Nontuberculous Respiratory Diseases. *Am. Rev. Resp. Dis.*, **85**, 762–8.

Haslan, P.L., Turton, C.W.G., Heard, B., Lukoszek, A., Collins, J.V., Salisbury, A.J. and Turner-Warwick, M. (1980), Bronchoalveolar lavage in pulmonary fibrosis: comparison of cells obtained with lung biopsy and clinical features. *Thorax*, **35**, 9–18.

Hayes, J.A. (1986), *Biopsy Pathology of the Lung*, Chapman and Hall, London.

Heard, B.E., Khatchatourov, V., Otto, H., Putov, N.V. and Sobin, L. (1979), The morphology of emphysema, chronic bronchitis, and bronchiectasis: definition, nomenclature, and classification. *J. Clin. Pathol.*, **32**, 882–92.

Hedemark, L.L., Kronenberg, R.S., Rasp, F.L., Simmons, R.L. and Peterson, P.K. (1982), The value of bronchoscopy in establishing the etiology of pneumonia in renal transplant recipients. *Am. Rev. Resp. Dis.*, **126**, 981–5.

Henderson, W.J., Gough, J. and Harse, J. (1970), Identification of mineral particles in pneumoconiotic lungs. *J. Clin. Pathol.*, **23**, 104–9.

Heppleston, A.G. (1979), Silica and asbestos: contrasts in tissue response. *Ann. N. Y. Acad. Sci.*, **330**, 725–44.

Hogg, J.C. (1982), Pathophysiology of asthma. In *Advances in Assessment and Therapy of Asthma* (eds S.W. Epstein and E.W. Middleton), *Chest*, **82** (suppl.), 8s–12s.

Hook, G.E.R., Bell, D.Y., Gilmore, L.B., Nadeau, D., Reasor, M.J. and Talley, F.A. (1978), Composition of bronchoalveolar lavage effluents from patients with pulmonary alveolar proteinosis. *Lab. Invest.*, **39**, 342–57.

Hunninghake, G.W., Gadek, J.E., Kawanami, O, Ferrans, V.J. and Crystal, R.G. (1979), Inflammatory and immune processes in the human lung in health and disease: evaluation by bronchoalveolar lavage. *Am. J. Pathol.*, **97**, 149–90.

Ito, M., Takeuchi, N., Ogura, T., Masuno, T., Hotta, H., Sakatani, M., Nishikawa, H., Yoshimoto, T. and Yamamura, Y. (1978), Pulmonary alveolar proteinosis: analysis of pulmonary washings. *Brit. J. Dis. Chest*, **72**, 313–20.

Jelihovsky, T. (1983), The structure of bronchial plugs in mucoid impaction, bronchocentric granulomatosis and asthma. *Histopathol.*, **7**, 153–67.

Johnson, F.B. (1972), Crystals in pathologic specimens. In *Pathology Annual 1972* (ed. S.C. Sommers), Appleton-Century-Crofts, New York, pp. 321–44.

Jones, A.W. (1978), Bleomycin lung damage: the pathology and nature of the lesions. *Brit. J. Dis. Chest*, **72**, 321–6.

Karr, R.M. (1980), Mechanisms of immune injury. *Chest*, **78** (suppl.), 388–92.

Karkinen-Jääskeläinen, M., Määttä, K., Pasila, M. and Saxén, L. (1982), Pulmonary berylliosis: report on a fatal case. *Brit. J. Dis. Chest*, **76**, 290–7.

Kartagener, M. (1933), Zur Pathogeneses der Bronchiektasien. I. Mitteilung: Bronchiektasien bei Situs viscerum inversus. *Beiträge klinik. Tuberkul.*, **83**, 489–501.

Katzenstein, A.A. and Askin, F.B. (1980), Interpretation and significance of pathologic findings in transbronchial lung biopsy. *Am. J. Surg. Pathol.*, **4**, 223–34.

Keeling, P.L., Pratt, I.S., Aldridge, W.N. and Smith, L.L. (1981), The enhancement of Paraquat toxicity in rats by 85% oxygen: lethality and cell-specific lung damage. *Brit. J. Exp. Path.*, **62**, 643–54.

Keenan, K.P., Wilson, T.S. and McDowell, E.M. (1983), Regeneration of hamster tracheal epithelium after mechanical injury. *Virch. Arch. (Cell Pathol.)*, **43**, 213–40.

Khan, Z.U., Sandhu, R.S., Randhawa, H.S., Menon, M.P.S. and Dusaj, I.S. (1976), Allergic bronchopulmonary aspergillosis: a study of 46 cases with special reference to laboratory aspects. *Scand. J. Resp. Dis.*, **57**, 73–87.

Kleinerman, J., Green, F., Harley, R.A., Lapp, N.L., Laqueur, W., Naeye, R.L., Pratt, P., Taylor, G., Wiot, J. and Wyatt, J. (1979), Pathology standards for coal worker's pneumoconiosis. Report of the Pneumoconiosis Committee of the College of American Pathologists to the National Institute for Occupational Safety and Health. *Arch. Pathol. Lab. Med.*, **103**, 375–432.

Koss, L.G. (1979), The respiratory tract in the absence of cancer. In *Diagnostic Cytology and Its Histopathologic Bases*, 3rd edn, J.B. Lippincott, Philadelphia, pp. 595–9.

Koss, L.G., Melamed, M.R. and Majer, K. (1965), The effect of Busulfan on human epithelia. *Am. J. Clin. Pathol.*, **44**, 385–97.

Krous, H.F. and Hamlin, W.B. (1973), Pulmonary toxicity due to Bleomycin. Report of a case. *Arch. Pathol.*, **95**, 407–10.

Kupke, K.G., Pickett, J.P., Ingram, R., Griffis, D.P., Linton, R.W. and Shelburne, J.D. (1983), Correlative light, electron, and ion microscopy on a single histologic section. *J. Microsc.*, **131**, RP1–RP2.

Lapenas, D.J., Davis, G.S., Gale, P.N. and Brody, A.R. (1982), Mineral dusts as etiologic agents in pulmonary fibrosis: the diagnostic role of analytical scanning electron microscopy. *Am. J. Clin. Pathol.*, **78**, 701–6.

Lauver, G.L., Hasan, F.M., Morgan, R.B. and Campbell, S.C. (1979), The usefulness of fiberoptic bronchoscopy in evaluating new pulmonary lesions in the compromised host. *Am. J. Med.*, **66**, 580–5.

Lee, R.J. and Fisher, R.M. (1979), Identification of fibrous and nonfibrous amphiboles in the electron microscope. *Ann. N. Y. Acad. Sci.*, **330**, 645–59.

Leff, A. (1982), Pathogenesis of asthma. Neurophysiology and pharmacology of bronchospasm. *Chest*, **81**, 224–9.

Leineweber, J.P. (1981), Fiber toxicology. *J. Occup. Med.*, **23**, 431–4.

Lewis, F.H., Beals, T.F., Carey, T.E., Baker, S.R. and Mathews, K.P. (1983), Ultrastructural and functional studies of cilia from patients with asthma, aspirin intolerance, and nasal polyps. *Chest*, **83**, 487–90.

Leyden, E. (1872), Zur Kenntniss des Bronchial-Asthma. *Virch. Arch. (Pathol. Anat.)*, **54**, 324–44.

Liebow, A.A. and Carrington, C.B. (1969), The eosinophilic pneumonias. *Med.*, **48**, 251–85.

Luna, M.A., Bedrossian, C.W.M., Lichtiger, B. and Salem, P.A. (1972), Interstitial pneumonitis associated with Bleomycin therapy. *Am. J. Clin. Pathol.*, **58**, 501–10.

Lundgren, R. and Stjernberg, N.L. (1981), Tracheobronchopathia osteochondroplastica. A clinical bronchoscopic and spirometric study. *Chest*, **80**, 706–9.

Mark, E.J. (1981), The second diagnosis: the role of the pathologist in identifying pneumoconioses in lungs excised for tumors. *Human Pathol.*, **12**, 585–7.

Mark, G.J., Monroe, C.B. and Kazemi, H. (1979), Mixed pneumoconiosis. Silicosis, asbestosis, talcosis and berylliosis. *Chest*, **75**, 726–8.

Martin, R.J., Coalson, J.J., Rogers, R.M., Horton, F.O. and Manous, L.E. (1980), Pulmonary alveolar proteinosis: the diagnosis by segmental lavage. *Am. Rev. Resp. Dis.*, **121**, 819–25.

Mason, G.R., Abraham, J.L., Hoffman, L., Cole, S., Lippmann, M. and Wasserman, K. (1982), Treatment of mixed-dust pneumoconiosis with whole lung lavage. *Am. Rev. Resp. Dis.*, **126**, 1102–7.

Mathews, K.P. (1982), Respiratory atopic disease. *J. Am. Med. Assoc.*, **248**, 2587–610.

McCook, T.A., Kirks, D.R., Morten, D.F., Osborne, D.R., Spock, A. and Pratt, P.C.

(1981), Pulmonary alveolar proteinosis in children. *Am. J. Radiol.*, **137**, 1023–7.

McCrea, E.S., Diaconis, J.N., Wade, J.C. and Johnston, C.A. (1981), Bleomycin toxicity simulating metastatic nodules to the lungs. *Cancer*, **48**, 1096–100.

McLarty, J.W., Greenberg, S.D., Hurst, G.A., Spivey, C.G., Seitzman, L.H., Hieger, L.R., Farley, M.L. and Mabry, L.C. (1980), The clinical significance of ferruginous bodies in sputa. *J. Occup. Med.*, **22**, 92–6.

Michael, J.R. and Rudin, M.L. (1981), Acute pulmonary disease caused by Phenytoin. *Ann. Intern. Med.*, **95**, 452–4.

Middleton, E., Jr., Atkins, F.M., Fanning, M. and Georgitis, J.W. (1981), Cellular mechanisms in the pathogenesis and pathophysiology of asthma. In *Symposium on Clinical Allergy. Med. Clin. No. Am.*, **65**, 1013–31.

Miller, A., Langer, A.M., Teirstein, A.S. and Selikoff, I.J. (1975), 'Nonspecific' interstitial pulmonary fibrosis. Association with asbestos fibers detected by electron microscopy. *New Engl. J. Med.*, **292**, 91–3.

Miro, J.M., Moreno, A., Coca, A., Sequru, F. and Soriano, E. (1982), Pulmonary alveolar microlithiasis with an unusual radiological pattern. *Brit. J. Dis. Chest*, **76**, 91–6.

Mitchell, R.E. and Bury, R.G. (1975), Congenital bronchiectasis due to deficiency of bronchial cartilage (Williams-Campbell syndrome). *J. Ped.*, **87**, 230–4.

Modin, B.E., Greenberg, S.D., Buffler, P.A., Lockhart, J.A., Seitzman, L.H. and Awe, R.J. (1982), Asbestos bodies in a general hospital/clinic population. *Acta Cytol.*, **26**, 667–70.

Nash, G. (1972), Necrotizing tracheobronchitis and bronchopneumonia consistent with Herpetic infection. *Human Pathol.*, **3**, 283–91.

Nash, G. (1982), Pathologic features of the lung in the immunocompromised host. *Human Pathol.*, **13**, 841–58.

Naylor, B. (1962), The shedding of the mucosa of the bronchial tree in asthma. *Thorax*, **17**, 69–72.

Naylor, B. (1977), Regarding cyanophilic bodies, toxoplasma cysts and ferruginous bodies. *Acta Cytol.*, **21**, 490–1.

Naylor, B. and Railey, C. (1964), A pitfall in the cytodiagnosis of sputum in asthmatics. *J. Clin. Pathol.*, **17**, 84–9.

Nelsen, N. (1980), Beryllium and beryllium compounds. In *On the Evaluation of the Carcinogenic Risk of Chemicals to Humans*, Vol. 23. International Agency for Research on Cancer (IARC), Lyon, pp. 143–204.

Olsen, A.M. (1942), Bronchiectasis and dextracardia: observations on the aetiology of bronchiectasis. *Amer. Rev. Resp. Dis.*, **47**, 435–9.

Orwoll, E.S., Kiessling, P.J. and Patterson, J.R. (1978), Interstitial pneumonia from Mitomycin. *Ann. Intern. Med.*, **89**, 352–5.

Patterson, R. and Goldstein, R.A. (1982), Occupational immunologic lung disease. *J. Allergy Clin. Immunol.*, **70**, 1–72.

Pepys, J. (1982), Occupational asthma: an overview. *J. Occup. Med.*, **24**, 534–8.

Perlow, G.M., Jain, B.P., Pauker, S.G., Zarren, H.S., Wistran, D.C. and Epstein, R.L. (1981), Tocainide-associated interstitial pneumonitis. *Ann. Intern. Med.*, **94**, 489–90.

Pickett, J.P., Ingram, P. and Shelburne, J.D. (1980), Identification of inorganic particulates in a single histologic section using both light microscopy and x-ray microprobe analysis. *J. Histotechnol.*, **3**, 155–8.

Podall, L.N. and Winkler, S.S. (1974), Busulfan lung. Report of two cases and review of the literature. *Am. J. Roen. Rad. Ther. Nucl. Med.*, **120**, 151–6.

Pounder, D.J. and Pieterse, A.S. (1982), Tracheopathia osteoplastica: report of four cases. *Pathol.*, **14**, 429–33.

Prakash, U.B.S., Barham, S.S., Rosenow, E.C., III, Brown, M.L. and Payne, W.S. (1983), Pulmonary alveolar microlithiasis. A review including ultrastructural and pulmonary function studies. *Mayo Clin. Proc.*, **58**, 290–300.

Primer, G. (1979), Tracheobronchopathia osteochondroplastica. *Prax. Pneumol.*, **33**, 1060–3.

Rall, D.P. (1977), Asbestos. In *Monographs on the Evaluation of Carcinogenic Risk of Chemical to Man*, Vol. 14. International Agency for Research on Cancer (IARC), Lyon.

Reed, C.E. and deShazo, R. (1982), Immunologic aspects of granulomatous and interstitial lung diseases. *J. Am. Med. Assoc.*, **248**, 2683–91.

Reid, L. (1954), Pathology of chronic bronchitis. *Lancet*, **i**, 275–8.

Reid, L. (1960), Measurement of the bronchial mucous gland layer: a diagnostic yardstick in chronic bronchitis. *Thorax*, **15**, 132–41.

Reynolds, H.Y., Fulmer, J.D., Kazmierowski, J.A., Roberts, W.C., Frank, M.M. and Crystal, R.G. (1977), Analysis of cellular and protein content of broncho-alveolar lavage fluid from patients with idiopathic pulmonary fibrosis and chronic hypersensitivity pneumonitis. *J. Clin. Invest.*, **59**, 165–75.

Riley, D.J., Mackenzie, J.W., Uhlman, W.E. and Edelman, N.J. (1975), Allergic bronchopulmonary aspergillosis: evidence of limited tissue invasion. *Am. Rev. Resp. Dis.*, **111**, 232–6.

Roeckel, I.E. (1973), Pathologic alterations in the lung following use of immuno-suppressant agents. *Ann. Clin. Lab. Sci.*, **3**, 212–18.

Roggli, V.L., Greenberg, S.D., McLarty, J.W., Hurst, G.A., Heiger, L.R., Farley, M.L. and Mabry, L.C. (1980a), Comparison of sputum and lung asbestos body counts in former asbestos workers. *Am. Rev. Resp. Dis.*, **122**, 941–5.

Roggli, V.L., Greenberg, S.D., Seitzman, L.H., McGavran, M.H., Hurst, G.A., Spivey, C.G., Nelson, K.G. and Hieger, L.R. (1980b), Pulmonary fibrosis, carcinoma, and ferruginous body counts in amosite asbestos workers. A study of six cases. *Am. J. Clin. Pathol.*, **73**, 496–503.

Roggli, V.L. and Shelburne, J.D. (1982), New concepts in the diagnosis of mineral pneumoconioses. In *Seminars in Respiratory Medicine*, Vol. 4, Thieme-Stratton, New York, pp. 138–48.

Rosen, P., Melamed, M. and Savino, A. (1972), The 'ferruginous-body' content of lung tissue: a quantitative study of 86 patients. *Acta Cytol.*, **16**, 207–11.

Rosen, S.H., Castleman, B., Liebow, A.A., Enzinger, F.M. and Hunt, R.T.N. (1958), Pulmonary alveolar proteinosis. *New Engl. J. Med.*, **258**, 1123–42.

Rosenberg, M., Patterson, R., Mintzer, R., Cooper, B.J., Roberts, M. and Harris, K.E. (1977), Clinical and immunologic criteria for the diagnosis of allergic bronchopulmonary aspergillosis. *Ann. Intern. Med.*, **86**, 405–14.

Rossiter, S.J., Miller, D.C., Churg, A.M., Carrington, C.B. and Mark, J.B.O. (1979), Open lung biopsy in the immunosuppressed patient, is it really beneficial? *J. Thorac. Cardiov. Surg.*, **77**, 338–45.

Roswit, B. and White, D.C. (1977), Severe radiation injuries of the lung. *Am. J. Roent.*, **129**, 127–36.

Rubin, E., Weisbrod, G.L. and Sanders, D.E. (1980), Pulmonary alveolar proteinosis. Relationship to silicosis and pulmonary infection. *Radiol.*, **135**, 35–41.

Sakula, A. (1968), Tracheobronchopathia osteoplastica. Its relationship to primary tracheobronchial amyloidosis. *Thorax*, **23**, 105–10.

Samter, M. and Beers, R.F., Jr. (1968), Intolerance to aspirin. Clinical studies and consideration of its pathogenesis. *Ann. Intern. Med.*, **68**, 975–83.

Sanerkin, N.G. and Evans, D.M.D. (1965), The sputum in bronchial asthma: pathognomonic patterns. *J. Pathol. Bact.*, **89**, 535–41.

Schatz, M., Wasserman, S. and Patterson, R. (1981), Eosinophils and immunologic lung disease. In *Symposium on Clinical Allergy. Med. Clin. No. Am.*, **65**, 1055–71.

Schlueter, D.P. (1982), Infiltrative lung disease hypersensitivity pneumonitis. *J. Allergy Clin. Immunol.*, **70**, 50–5.

Shelburne, J.D., Wisseman, C.L., Broda, K.R., Roggli, V.L. and Ingram, P. (1983), Lung – nonneoplastic conditions. In *Diagnostic Electron Microscopy*, Vol. 4 (eds B.F. Trump and R.T. Jones), Wiley, New York, pp. 475–538.

Sieniewicz, D.J. and Nidecker, A.C. (1980), Conglomerate pulmonary disease: a form of talcosis in intravenous methadone abusers. *Am. J. Roent.*, **135**, 697–702.

Sluis-Cremer, G.K. (1980), Active pulmonary tuberculosis discovered at postmortem examination of the lungs of black miners. *Brit. J. Dis. Chest*, **74**, 374–8.

Sly, R.M. (1982), Pathogenesis of asthma. *Ann. Allergy*, **49**, 16–19.

Smith, L.J. (1981), Bronchoalveolar lavage today. *Chest*, **80**, 251–2.

Snider, D.E., Jr. (1978), The relationship between tuberculosis and silicosis. *Am. Rev. Resp. Dis.*, **118**, 455–60.

Snider, G.L. (1981), Pathogenesis of emphysema and chronic bronchitis. In *Symposium on Obstructive Lung Diseases* (ed. R.A. Matthay), *Med. Clin. No. Am.*, **65**, W.B. Saunder, Philadelphia, pp. 647–65.

Sostman, H.D., Matthay, R.A. and Putnam, C.E. (1977), Cytotoxic drug-induced lung disease. *Am. J. Med.*, **62**, 608–15.

Stellman, J.L., Spicer, J.E. and Cayton, R.M. (1982), Morbidity from chronic asthma. *Thorax*, **37**, 218–21.

Stenius, B.S.M. and Lemola, M. (1976), Hypersensitivity to acetylsalicylic acid (ASA) and tartrazine in patients with asthma. *Clin. Allergy*, **6**, 119–29.

Surgeon General of the United States (1982) Office on Smoking and Health, The health consequence of smoking: cancer. A Report of the Surgeon General. Rockville, Maryland, Public Health Service, US Department of Health and Human Services.

Szwed, J.J. (1970), Pulmonary angiothrombosis caused by 'Blue Velvet' addiction. *Ann. Intern. Med.*, **73**, 771–4.

Takizawa, T. and Thurlbeck, W.M. (1971), Muscle and mucous gland size in the major bronchi of patients with chronic bronchitis, asthma, and asthmatic bronchitis. *Am. Rev. Resp. Dis.*, **104**, 331–6.

Tao, L.-C. (1978), Microliths in sputum specimens and their relationship to pulmonary microlithiasis. *Am. J. Clin. Pathol.*, **69**, 482–5.

Taylor, A.J.N. (1980), Occupational asthma. *Thorax*, **35**, 241–5.

Teja, K., Cooper, P.H., Squires, J.E. and Schnatterly, P.T. (1981), Pulmonary alveolar proteinosis in four siblings. *New Engl. J. Med.*, **305**, 1390–2.

Thurlbeck, W.M., Henderson, J.A., Fraser, R.G. and Bates, D.V. (1970), Chronic obstructive lung disease. A comparison between clinical, roentgenologic, functional and morphologic criteria in chronic bronchitis, emphysema, asthma and bronchiectasis. *Med.*, **49**, 81–147.

Thurlbeck, W.M. and Thurlbeck, S.M. (1976), Pulmonary effects of Paraquat poisoning. *Chest*, **70**, 276–80.

Tomashefski, J.F., Jr. (1982), Benign endobronchial mesenchymal tumors. Their relationship to parenchymal pulmonary hamartomas. *Am. J. Surg. Pathol.*, **6**, 531–40.

Tomashefski, J.F., Jr. and Hirsch, C.S. (1980), The pulmonary vascular lesions of intravenous drug abuse. *Human Pathol.*, **11**, 133–45.

Torgersen, J. (1949), Genetic factors in visceral asymmetry and in the development and pathologic changes of lungs, heart and abdominal organs. *Arch. Pathol.*, **47**, 566–93.

Tryka, A.F., Skornik, W.A., Godleski, J.J. and Brain, J.D. (1982), Potentiation of Bleomycin-induced lung injury by exposure to 70% oxygen. Morphologic assessment. *Am. Rev. Resp. Dis.*, **126**, 1074–9.

Van Nierop, M.A.M.F., Wagenaar, Sj.Sc., Van den Bosch, J.M.M. and Westermann, C.J.J. (1983), Tracheobronchopathia osteochondroplastica. *Europ. J. Resp. Dis.*, **64**, 129–33.

Wagner, J.C. (1980), The biological effects of mineral fibers. In International Agency for Research on Cancer (IARC) Scientific Publication no. 30, Lyon.

Walker, K.R. and Fullmer, C.D. (1970), Progress report on study of respiratory spirals. *Acta Cytol.*, **14**, 396–8.

Wall, C.P., Gaensler, E.A., Carrington, C.B. and Hayes, J.A. (1981), Comparison of transbronchial and open biopsies in chronic infiltrative lung disease. *Am. Rev. Resp. Dis.*, **123**, 280–5.

Ward, P.A., Senior, R.M. and Cole, S. (1978), The immunopathologic basis of hypersensitivity pneumonitis. In *The Lung Structure, Function and Disease* (eds W.M. Thurlbeck and M.A. Abell), Williams and Wilkins, Baltimore, pp. 88–95.

Warnock, M.L. and Churg, A.M. (1980), Asbestos bodies. *Chest*, **77**, 129–30.

Wayne, K.S. and Taussig, L.M. (1976), Probable familial congenital bronchiectasis due to cartilage deficiency (Williams-Campbell syndrome). *Am. Rev. Resp. Dis.*, **114**, 15–22.

Weiss, R.B. and Muggia, F.M. (1980), Cytotoxic drug-induced pulmonary disease: update 1980. *Am. J. Med.*, **68**, 259–66.

Whitaker, D. (1978), Asbestos bodies in sputum. *Acta Cytol.*, **22**, 443–4.

Whitcomb, M.E. (1973), Drug-induced lung disease. *Chest*, **63**, 418–22.

Whitwell, F. (1952), A study of the pathology and pathogenesis of bronchiectasis. *Thorax*, **7**, 213–39.

Whitwell, F., Scott, J. and Grimshaw, M. (1977), Relationship between occupations and asbestos-fibre content of the lungs of patients with pleural mesothelioma, lung cancer and other diseases. *Thorax*, **32**, 377–86.

Williams, H. and Campbell, P. (1960), Generalized bronchiectasis associated with deficiency of cartilage in the bronchial tree. *Arch. Dis. Child.*, **35**, 182–91.

Williams, W.J. (1958), A histological study of the lungs in 52 cases of chronic beryllium disease. *Brit. J. Indust. Med.*, **15**, 84–91.

Wright, E.P., Holmberg, K., Houston, J., Morrison, I.M. and Roberts, C. (1983), Pulmonary actinomycosis simulating a bronchial neoplasm. *J. Infect.*, **6**, 179–81.

Young, R.H., Sandstrom, R.E. and Mark, G.J. (1980), Tracheopathia osteoplastica. Clinical, radiologic, and pathological correlations. *J. Thorac. Cardiovasc. Surg.*, **79**, 537–41.

Ziskind, M., Jones, R.N. and Weill, H. (1976), Silicosis. *Am. Rev. Resp. Dis.*, **113**, 643–65.

6 Granulomatous reactions

6.1 Definition of granuloma

Granulomatous reactions are inflammatory responses to a variety of specific pathogens, particulate materials and some nonspecific irritants. Sometimes the etiology is unknown. In those lesions in which the etiology has been established, a common factor is the presence of a sustained tissue irritant which is poorly degraded by the defense mechanisms of the host. The irritant may persist because it is only slowly dissolved or degraded by enzymes or because it is capable of replication within the tissue. There is evidence that granulomas persist only as long as the irritant is present (Adams, 1975) and granulomatous inflammations serve to sequester the irritant. It is attractive to propose that under all of these conditions there is a slow but continuing antigenic stimulus responsible for the reaction, but this has not been proven. A number of excellent reviews are available for a more detailed examination of granulomatous reactions (Adams, 1976; Siltzbach, 1976; Spector, 1976; Epstein, 1977; Boros, 1978; Spector, 1980; Williams and Davies, 1980; Spector, 1982).

The morphological key to granulomatous reactions is the formation of granulomas (Fig. 6.1). Granulomas are organized groups of inflammatory cells, the principal of which is the macrophage and its derivatives, the epithelioid cell and the multinucleated giant cell. Lymphocytes, leukocytes and fibrocytes play variable roles in the development, organization, and ultimate fate of the granuloma (James and Neville, 1977; Cain and Kraus, 1982; Müller-Hermelink *et al.*, 1982). The granuloma is more or less spherical with the macrophages localized centrally and surrounded by lymphocytes, leukocytes and fibrocytes. Granulomas vary in size from those formed by only a few macrophages (and therefore hardly recognizable) to large coalescent nodules, several centimeters in diameter.

Although individual granulomas are small enough to be contained completely within the tissue of a fiberoptic bronchoscope mucosal or transbronchial biopsy (Mitchell *et al.*, 1980; Armstrong *et al.*, 1981; Wallace *et al.*, 1981; Kataria *et al.*, 1982), incomplete recovery, fragmentation and mechanical distortion may make recognition difficult. Furthermore, the morphological distinctions between types of granulomatous lesions are

192

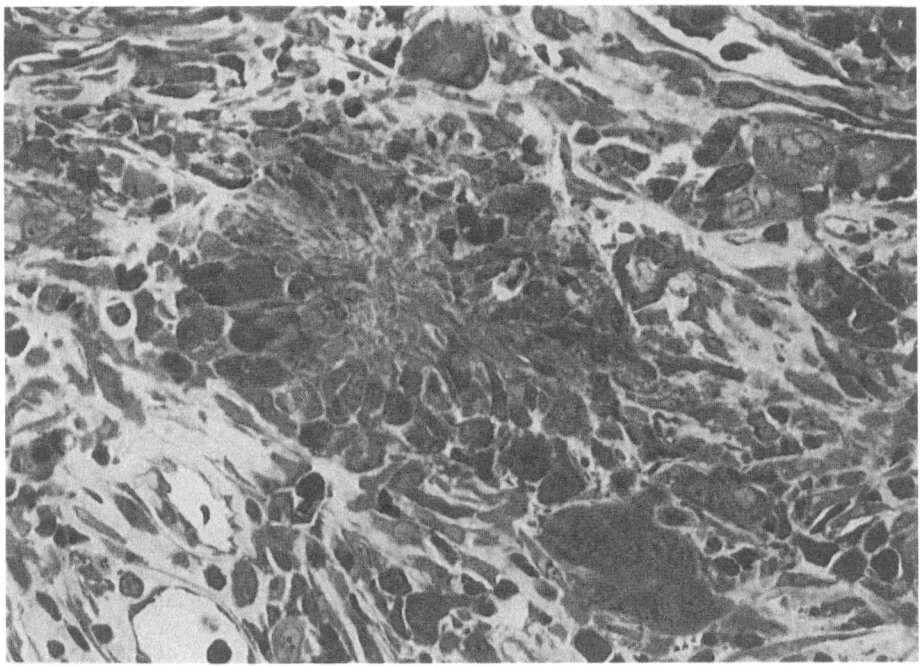

Fig. 6.1 Granuloma. Organized macrophages, epithelioid cells and multinucleated giant cells form a spherical cluster, which when cut in section gives this characteristic round appearance with somewhat radial symmetry. (Epon/Araldite section stained with toluidine blue: × 470.)

often subtle, even under ideal circumstances, and may be unrecognizable in the small biopsies. For these reasons the surgical pathologist (and the clinician) should not expect to be able to be very specific in the final diagnosis. In this chapter we will present some of the microscopically characteristic features of the more important granulomatous reactions, to assist in their recognition. If the specimen does not allow a definite diagnosis, a more substantial biopsy should be obtained, preferably an open wedge biopsy.

Most granulomatous reactions which are accessible to the fiberoptic bronchoscope are infectious (Katzenstein and Askin, 1980; Ulbright and Katzenstein, 1980; Nash, 1982; Churg, 1983). Histological diagnosis relies upon identification of the micro-organism (Chapter 4), which usually requires multiple sections and special stains. Those few caused by particulate inorganic materials are diagnosed by discovery and identification of the material and by inquiry into possible environmental exposure (Section 5.8). The remaining granulomatous lesions are caused by as of yet

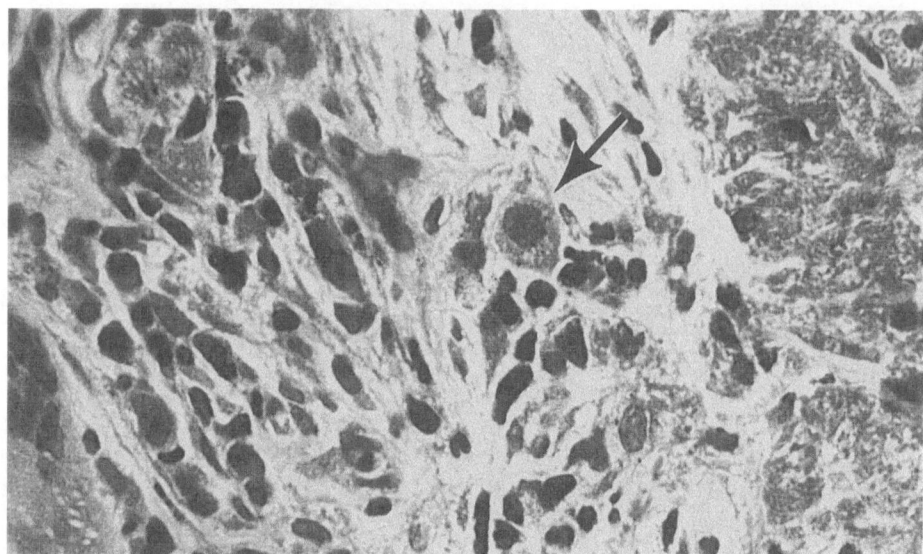

Fig. 6.2   Macrophage in granulomatous reaction (arrow). The cell appears discrete from its neighbors and has particulate material in the cytoplasm and an eccentric nucleus. (Paraffin section stained with hematoxylin and eosin: × 740.)

unrecognized 'agents'. Although relatively rare, the diseases in the last group each have different clinical significance and their specific diagnosis is essential to the appropriate handling of individual patients (Cole *et al.*, 1983). Particularly when the specimen is scanty it should be remembered that granulomas or at least reactions mimicking granulomas have been reported as reactions to neoplasms (Gregorie *et al.*, 1962).

6.2   The cellular components of the granulomatous reaction

The macrophage is the principal (and essential) cellular component of the granuloma. After considerable investigation (Lasser, 1983) it is now accepted that these cells are derived from monocyte precursors of the bone marrow and are part of the mononuclear phagocyte system of van Furth *et al.* (1972). The alveolar macrophage is part of this system (van Furth, 1980) and there may also be resident cells in the pulmonary interstitium

Fig. 6.3   Epithelioid cells. (a) Mixture of epithelioid and other inflammatory cells including two cells in mitosis (arrows). (b) Organized epithelioid cells in a granuloma. The cells are elongated, tend to blend together and have abundant eosinophilic cytoplasm. (Paraffin sections stained with hematoxylin and eosin: × 710.)

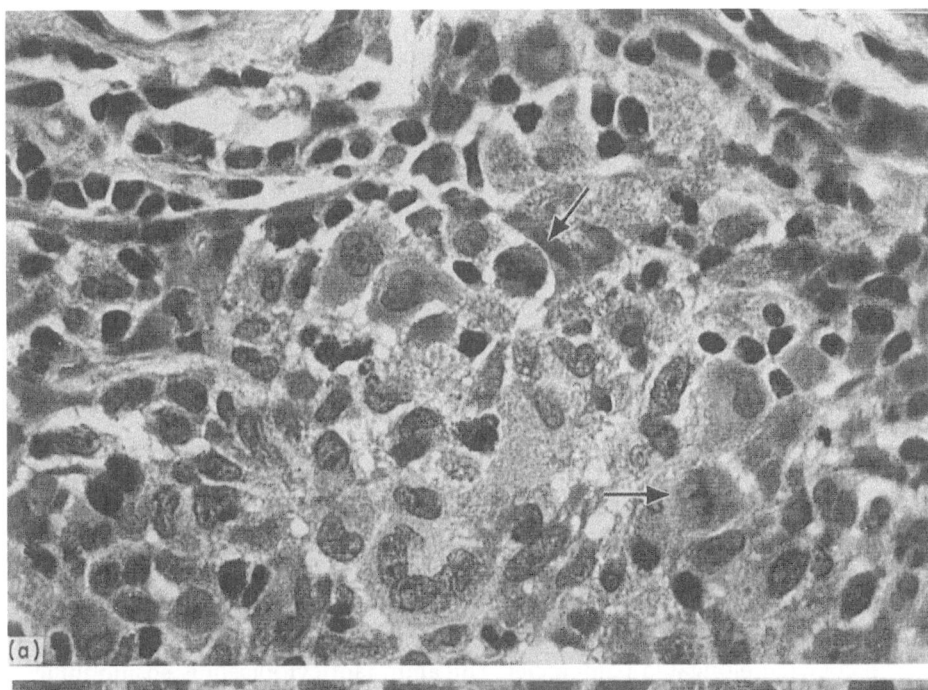

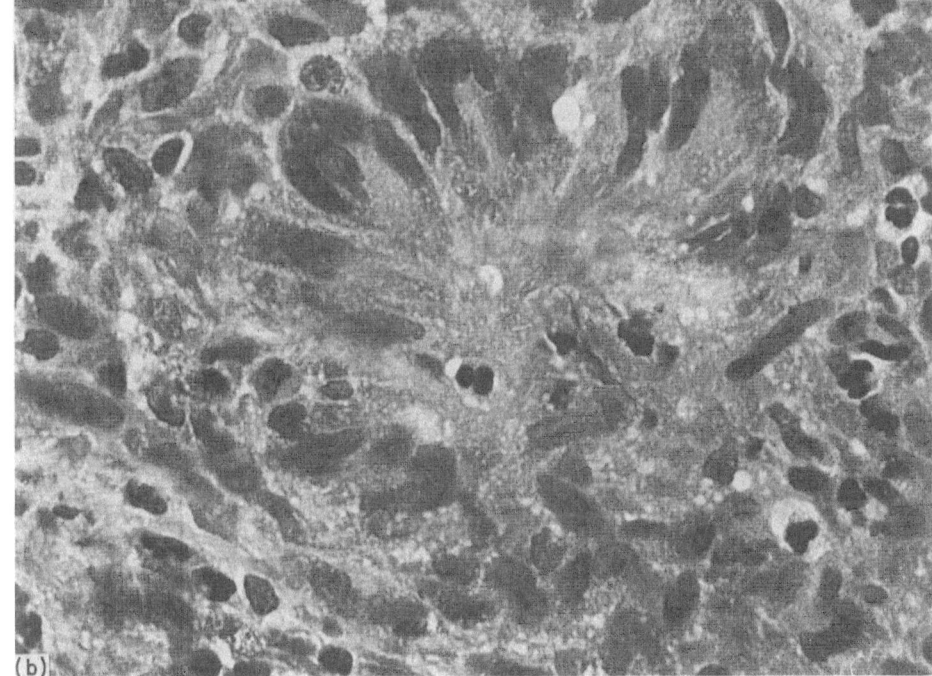

(Bowden and Adamson, 1980). Most of the macrophages which join in the development and maintenance of granulomas are derived from monocytes circulating in the blood (Epstein, 1977; Spector, 1982; van Furth and van Oud Albas, 1982). Macrophages are motile and phagocytic and tend to be discrete round cells with eccentrically located nuclei and a moderate amount of cytoplasm (Fig. 6.2). (The term histiocyte is used by some to mean tissue macrophage. However, it is also used for other cells not necessarily of the mononuclear phagocyte system.) It is known that macrophages participate in the presentation of some antigens to T lymphocytes (Unanue, 1975), but it is probably their phagocytic activity which is important in the early development of granulomas (Boros, 1978; Spector, 1982). Macrophages synthesize lysosomal enzymes which are largely responsible for the destruction/dissolution of the inciting agent and may result in necrosis within the granuloma. As long as the phagocytosed material is not totally degraded, the granuloma is maintained by the constant immigration of new macrophages and the proliferation of existing ones.

Epithelioid cells are functionally altered macrophages (Sutton and Weiss, 1966; Epstein and Krasnobrod, 1968; Papadimitriou and Spector, 1971; Spector, 1976). These cells are larger than macrophages and have somewhat elongated pale nuclei. The abundant cytoplasm is eosinophilic (Fig. 6.3). The cells are closely adherent and by light microscopy adjacent cells appear to blend together. By electron microscopy this is shown to be the result of close interdigitation of the numerous surface ruffles characteristic of these cells (Williams *et al.*, 1970; Papadimitriou *et al.*, 1973; Adams, 1974; Spector, 1976). All ultrastructural studies suggest that the cytoplasmic apparatus is organized for synthetic activity. The exact nature of the synthesized product is unknown, and the principal function of the epithelioid cell remains speculative. Phagocytic ability is either absent or minimized and one key to the identification of these cells in mixed inflammatory reactions is their lack of phagocytosed material. The stimulus for macrophage evolution to epithelioid cell is controversial and may be variable. The changes can at least experimentally be spontaneous, leading Spector (1976) to propose that macrophages which have accumulated at a site of activity but are unable to find material to engulf change into epithelioid cells. Müller-Hermelink *et al.* (1982) suggest that T lymphocytes stimulate the development and organization of epithelioid cells. Epithelioid cells can divide, producing macrophages (Spector, 1976). Otherwise their life span is limited to several weeks. Studies have demonstrated that the surface receptors for the Fc portion of IgG, C_3 and lymphocytes, characteristic of macrophages (Groopman and Golde, 1981), are lost (or masked) on epithelioid cells (Mariano *et al.*, 1976; Ridley *et al.*, 1978).

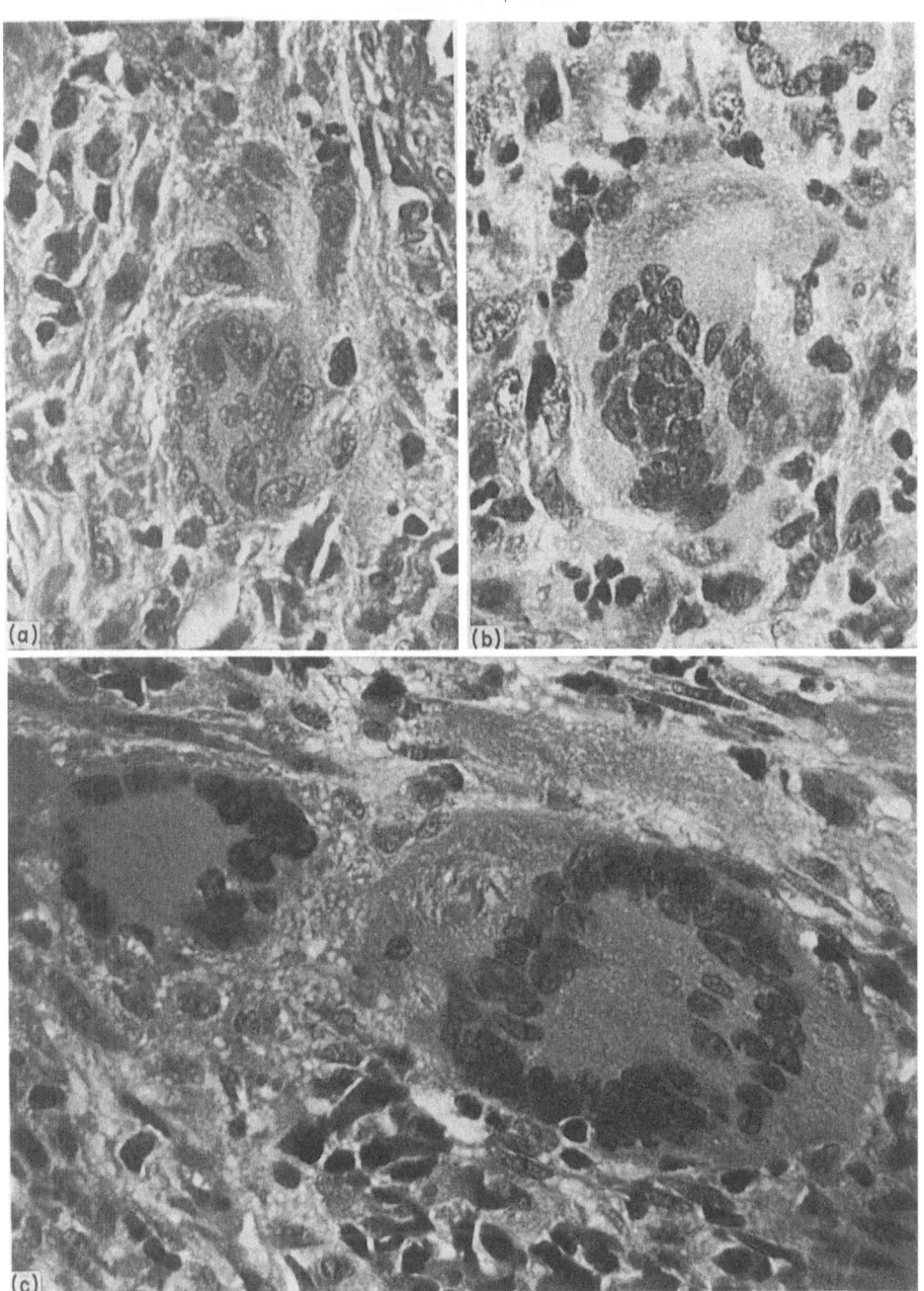

Fig. 6.4 Multinucleated giant cells. (a) Unorganized giant cell early in its formation. (b) More developed giant cell with nuclei organized at one pole of the syncythium. The nuclei tend to be oriented with their long axes in the same direction. (c) Two very organized giant cells with their nuclei distributed in a ring. (Paraffin sections stained with hematoxylin and eosin: × 740.)

Multinucleated giant cells are easily recognized components of most granulomatous reactions (Fig. 6.4). It is now accepted that these form by the fusion of macrophages and/or epithelioid cells (Chambers, 1978). Specifically in granulomatous reactions they are formed by the fusion of macrophages (Sutton and Weiss, 1966; Spector, 1976; Cain and Kraus, 1982). Ultrastructurally they have an active appearing cytoplasm with a large number of mitochondria, abundant endoplasmic reticulum and Golgi apparatus. They are capable of synchronous nuclear division (Mariano and Spector, 1974). At least some multinucleated giant cells are formed by the continuous fusion of newly arriving macrophages. The surface of multinucleated cells is similar to that of epithelioid cells, covered with numerous ruffles. Unlike epithelioid cells, multinucleated giant cells may contain phagocytosed material or micro-organisms. Whether this phago-cytosis occurs prior to the formation of the giant cell or after is not known. There is some evidence that without the fusion of new macrophages, multinucleated giant cells would have a short life span of about one week (Mariano and Spector, 1974; Epstein, 1977). The function of multinucle-ated giant cells in granulomas remains a matter of conjecture.

It has been traditional to subdivide multinucleated giant cells into two types based on the location of the nuclei. The foreign body type has randomly distributed nuclei (Fig. 6.4a) while the Langhans' type has nuclei organized either at one 'pole' of the cell (Fig. 6.4b) or spaced peripherally (Fig. 6.4c). Accumulated evidence has shown that these are different degrees of orderly arrangement and not really different cell types. Lan-ghans' giant cells develop through a stage of foreign body configuration; then as the cytoskeleton develops and the overall distribution of cellular components becomes more organized the Langhans' form evolves. Cain and Kraus (1982) studied the sequence of maturation or ordering of the multinuclear cell using immunofluorescent markers for components of the cytoskeleton. Pathologists will probably continue to use the terms Lang-hans' and foreign body giant cells because it is so convenient; what is important is not to equate diagnostic significance to these structural changes.

Several histologically distinctive inclusions can be seen in multinucle-ated giant cells (Fig. 6.5). Schaumann (1941) described certain 'peculiar corpuscles' which subsequently have been termed Schaumann's bodies (Fig. 6.5a). These are cytoplasmic densely basophilic inclusions, sometimes with a roughly spherical shape but often with a more convoluted form likened to a conch shell. Schaumann or conchoid bodies are built up by the successive deposition of material containing calcium and iron and, when sectioned, display a multilaminar appearance. They are rather similar to microliths (which are, however, usually extracellular) and cor-pora amylacea (which are eosinophilic) except that these two structures

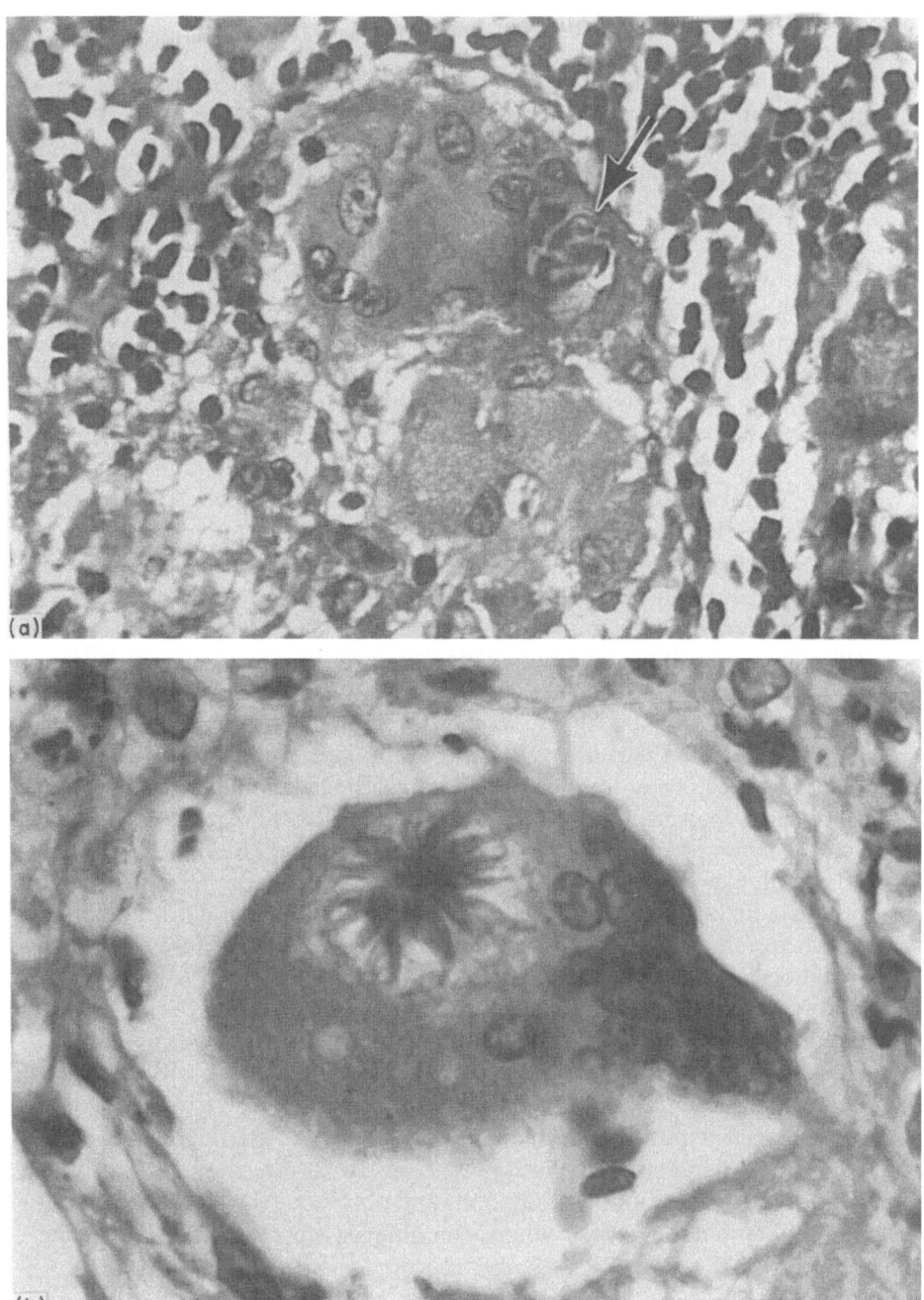

Fig. 6.5 Distinctive inclusion bodies in multinucleated giant cells. (a) Schaumann (conchoid) body. In this section the body (arrow), which contains iron and calcium salts, has become fragmented during sectioning. (b) Asteroid body. The brightly eosinophilic cytoplasmic inclusion is a condensation of organized cytoskeleton. (Paraffin sections stained with hematoxylin and eosin: × 760.)

tend to have smooth outlines. A Schaumann body is thought to be a reactive intracellular encrustation of a particulate nidus because particulate material is present at the center (Longcope and Freiman, 1952; Rasmussen and Caulfield, 1960; Williams, 1960; Uehlinger, 1963; Zak, 1964; Kraus, 1980; Wang et al., 1981). Since these bodies enlarge with time, they are variable in size from barely detectible to those larger than nuclei. They can be multiple.

Asteroid bodies (Fig. 6.5b) are eosinophilic, star-shaped, cytoplasmic cytoskeletal structures. In well-developed Langhans' giant cells the cytoplasmic focus of organization is called the cytosphere, composed of centrioles and radially arranged microtubules and microfilaments. These components become condensed and the distinctive asteroid body is the expression of this aggregation (Cain and Kraus, 1983). In some multinucleated giant cells associated with granulomas there are also less easily distinguished perinuclear vesicular inclusions called microcentrosomes. The Schaumann body, asteroid body and vesicular inclusions are seen more frequently in sarcoidosis but are not diagnostically useful since they are also seen in other granulomatous reactions (Longcope and Freiman, 1952; Williams, 1960; Uehlinger, 1963).

Lymphocytes have been shown to be directly involved in granulomatous inflammation and specifically in the development of granulomas (Hunninghake et al., 1980; Crystal et al., 1981; James and Williams, 1982). They are specifically involved in the accelerated granulomas which develop in hypersensitivity, and they produce lymphokines which will activate macrophages (a process that may be important in the early process of granulomatous reactions). T lymphocytes are usually present in large numbers in well-organized granulomas. On the other hand granulomas which develop in response to foreign bodies may have few associated lymphocytes. For a review see Boros (1978).

Polymorphonuclear leukocytes are probably involved in nearly all granulomatous lesions at their onset and may be a conspicuous component of certain fully developed reactions. Eosinophils are associated with parasitic-induced granulomas and antigen-antibody complex reactions. Fibrocytes and collagen deposition are features of some of the granulomatous reactions. As can be seen in Section 6.5 and Table 6.1, the association of lymphocytes, neutrophils, eosinophils and fibrosis can be an aid in refining the differential diagnoses when granulomas are present in bronchial biopsies.

6.3 Types of necrosis in granulomas

Necrosis may occur in granulomas or may be associated with granulomatous reactions. Caseous necrosis, equated with infectious granulomas

Table 6.1 Morphological characteristics of granulomatous reactions in bronchial biopsies

Disease entity	Morphology of granulomas	Necrosis	Giant cell inclusions	Lymphocytes	Neutrophils	Eosinophils	Fibrosis	Vessel involvement	Microorganism
Infectious	Complex Many giant cells Epithelioid cells Confluent	Caseous	Intra- or extracellular organisms	Abundant	Early	Usually not	End stage may calcify	May have perivascular lymphs	Positive
Foreign body	Mature	No	May contain the particles	Minimal	Early	No	Yes	Small vessels when 2° to IV abuse	No
Silicosis	Nodules Giant cells early	Of macrophages but not conspicuous	Birefringent particles usually extracellular	Early	Early	No	Extensive nodules	No	No
Sarcoidosis	Epithelioid Compact	Minimal except in rare necrotizing type	Frequent: asteroid, and Schaumann bodies	Minimal	No	No	Surrounding nodules	No	No
Berylliosis	Epithelioid Non-necrotizing	Minimal	Frequent: asteroid, and Schaumann bodies	Abundant interstitial	No	No	Late	No	No
Wegener's granulomatosis	Poorly organized Necrosis Angiocentric	Extensive particularly of arteries and veins	Not reported	Abundant	Yes	Rare	?	Destructive of arteries and veins	No
Bronchocentric granulomatosis	Pallisading Epithelioid cells Noncaseous	Yes, bronchial walls	Not reported	Abundant	Yes	Abundant	Yes	Yes Veins spared	Septate hyphae

formed in response to *M. tuberculosis* but seen in other infections as well, appears coincident with the onset of immunological sensitivity (Dannenberg, 1968). Eosinophilic, granular necrotic debris accumulates in the center of the developing granuloma (Fig. 6.6). As these granulomas coalesce the caseous material increases to form large deposits of 'cheezy' material visible to the unaided eye. It is the macroscopic character of this material which is the source of the term caseous. Tubercle bacilli and the yeast forms of *H. capsulatum* can be demonstrated within the necrotic debris. Fibrinoid necrosis, such as that seen in Wegener's granulomatosis, has a rich eosinophilic hyaline appearance and is associated more with the blood vessels than the granuloma itself (Fig. 6.7). Purulent necrosis can also be seen in these granulomatous reactions.

6.4 Classification

When morphologically recognizable entities are found to have a variety of causes there are often many systems developed to categorize the types. The granulomatous reactions are no exception. Each of those systems

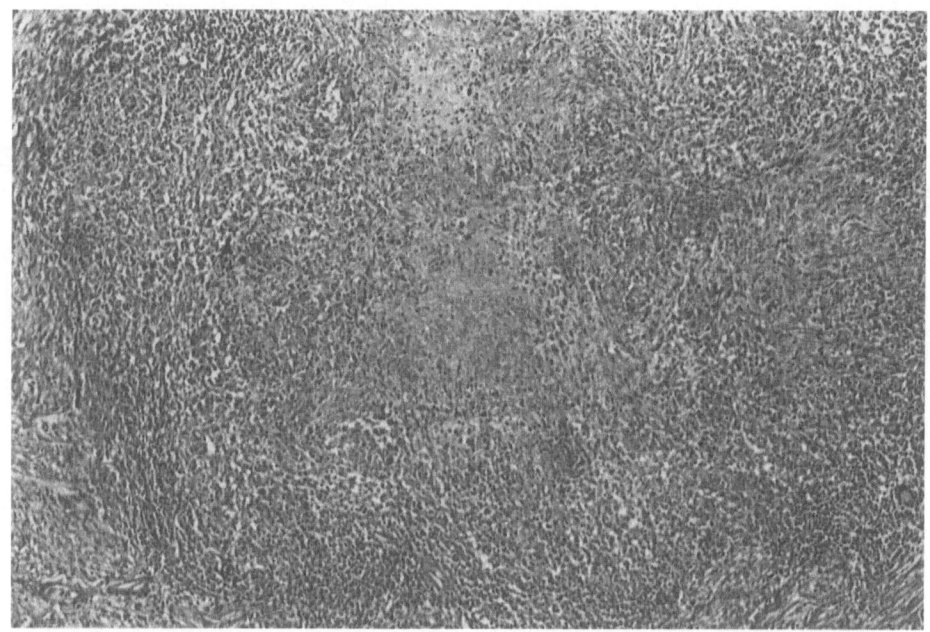

Fig. 6.6 Caseous necrosis in the center of several coalescing tuberculous granulomas. The eosinophilic granular but acellular focus of necrosis is surrounded by granulomas with large numbers of lymphocytes. (Paraffin section stained with hematoxylin and eosin: × 70.)

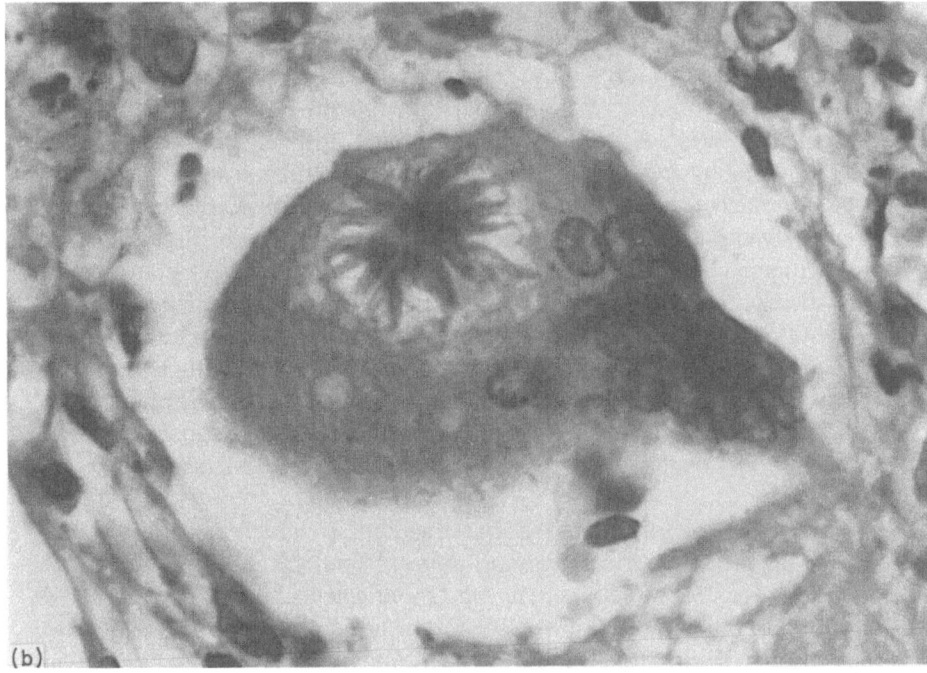

(b)

Fig. 6.7 Fibrinoid necrosis. Wegener's granulomatosis. Biopsy includes a moderate-sized vessel totally obliterated by necrotizing granulomatous reaction with focal fibrinoid necrosis associated with the vessel wall (arrows). (Paraffin section stained with hematoxylin and eosin: × 80.)

proposed to date have advantages and disadvantages. It is the ultimate goal of the pathologist to identify the specific agent responsible for the lesion they are seeing. Nevertheless, a classification of granulomatous lesions by etiology becomes a cumbersome listing of diseases, and there remain some entities with no known etiology. What is needed is a manageable classification which will facilitate our understanding and/or description of the reactions. A useful subdivision separates the reactions into those centered around blood vessels (angiocentric) and those centered around bronchi (bronchocentric). This is particularly helpful with large specimens such as open lung biopsies, lobectomies and autopsies. It also allows some meaningful subcategorizations and has significance as to the mechanisms of the disease processes. Unfortunately, it is of little value in the bronchial specimens, since the overall anatomical pattern is rarely discernible in the small tissue fragments.

A traditional approach to the classification of these lesions used the various types of necrosis (or lack thereof) to separate the groups. Caseous, fibrinoid, etc., are recognizable histologically, but there is such a mixture of diseases and so much overlap of specific etiologies that this system is now used only in a descriptive sense.

Spector (1976), observing the cellular dynamics in granuloma, separated them into *high turnover*, with massive daily replenishment of macrophages and many epithelioid cells and giant cells, and *low turnover*, with a relatively stable population of macrophages, epithelioid and giant cells. This approach has done much to alter our concept of the granuloma, previously viewed as a semipermanent structure, and correctly emphasized the dynamic changes which occur even in the low turnover granulomas. The disadvantages of this classification are its oversimplicity and the inability of surgical pathologists to see such cellular dynamics in biopsy tissue. Subsequent studies have also demonstrated that high and low turnover lesions can be found in a single disease such as sarcoidosis in which early granulomas are high turnover, whereas late stage lesions tend to be low turnover (van der Gaag *et al.*, 1983; van Maarsseveen *et al.*, 1983).

Warren (1976) formulated a classification in which he stressed the current state of immunological and pathophysiological understanding of granulomatous reactions. *Immunologic granulomas*, either of cell mediated or antibody mediated type, were distinguished because prior exposure to the causative agent altered the response. *Nonimmunological granulomas*, in which prior challenge did not alter subsequent reactions, were subdivided into *inactive*, with a rapidly developing lesion which quickly becomes quiescent, and *active*, with chronicity caused by continuous immigration of new macrophages. This classification does very little for the surgical pathologist since morphological features are not stressed and often do not correlate. However, it does help understand the apparently heterogeneous group of diseases associated with granulomatous tissue reactions. The subtypes were based on well-documented experimental models (Warren, 1976). However, in practice the distinctions blur somewhat and the immunological group in particular may have clinical entities with mixed cell mediated and antibody mediated reactions.

Table 6.2 lists some of the more frequently encountered granulomatous lesions in bronchial biopsy material, categorized by each of the classification systems mentioned above.

6.5   The granulomatous reactions of specific diseases

All diseases reviewed in this section are discussed in more detail in Chapters 4, 8 or 11. In this section we will focus attention on the granulomatous lesions and those characteristics which help to refine the differential diagnoses.

Table 6.2 Classification for pulmonary granulomatous reactions

	Necrosis	Location	Spector's high/low turnover	Warren's immunology	Adams' morphology
Infectious	Yes	Bronchocentric interstitial	High	Immunological (cell mediated) (? antibody mediated)	Complex
Foreign body	No	Small vessels interstitial	Low or high	Nonimmunological (inactive)	Mature
Silicosis	Early—yes Later—no	Alveolar	High	Nonimmunological (active)	Epithelioid
Berylliosis	No	Alveolar	High	Immunological (cell mediated)	Epithelioid
Sarcoidosis	No (rarely)	Bronchocentric interstitial	High → low	Immunological (?)	Epithelioid
Wegener's granulomatosis	Yes	Angiocentric	High	Unknown	—
Bronchocentric granulomatosis	Yes	Bronchocentric	Unknown	Immunological (cell mediated)	Epithelioid

6.5.1　Foreign bodies

Most foreign materials causing granulomatous reactions in bronchial specimens result from deliberate intravenous injection of drugs which were
manufactured in tablet form for *oral* use. The most frequent intravenously
abused oral drugs are: methylphenidate (Ritalin®), phenmetrazine (Pre-
ludin®), pentazocaine (Talwin®) and methadone (Pare *et al.*, 1979; Tomashefski *et al.*, 1981; Radow *et al.*, 1983). The particular drug(s) which
is abused tends to be faddish and varies with locale and period. Tablets
are usually crushed in water, heated, and strained through cigarette filters
or clothing before injection. Manufacturers have added various materials
to these tablets to facilitate fabrication and maintain cohesiveness. These
fillers include microcrystalline cellulose, talc and corn starch. The first two
can evoke a granulomatous reaction. Intravenously injected material
lodges in the pulmonary vasculature and causes an angiothrombosis or
veno-occlusive disease (Szwed, 1970; Crissman *et al.*, 1980; Tomashefski
and Hirsch, 1980). Clinically these patients usually present with dyspnea
(after injecting from 2000 to 50 000 tablets), although their chest x-rays
may be unremarkable (Pare *et al.*, 1979; Waller *et al.*, 1980). Microcrystalline cellulose is a 10–25 μm diameter, pale gray, PAS-positive, diastase-
resistant, birefringent crystal (Fig. 6.8a). Talc is a plate-like crystal which
is birefringent, particularly when viewed on edge, and appears gray or
refractile in H&E-stained sections (Fig. 6.8b). Natural clothing fibers such
as cotton or wool are also capable of eliciting a granulomatous reaction.
These fibers are also birefringent. Histologically the granulomas are associated with small blood vessels and intra- or extracellular particles are
readily seen with polarizing microscopy (Section 5.8). There are usually
only a few lymphocytes and neutrophils associated with the macrophages
and multinucleated giant cells surrounding the involved vessels. Fibrosis
is usually present by the time the patients become symptomatic.

Foreign particulate material causing granulomatous lesions in the bronchial wall may also arrive by inhalation of dusts or embolization from
implanted surgical prosthetic material (Berner *et al.*, 1981; Robinson *et al.*,
1981). Silica and beryllium are special cases and are discussed in Sections
6.5.3 and 6.5.5.

6.5.2　Infectious granulomatous reactions

For a discussion of the various micro-organisms which can cause granulomatous lesions see Chapter 4. Tuberculosis is the classic delayed type
hypersensitivity granulomatous reaction. The granulomas may be found
in the bronchial wall, although the principal site of activity is usually the
alveolar spaces (Ulbright and Katzenstein, 1980; Dannenberg, 1982).

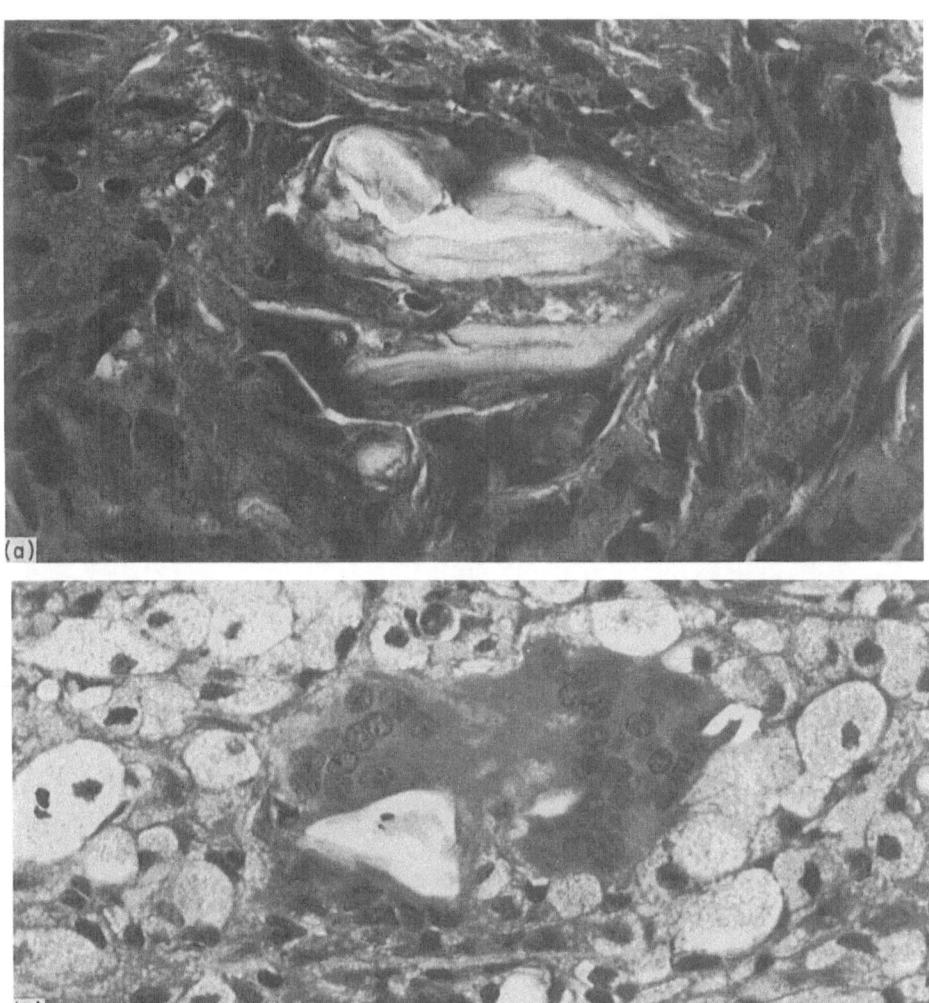

Fig. 6.8 Foreign body inclusions. (a) Microcrystalline cellulose particles in giant cells. This material is used in the manufacture of tablets intended for oral use. (b) Plate-like particle, probably talc, within a multinucleated giant cell. The sections are from bronchial tissue of drug addicts with diffuse pulmonary disease secondary to the chronic intravenous injection of crushed tablets. Slightly crossed polarizing filters were used to enhance the foreign material in these photomicrographs. (Paraffin sections stained with hematoxylin and eosin: × 710.)

Consequently diagnostic material is more likely to be present when both endobronchial and transbronchial biopsies are obtained (Katzenstein and Askin, 1980; Wallace *et al.*, 1981). The granulomas are usually well formed and typically confluent, with easily recognized epithelioid cells and necrotic centers (Fig. 6.9). Lymphocytes are usually present in the adjacent tissue. Caseous necrosis is characteristic but many cases of subsequently proven tuberculous lesions have little or no necrosis in their granulomas (Katzenstein and Askin, 1980; Ulbright and Katzenstein, 1980; Wallace *et al.*, 1981). Finding characteristic acid-fast bacilli establishes the diagnosis of tuberculosis but they are not always present (Burk *et al.*, 1978; Katzenstein and Askin, 1980; Wallace *et al.*, 1981; So *et al.*, 1982). There may be a lymphocytic vasculitis associated with the reaction but it is rarely necrotizing; neither are granulomas specifically present in the vessel walls (Koss *et al.*, 1980; Ulbright and Katzenstein, 1980). Giant cells are a conspicuous component of these granulomas and both asteroid and Schaumann bodies may occasionally be seen (Williams, 1960). Fibrosis is the ultimate fate of this reaction in the bronchial wall.

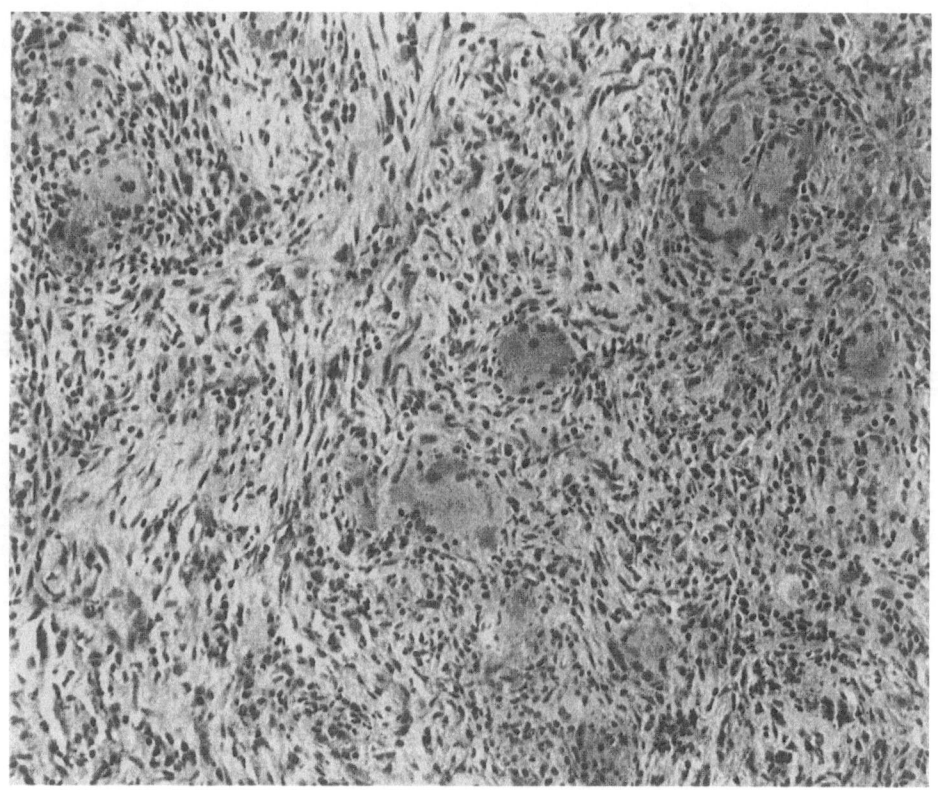

Fig. 6.9 Infectious granulomas. Blastomycosis. Numerous small granulomas are scattered throughout a background of lymphocytes and fibrocytes. (Paraffin section stained with hematoxylin and eosin: × 100.)

Nontuberculous mycobacteria can evoke a granulomatous reaction although it tends not to be caseous (Gribetz *et al.*, 1981; Müller-Hermelink *et al.*, 1982; Scully *et al.*, 1983). The granulomas of histoplasmosis are very similar to tuberculosis (Ulbright and Katzenstein, 1980; Zollinger and Ohnacker, 1980; Goodwin *et al.*, 1981). Infections with aspergillus (Churg, 1983; George *et al.*, 1983), coccidioides (Straub and Schwarz, 1962), cryptococcus (Hatcher *et al.*, 1971; Baker, 1976; Ulbright and Katzenstein, 1980), blastomyces (Schwarz and Salfelder, 1977) and extremely rarely pneumocystis (LeGolvan and Heidelberger, 1973; Cruickshank, 1975) can evoke a granulomatous reaction, usually with many giant cells. With the exception of pneumocystis granulomas, most of these reactions contain abundant lymphocytes.

Katzenstein *et al.* (1975) described a granulomatous reaction involving distal bronchial walls, with necrosis and a heavy leukocytic infiltrate with conspicuous eosinophils. Many of these cases of *bronchocentric granulomatosis* have been associated with colonized aspergillus and/or the patients have a positive skin reaction to injected aspergillus antigen. The reaction is similar to the hypersensitivity pneumonias (Section 5.7). Unlike most hypersensitivity pneumonias which are localized in alveoli, these cases frequently have granulomas in the walls of more proximal bronchi (Edwards, 1982). Unfortunately the term bronchocentric granulomatosis is also used in a descriptive sense by some (meaning localized to bronchi). As commented above many of the infectious granulomatous reactions are bronchocentric in this descriptive sense. Churg (1983) has suggested calling those cases with hypersensitivity to aspergillus *allergic bronchopulmonary aspergillosis* and reserving the term bronchocentric granulomatosis for those cases where an etiology is not found.

6.5.3 Silicosis

Silica crystals 1–3 μm in length, inhaled in large amounts, result in nodular pulmonary lesions (deShazo, 1982) (Section 5.8.2). The mature silicotic nodule is composed of fibrocytes and layers of collagen organized around a central hyalinized core (Kleinerman *et al.*, 1979). Nodules are circumscribed and are predominantly interstitial, although peribronchial nodules are frequently seen. The shape of these nodules is reminiscent of the granuloma and experimental models demonstrate the granulomatous nature of the reaction. Particulate silica is phagocytized by alveolar macrophages, which then destroy the cells by a direct cytotoxic effect of small amounts of solubilized silica (Marks and Nagelschmidt, 1959). The remaining undissolved silica is then liberated into the alveolar space where it can be rephagocytosed, the process repeating itself numerous times

(Heppleston, 1962). Multinucleated giant cells are formed and fibrosis with abundant collagen deposition follows (Heppleston, 1979).

Histologically the nodules are quite distinctive (Fig. 5.11) and the remaining particles of silica are easily seen in the polarized light microscope as birefringent triangular spicules. However, Craighead and Vallyathan (1980) have shown that in some nodules the silica is so small that only electron microscopic analysis is capable of detecting the particles. In a study of sarcoidosis, Longcope and Freiman (1952) found birefringent material in some of the specimens and suggested that these might in fact be silicotic rather than late stage sarcoid nodules.

6.5.4   Sarcoidosis

Much has been written about this disease, both because it is a universal diagnostic problem and because its etiology remains obscure. The disease itself is discussed in more detail in Chapter 8. Here we will concentrate on the granulomatous reaction *per se*. It should be pointed out from the onset that the histological lesions are not diagnostic unto themselves but are frequently essential to the diagnosis (Mitchell and Scadding, 1974; Mitchell *et al.*, 1977; Selroos, 1981).

Various terms are used to describe the sarcoid granuloma: hard, sharply circumscribed, tightly packed and epithelioid (Fig. 6.10) (Mitchell *et al.*, 1977; Casuccio and Yanagisawa, 1981; Crystal *et al.*, 1981; Cain and Kraus, 1982). Multinucleated giant cells are frequently seen and may be numerous, although Williams *et al.* (1970) suggest that tuberculous granulomas characteristically have more. Cytoplasmic inclusions of various types are characteristic of sarcoid multinucleated giant cells (Longcope and Freiman, 1952; Williams, 1960; Uehlinger, 1963; Nessan *et al.*, 1981). Nessan *et al.* also found birefringent crystals which they suspected to be calcium oxalate. The various inclusion bodies are described in Section 6.2. Some investigators describe a central follicle of closely packed epithelioid cells and macrophages with a peripheral zone of loosely arranged mononuclear cells, apparently entering or leaving the follicle (Soler *et al.*, 1976). Although the characteristic sarcoid granuloma is noncaseating, central necrosis described as eosinophilic or fibrinoid is seen rarely (Mitchell and Scadding, 1974; Nessan *et al.*, 1981; Cain and Kraus, 1982). Lymphocytes of both T and B types are present in the reactions although their relative numbers vary with the progression of the granulomas (Daniele *et al.*, 1980; Crystal *et al.*, 1981).

Chronic berylliosis produces granulomas very similar to those of sarcoidosis (Williams, 1958; Freiman and Hardy, 1970; Sprince *et al.*, 1976). Schaumann and asteroid bodies are both more frequently seen in beryllium-induced granulomas than in sarcoidosis (Williams, 1960). There tends to be a more intense lymphocytic infiltrate in chronic berylliosis than in sarcoidosis and the granulomas are less circumscribed (Freiman and Hardy, 1970; Mitchell *et al.*, 1977; Williams, 1980).

In the J. Burns Amberson lecture, Liebow (1973) described a group of patients who had aggregated sarcoid-like granulomas with necrosis and a vasculitis. Subsequent reviews have generally placed these lesions in the group of pulmonary vasculitides (Saldana *et al.*, 1977; Edwards, 1982; Fulmer and Kaltreider, 1982; Cole *et al.*, 1983). Despite several distinctive features including necrosis, an intense vasculitis and less well circumscribed granulomas (Churg *et al.*, 1979; Koss *et al.*, 1980), Churg (1983) has presented convincing arguments that this is a varient of sarcoidosis and not a separate disease.

In concluding this discussion of the distinguishing features of the sarcoid granuloma it should be remembered that most investigators who have had the opportunity to review large series of cases caution that every means to discover specific etiologic agents must be exhausted and the

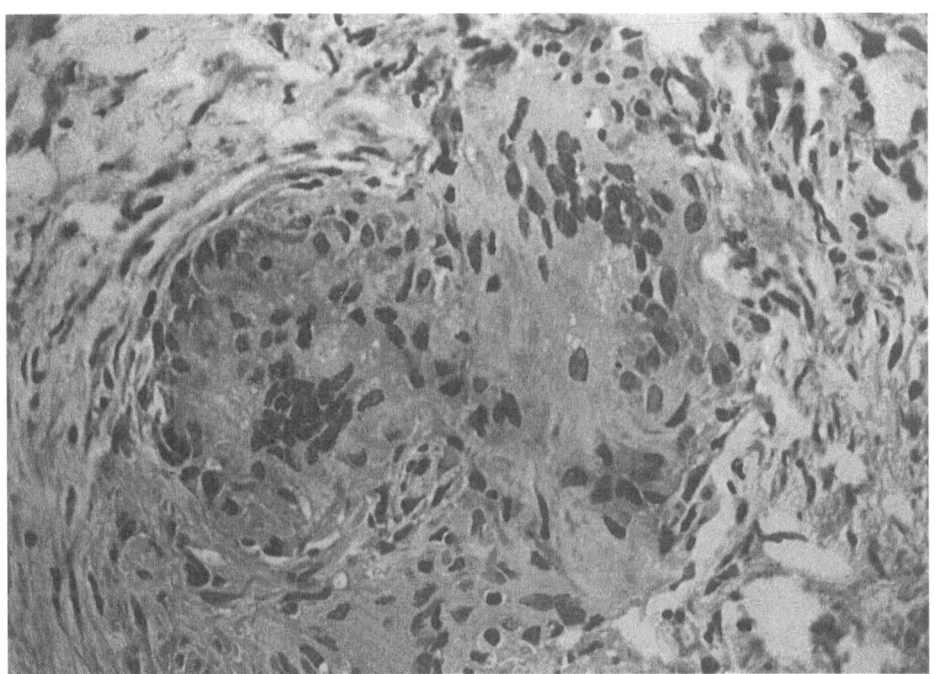

Fig. 6.10   Sarcoid granulomas. Bronchial biopsy with two well-formed epithelioid granulomas with developing outer rims of fibrocytes and collagen. There is a hyaline appearance to these reactions. Necrosis is rarely seen in the fully developed granulomas. (Paraffin section stained with hematoxylin and eosin: × 470.)

clinical picture analyzed before reaching the conclusion that a lesion is sarcoidosis (Mitchell and Scadding, 1974; Mitchell *et al.*, 1977; Nessan *et al.*, 1981; Williams, 1982). The pathological diagnosis of sarcoidosis frequently stops all clinical attempts to search for specific causes (often treatable) of the patient's illness.

6.5.5 Berylliosis

Berylliosis is a far less common cause of granulomatous pulmonary reaction than any other considered in this chapter. A more extensive discussion of the disease can be found in Section 5.8.4. Chronic forms evoke granulomas which are histologically very similar to those of sarcoidosis (Williams, 1958; Freiman and Hardy, 1970; Mitchell *et al.*, 1977; Williams, 1980). The lesions have more associated lymphocytes and the multinucleated giant cell inclusion bodies (asteroid, Schaumann or conchoid) are seen with greater frequency than in sarcoidosis (Williams, 1960; Freiman and Hardy, 1970). Nevertheless only direct analysis for beryllium or a positive exposure history from the patient will distinguish these cases, and only continuing surveillance will allow recognition (Sprince *et al.*, 1976; Tanaka *et al.*, 1983).

6.5.6 Wegener's granulomatosis

Wegener's granulomatosis is a multisystem disease characterized by necrotizing vasculitis with granulomas. For a general discussion see Chapter 8. The differential diagnosis is not with those lesions dominated by granuloma (discussed above) but with the vasculidites. Since we are discussing the granuloma at this time we will emphasize that component of the reaction. There is considerable variability in the intensity and extent of individual lesions in a patient at a given time. The lesions tend to be nodular and scattered throughout the lungs. Although these are important differential features, neither is discernible in bronchial biopsy specimens. Necrosis is a dominant feature with a full range of inflammatory cellular infiltrates, including macrophages. Unfortunately the macrophages tend to be scattered and not as organized (and are therefore less easily recognized) than in the reactions of the diseases already discussed in this chapter. Epithelioid cells often palisade around arteries or veins (Fig. 6.11) and around foci of necrosis, which can be shown with elastic stains (which identify the fragmented elastic lamina) to be destroyed vessels. The necrosis has a brightly eosinophilic hyaline character (fibrinoid), particularly in the early stages of vascular damage. Multinucleated giant cells are frequently seen, either randomly scattered or spaced around degenerating

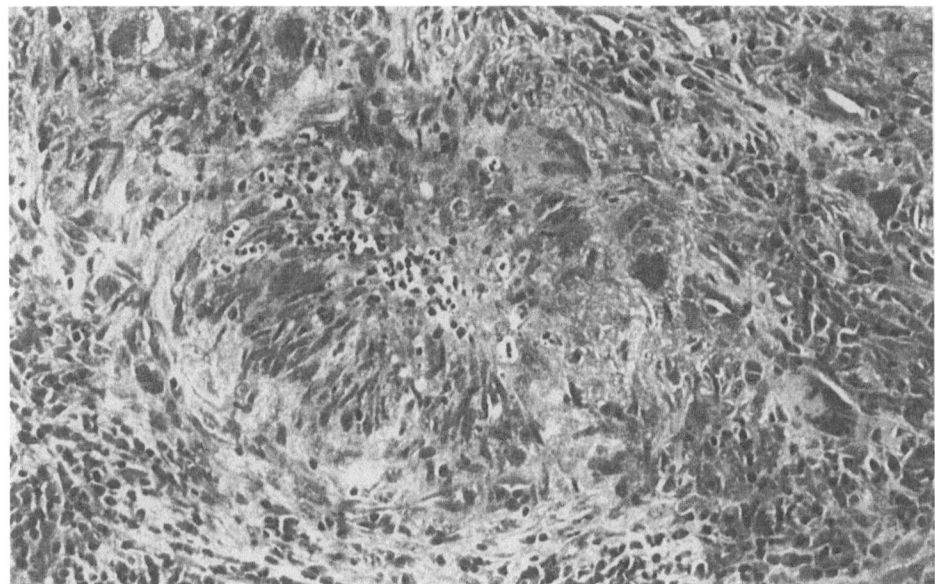

Fig. 6.11 Wegener's granulomatosis. Pallisading epithelioid cells are organized around a necrotic focus containing numerous polymorphonuclear leukocytes. Many lymphocytes, macrophages and plasma cells surround the granuloma. Several multinucleated giant cells are forming around the lesion. (Paraffin section stained with hematoxylin and eosin: × 200.)

vessels (Liebow, 1973; Koss *et al.*, 1980; Casuccio and Yanagisawa, 1981; Churg, 1983; Cole *et al.*, 1983; Fauci *et al.*, 1983). Histologically the differential diagnosis should include infectious granulomatous diseases, allergic granulomatous angiitis (Churg-Strauss syndrome), lymphomatoid granulomatosis and hypersensitivity angiitis (Veevaete *et al.*, 1976; Edwards, 1982; Kornblut *et al.*, 1982). With the exception of those with infectious etiologies these are all very rare causes of necrotizing bronchial granulomatous lesions.

The lymphoid infiltrate of lymphomatoid granulomatosis is cytologically atypical. Allergic granulomatous angiitis and hypersensitivity angiitis are characterized by conspicuous eosinophils in the infiltrate. Endobronchial biopsies are rarely capable of distinguishing these differences. In fact the diagnosis of Wegener's granulomatosis is difficult if not impossible to establish by the endobronchial approach because the most definitive and distinctive pattern of granulomatous angiitis and phlebitis, seen in the parenchymal vessels adjacent to the necrotic nodule, is rarely seen because the specimen is very small.

6.5.7   Granulomatous reactions with conspicuous eosinophils

A group of rare disorders should be considered when the leukocytic infiltrate associated with a granulomatous reaction contains many eosinophils. In particular, granulomas associated with certain infectious agents and parasitic infections are accompanied by numerous eosinophils. Extrinsic allergic alveolitis (hypersensitivity pneumonitis) may involve bronchial and peribronchial tissues with granulomas (Section 5.7), although the lesions are primarily in alveoli. Hypersensitivity reactions to drugs may include arteritis with occasional granulomas. Churg and Strauss (1951) described a clinical syndrome of asthma, circulating hypereosinophilia and a systemic granulomatous arteritis which frequently involves lung. Each of these are extremely rare disorders and although each has characteristics which might allow histological differentiation such discrimination requires larger specimens than are available in the bronchial biopsy. (For further discussion see Liebow and Carrington, 1969; Liebow, 1973; Veevaete et al., 1976; Koss et al., 1981; Edwards, 1982; Fulmer and Kaltreider, 1982; Kornblut et al., 1982; Churg, 1983; Cole et al., 1983.)

The proliferative disorders collectively termed histiocytosis X may involve the lung and are rarely sampled in bronchial biopsy. Particularly the entity eosinophilic granuloma may include a pulmonary 'granulomatous' reaction with numerous eosinophils. These diseases are characterized by proliferating 'histiocytes' which have been identified as Langerhans' cells (not to be confused with the Langhans' type of multinucleated giant cell). The proliferating cell is ultrastructurally distinctive because of the cytoplasmic structures called either Langerhans' or Birbeck's granules (Shelburne et al., 1983). The cellular proliferations are not granulomas. For further discussion see Chapter 8.

6.5.8   Lymphomatoid granulomatosis

This disease is now considered to be a lymphoproliferative disorder characterized by atypical lymphoreticular cells with tissue necrosis. The associated reaction tends to be angiocentric and granulomatous and may resemble Wegener's granulomatosis or the infectious granulomatoses. The histological distinction is based on the recognition of the atypical lymphoid cells which are not seen in the other granulomatous disease. Chapters 8 and 11 contain additional comments.

6.6   Summary

Second only to the finding of neoplasm, the detection of granuloma is a significant observation. Granuloma in bronchial biopsy specimens should set in operation a spectrum of analyses to determine, if possible, the specific etiology. This analysis should include clinical information on the extent of the patient's disease process, pre-existing disease, environmental and work exposures and constitution signs. It requires the use of special tissue stains to visualize and identify micro-organisms, polarizing filters to detect birefringent particles and possibly specialized equipment such as electron microprobe or x-ray analysis to detect and identify material not visible in the light microscope (Section 5.8.6). The importance of correctly identifying the etiology is a consequence of the heterogeneity of the diseases which may have granulomas as a morphological manifestation and the diversity of specifically required therapies for many of these diseases. The surgical pathologist should not be satisfied with the analysis until a diagnosis is found which fits both the clinical picture and the morphological characteristics. Above all, if the bronchial specimen proves inadequate for a specific (meaningful) diagnosis, additional specimens, usually open lung biopsy, should be requested. A coordinated approach to the selection and processing of additional material can be advantageous to the patient, the physician and the pathologist.

References

Adams, D.O. (1974), The structure of mononuclear phagocytes differentiating *in vivo*. I. Sequential fine and histologic studies of the effect of *Bacillus Calmette-Guerin* (BCG). *Am. J. Pathol.*, **76**, 17–48.

Adams, D.O. (1975), The structure of mononuclear phagocytes differentiating *in vivo*. II. The effect of *Mycobacterium tuberculosis. Am. J. Pathol.*, **80**, 101–16.

Adams, D.O. (1976), The granulomatous inflammatory response. A review. *Am. J. Pathol.*, **84**, 164–91.

Armstrong, J.R., Radke, J.R., Eichenhorn, M.S., Kvale, P.A. and Popovich, J., Jr. (1981), Endoscopic findings in sarcoidosis. Characteristics and correlations with radiographic staging and bronchial mucosal biopsy yield. *Ann. Otol.*, **90**, 339–43.

Baker, R.D. (1976), The primary pulmonary lymph node complex of cryptococcosis. *Am. J. Clin. Pathol.*, **65**, 83–92.

Berner, A., Gylseth, B. and Levy, F. (1981), Talc dust pneumoconiosis. A case report. *Acta Path. Microbiol. Scand. Sect. A*, **89**, 17–21.

Boros, D.L. (1978), Granulomatous inflammations. *Prog. Allergy*, **24**, 183–267.

Bowden, D.H. and Adamson, I.Y.R. (1980), Role of monocytes and interstitial cells in the generation of alveolar macrophages. I. Kinetic studies of normal mice. *Lab. Invest.*, **42**, 511–17.

Burk, J.R., Viroslav, J. and Bynum, L.J. (1978), Miliary tuberculosis diagnosed by fibreoptic bronchoscopy and transbronchial biopsy. *Tubercle*, **59**, 107–9.

Cain, H. and Kraus, B. (1982), Cellular aspects of granulomas. *Path. Res. Pract.*, **17**, 13–37.

Cain, H. and Kraus, B. (1983), Immunofluorescence microscopic demonstration of vimentin filaments in asteroid bodies of sarcoidosis. A comparison with electron microscopic findings. *Virchows Arch. (Cell Pathol.)*, **42**, 213–26.

Casuccio, J.R. and Yanagisawa, E. (1981), Disease of obscure etiology: sarcoidosis, Wegener's granulomatosis, and midline granuloma. *Otolaryngol. Cl. No. Am.*, **14**, 331–45.

Chambers, T.J. (1978), Multinucleate giant cells. *J. Pathol.*, **126**, 125–48.

Churg, A. (1983), Pulmonary angiitis and granulomatosis revisited. *Human Pathol.*, **14**, 868–83.

Churg, A., Carrington, C.B. and Gupta, R. (1979), Necrotizing sarcoid granulomatosis. *Chest*, **76**, 406–13.

Churg, J. and Strauss, L. (1951), Allergic granulomatosis, allergic angiitis and periarteritis nodosa. *Am. J. Pathol.*, **27**, 277–302.

Cole, S.R., Johnson, K.J. and Ward, P.A. (1983), Pathology of sarcoidosis, granulomatous vasculitis, and other idiopathic granulomatous diseases of the lung. In *Sarcoidosis and Other Granulomatous Diseases of the Lung* (ed. B.L. Fanburg), Marcel Dekker, New York, pp. 149–202.

Craighead, J.E. and Vallyathan, N.V. (1980), Cryptic pulmonary lesions in workers occupationally exposed to dust containing silica. *J. Am. Med. Assoc.*, **244**, 1939–41.

Crissman, J.D., Koss, M. and Carson, R.P. (1980), Pulmonary veno-occlusive disease secondary to granulomatous venulitis. *Am. J. Surg. Pathol.*, **4**, 93–9.

Cruickshank, B. (1975), Pulmonary granulomatous pneumocystosis following renal transplantation. Report of a case. *Am. J. Clin. Pathol.*, **63**, 384–90.

Crystal, R.G., Roberts, W.C., Hunninghake, G.W., Gadek, J.E., Fulmer, J.D. and Line, B.R. (1981), Pulmonary sarcoidosis: disease characterized and perpetuated by activated lung T-lymphocytes. *Ann. Intern. Med.*, **94**, 73–94.

Daniele, R.P., Dauber, J.H. and Rossman, M.D. (1980), Immunologic abnormalities in sarcoidosis. *Ann. Intern. Med.*, **92**, 406–16.

Dannenberg, A.M., Jr. (1968), Cellular hypersensitivity and cellular immunity in the pathogenesis of tuberculosis: specificity, systemic, and local nature and associated macrophage enzymes. *Bacteriol. Rev.*, **32**, 85–102.

Dannenberg, A.M., Jr. (1982), Pathogenesis of pulmonary tuberculosis. *Am. Rev. Respir. Dis.* (Koch Centennial Supplement), **125**, 25–30.

deShazo, R. (1982), Current concepts about the pathogenesis of silicosis and asbestosis. *J. Allergy Clin. Immunol.*, **70**, 41–9.

Edwards, C.W. (1982), Vasculitis and granulomatosis of the respiratory tract. *Thorax*, **37**, 81–7.

Epstein, W.L. (1977), Granuloma formation in man. In *Pathobiology Annual*, Vol. 7 (ed. H.L. Ioachim), Appleton-Century-Crofts, New York, pp. 1–30.

Epstein, W.L. and Krasnobrod, H. (1968), The origin of epithelioid cells in experimental granulomas of man. *Lab. Invest.*, **18**, 190–5.

Fauci, A.S., Haynes, B.F., Katz, P. and Wolff, S.M. (1983), Wegener's granulomatosis: prospective clinical and therapeutic experience with 85 patients for 21 years. *Ann. Intern. Med.*, **98**, 76–85.

Freiman, D.G. and Hardy, H.L. (1970), Beryllium disease. The relation of pulmonary pathology to clinical course and prognosis based on a study of 130 cases from the U.S. Beryllium Case Registry. *Human Pathol.*, **1**, 25–44.

Fulmer, J.D. and Kaltreider, H.B. (1982), The pulmonary vasculitides. *Chest*, **82**, 615–24.

George, P.J.M., Boffa, P.B.J., Naylor, C.P.E. and Higenbottam, T.W. (1983), Necrotizing pulmonary aspergillosis complicating the management of patients with obstructive airways disease. *Thorax*, **38**, 478–80.

Goodwin, R.A., Loyd, J.E. and DesPrez, R.M. (1981), Histoplasmosis in normal hosts. *Medicine*, **60**, 231–66.

Gregorie, H.B., Jr., Othersen, H.B., Jr. and Moore, M.P., Jr. (1962), The significance of sarcoid-like lesions in association with malignant neoplasms. *Am. J. Surg.*, **104**, 577–86.

Gribetz, A.R., Damsker, B., Bottone, E.J., Kirschner, P.A. and Teirstein, A.S. (1981), Solitary pulmonary nodules due to nontuberculous mycobacterial infection. *Am. J. Med.*, **70**, 39–43.

Groopman, J.E. and Golde, D.W. (1981), The histocytic disorders: pathophysiologic analysis. *Ann. Intern. Med.*, **94**, 95–107.

Hatcher, C.R., Jr., Sehdeva, J., Waters, W.C., III, Schulze, V., Logan, W.D., Jr., Symbas, P. and Abbott, O.A. (1971), Primary pulmonary cryptococcosis. *J. Thorac. Cardiovasc. Surg.*, **61**, 39–49.

Heppleston, A.G. (1962), The disposal of dust in the lungs of silicotic rats. *Am. J. Pathol.*, **40**, 493–506.

Heppleston, A.G. (1979), Silica and asbestos: contrasts in tissue response. *Ann N.Y. Acad. Sci.*, **330**, 725–44.

Hunninghake, G.W., Gadek, J.E., Young, R.C., Jr., Kawanami, O., Ferrans, V.J. and Crystal, R.G. (1980), Maintenance of granuloma formation in pulmonary sarcoidosis by T lymphocytes within the lung. *New Engl. J. Med.*, **302**, 594–8.

James, D.G. and Neville, E. (1977), Pathobiology of sarcoidosis. In *Pathobiology Annual*, Vol. 7 (ed. A.L. Ioachim), Appleton-Century-Crofts, New York, pp. 31–62.

James, D.G. and Williams, W.J. (1982), Immunology of sarcoidosis. *Am. J. Med.*, **72**, 5–8.

Kataria, Y.P., Shaw, R.A. and Campbell, P.B. (1982), Sarcoidosis: an overview, II. *Clin. Notes Respir. Dis.*, **20**, 3–15.

Katzenstein, A.A. and Askin, F.B. (1980), Interpretation of and significance of pathologic findings in transbronchial lung biopsy. *Am. J. Surg. Pathol.*, **4**, 223–34.

Katzenstein, A.-L., Liebow, A.A. and Friedman, P.J. (1975), Bronchocentric granulomatosis, mucoid impaction, and hypersensitivity reactions to fungi. *Am. Rev. Respir. Dis.*, **111**, 497–537.

Kleinerman, J., Green, F., Harley, R.A., Lapp, N.L., Laqueur, W., Naeye, R.L., Pratt, P., Taylor, G., Wiot, J. and Wyatt, J. (1979), Pathology standards for coal worker's pneumoconiosis. *Arch. Pathol. Lab. Med.*, **103**, 375–432.

Kornblut, A.D., deFries, H.O., Wolff, S.M. and Fauci, A.S. (1982), Wegener's granulomatosis. *Otolaryngol. Cl. No. Am.*, **15**, 673–83.

Koss, M.N., Antonovych, T. and Hochholzer, L. (1981), Allergic granulomatosis (Churg-Strauss syndrome). Pulmonary and renal morphologic findings. *Am. J. Surg. Pathol.*, **5**, 21–8.

Koss, M.N., Hochholzer, L., Feigin, D.S., Garancis, J.C. and Ward, P.A. (1980), Necrotizing sarcoid-like granulomatosis: clinical, pathologic, and immunopathologic findings. *Human Pathol.*, **11**, 510–19.

Kraus, B. (1980), Mehrkernige Riesenzellen in Granulomen. *Verh. Dtsch. Ges. Path.*, **64**, 103–25.

Lasser, A. (1983), The mononuclear phagocytic system: a review. *Human Pathol.*, **14**, 108–26.

LeGolvan, D.P. and Heidelberger, K.P. (1973), Disseminated granulomatous *Pneumocystis carinii* pneumonia. *Arch. Pathol.*, **95**, 344–8.

Liebow, A.A. (1973), The J. Burns Amberson Lecture: pulmonary angiitis and granulomatosis. *Am. Rev. Respir. Dis.*, **108**, 1–18.

Liebow, A.A. and Carrington, C.B. (1969), The eosinophilic pneumonias. *Medicine*, **48**, 251–85.

Longcope, W.T. and Freiman, D.G. (1952), A study of sarcoidosis based on a combined investigation of 160 cases including 30 autopsies from the Johns Hopkins Hospital and Massachusetts General Hospital. *Medicine*, **31**, 1–132.

Mariano, M., and Spector, W.G. (1974), The formation and properties of macrophage polykaryons (inflammatory giant cells). *J. Pathol.*, **113**, 1–19.

Mariano, M., Nikitin, T. and Malucelli, B.E. (1976), Immunological and nonimmunological phagocytosis by inflammatory macrophages, epithelioid cells and macrophage polykaryons from foreign body granulomata. *J. Pathol.*, **120**, 151–60.

Marks, J. and Nagelschmidt, G. (1959), Study of the toxicity of dust with use of the *in vitro* dehydrogenase technique. *A.M.A. Arch. Indust. Health*, **20**, 383–9.

Mitchell, D.N. and Scadding, J.G. (1974), Sarcoidosis. *Am. Rev. Respir. Dis.*, **110**, 774–802.

Mitchell, D.N., Scadding, J.G., Heard, B.E. and Hinson, K.F.W. (1977), Sarcoidosis: histopathological definition and clinical diagnosis. *J. Clin. Pathol.*, **30**, 395–408.

Mitchell, D.M., Mitchell, D.N., Collins, J.V. and Emerson, C.J. (1980), Transbronchial lung biopsy through fibreoptic bronchoscope in diagnosis of sarcoidosis. *Brit. Med. J.*, **280**, 679–81.

Müller-Hermelink, H.K., Kaiserling, E. and Sonntag, H.G. (1982), Modulation of epithelioid cell granuloma formation to apathogenic Mycobacteria by cyclosporin. *A. Path. Res. Pract.*, **175**, 80–96.

Nash, G. (1982), Pathologic features of the lung in the immunocompromised host. *Human Pathol.*, **13**, 841–58.

Nessan, V.J., Malin, J. and Parks, S.D. (1981), Sarcoidosis: a clinical, roentgenographic and pathological survey. *West. J. Med.*, **135**, 353–9.

Papadimitriou, J.M., Finlay-Jones, J-M. and Walters, M.N. (1973), Surface characteristics of macrophages, epithelioid and giant cells using scanning electron microscopy. *Exp. Cell Res.*, **76**, 353–62.

Papadimitriou, J.M. and Spector, W.G. (1971). The origin, properties and fate of epithelioid cells. *J. Pathol.*, **105**, 187–203.

Pare, J.A.P., Fraser, R.G., Hogg, J.C., Howlett, J.G. and Murphy, S.B. (1979), Pulmonary 'mainline' granulomatosis; talcosis of intravenous methadone abuse. *Medicine*, **58**, 229–39.

Radow, S.K., Nachamkin, I., Morrow, C., Fairman, R.P., Fratkin, M., Rodriquez, G.E. and Glauser, F.L. (1983), Foreign body granulomatosis. Clinical and immunologic findings. *Am. Rev. Respir. Dis.*, **127**, 575–80.

Rasmussen, P. and Caulfield, J.B. (1960), The ultrastructure of Schaumann bodies in the golden hamster. *Lab. Invest.*, **9**, 330–8.

Ridley, M.J., Ridley, D.S. and Turk, J.L. (1978), Surface markers on lymphocytes and cells of the mononuclear phagocyte series in skin sections in leprosy. *J. Pathol.*, **125**, 91–8.

Robinson, M.J., Nestor, M. and Rywlin, A.M. (1981), Pulmonary granulomas secondary to embolic prosthetic valve material. *Human Pathol.*, **12**, 759–62.

Saldana, M.J., Patchefsky, A.S., Israel, H.I. and Atkinson, G.W. (1977), Pulmonary angiitis and granulomatosis. The relationship between histological features, organ involvement, and response to treatment. *Human Pathol.*, **8**, 391–409.

Schaumann, J. (1941), On the nature of certain peculiar corpuscles present in the tissue of lymphogranulomatosis benigna. *Acta Medica Scand.*, **106**, 239–53.

Schwarz, J. and Salfelder, K. (1977), Blastomycosis. A review of 152 cases. In *Current Topics in Pathology*, Vol. 65, Springer-Verlag, Berlin, pp. 165–200.

Scully, R.E., Mark, E.J. and McNeely, B.U. (1983), Case records of the Massachusetts General Hospital. Weekly clinicopathological exercises. *New Engl. J. Med.*, **308**, 949–57.

Selroos, O. (1981), The diagnosis of sarcoidosis. *Europ. J. Respir. Dis.*, **62**, 219–22.

Shelburne, J.D., Wissemann, C.L., Broda, K.R., Roggli, V.L. and Ingram, P. (1983), Lung – nonneoplastic conditions. In *Diagnostic Electron Microscopy*, Vol. 4 (eds B.F. Trump and R.T. Jones), Wiley, New York, pp. 475–538.

Siltzbach, L.E. (1976) (ed.), Seventh International Conference on Sarcoidosis and other Granulomatous Disorders. *Ann. N.Y. Acad. Sci.*, **278**, 1–751.

So, S.Y., Lam, W.K. and Yu, D.Y.C. (1982), Rapid diagnosis of suspected pulmonary tuberculosis by fiberoptic bronchoscopy. *Tubercle*, **63**, 195–200.

Soler, P., Basset, F., Bernaudin, J.F. and Chretien, J. (1976), Morphology and distribution of the cells of a sarcoid granuloma: ultrastructural study of serial sections. *Ann. N.Y. Acad. Sci.*, **278**, 147–58.

Spector, W.G. (1976), Epithelioid cells, giant cells and sarcoidosis. *Ann. N.Y. Acad. Sci.*, **278**, 3–6.

Spector, W.G. (1980), Die Morphologie, Kinetick and Schicksal der Granulome. *Verh. Dtsch. Ges. Path.*, **64**, 21–4.

Spector, W.G. (1982), Experimental granulomas. *Path. Res. Pract.*, **175**, 110–17.

Sprince, N.L., Kazemi, H. and Hardy, H.L. (1976), Current (1975) problem of differentiating between beryllium disease and sarcoidosis. *Ann. N.Y. Acad. Sci.*, **278**, 654–64.

Straub, M. and Schwarz, J. (1962), Histoplasmosis, coccidioidomycosis and tuberculosis: a comparative pathological study. *Path. Microbiol.*, **25**, 421–77.

Sutton, J.S. and Weiss, L. (1966), Transformation of monocytes in tissue culture into macrophages, epithelioid cells, and multinucleated giant cells. An electron microscopic study. *J. Cell Biol.*, **28**, 303–32.

Szwed, J.J. (1970), Pulmonary angiothrombosis caused by blue velvet addiction. *Ann Int. Med.*, **73**, 771–4.

Tanaka, S., Smith, A.B., Halperin, W. and Mullan, R.J. (1983), Beryllium disease. Necessity for continuing surveillance. *Chest*, **84**, 312.

Tomashefski, J.F., Jr. and Hirsch, C.S. (1980), The pulmonary vascular lesions of intravenous abuse. *Human Pathol.*, **11**, 133–45.

Tomashefski, J.F., Jr., Hirsch, C.S. and Jolly, P.N. (1981), Microcrystalline cellulose pulmonary embolism and granulomatosis. A complication of illicit intravenous injection of pentazocine tablets. *Arch. Pathol. Lab. Med.*, **105**, 89–93.

Uehlinger, E. (1963), The sarcoid tissue reaction. The origin and significance of inclusion bodies. Differential diagnosis with particular delineation from tuberculosis. *Acta Medica Scand. Suppl.*, **425**, 7–13.

Ulbright, T.M. and Katzenstein, A.A. (1980), Solitary necrotizing granulomas of the lung. Differentiating features and etiology. *Am. J. Surg. Pathol.*, **4**, 13–28.

Unanue, E.R. (1975), The regulation of the immune response by macrophages. In *Mononuclear Phagocytes in Immunity, Infection and Pathology* (ed. R. van Furth), Blackwell, Oxford, p. 721.

van der Gaag, R.D., van Maarsseveen, A.C.M.Th., Broekhuizen-Davies, J.M. and Stam, J. (1983), Application of *in vitro* techniques to determine proliferation in human sarcoid lymph nodes. *J. Pathol.*, **139**, 239–45.

van Furth, R. (1980), The mononuclear phagocyte system. *Verh. Dtsch. Ges. Pathol.*, **64**, 1–11.

van Furth, R., Cohn, Z.A., Hirsch, J.G., Humphrey, J.H., Spector, W.G. and Langevoort, H.L. (1972), The mononuclear phagocyte system: a new classification of macrophages, monocytes, and their precursor cells. *Bull. WHO*, **46**, 845–52.

van Furth, R. and van Oud Albas, A.B. (1982), The current view on the origin of pulmonary macrophages. *Path. Res. Pract.*, **175**, 38–49.

van Maarsseveen, A.C.M.Th., Veldhuizen, R.W., Stam, J., Alons, C.L. and Mullink,

H. (1983), A quantitative histomorphologic analysis of lymph node granulomas in sarcoidosis in relation to radiological stage I and II. *J. Pathol.*, **139**, 441–53.

Veevaete, F., van der Straeten, M., del Vos, M. and Roels, H. (1976), Allergic granulomatous angiitis. *Scand. J. Respir. Dis.*, **59**, 287–96.

Wallace, J.M., Deutsch, A.L., Harrell, J.H. and Moser, K.M. (1981), Bronchoscopy and transbronchial biopsy in evaluation of patients with suspected active tuberculosis. *Am. J. Med.*, **70**, 1189–94.

Waller, B.F., Brownlee, W.J. and Roberts, W.C. (1980), Self-induced pulmonary granulomatosis. A consequence of intravenous injections of drugs intended for oral use. *Chest*, **78**, 90–4.

Wang, N.-S., Schraufnagel, D.E. and Sampson, M.G. (1981), The tadpole-shaped structures in human non-necrotizing granulomas. *Am. Rev. Respir. Dis.*, **123**, 560–4.

Warren, K.S. (1976), A functional classification of granulomatous inflammation. *Ann. N.Y. Acad. Sci.*, **278**, 7–18.

Williams, W.J. (1958), A histological study of the lungs in 52 cases of chronic beryllium disease. *Brit. J. Indust. Med.*, **15**, 84–91.

Williams, W.J. (1960), The nature and origin of Schaumann bodies. *J. Pathol. Bact.*, **79**, 193–201.

Williams, W.J. (1980), Granulomas in sarcoidosis and chronic beryllium disease. *Verh. Dtsch. Ges. Pathol.*, **64**, 177–80.

Williams, W.J. (1982), Aetiology of sarcoidosis. *Path. Res. Pract.*, **175**, 1–12.

Williams, W.J. and Davies, B.H. (1980), *Proceedings of the 8th International Conference on Sarcoidosis and other Granulomatous Diseases*, Alpha and Omega, Cardiff.

Williams, W.J., James, E.M.V., Erasmus, D.A. and Davies, T. (1970), The fine structure of sarcoid and tuberculous granulomas. *Postgrad. Med. J.*, **46**, 496–500.

Zak, F. (1964), Contribution to the origin, development and experimental production of laminated calcinosiderotic Schaumann bodies. *Acta Medica Scand. Suppl.*, **425**, 21–4.

Zollinger, H.U. and Ohnacker, H. (1980), Multiple asymptomatic pulmonary nodules. *Pathol. Res. Pract.*, **169**, 109–12.

7 Ciliary abnormalities

7.1 Introduction

Cilia extend from the apical surfaces of ciliated cells into the airway. Each cilium is made up of many components and a defect in any of the constituent elements will likely lead to failure of ciliary movement. Ciliary abnormalities are of two main types: *acquired lesions*, which result from sublethal injury to the ciliated cells, and *inborn genetic errors*. In most cases it is possible to determine whether or not a patient has an acquired or genetic defect. In this regard the patient history is very helpful. Furthermore, genetic defects affect all of the cilia permanently, whereas acquired defects usually affect a proportion of the cilia during or for some time following the insult. However, discrimination between genetic and acquired defects is complicated by the fact that symptoms induced by the former, such as lack of mucociliary clearance, often lead to chronic inflammation which may readily induce multiple and widespread acquired defects in the cilia (Cornillie *et al.*, 1984). This was likely in the case reported by Howell *et al.* (1980) when, in addition to a lack of dynein arms (a genetic defect), numerous apparently acquired defects were also seen in the cilia of a 12-year-old boy who had repeated respiratory tract infections. Likewise, genetically abnormal cilia were described in patients who developed bronchiectasis, yet numerous seemingly acquired ciliary lesions were also noted, superimposed upon the genetic defects (Wakefield and Waite, 1980). No specific axonemal defects which could be genetically derived and not simply the result of the insult due to recurrent infections or medications have been found in patients with cystic fibrosis (Kollberg *et al.*, 1978; Katz and Holsclaw, 1980; Robertson, 1982; see also Section 8.2).

Normal ciliary structure is shown in Fig. 7.1. At the base of each cilium is a basal body which lies in the apical cytoplasm of the ciliated cell. Nine sets of vertically oriented paired microtubules (microtubular doublets) extend upwards from the basal body, are evenly spaced around the perimeter of the cilium and surround a central set of two separated and vertically oriented microtubules. A cylindrical sheath surrounds the two central microtubules. The microtubules are composed of tubulin. Extend-

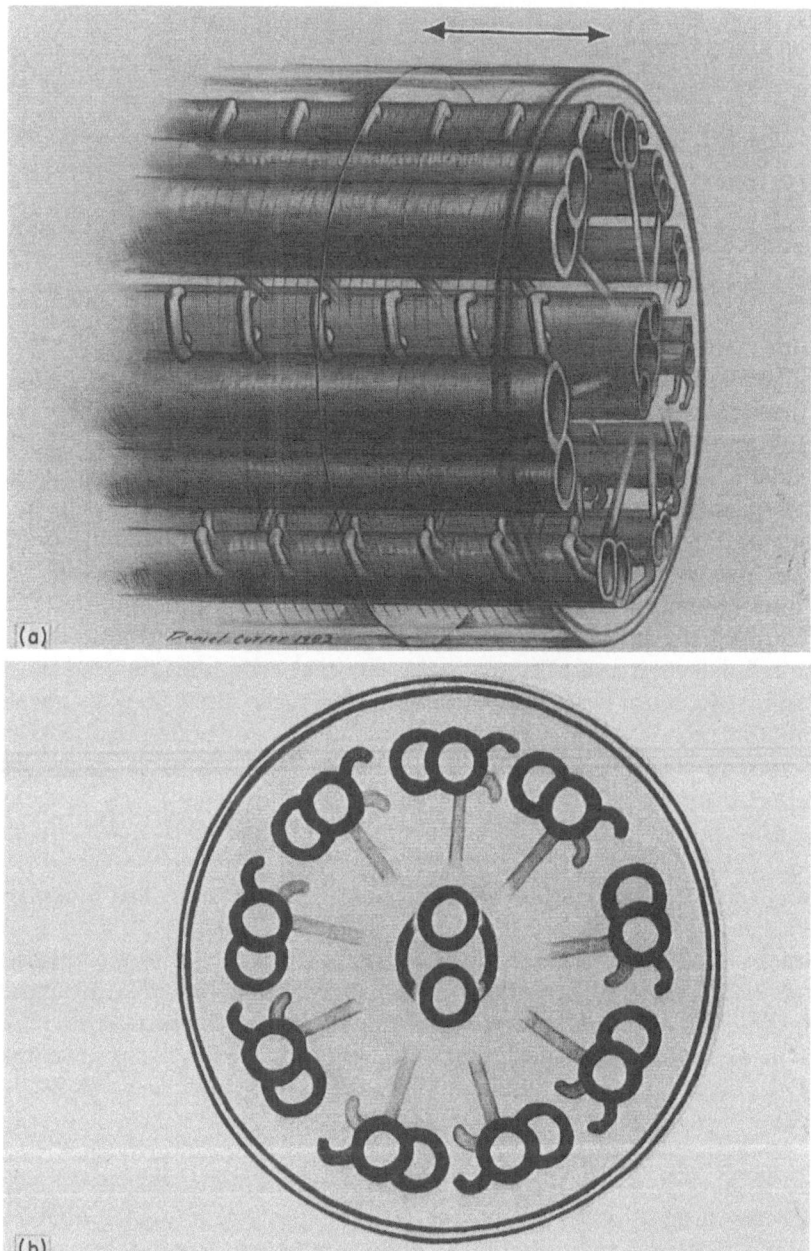

Fig. 7.1 Drawings of the axonemal components of the cilium. The orientation used here is that most commonly shown in drawings and published micrographs with the dynein arms extending out clockwise. This is the view as seen from within

ing from each pair of peripheral microtubules are a row of inner and a row of outer dynein arms. At least a portion of these arms have ATPase activity and are considered essential for ciliary movement (Gibbons and Rowe, 1965; Sleigh, 1977; Warner *et al.*, 1977). The angle between the dynein arms and the microtubular doublet changes with the dynamics of ciliary motion (Goodenough and Heuser, 1982). Radial spokes extend between the two central microtubules and the peripheral circle of microtubular doublets. This microtubular apparatus, called the axoneme, lies in an extension of the cell cytoplasm and the entire cilium is enclosed by a specialization of the apical cell membrane, the ciliary membrane (Figs 7.1, 7.2, 7.6a).

Individual cilia can be seen by light microscopy and their motility can be observed particularly well with phase optics (Veerman *et al.*, 1980a; Pederson and Mygind, 1980). However, their axonemal structures cannot be resolved. Therefore, detection of ciliary structural abnormalities requires electron microscopic examination. Because of the high magnification and resolution necessary to identify the individual components of the cilium, the thickness and orientation of the sections are critical. Ultrathin silver-gray sections and perfect ciliary orientation, 90° to the ciliary shaft, are essential to obtain distinct images of axonemal elements in the micrographs. The effect of slightly oblique cuts through cilia can be seen in randomly sectioned cilia which happen to be located adjacent to the more perfectly sectioned cilia being pictured (Figs 7.2b, 7.3, 7.5c, 7.6). Further comments on this are found at the end of the chapter.

7.2 Acquired abnormalities

Respiratory ciliated cells are highly susceptible to many different types of injury. Following an insult, ciliated cells will be lethally or sublethally injured. Dead and some sublethally injured ciliated cells slough from the bronchial epithelium but, depending on the severity of the insult, varying

---

the cell looking out toward the tip of the cilium. (a) Three dimensional configuration of those components visible in electron microscopic images. Nine joined pairs of radially arranged microtubules (doublets) are evenly spaced around the perimeter. Extending from each pair of microtubules are the dynein arms, an outer and an inner row, uniformly spaced along one side of each doublet and extending toward the adjacent doublet. The angle between the dynein arms and the microtubules changes with the dynamics of ciliary motility. Radial spokes extend from the doublets towards the center of the axoneme. A central set of two separated microtubules is surrounded by a central tubular sheath. An extension of the apical cell membrane encloses these structures. The double-ended arrow represents the thickness of a typical thin section. (b) Two dimensional representation of the cross-section of these components as seen in an idealized electron micrograph.

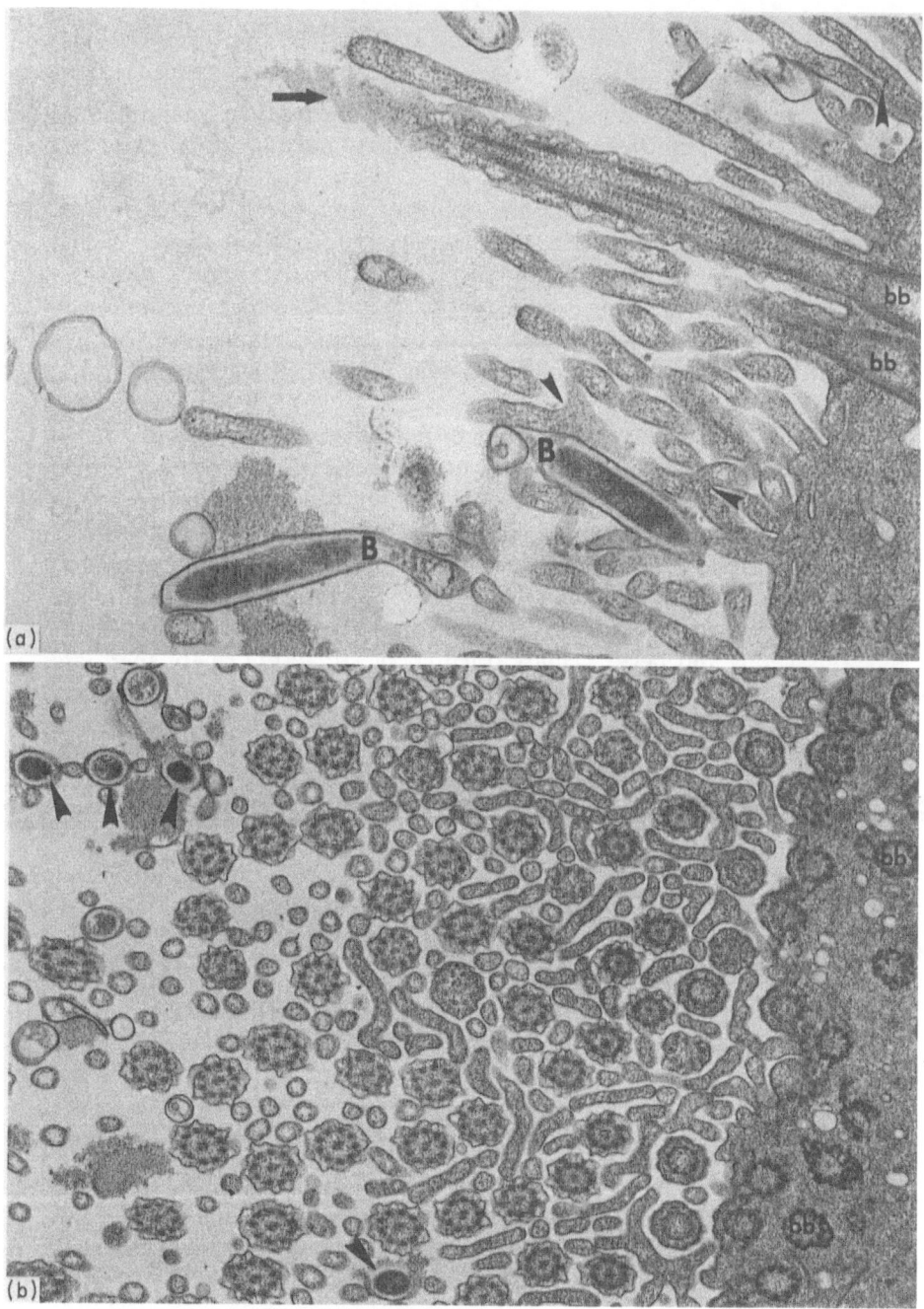

Fig. 7.2 (a) Apical portion of the ciliated cell in human bronchus. Microtubules run longitudinally in the cilium from basal body (bb) to near ciliary tip (arrow). Microvilli are slender and branched (arrowheads). Bacterial rods (B) have a characteristic morphology different from that of cilia. (× 32 000) (b) Same specimen. Cilia are cut in cross-section and the 9 + 2 microtubular pattern is clear. Basal bodies (bb) are cut in cross-section in the apical cytoplasm. Bacterial rods, cut in cross-section, show dense internal structure (arrowheads). (× 22 000)

numbers of sublethally injured cells will remain viable (Chapter 9). Some cilia of the sublethally injured cells will acquire various types of abnormalities. The clinical significance of these abnormalities is unknown. However, it has been established that inhalation of irritants such as cigarette smoke, sulfur dioxide, formaldehyde, mucolytic drugs and even commercial hairspray impairs movement of the mucociliary escalator by altering the viscosity of the mucus and diminishing or paralyzing the ciliary beats (Asmundsson and Kilburn, 1973; Wanner, 1977; Last, 1982; Roomans et al., 1983). Therefore, it is likely that pathologically altered cilia contribute in some degree to the diminished movement of mucus, thereby impairing clearance of irritants and particulates, including microorganisms and carcinogenic substances.

Acquired ciliary abnormalities of various types are very common in human bronchial epithelium (Afzelius, 1979; Afzelius, 1981). Abnormalities include disorganized axonemes and axonemes with extra or missing microtubules; swollen cilia composed of a single axoneme surrounded by excess cytoplasm or cytoplasmic projections in the form of wing-like folds; abnormal basal bodies; compound cilia (Fig. 7.3), also called fused cilia, megacilia and multicilia; and internalized cilia with and without their ciliary membranes (Fig. 7.4). Such abnormalities are seen in adults (Ailsby and Ghadially, 1973; Miskovits et al., 1974; Kondrádová et al., 1975; McDowell et al., 1976; Torikata et al., 1976; Wakefield and Waite, 1980; Katz and Holsclaw, 1980) and in children (Cutz et al., 1978; Howell et al., 1980; Corbeel et al., 1981; Rutland et al., 1982a; Cornillie et al., 1984). Although most commonly described in patients with overt bronchial disease and/or who smoke, ciliary abnormalities of various types, including microtubular abnormalities and compound cilia, have been reported in nonsmoking adults (Fox et al., 1981), in children (Wisseman et al., 1981) and in dogs (Wilsman et al., 1982) without chronic respiratory disease. In the study by Fox et al. (1981) there were no differences between the number of abnormalities, either of compound cilia or of microtubular structures, in smokers and nonsmokers, in patients with or without lung carcinoma, or in those with and without evidence of chronic infection. Furthermore, ciliary abnormalities were sometimes focal and showed marked variations in different sites of the bronchial tree of a single patient. Nevertheless, animal experiments indicate that many (if not all) of these ciliary alterations are nonspecific reactions of the ciliated cells to sublethal injury (Fig. 7.5). This is consistent with reports that abnormal cilia are commonly seen concurrent with various inflammatory states and other conditions that irritate the delicate mucociliary epithelium (Cornillie et al., 1984). Moreover, in some children who suffered from chronic airway infections, ciliary abnormalities regressed following antibiotic treatments (Corbeel et al., 1981) and repeated sampling of ciliated mucosa from the

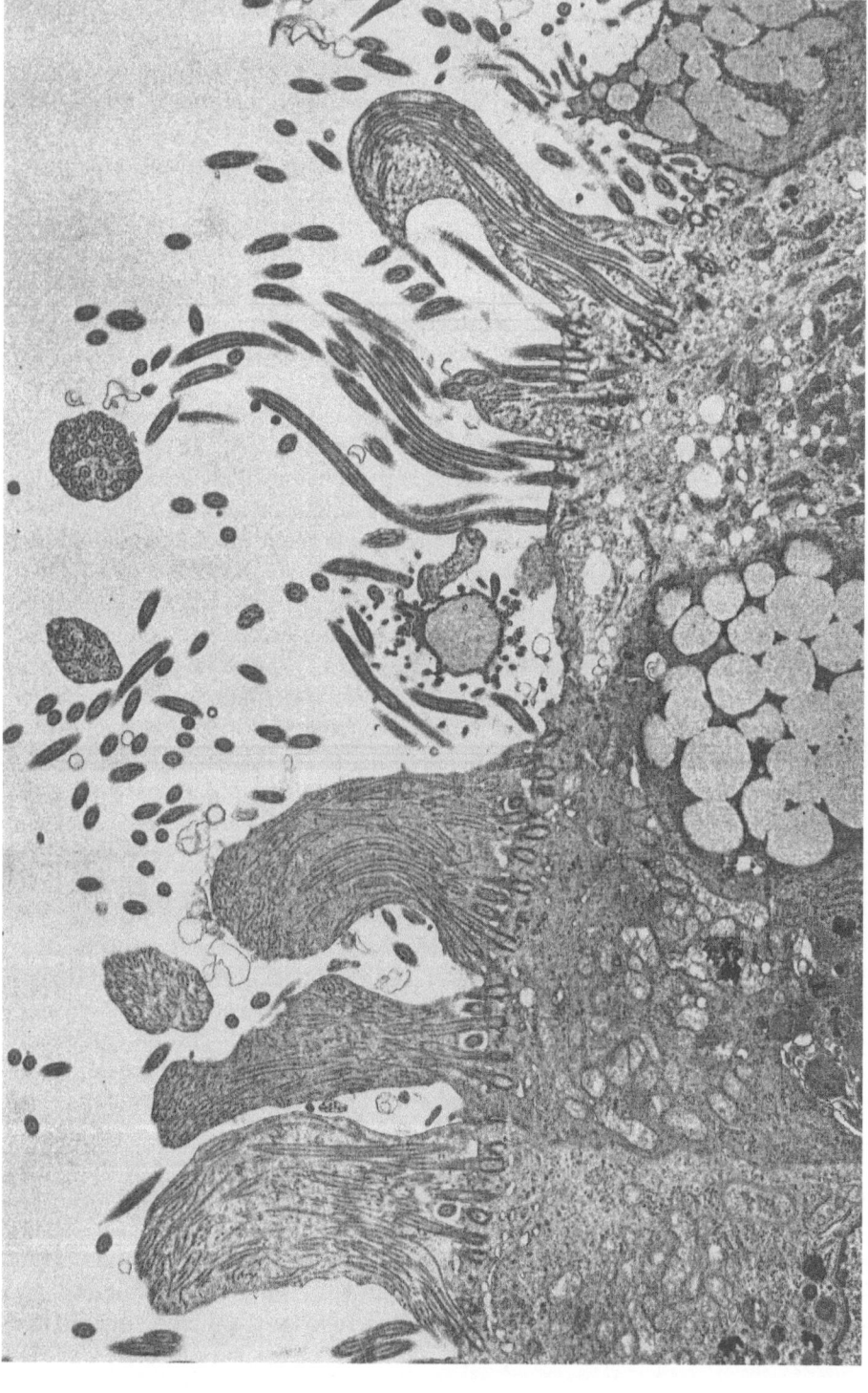

same individual, made possible by less traumatic techniques of nasal brushing (Rutland and Cole, 1980; Rutland et al., 1982b), further suggested that acquired ciliary abnormalities are transitory (Rutland et al., 1982a).

Axonemes with extra or missing microtubules have been described in patients with recurring infections (Howell et al., 1980; Rutland et al., 1982a), bronchiectasis (Wakefield and Waite, 1980), cystic fibrosis (Katz and Holsclaw, 1980) and in a young boy without chronic respiratory disease (Wisseman et al., 1981).

Cilia with excess cytoplasm usually occur singly, surrounded by cilia of normal size. They may have a normal axonemal 9 + 2 pattern or the microtubular doublets may be in disarray (McDowell et al., 1976). They have been seen in animals following nitrogen dioxide inhalation (Ranga and Kleinerman, 1981) and mechanical trauma. Swelling of the ciliary tips has been described following exposure to ionizing radiation (Baldetorp et al., 1977) and rather bizarre swollen ciliary tips were induced in porcine nasal mucosa by Bordetella bronchiseptica (Duncan and Ramsey, 1965). Shrunken cilia have also been described. It has been suggested that cilia shrink and become electron dense upon exposure to hypertonic fluids (Afzelius, 1979). Shrunken cilia must not be confused with contaminating bacterial rods which may be cut longitudinally (Fig. 7.2a) or in cross-section (Fig. 7.2b). Bacteria are rarely seen in human bronchi but they are said to be quite common in rat trachea (Afzelius, 1979).

Compound cilia (Figs 7.3, 7.5c) consist of multiple axonemal shafts enclosed within an apical extension of the ciliated cell. They arise following sublethal injury when the apical membrane blebs out focally and encloses several axonemes. They may also arise by fusion of adjacent cilia. Compound cilia have been reported in smokers (Ailsby and Ghadially, 1973; McDowell et al., 1976) and nonsmokers (Torikata et al., 1976; Fox et al., 1981; Wisseman et al., 1981) and in patients with chronic bronchitis, asthma, bronchiectasis, cystic fibrosis, Kartagener's syndrome, viral and bacterial pneumonias and pneumonia with asthma (Miskovits et al., 1974; Cutz et al., 1978; Katz and Holsclaw, 1980; Wakefield and Waite, 1980; Cornillie et al., 1984). As many as 40 axonemes have been described in one compound cilium (Torikata et al., 1976). Compound cilia have also been described in the tracheobronchial ciliated cells of animals following mechanical trauma (Keenan et al., 1983), nitrogen dioxide inhalation (Ranga and Kleinerman, 1981), application of mucolytic drugs (Roomans

Fig. 7.3 Bronchial epithelium from patient with epidermoid carcinoma. This specimen was far removed from the tumor. Compound cilia are numerous, with multiple axonemes in large cytoplasmic processes. Reproduced with permission from McDowell et al. (1978), Morphogenesis and classification of lung cancer. In *Pathogenesis and Therapy of Lung Cancer*, Marcel Dekker, New York.

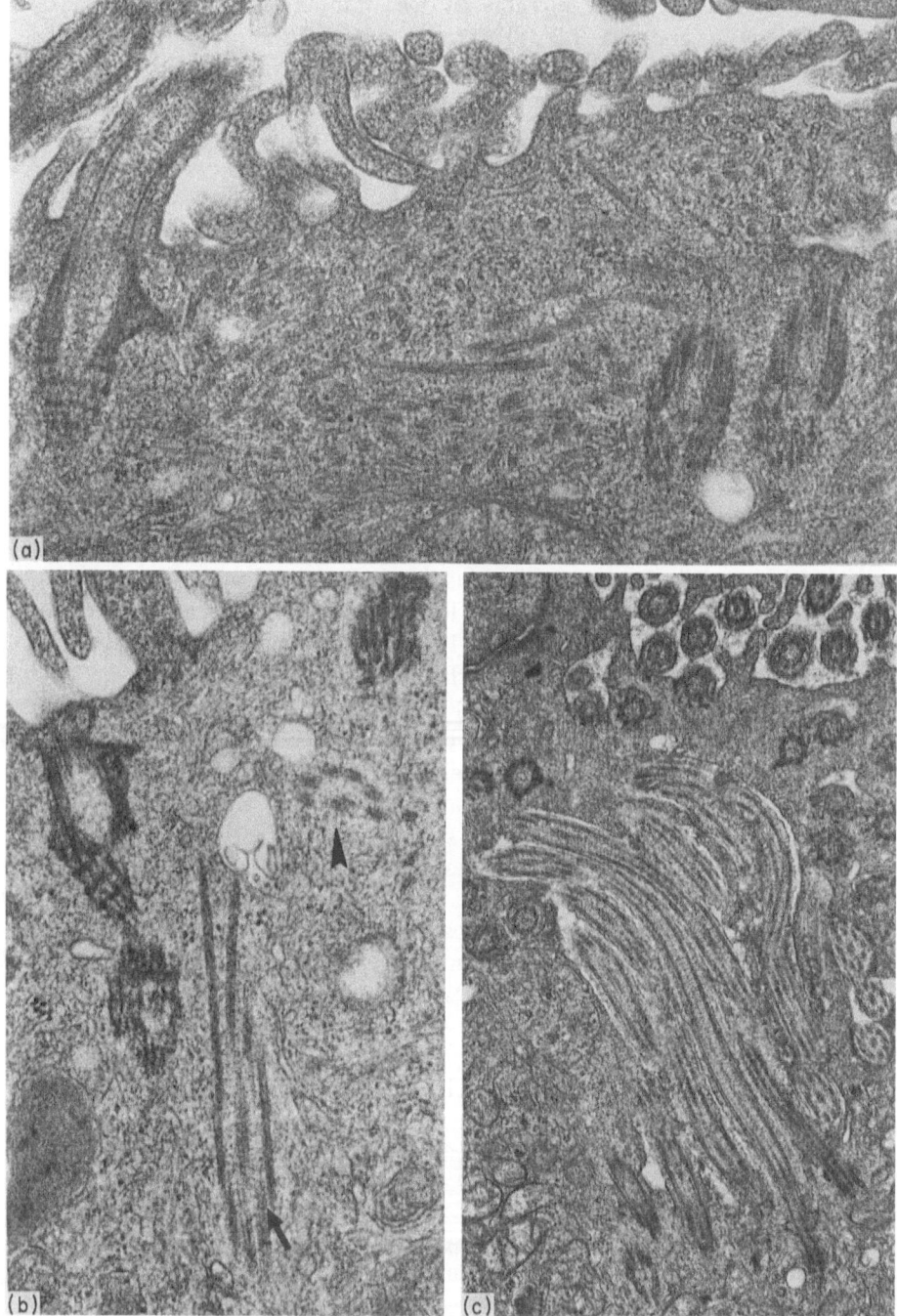

et al., 1983) and instillation of elastase (Lungarella *et al.*, 1980) or dilute aqueous formalin (Fig. 7.5c).

Another common reaction of ciliated cells to sublethal injury is internalization of their cilia (Figs 7.4, 7.5a, b). This can occur in at least two different ways. One is that the ciliary basal bodies retract into the apical cytoplasm and pull their axonemes into the cytoplasm of the cell (Figs 7.4b, 7.5a, b). This causes numerous microtubules in single and doublet configurations to accumulate in the apical cytoplasm in disarray (Figs 7.4a, 7.5a). In this case the internalized axonemes are *not* surrounded by a ciliary membrane. This abnormality has been described in human bronchi in smokers and nonsmokers (McDowell *et al.*, 1976; Torikata *et al.*, 1976; Wakefield and Waite, 1980), in patients with pneumonia (Cornillie *et al.*, 1984) and in hamsters following mechanical injury (McDowell *et al.*, 1979; Keenan *et al.*, 1983). Internalized axonemes were also seen in tracheal ciliated cells of animals in vitamin A deficiency (Wong and Buck, 1971) and following intratracheal instillation of carcinogens (Harris *et al.*, 1974; Reznik-Schüller, 1975) or inhalation of hyperbaric oxygen (Torikata *et al.*, 1976).

Internalization of basal bodies and the axonemal shafts superficially resembles ciliary development and could easily be mistaken for it. However, in ciliary development the formation of fibrogranular complexes precedes development of the basal bodies which become dispersed in the apical cytoplasm of preciliated cells. The newly formed basal bodies move apically *before* the ciliary axonemes are formed and disorganized axonemal structures are not observed in the apical cytoplasm of preciliated cells (Fig. 9.6). Therefore, if basal bodies *and* axonemal microtubules are seen together in disarray it can be assumed that injury has occurred with subsequent internalization of the cilia into the apical cytoplasm. Whether axonemal reabsorption is a reversible change in mammalian ciliated cells is presently unknown; however, the process is reversible in ciliated protozoa (Bloodgood, 1974; Calzone and Gorovsky, 1982).

Cilia may also be internalized when the apical membrane (which bears the cilia) invaginates into the cell so that the cilia, still surrounded by the ciliary membrane, project into a membrane-bounded cytoplasmic cavity (Fig. 7.4c). Cilia internalized in this way have been described in human

---

Fig. 7.4 Electron micrographs of human bronchial epithelium. Reproduced with permission from McDowell *et al.* (1976). (a) Numerous intracytoplasmic microtubular doublets are in disarray in the apical cytoplasm. These derive from internalized cilia. Note that cilia are absent immediately above the internalized microtubules but are present at left. (b) Intracytoplasmic axonemes in longitudinal (arrow) and cross-section (arrowhead). (× 61 000) (c) Several cilia, each surrounded by the ciliary membrane, lie in an intracytoplasmic cavity. (× 14 000)

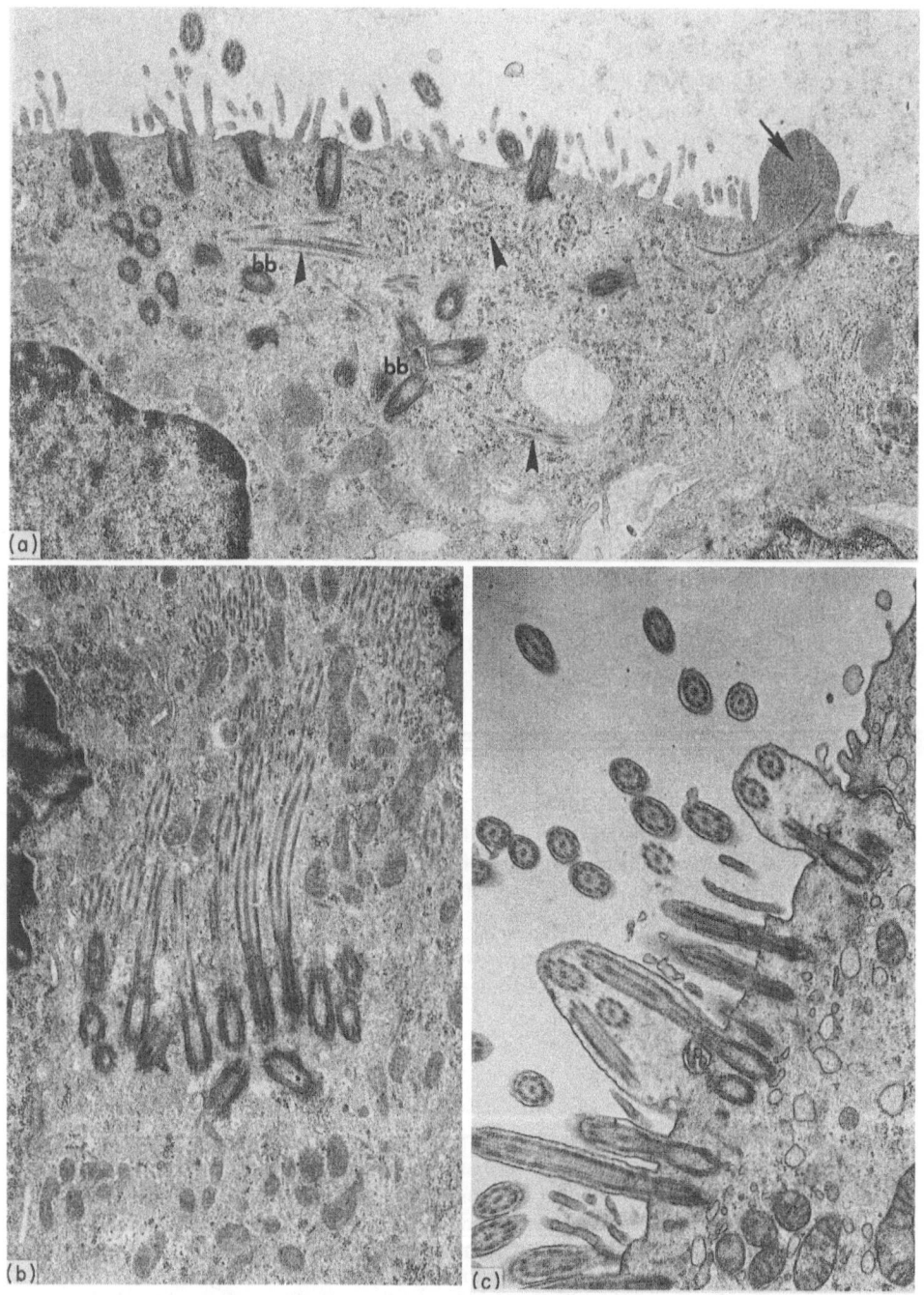

(McDowell *et al.*, 1976; Cornillie *et al.*, 1984) and hamster bronchi (Becci *et al.*, 1978), in guinea pigs exposed to hyperbaric oxygen (Torikata *et al.*, 1976) and in hamsters dosed intratracheally with carcinogens (Harris *et al.*, 1974).

Because acquired ciliary defects are seen so commonly and may occur in normal subjects, they have little or no diagnostic value. Moreover, the reported focal distributions of abnormalities in some patients and the apparent transient nature of the defects caution against attributing much significance to a single biopsy specimen (Fox *et al.*, 1981; Rutland *et al.*, 1982a).

7.3 Genetic defects

In 1933, Kartagener reported on a small group of individuals who had situs inversus, bronchiectasis and chronic sinusitis. Additional cases, some of whom also had nasal polyps, were described in a subsequent report (Kartagener and Horlacher, 1935). Some parents and siblings had recurrent respiratory disease; however, they generally lacked the full triad of Kartagener's syndrome. Since that time several hundred cases have been documented. Case analyses in Europe and the United States suggest that 1 out of between 30 000 and 70 000 individuals have Kartagener's triad (Olsen, 1942; Torgersen, 1947, 1949, 1950; Amjad *et al.*, 1974). Situs inversus occurs in about 1 out of 10 000 individuals (Torgersen, 1950) and bronchiectasis, which is seen in only about 0.5% of the general patient population, is seen in 17–23% of individuals with situs inversus (Olsen, 1942; Torgersen, 1949). Most of the people with Kartagener's triad have total situs inversus with dextrocardia and transposition of abdominal organs. In males, the right testicle is lower than the left (Rott, 1979). It is generally accepted that the pattern of inheritance is an autosomal recessive characteristic. Although bronchiectasis may be severe, resulting in surgical resection(s) of the affected lobes, the life expectancy of these people is not significantly impaired (Eliasson *et al.*, 1977; Rott, 1979).

In an infertility clinic in Sweden, Afzelius and co-workers recognized a small group of men who had immotile sperm without light microscopic abnormality. Ultrastructural examination revealed that the axonemes in

---

Fig. 7.5 Electron micrographs of hamster tracheal epithelium. (a) Sublethally injured ciliated cell near wound margin, 6 hours following mechanical injury. Note microtubules in apical bleb (arrow), internalized axonemes (arrowhead) and internalized basal bodies (bb). ($\times$ 11 000) (b) Numerous cilia with their basal bodies are internalized in a sublethally injured ciliated cell, 20 hours following mechanical injury. ($\times$ 13 000) (c) Compound cilia, 6 hours after intratracheal instillation of 1% formaldehyde in water. ($\times$ 13 000)

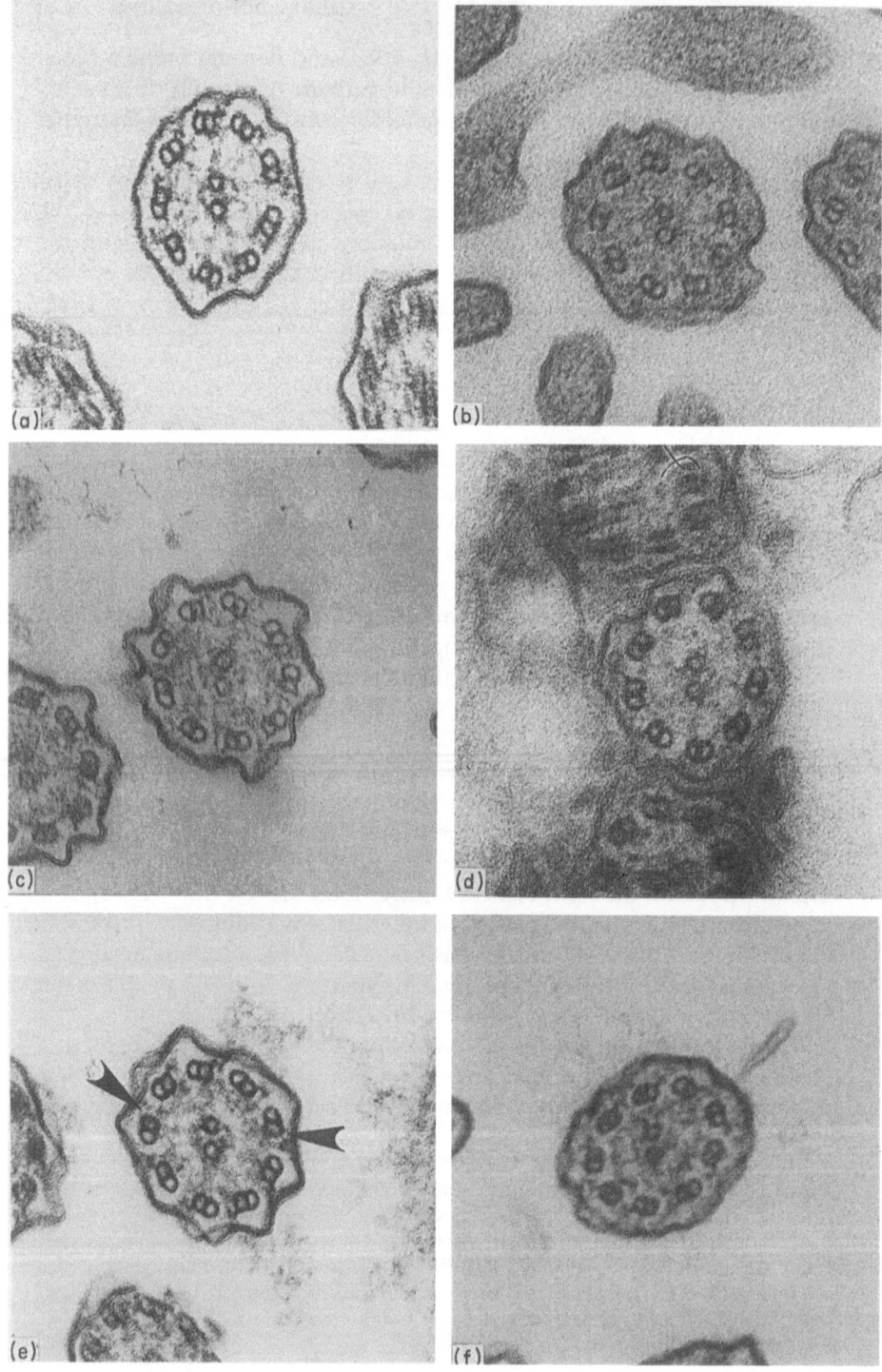

these sperm lacked the dynein arms (Afzelius *et al.*, 1975; Afzelius, 1976). The axonemal structures of the respiratory cilia were affected similarly (Fig. 7.6b), interfering with mucociliary clearance, and thereby causing chronic respiratory diseases. The dynein arms are known to have ATPase activity and are essential for ciliary movement (Section 7.1). Some of these men had Kartagener's syndrome and it was postulated that the absence of dynein arms was inherited. They concluded that in Kartagener's syndrome embryonic ciliated cells would also lack dynein arms and cause a failure of the normal visceral rotation, resulting in situs inversus in some individuals (theoretically 50%).

Other specific axonemal defects were subsequently observed in Kartagener's syndrome including absent (or nonimaged) radial spokes (Sturgess *et al.*, 1979; Schneeberger *et al.*, 1980; Corkey *et al.*, 1981; Kondrádová *et al.*, 1982; Herzon, 1983) and 'stubby' dynein arms (Waite *et al.*, 1978;

Fig. 7.6 Transmission electron micrographs of human respiratory cilia. In these six individual cilia which were sectioned perpendicular to their long axis, the axonemes have been arranged so that the central pair of microtubules is oriented in the same direction. In normal individuals there is a uniformity of this orientation among all the axonemes from a single cell. Conformity of orientation is not always seen in the axonemes of individuals with the immotile (dyskinetic) cilia syndrome. All dynein arms extend from the doublets in a clockwise direction. This is the view as seen from the cell looking 'upward'. They would extend counterclockwise if viewed from above the cell, looking 'down' upon the cilia. The radial spokes and central tubular sheath are somewhat visible in most of the micrographs. There is no reason to believe that they are absent in the others; they are simply not adequately imaged. Notice that the inner dynein arms are rarely imaged in any of the micrographs, including those from normal individuals. (a) Axoneme of a normal individual used as a control in a study of ciliary abnormality. (b) Classical pattern of complete lack of dynein arms in an axoneme from a young adult male with Kartagener's triad. All of the axonemes examined from this man showed an identical pattern. (c) Seven-year-old male with Kartagener's triad with the axonemal pattern of uniformly 'stubby' outer dynein arms. It has not been established if this form of genetic defect is caused by shortening of the arms by deletion of some of their macromolecular components or by a fixed acute angle of the arms (as they extend from the doublets), which would result in a foreshortened profile. (d) Axoneme from an 18-year-old female with bronchiectasis, sinusitis and recurring otitis media, but with a normal orientation of the heart and visceral organs. The cilia were all immotile in phase microscopy and could not be activated with the addition of ATP or ATPase. This defines the immotile (dyskinetic) cilia syndrome. The outer dynein arms are either stubby or absent, as was the finding in all other axonemes viewed. (e) Young adult with only rare respiratory infections, no bronchiectasis, sinusitis or situs inversus. Many outer dynein arms are normal; however, occasional doublets totally lack dynein arms (arrows). This was seen in many other axonemes from this person. (f) Adult male with Kartagener's triad whose axonemes appeared normal. All the outer dynein arms are visible in this axoneme. The cilia from this individual were motile. (× 110 000)

Jahrsdoerfer *et al.*, 1979; Forrest *et al.*, 1979; Kondrádová *et al.*, 1982; Woodring *et al.*, 1982; Lewis *et al.*, 1983) (Fig. 7.6c). Other less frequently found abnormalities in documented Kartagener's syndrome include prominent outer dynein arms (Kondrádová *et al.*, 1982), absent inner arms with unusually prominent outer arms (Forrest *et al.*, 1979), or lack of inner arms (Neustein *et al.*, 1980; Sturgess and Peter Turner, 1982).

The subject is further complicated by the following observations. Some patients with Kartagener's triad have ultrastructurally normal outer and inner dynein arms (Fig. 7.6f) (Herzon and Murphy, 1980). Although theoretically a genetic defect should be present in all structures, a number of patients with Kartagener's have some but not all dynein arms within an axoneme or some axonemes with all normal dynein arms (Jahrsdoerfer *et al.*, 1979; Pedersen and Mygind, 1980; Kondrádová *et al.*, 1982). Although immotility of sperm is required for the immotile-cilia syndrome, there are reports of five male Kartagener's triad patients fathering twelve children (Rott, 1979). Nine females with Kartagener's in the same review gave birth to eighteen children; however, the effect of immotile cilia on female fertility is less definitive than in the male (Afzelius and Eliasson, 1983). Moreover, microscopic observation of respiratory epithelium in eleven individuals with Kartagener's triad showed that all cases had motile cilia; in some only one third of the ciliated cells observed had motility whilst in other cases all of the cells observed had normal motile cilia (Pedersen and Mygind, 1980). It should also be noted that normal individuals may apparently lack some dynein arms (Fox and Bull, 1979; Fox *et al.*, 1980; Lewis *et al.*, 1983) (Fig. 7.6e).

Additional study indicated that not all individuals with normally appearing but immotile sperm and chronic respiratory diseases had the full triad of Kartagener's syndrome (Fig. 7.6d). Therefore, the group at the Karolinska Institute proposed the term immotile-cilia syndrome, with a subclass of those with the Kartagener's triad (Eliasson *et al.*, 1977). All of these would be genetic and have abnormalities of their axonemes. With the observation of some visible ciliary activity in similar patients, the terms ciliary dysfunction (Pedersen and Mygind, 1980; Veerman *et al.*, 1980a) and dyskinetic cilia syndrome (Corkey *et al.*, 1981) were proposed as more accurate (Veerman *et al.*, 1980b; Sleigh, 1981).

It is difficult to overlook the presence of situs inversus, but since those individuals with inherited dynein arm defects who did not have Kartagener's triad were not readily apparent using routine medical examination, and because these individuals if diagnosed early could be treated aggressively for their recurrent infections and presumably reduce the progression to severe bronchiectasis, there was a flurry of interest in ultrastructural examination of cilia. With the less-selective choice of individuals examined it became apparent that the nature of the ciliary abnormalities was often more complex than the presence or absence of dynein arms and a large number of ultrastructural abnormalities were found, not only in patients with recurrent respiratory infections, but also in 'normal' children (Section 7.2).

Microtubular disarray is a relatively common nonspecific acquired abnormality of cilia (McDowell *et al.*, 1976; Pedersen and Mygind, 1980; Sturgess *et al.*, 1980; Afzelius, 1981; Corkey *et al.*, 1981; Wisseman *et al.*, 1981; Lewis *et al.*, 1983). Comments on the radial spokes were not included in these reports, although problems of arrangement of the microtubules could result from lack of radial spokes (Sturgess *et al.*, 1979; Sturgess *et al.*, 1980; Kondrádová *et al.*, 1982). However, at this stage of our knowledge, microtubular disarray should *not* be considered a genetic abnormality, unless there is definite proof of absence of radial spokes.

There are recent reports of individuals with recurrent respiratory infections and immotile sperm (when looked for in males), in which the cilia are said to lack axonemal structures (Baccetti *et al.*, 1980; Fonzi *et al.*, 1982) or in which the cilia are completely absent (aplasia). In one case of ciliary aplasia, columnar cells were present which bore long surface microvilli and fibrogranular complexes in their apical cytoplasm (Götz and Stockinger, 1983). These cells resembled preciliated cells (Section 3.2.3). In another case the nonciliated columnar cells bore slender microvilli with well-developed actin cores (Gordon and Kattan, 1984).

As we learn more about the molecular and functional structure of cilia it is becoming evident that much of the apparent confusion may be clarified with more complete analysis. Normal ciliary motility requires cranial direction of beat, universal synchronization and movement of the effective and recovery strokes in the same plane (Herzon, 1983). Each outer dynein arm is composed of 5 subunits, all of which directly participate in the dynamics of ciliary movement (Goodenough and Heuser, 1982). Defects in the dynein arm(s), radial spokes (or spoke heads), central microtubules and the central tubular sheath may each cause paralysis of the cilium (Schneeberger *et al.*, 1980). Any one, all or combinations of these abnormalities could be effected by specific genetic defects. Individuals with immotile (dyskinetic) cilia, recurrent respiratory infections, male sterility with normal light microscopic sperm morphology and situs inversus represent a heterogeneous genetic population. Future studies using higher resolution ultrastructural techniques, isolation of specific protein components, examination of motility and reaction to addition of ATP and/or ATPase will be necessary to learn more about each potential defect and clarify the situation. During the work-up of many of the patients reported in the papers cited above, some type of test for mucociliary clearance was performed (Camner *et al.*, 1975) which usually demonstrated a significant reduction or lack of clearance. However, very few investigators have directly observed ciliary movement microscopically and none has used the exquisite high resolution techniques of quick-freeze deep-etch replication needed to clarify the fine detail of dynein arms as used by Goodenough and Heuser (1982).

Scanning electron microscopic examination of respiratory ciliated epithelium from individuals with Kartagener's triad or the broader group of patients with immotile (dyskinetic) cilia syndrome fails to discern any outward sign of abnormal axonemal structure. However, in a few cases the cilia from individual cells do not have the usual uniform orientation and present as a disorganized tangle (Fig. 7.7) (Veerman *et al.*, 1980a). This could be related to the observation that in cilia from some patients with Kartagener's triad, there is a lack of the expected uniformity of the axonemal radial orientation (best seen by comparing the plane of the central separated microtubules in cilia from an individual cell). In normal persons all of the cilia from a given cell have a uniform radial orientation of the central microtubules (and presumably the whole axoneme), which is probably required for effective ciliary beat.

It is not difficult to identify individuals with Kartagener's triad and it is possible to distinguish individuals with 'immotile-cilia syndrome' in males if normal appearing but immotile sperm are seen. Ciliary dyskinesis can be observed in the light microscope with special lighting; however, the sophisticated equipment required is available in only a few laboratories. Routine transmission microscopy, as available in many diagnostic facilities, is generally inadequate to define the specific defects which might be genetic in origin. Inspection of micrographs in published case reports, some from very competent electron microscopy laboratories, attests to the difficulties of this type of study, even allowing for some loss of detail in the published plates. Inner dynein arms are frequently not imaged, and the clarity of the outer arms is variable. Radial spokes are poorly imaged in nearly all published case reports, and the central tubular sheath is difficult to discern even in the highest resolution micrographs.

The dynein arms and radial spokes, unlike the microtubular components of the axoneme, are not vertically continuous (Fig. 7.1). Depending on the thickness of the thin section, as well as the orientation of these structures within the axoneme, which change with the dynamics of ciliary movement

---

Fig. 7.7 Scanning electron micrographs of respiratory ciliated cells. (a) From a normal individual with the characteristic parallel alignment of cilia from the cell. (b) From a patient with Kartagener's syndrome. The cilia from this cell are disorganized, appearing as a tangle. Preliminary observations suggest that this may be characteristic of at least some of the types of genetically defective cilia. The appearance of individual cilia is indistinguishable from those of normal persons. (Horizontal field width = 12 μm.)

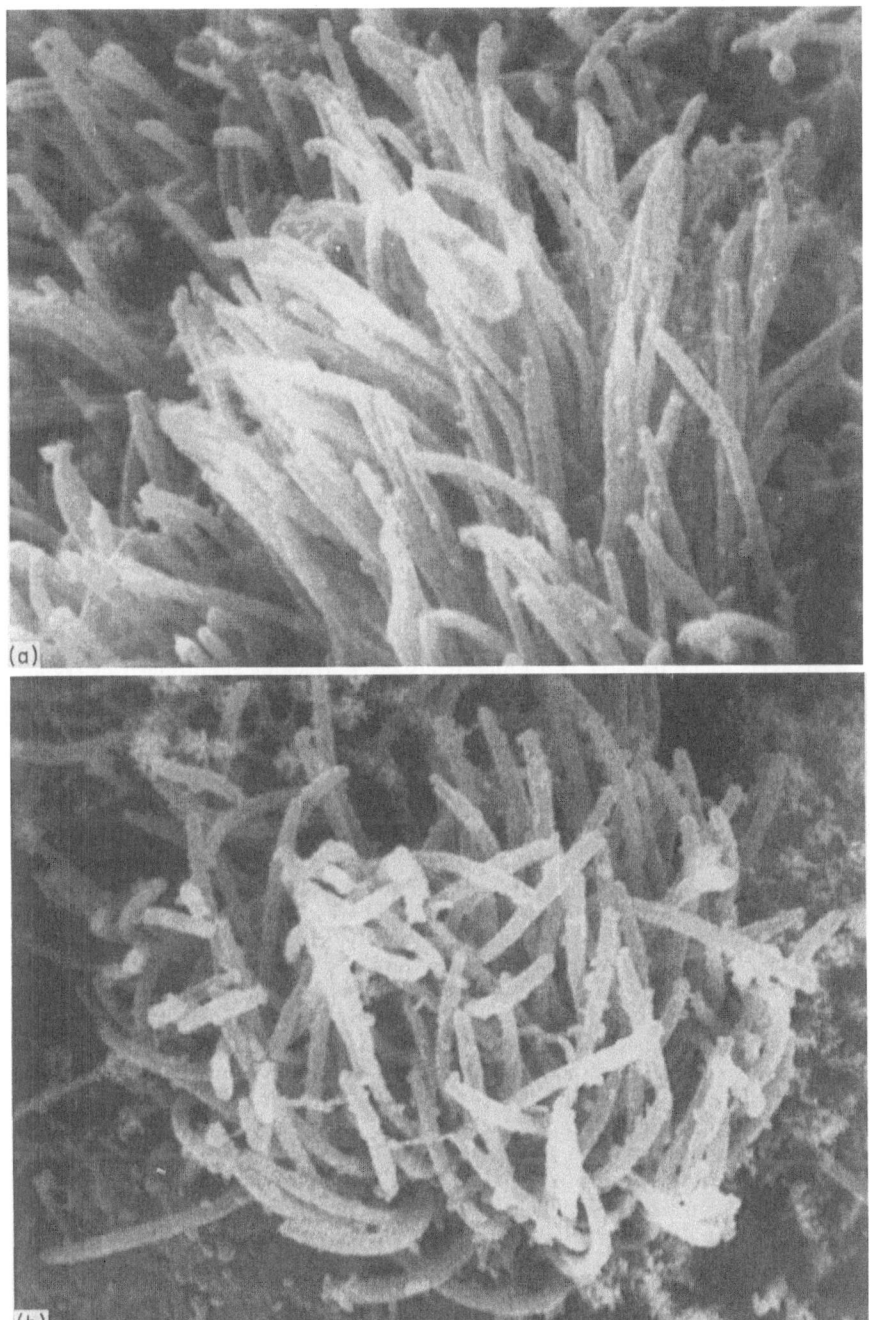

(a)

(b)

(Goodenough and Heuser, 1982), the characteristics of the arms and spokes may appear 'abnormal' in micrographs even if the microtubules are perfectly cross-sectioned. Except for total lack of axonemes or total absence of dynein arms in each and every axoneme, most diagnostic electron microscopy units should exercise caution in over-interpreting 'abnormalities' of axonemal fine structure in patients with recurrent upper respiratory infections suspected clinically of having *genetic* ciliary defects.

References

Afzelius, B.A. (1976), A human syndrome caused by immotile cilia. *Science*, **193**, 317–19.

Afzelius, B.A. (1979), The immotile-cilia syndrome and other ciliary diseases. *Int. Rev. Exp. Path.*, **19**, 1–43.

Afzelius, B.A. (1981), 'Immotile-cilia' syndrome and ciliary abnormalities induced by infection and injury. *Am. Rev. Resp. Dis.*, **124**, 107–9.

Afzelius, B.A. and Eliasson, R. (1983), Male and female infertility problems in the immotile-cilia syndrome. *Eur. J. Resp. Dis.*, **64**, suppl. 127, 144–7.

Afzelius, B.A., Eliasson, R., Johnsen, Ø. and Lindholmer, C. (1975), Lack of dynein arms in immotile human spermatozoa. *J. Cell Biol.*, **66**, 225–32.

Ailsby, R.L. and Ghadially, F.N. (1973), Atypical cilia in human bronchial mucosa. *J. Pathol.*, **109**, 75–8.

Amjad, H., Richburg, F.D. and Adler, E. (1974), Kartagener syndrome. Case report in an elderly man. *J. Am. Med. Assoc.*, **227**, 1420–2.

Asmundsson, T. and Kilburn, K.H. (1973), Mechanisms of respiratory tract clearance. In *Sputum. Fundamentals and Clinical Pathology* (ed. M.J. Dulfano), Charles C. Thomas, pp. 107–80.

Baccetti, B., Burrini, A.G. and Pallini, V. (1980), Spermatozoa and cilia lacking axoneme in an infertile man. *Andrologia*, **12**, 525–32.

Baldetorp, L., van Mecklenburg, C. and Håkansson, C.H. (1977), Ultrastructural alterations in ciliary cells exposed to ionizing radiation. A scanning and transmission electron microscopic study. *Cell Tiss. Res.*, **180**, 421–31.

Becci, P.J., McDowell, E.M. and Trump, B.F. (1978), The respiratory epithelium. II. Hamster trachea, bronchus and bronchioles. *J. Natl Cancer Inst.*, **61**, 551–61.

Bloodgood, R.A. (1974), Resorption of organelles containing microtubules. *Cytobios*, **9**, 143–61.

Calzone, F.J. and Gorovsky, M.A. (1982), Cilia regeneration in Tetrahymena. A simple reproducible method for producing large numbers of regenerating cells. *Exp. Cell Res.*, **140**, 471–6.

Camner, P., Mossberg, B. and Afzelius, B.A. (1975), Evidence for congenitally nonfunctioning cilia in the tracheobronchial tract in two subjects. *Am. Rev. Resp. Dis.*, **112**, 807–9.

Corbeel, L., Cornillie, F., Lauweryns, J., Boel, M. and Van Den Berghe, G. (1981), Ultrastructural abnormalities of bronchial cilia in children with recurrent airway infections and bronchiectasis. *Arch. Dis. Child.*, **56**, 929–33.

Corkey, C.W.B., Levison, H. and Turner, J.A.P. (1981), The immotile cilia syndrome: a longitudinal survey. *Am. Rev. Resp. Dis.*, **124**, 544–8.

Cornillie, F.J., Lauweryns, J.M. and Corbeel, L. (1984), Atypical bronchial cilia in children with recurrent respiratory tract infections. A comparative ultrastructural study. *Path. Res. Pract.*, **178**, 595–604.

Cutz, E., Levison, H. and Cooper, D.M. (1978), Ultrastructure of airways in children with asthma. *Histopathol.*, **2**, 407–21.

Duncan, J.R. and Ramsey, F.K. (1965), Fine structural changes in the porcine nasal ciliated epithelial cell produced by *Bordetella bronchiseptica* rhinitis. *Amer. J. Pathol.*, **47**, 601–12.

Eliasson, R., Mossberg, B., Camner, P. and Afzelius, B.A. (1977), The immotile-cilia syndrome. A congenital ciliary abnormality as an etiologic factor in chronic airway infections and male sterility. *New Engl. J. Med.*, **297**, 1–6.

Fonzi, L., Lungarella, G. and Palatresi, R. (1982), Lack of kinocilia in the nasal mucosa in the immotile-cilia syndrome. *Eur. J. Resp. Dis.*, **63**, 558–63.

Forrest, J.B., Rossman, C.M., Newhouse, M.T. and Ruffin, R. (1979), Activation of nasal cilia in immotile cilia syndrome. *Amer. Rev. Resp. Dis.*, **120**, 511–15.

Fox, B. and Bull, T.B. (1979), Electron microscopic structure of human cilia: what is normal? *J. Clin. Pathol.*, **32**, 969–70.

Fox, B., Bull, T.B. and Arden, G.B. (1980), Variations in the ultrastructure of human nasal cilia including abnormalities found in retinitis pigmentosa. *J. Clin. Pathol.*, **33**, 327–35.

Fox, B., Bull, T.B., Makey, A.R. and Rawbone, R. (1981), The significance of ultrastructural abnormalities of human cilia. *Chest*, **80**, suppl., 796–9.

Gibbons, I.R. and Rowe, A.J. (1965), Dynein: a protein with adenosine triphosphatase activity from cilia. *Science*, **149**, 424–6.

Goodenough, U.W. and Heuser, J.E. (1982), Substructure of the outer dynein arm. *J. Cell Biol.*, **95**, 798–815.

Gordon, R.E. and Kattan, M. (1984), Absence of cilia and basal bodies with predominance of brush cells in the respiratory mucosa from a patient with immotile cilia syndrome. *Ultrastruct. Pathol.*, **6**, 45–9.

Götz, M. and Stockinger, L. (1983), Aplasia of respiratory tract cilia. *Lancet*, **i**, 1283.

Harris, C.C., Kaufman, D.G., Jackson, F., Smith, J.M., Dedick, P. and Saffiotti, U. (1974), Atypical cilia in the tracheobronchial epithelium of the hamster during respiratory carcinogenesis. *J. Pathol.*, **114**, 17–19.

Herzon, F.S. (1983), Nasal ciliary structural pathology. *Laryngoscope*, **93**, 63–7.

Herzon, F.S. and Murphy, S. (1980), Normal ciliary ultrastructure in children with Kartagener's syndrome. *Ann. Otol. Rhin. Laryg.*, **89**, 81–3.

Howell, J.T., Schochet, S.S., Jr. and Goldman, A.S. (1980), Ultrastructural defects of respiratory tract cilia associated with chronic infections. *Arch. Pathol. Lab. Med.*, **104**, 52–5.

Jahrsdoerfer, R., Feldman, P.S., Rubel, E.W., Guerrant, J.L., Eggleston, P.A. and Selden, R.F. (1979), Otitis media and the immotile-cilia syndrome. *Laryngoscope*, **89**, 769–78.

Kartagener, M. (1933), Zur Pathogenese der Bronchiektasien. I. Mitteilung: Bronchiektasien bei Situs viscerum inversus. *Beitrage Klinik Tuberkul. (Pneumonol.-Pneumonol.)*, **83**, 489–501.

Kartagener, M. and Horlacher, A. (1935), Bronchiektasien bei Situs viscerum inversus. *Schweiz. Med., Wochenschr.*, **34**, 782–4.

Katz, S.M. and Holsclaw, D.S. (1980), Ultrastructural features of respiratory cilia in cystic fibrosis. *Am. J. Clin. Pathol.*, **73**, 682–5.

Keenan, K.P., Wilson, T.S. and McDowell, E.M. (1983), Regeneration of hamster tracheal epithelium after mechanical injury. IV. Histochemical, immunocytochemical and ultrastructural studies. *Virch. Arch. (Cell Pathol.)*, **43**, 213–40.

Kollberg, H., Mossberg, B., Afzelius, B.A., Philipson, K. and Camner, P. (1978), Cystic fibrosis compared with the immotile-cilia syndrome. A study of mucociliary clearance, ciliary ultrastructure, clinical picture and ventilatory function. *Scand. J. Resp. Dis.*, **59**, 297–306.

Kondrádová, V., Hloušková, Z. and Tománek, A. (1975), Atypical kinocilia in human epithelium from large bronchus. *Folia Morphol. (Praha)*, **23**, 293–5.

Kondrádová, V., Vávrová, V., Hloušková, Z., Copova, M., Tománek, A. and Houštěk, J. (1982), Ultrastructure of bronchial epithelium in children with chronic or recurrent respiratory disease. *Eur. J. Resp. Dis.*, **63**, 516–25.

Last, J.A. (1982), Mucus production and the ciliary escalator. In *Mechanisms in Respiratory Toxicology*, Vol. 1 (eds H. Witschi and P. Nettesheim), CRC Press, Boca Raton, Florida, pp. 247–68.

Lewis, F.H., Beals, T.F., Carey, T.E., Baker, S.R. and Mathews, K.P. (1983), Ultrastructural and functional studies of cilia from patients with asthma, aspirin intolerance and nasal polyps. *Chest*, **83**, 487–90.

Lungarella, G., Fonzi, L. and Pacini, E. (1980), Atypical cilia in rabbit bronchial epithelial cells induced by elastase: an ultrastructural study. *J. Pathol.*, **131**, 379–83.

McDowell, E.M., Barrett, L.A., Harris, C.C. and Trump, B.F. (1976), Abnormal cilia in human bronchial epithelium. *Arch. Pathol. Lab. Med.*, **100**, 429–36.

McDowell, E.M., Becci, P.J., Schürch, W. and Trump, B.F. (1979), The respiratory epithelium. VII. Epidermoid metaplasia of hamster tracheal epithelium during regeneration following mechanical injury. *J. Natl Cancer Inst.*, **62**, 995–1008.

Miskovits, G., Appel, J. and Szüle, P. (1974), Ultrastructural changes of ciliated columnar epithelium and goblet cells in chronic bronchitis biopsy material. *Acta Morph. Acad. Sci. Hung.*, **22**, 91–103.

Neustein, H.B., Nickerson, B. and O'Neal, M. (1980), Kartagener's syndrome with absence of inner dynein arms of respiratory cilia. *Am. Rev. Resp. Dis.*, **122**, 979–81.

Olsen, A.M. (1942), Bronchiectasis and dextrocardia: observations on the etiology of bronchiectasis. *Coll. Papers Mayo Clin.*, **34**, 764–5.

Pedersen, M. and Mygind, N. (1980), Ciliary motility in the 'immotile cilia syndrome'. First results of microphoto-oscillographic studies. *Brit. J. Dis. Chest*, **74**, 239–44.

Ranga, V. and Kleinerman, J. (1981), A quantitative study of ciliary injury in the small airways of mice: the effects of nitrogen dioxide. *Exp. Lung Res.*, **2**, 49–55.

Reznik-Schüller, H. (1975), Ciliary alterations in hamster respiratory tract epithelium after exposure to carcinogens and cigarette smoke. *Cancer Letters*, **1**, 7–13.

Robertson, B. (1982), Editorial. Ultrastructural abnormalities in young patients with recurrent respiratory infections. *Eur. J. Resp. Dis.*, **63**, 496–7.

Roomans, G.M., Tegner, H. and Toremalm, N.G. (1983), Acetylcysteine and its derivatives: functional and morphological effects on tracheal mucosa *in vitro*. *Eur. J. Resp. Dis.*, **64**, 416–25.

Rott, H.-D. (1979), Kartagener's syndrome and the syndrome of immotile cilia. *Human Genet.*, **46**, 249–61.

Rutland, J. and Cole, P.J. (1980), Noninvasive sampling of nasal cilia for measurement of beat frequency and study of ultrastructure. *Lancet*, **ii**, 564–5.

Rutland, J., Cox, T., Dewar, A., Cole, P. and Warner, J.O. (1982a), Transitory ultrastructural abnormalities of cilia. *Brit. J. Dis. Chest*, **76**, 185–8.

Rutland, J., Dewar, A., Cox, T. and Cole P. (1982b), Nasal brushing for the study of ciliary ultrastructure. *J. Clin. Pathol.*, **35**, 357–9.

Schneeberger, E.E., McCormack, J., Issenberg, H.J., Schuster, S.R. and Gerald, P.S. (1980), Heterogeneity of ciliary morphology in the immotile-cilia syndrome in man. *J. Ultrastr. Res.*, **73**, 34–43.

Sleigh, M.A. (1977), The nature and action of respiratory tract cilia. In *Respiratory defense mechanisms*, Part 1, Vol. 5 (eds J. Brain, D. Proctor and L. Reid), Marcel Dekker, New York, pp. 247–88.

Sleigh, M.A. (1981), Primary ciliary dyskinesia. *Lancet*, **ii**, 476.

Sturgess, J.M., Chao, J. and Turner, J.A.P. (1980), Transposition of ciliary microtubules. Another cause of impaired ciliary motility. *New Engl. J. Med.*, **303**, 318–22.

Sturgess, J.M., Chao, J., Wong, J., Aspin, N. and Turner, J.A.P. (1979), Cilia with defective radial spokes. A cause of human respiratory diseases. *New Engl. J. Med.*, **300**, 53–6.

Sturgess, J.M. and Turner, J.A.P. (1982), Pathology of cilia in human respiratory disease. *Lab. Invest.*, **46**, 81A.

Torgersen, J. (1947), Transposition of viscera-bronchiectasis and nasal polyps. A genetical analysis and a contribution to the problem of constitution. *Acta Radiol.*, **28**, 17–24.

Torgersen, J. (1949), Genetic factors in visceral asymmetry and in the development and pathologic changes of lungs, heart and abdominal organs. *Arch. Pathol.*, **47**, 566–93.

Torgersen, J. (1950), Situs inversus, asymmetry, and twinning. *Am. J. Hum. Genet.*, **2**, 361–70.

Torikata, C., Takeuchi, H., Yamaguchi, H. and Kageyama, K. (1976), Abnormal cilia in the bronchial mucosa. Case reports of non-smoking women with bronchogenic carcinomas and an experimental model in guinea-pigs. *Virch. Arch. A Path. Anat.*, **371**, 121–9.

Veerman, A.J.P., van Delden, L., Feenstra, L. and Leene, W. (1980a), The immotile cilia syndrome: phase contrast light microscopy, scanning and transmission electron microscopy. *Pediatr.*, **65**, 698–702.

Veerman, A.J.P., van der Baan, A., Weltevreden, E.F., Leene, W. and Feenstra, L. (1980b), Cilia: immotile, dyskinetic, dysfunctional. *Lancet*, **ii**, 266.

Waite, D., Steele, R., Ross, I., Wakefield, St.J., Mackay, J. and Wallace, J. (1978), Cilia and sperm tail abnormalities in Polynesian bronchiectatics. *Lancet*, **ii**, 132–3.

Wakefield, St.J. and Waite, D. (1980), Abnormal cilia in Polynesians with bronchiectasis. *Am. Rev. Resp. Dis.*, **121**, 1003–10.

Wanner, A. (1977), State of the art. Clinical aspects of mucociliary transport. *Am. Rev. Resp. Dis.*, **116**, 73–125.

Warner, F.D., Mitchell, D.R. and Perkins, C.R. (1977), Structural conformation of the ciliary ATPase dynein. *J. Mol. Biol.*, **114**, 367–84.

Wilsman, N.J., Farnum, C.E. and Reed, D.K. (1982), Variability of ciliary ultrastructure in normal dogs. *Am. J. Anat.*, **164**, 343–52.

Wisseman, C.L., Simel, D.L., Spock, A. and Shelburne, J.D. (1981), The prevalence of abnormal cilia in normal pediatric lungs. *Arch. Pathol. Lab. Med.*, **105**, 552–5.

Wong, Y.-C. and Buck, R.C. (1971), An electron microscopic study of metaplasia of the rat tracheal epithelium in vitamin A deficiency. *Lab. Invest.*, **24**, 55–66.

Woodring, J.H., Royer, J.M. and McDonagh, D. (1982), Kartagener's syndrome. *J. Am. Med. Assoc.*, **247**, 2814–16.

8 Systemic diseases with bronchial manifestations

The lung is frequently involved in systemic disease either as the primary site of the lesion or as an extension of processes which are occurring in other organs. Most of the pulmonary changes associated with these diseases are centered in the parenchyma; however, a few affect the bronchial tissues and the adjacent parenchyma which are reached by bronchial biopsy. Principal among these is sarcoidosis which has been mentioned in Chapter 6 but is discussed further here. The remaining examples are rather rare and the patient's underlying disease is generally known to the clinician at the time of bronchoscopy. More often than not the reason for the bronchoscopy in these cases is for diagnosis of other suspected secondary diseases and the expression of the systemic disease is a curiosity. Nevertheless, occasional biopsy material may suggest, to the observant pathologist, systemic disease previously unrecognized clinically.

8.1 Amyloidosis

Amyloid may be deposited locally or as a generalized process and in both forms may be found in any organ of the body (Kyle and Bayrd, 1975). Amyloidosis refers to the process, regardless of the location, nature of the deposits or etiology. Amyloid has a hyaline appearance, is eosinophilic and gives a bright orangish-red (salmon) color when somewhat thick sections are stained with Congo red. When examined with crossed polarizing filters the Congo-red-stained material gives an apple green color which is more specific for amyloid. Amyloid may be associated with multiple myeloma, in which case the deposits are monoclonal immunoglobulin light chains. Amyloid may also accumulate secondarily to a variety of chronic inflammatory situations; the most common being tuberculosis, rheumatoid arthritis and chronic osteomyelitis. In these cases the protein is not immunoglobulin or its subunits. In fact the proteinaceous nature of amyloid varies considerably between different patients and/or different clinical settings (Glenner, 1980). However, the material is relatively consistent within a single individual. Despite the variety, both the light microscopic and the ultrastructural characteristics are uniform

(Wright and Calkins, 1981). Kisilevsky (1983) has suggested that amyloid deposition may result from the coupled effects of increases in specific proteins and a decreased ability to degrade the protein.

The lung can be the site of amyloid deposition under a variety of situations (Prowse, 1958). Thompson and Citron (1983) classified amyloidosis of the lung into eight morphological types. Lung parenchyma may have *nodular* or *diffuse* amyloid deposition as a part of *systemic primary amyloidosis* (Sappington *et al.*, 1942; Mäkinen *et al.*, 1977; Celli *et al.*, 1978; Kanada and Sharma, 1979). Lung involvement is much more rare as a complication of *systemic secondary amyloidosis* (Lee and Johnson, 1975; Smith *et al.*, 1979). Although amyloid may be deposited in the bronchial wall and peribronchial vessels in these systemic conditions, bronchial biopsy material is often reported as being free of visible deposits.

In those cases where amyloidosis is confined to the lung the deposition can be dramatically different. *Localized secondary pulmonary amyloidosis* (associated with tuberculosis, hypergammaglobulinemia, carcinoids and other neoplasms) can occur with a diffuse or nodular parenchymal pattern or as tracheobronchial plaques or masses. In Thompson and Citron's series (1983), amyloidosis confined to the lung was about four times more likely to be of the primary form (not associated with other disease processes). Somewhat less than half of these *localized primary amyloidosis* cases had a parenchymal distribution with either a nodular or a diffuse alveolar pattern. The nodular form presents with solitary or multiple bilateral masses often interpreted on x-ray as neoplastic (Bierny, 1978; Desai *et al.*, 1979). Most reported cases had nondiagnostic bronchial biopsies (Saab *et al.*, 1974; Schoen *et al.*, 1980), although in one reported case the massive solitary nodule had extended through the bronchial wall (mimicking neoplasia) and was biopsied endobronchially (Thompson *et al.*, 1983).

The tracheobronchial forms of amyloid deposition are of most interest to us here because both their diagnosis and treatment rely on bronchial biopsy. In Thompson and Citron's series (1983), most cases occurred as multifocal submucosal plaques giving an irregular appearance at bronchoscopy similar to the submucosal spread of malignancies. In these cases the amyloid is described histologically as small submucosal nodules (Attwood *et al.*, 1972; Flemming *et al.*, 1980; Schraufnagel *et al.*, 1980; Balázs, 1983) or surrounding submucosal glands (Mainwaring *et al.*, 1969).

Within the bronchus the deposition can be concentric and can become symptomatic with obstruction. Most reported cases have been treated with piecemeal resections. Since about half of the cases have progression, these local resections may have to be repeated numerous times over years. Solitary, polypoid endobronchial amyloid masses are less common. They usually present with post-obstructive pneumonia and are treated by excision (Gottlieb and Gold, 1972; Rubinow *et al.*, 1978).

Amyloid deposition in the bronchial wall may be associated with inflammatory cells including plasma cells and occasionally multinucleated giant cells. There may be squamous metaplasia of the overlying epithelium or ulceration. The deposits may extend between the bronchial cartilage and into the adjacent parenchyma. Calcification and osseous metaplasia may occur in the lamina propria making the lesions histologically similar to tracheobronchopathia osteoplastica (Section 5.12). However, amyloid lesions are usually symptomatic, whereas tracheobronchopathia osteoplastica is rarely any problem to the patient. Amyloid lesions are often vascular and bleeding is a frequent problem at bronchoscopy. Several cases have had fatal endobronchial hemorrhage associated with biopsy or therapeutic excisions.

8.2   Cystic fibrosis

Cystic fibrosis is the most frequent lethal genetic syndrome of Caucasian children and accounts for much of the chronic pulmonary disease of childhood (Wood et al., 1976). It is transmitted as an autosomal recessive character. Although the nature of the abnormality is not known there is a generalized dysfunction of epithelia, expressed clinically as pancreatic exocrine insufficiency, increased chloride ion in sweat and chronic pulmonary disease. Symptoms present in early childhood. There is mucous plugging in the airways and recurring pulmonary infections. Approximately one half of the cases of bronchiectasis in children are complications of cystic fibrosis (Davis et al., 1983) (Section 5.4). In the past, most of the patients who were homozygous for this disease died in childhood, usually from pulmonary infections. With aggressive treatment the life expectancy has increased and more of these people are reaching adulthood (Kollberg, 1982).

The diagnosis is made clinically with the support of a sweat chloride test. Bronchial biopsy is not indicated. The full range of changes of chronic infections can be seen in bronchial mucosa, none of which is specific for cystic fibrosis. Boucher et al. (1983) have a good review of the current knowledge of the pathophysiology of this disease.

8.3   Goodpasture's syndrome

Goodpasture's syndrome is a rapidly fatal disease of kidney and lungs (Benoit et al., 1964). In the kidney there is a focal glomerulonephritis with crescents, while in the lung there is intra-alveolar hemorrhage. It was recognized early that this syndrome is the consequence of development of antiglomerular basement membrane antibodies which have cross reactivity with the basement membrane of alveolar septae (Koffler et al., 1969).

In the lung hemosiderin-laden macrophages accumulate in the alveolar spaces and the histological differential diagnosis is with idiopathic pulmonary hemosiderosis. Transbronchial biopsies, reacted with immunofluorescent labeled anti-IgG and complement, show a characteristic linear pattern in alveolar septae (an identical pattern is present in glomerular capillaries) (Abboud et al., 1978; Beechler et al., 1980). There is no ultrastructural evidence of the immunoglobulin deposition (Shelburne et al., 1983). Patients with idiopathic pulmonary hemosiderosis lack this deposition.

8.4   Eosinophilic granuloma (histiocytosis X)

A group of clinically recognizable diseases (Hand-Schüller-Christian syndrome, Letterer-Siwe syndrome and eosinophilic granuloma) have in common the proliferation of 'histiocytic' cells. These diseases are collectively called histiocytosis X (Lichenstein, 1953). While some have argued that the group is so diverse both in morphological appearance and behavior that to simply designate them as histiocytosis X is to ignore their heterogeneity (Lieberman et al., 1969), others have taken large series of cases and attempted to make prognostically meaningful groups by other criteria (Greenberger et al., 1981). Despite their variable patterns it is clear that very young children with this proliferative disorder have a poor prognosis.

The proliferating cells, often called 'histiocytes', have been shown ultrastructurally to resemble the Langerhans' cells which normally inhabit the lower levels of the epidermis and which may have a wider distribution. They have characteristic cytoplasmic structures called Langerhans' granules which originate as modified invaginations of the plasma membrane (Fig. 8.1). The cells are believed to be derived from bone marrow precursors and apparently play a role in some inflammatory reactions (Silverberg-Sinakin et al., 1978; Tamaki et al., 1980). They may be a form of tissue macrophage similar to the Kupffer cell (Groopman and Golde, 1981).

Langerhans' cells, identified ultrastructurally, have been observed in lung tissue in association with usual interstitial pneumonitis (UIP), diffuse interstitial pneumonia (DIP) and bronchoalveolar carcinoma, as well as in the proliferative histiocytosis X. Langerhans' cells have also been identified in the lung parenchymal reactions of sarcoidosis, hypersensitivity pneumonitis and a variety of other inflammatory reactions (Basset et al., 1976).

Lung involvement with the proliferative lesions can occur either as a part of systemic histiocytosis X, or as an isolated pulmonary disease. Pulmonary extension of the systemic disease is uncommon (Lieberman et al., 1969; Carlson et al., 1976; Wester et al., 1982) although Greenberger et al. (1981) reported 45% of their systemic cases had lung involvement.

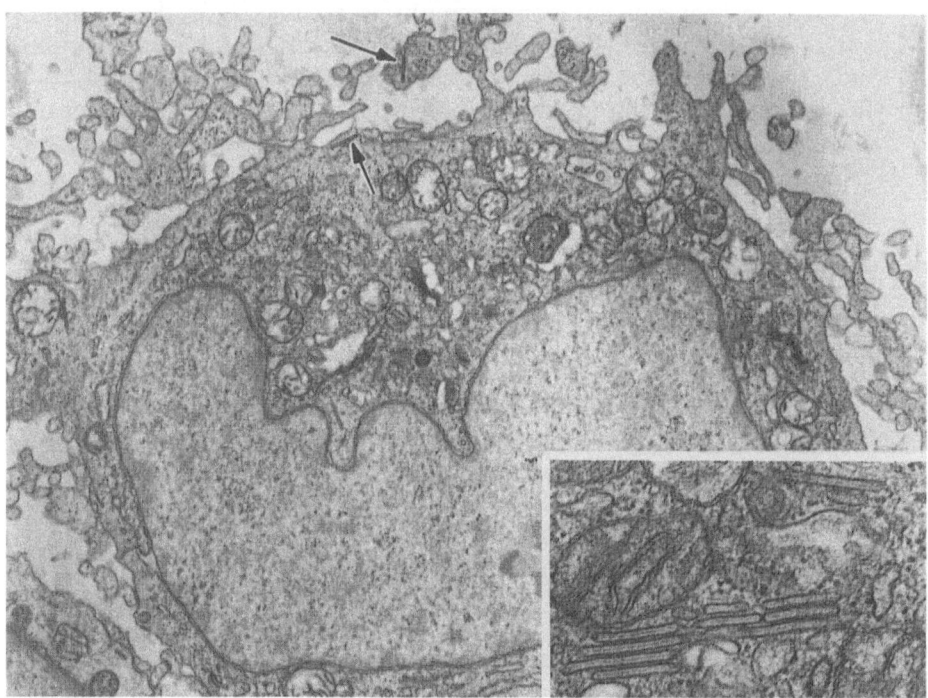

Fig. 8.1   Langerhans' cell in eosinophilic granuloma of lung. The surface of the cell has irregular processes. The characteristic Langerhans' granules appear to arise from the plasma membrane (arrows). (× 10 700) *Inset*: At higher magnification a group of Langerhans' granules with a central irregular beaded core which in this profile gives the appearance of a 'zipper'. (× 44 300) (Electron micrographs.)

The isolated form is frequently called eosinophilic granuloma of lung (Friedman *et al.*, 1981) or pulmonary histiocytosis X (Smith *et al.*, 1974; Basset *et al.*, 1978; Huhn *et al.*, 1981). There is a reticular nodular roentenographic pattern. The lesions consist of proliferating Langerhans' cells with variable numbers of associated eosinophils, plasma cells, lymphocytes and rare multinucleated giant cells (Fig. 8.2). The proliferating Langerhans' cells are similar to epithelioid cells in size, shape and nuclear characteristics and, like epithelioid cells, they do not contain phagocytized material. Unlike epithelioid cells their cytoplasm is less eosinophilic and individual cells are more discrete, rather than blending together. That epithelioid cells blend together is a reflection of the extensive surface ruffles which characteristically intertwine between adjacent cells. In contrast, the Langerhans' cells have less numerous irregular surface projections (Fig. 8.1). In older lesions foamy cells may become conspicuous. These are lipid-laden macrophages and not the Langerhans' cells. Hemorrhage may be significant and phagocytized hemosiderin may accumulate

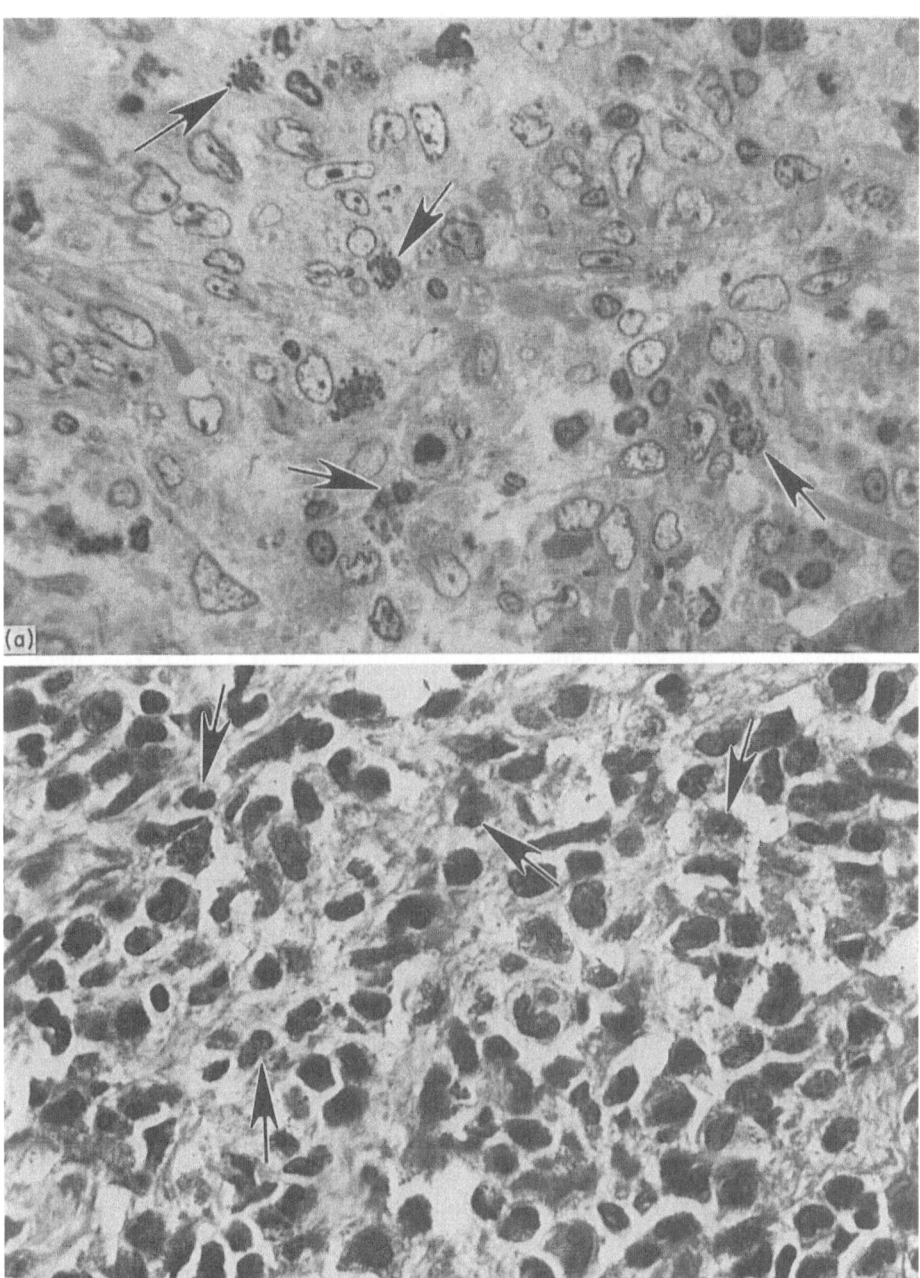

Fig. 8.2 Eosinophilic granuloma of lung. Diffuse proliferation of large individual Langerhans' cells admixed with neurophils, eosinophils (arrows) and lymphocytes. (a) Epon/Araldite embedded section stained with toluidine blue. (× 710) (b) Paraffin section stained with hematoxylin and eosin. (× 710)

in macrophages. Charcot-Leyden crystals may be present in the extracellular debris (Section 5.6).

Most cases of adult pulmonary histiocytosis X (eosinophilic granuloma) progress with eventual fibrosis (Lewis, 1964; Basset *et al.*, 1978), although spontaneous remissions are known (Smith *et al.*, 1974; Friedman *et al.*, 1980).

Transbronchial biopsy may provide diagnostic tissue but most cases require open lung biopsy for a definitive diagnosis (Basset *et al.*, 1978). This group and others have suggested bronchioalveolar lavage as a diagnostic approach using the electron microscope to identify the Langerhans' cells (Kullberg *et al.*, 1982; Verea-Hernando *et al.*, 1982).

8.5   Lymphomatoid granulomatosis

Liebow *et al.* (1972) first described lymphomatoid granulomatosis as a multisystem disease characteristically involving the lung and histologically resembling Wegener's granulomatosis. The disease is characterized by an infiltrate of atypical lymphoreticular cells in a variety of organs but usually in lungs, skin and the central nervous system. The infiltrates tend to be angiocentric and granulomas may develop (Fig. 8.3). Unlike Wegener's granulomatosis, involvement of the kidney and upper airways is uncommon. As additional cases have been followed and with a more complete immunological analysis, this disease was found to be associated with significant immunological deficiencies and many cases progress to lymphoma (Fauci *et al.*, 1982; Sordillo *et al.*, 1982). Because the characteristic lesion is angiocentric and composed of a mixed infiltrate of atypical lymphoid cells, macrophages and neutrophils with necrosis, involved vessels in cross-section resemble granulomas. In longitudinal sections, however, the lesions are linear and branching. Unlike Wegener's granulomatosis, well-formed epithelioid granulomas of the immunological type are not characteristic of this disease. The atypical lymphoid cells, which are the principal cellular component, are occasionally large and could be mistaken for epithelioid cells; however, their nuclei are extremely pleomorphic. There is a growing consensus that lymphomatoid granulomatosis is an expression of an immunological derangement associated with a lymphoma (often occult) (Churg, 1983; Colby and Carrington, 1983; Kradin and Mark, 1983). The granulomatous reaction is compared to other reactions with granuloma in Section 6.5.8. Further discussion will be found in Chapter 11.

8.6   Rheumatoid disease and Caplan's syndrome

Although more attention has been focused on the articular manifestations of rheumatoid disease, the lung is specifically involved in some patients.

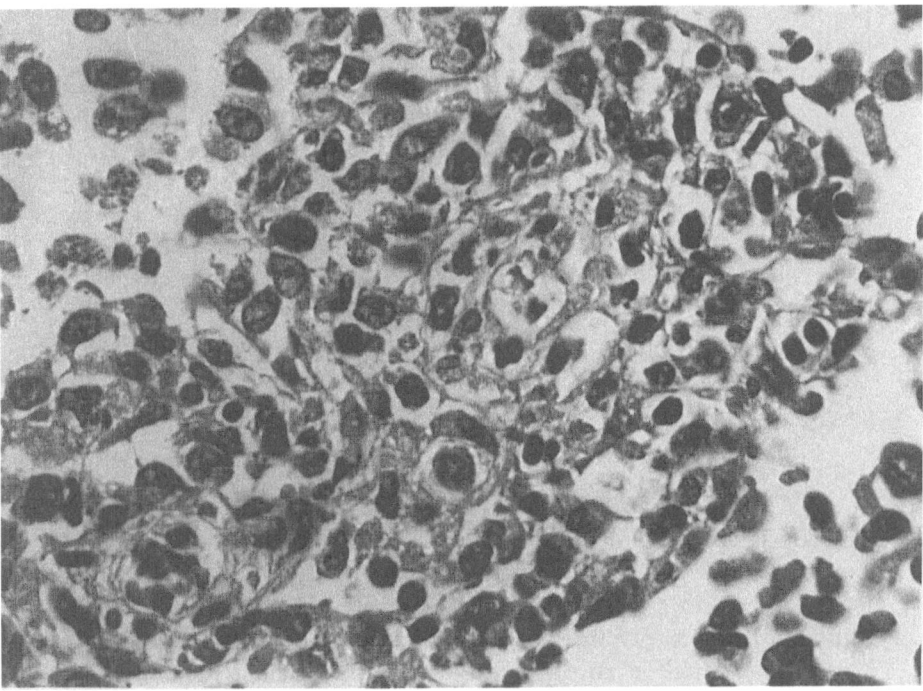

Fig. 8.3   Lymphomatoid granulomatosis. An atypical lymphoid infiltrate in lung, probably initially centered around a small vessel. (Paraffin section stained with hematoxylin and eosin: × 710.)

Depending on the techniques used to evaluate pulmonary changes, reports have shown that between 30 and 80% of patients with rheumatoid disease have histological alterations in their lungs (Cervantes-Perez *et al.*, 1980; Scott *et al.*, 1981). The most common and the least specific changes are diffuse interstitial inflammatory infiltrates with fibrosis and vessel wall thickening. Necrobiotic nodules (their extreme form known as Caplan's nodules) and necrobiotic pleuritis are rare but recognizable expressions of this disease. There is a greater risk for pulmonary involvement in patients with high rheumatoid factor titers (Turner-Warwick and Evans, 1977; Scott *et al.*, 1981) and in males (Macfarlane *et al.*, 1978). The pulmonary lesions may precede recognizable joint disease (Walker and Wright, 1968; Macfarlane *et al.*, 1978; Johnson *et al.*, 1982).

Necrobiotic lung nodules tend to be subpleural and are identical to those seen in the subcutis. They consist of central fibrinoid necrosis surrounded by pallisading macrophages which merge with a granulation tissue reaction. The lesions are quite well circumscribed but may enlarge and/or coalesce (Hunninghake and Fauci, 1979). Extension into the pleura is followed by pleuritis; extension into the bronchi produces bronchopleural fistula. In 1953 Caplan described the radiological pattern of rapidly progressing mass lesions in the lungs of coal-miners, who also had rheumatoid arthritis. The lesions may also occur in silicotic lungs (Chapter 5) and the mineral dusts are present within these large masses, which are essentially large necrobiotic cavities. For a more detailed account of this conglomeration of tissue reactions (which may also be associated with certain HLA types) see the case reviews of Gough et al. (1955), Caplan et al. (1962) and Darke et al. (1983).

Transbronchial biopsy of necrobiotic nodules has been reported (Turner-Warwick and Evans, 1977; Petrie et al., 1980; Johnson et al., 1982), although in biopsy the lesion may appear to be nonspecific necrotic tissue and the rheumatoid nature of the reaction may be overlooked without an accompanying clinical history.

8.7 Sarcoidosis

Sarcoidosis is a systemic disease manifested by the formation of granulomas, particularly in lung, pulmonary hilar lymph nodes and skin (James, 1976; James and Neville, 1977; Kataria et al., 1982; Cole et al., 1983). Although there is a characteristic histological pattern, the disease is not diagnosed without a constellation of findings which include clinical, roentgenographic and histological features, occasionally with the support of a skin reaction to injected material (the Kveim test) (Mitchell and Scadding, 1974; Selroos, 1981). Reflecting the complexity of making the diagnosis and the difficulty in comparing results of studies based on different diagnostic criteria, a committee chaired by James et al. (1976b) defined sarcoidosis as

A multisystem granulomatous disorder of unknown etiology, most commonly affecting young adults and presenting most frequently with bilateral hilar lymphadenopathy, pulmonary infiltrates, and skin or eye lesions. The diagnosis is established most securely when clinicoradiographic findings are supported by histological evidence of widespread noncaseating epithelioid-cell granulomas in more than one organ or a positive Kveim-Siltzbach skin-test.

The disease occurs world wide, affecting blacks somewhat more frequently than whites. Most patients are young adults when they present, there is no sex difference and prognosis is very good (James et al., 1976a; Nessan et al., 1981; Kataria et al., 1982). Although speculation has been great and quests intensive, sarcoidosis is currently defined by the absence of a discernible etiological agent(s) (Williams, 1982).

Histologically the lesions of sarcoidosis are well-circumscribed, small granulomas with conspicuous epithelioid cells and characteristically without central necrosis (Fig. 8.4). There are lymphocytes in and around the granulomas as well as macrophages and multinucleated giant cells. In lung, the granulomas tend to be numerous and can be found in peribronchial, subpleural, interlobular alveolar septae and perivascular tissue. They are also present in the lamina propria of the bronchi (Soler *et al.*, 1976; Crystal *et al.*, 1981; Cole *et al.*, 1983). Schaumann and asteroid bodies are often present in the multinucleated cells (Section 6.2) (Longcope and Freiman, 1952; Uehlinger, 1963). Early granulomas have more numerous macrophages and epithelioid cells, whereas aging granulomas become increasingly fibrotic with a concentric hyalinized collagen. Aging granulomas seldom calcify. For a general discussion of granulomas and their differential diagnosis see Chapter 6.

The histological confirmation of sarcoidosis has improved considerably with the use of the fiberoptic bronchoscope (Kataria *et al.*, 1982). Both endobronchial and transbronchial biopsies may contain the characteristic granulomas (Koerner *et al.*, 1975; Koontz *et al.*, 1976; Teirstein *et al.*, 1976; Koontz, 1978; Poe *et al.*, 1979; Mitchell *et al.*, 1980; Rohatgi *et al.*, 1981; Valenti *et al.*, 1982). Although transbronchial biopsy gives greater diagnostic yield than endobronchial biopsy, the combination of both improves the diagnostic yield (Mall, 1980; Armstrong *et al.*, 1981). Moreover, multiple bronchoscopic biopsies also increase the yield (Gilman and Wang, 1980; Roethe *et al.*, 1980; Nessan *et al.*, 1981). Bronchial biopsies have a potentially greater diagnostic yield than cervical lymph node or skin biopsies (Wiman and Hornblad, 1979). For a discussion of the value of bronchial biopsy in asymptomatic individuals with minimal clinical evidence of sarcoidosis see the interchange between Koontz and Dines in 1979.

Because of the difficulty in reaching a specific diagnosis of sarcoidosis, various ancillary tests have been suggested. The Kveim skin test (which is positive when noncaseating granulomas develop in the subcutaneous tissue following injection of extracts from patients with known sarcoidosis) has a mixed reputation (James and Neville, 1977; Selroos, 1981; Kataria *et al.*, 1982; Pierard *et al.*, 1982). This test suffers from inconsistency in the nature of the injected material (which is a relatively crude extract) and the necessity to biopsy the injected site to verify the development of granulomas. Elevated serum angiotensin-converting enzyme levels in sarcoidosis were felt to be specific; however, broader testing has shown that other diseases may also cause elevations of the enzyme in serum (Lieberman, 1976; Selroos *et al.*, 1981; Parrish *et al.*, 1982) and the elevation may be related to treatment rather than the disease itself (Davies, 1983).

Bronchoalveolar lavage has been used as both an investigative and a diagnostic tool in sarcoidosis (Hunninghake *et al.*, 1979b; Crystal *et al.*,

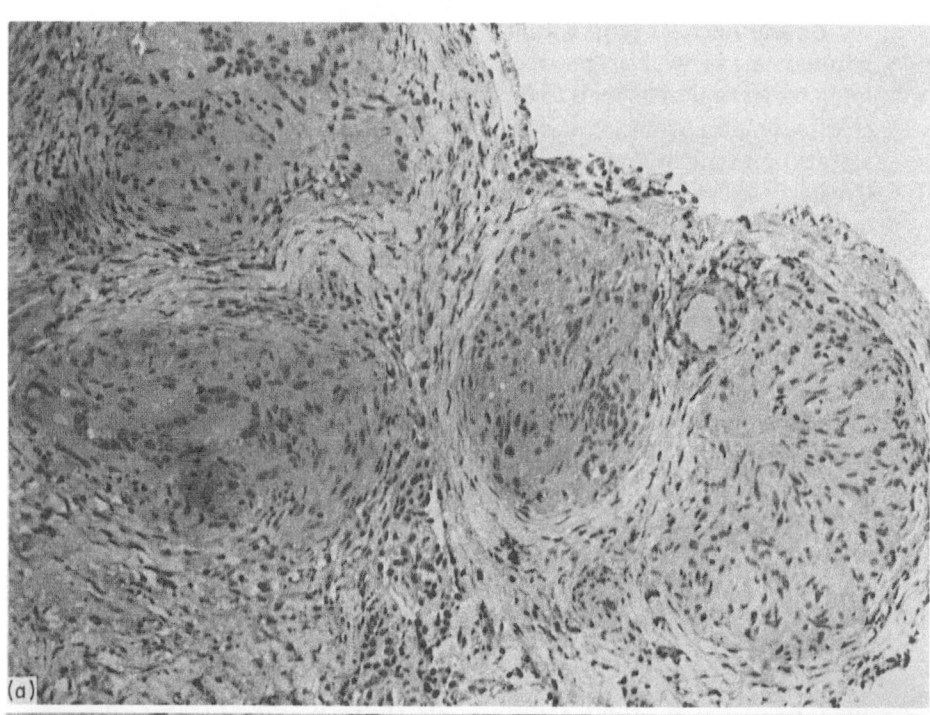

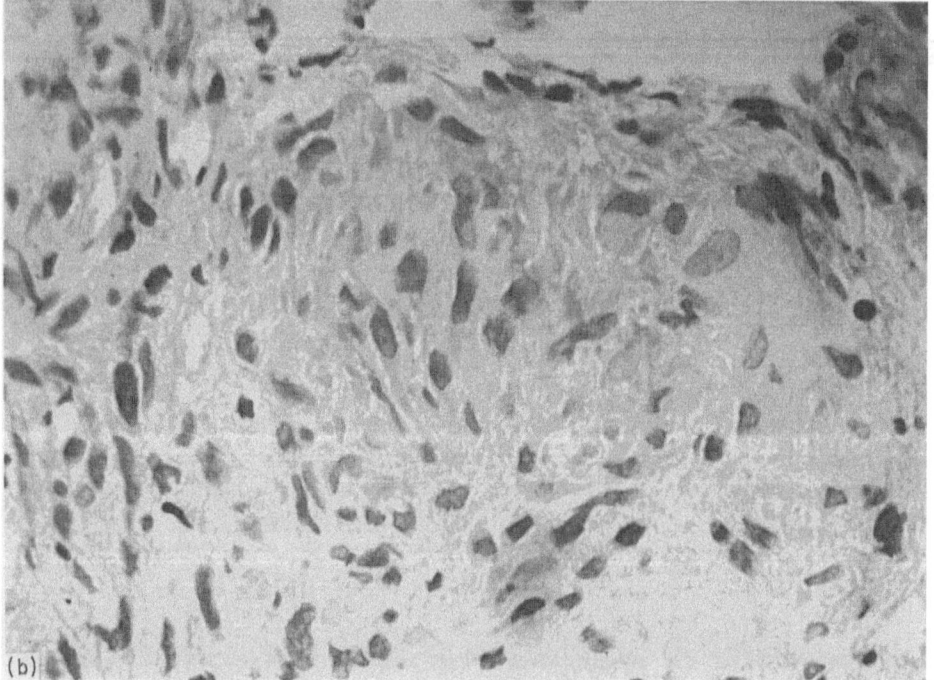

1981; Godard *et al.*, 1981; Roth *et al.*, 1981; Arnoux *et al.*, 1982; Valenti *et al.*, 1982; Cantin *et al.*, 1983; Martin *et al.*, 1983). This technique shows most value as a tool to help understand the immunological reactions in sarcoidosis. It was known that patients with sarcoidosis often have anergy, expressed by failure to react to hypersensitivity skin tests. When it was found that sarcoid patients had lower percentages of circulating T lymphocytes it was suggested that the disease was the result of a defective immunological state. More recent investigations have shown that there is an increase in both absolute and relative numbers of T lymphocytes in the lung tissues of sarcoid patients (Hunninghake *et al.*, 1979a; Crystal *et al.*, 1981; Reed and deShazo, 1982; Davies, 1983) and specifically in the T-helper to T-suppressor ratios (Hunninghake and Crystal, 1981; James and Williams, 1982; Martin *et al.*, 1983). It was then suggested that the decrease in circulating T lymphocytes may be the result of a pooling of this lymphocyte subset in the granulomatous lesions and that the anergy may be a reflection of this sequestration (Hunninghake *et al.*, 1979a; Davies *et al.*, 1982; James and Williams, 1982). Unfortunately, the increase in helper T lymphocytes in bronchoalveolar lavage cannot be used to diagnose sarcoidosis since a similar increase was found in a patient with infectious granulomatous disease (Martin *et al.*, 1983).

One of the characteristics of sarcoid granulomas is the lack of necrosis. However, Liebow (1973) described a series of eleven patients who had sarcoid-like lesions, except that there was a concomitant vasculitis and necrosis, sometimes even becoming cavitary. The granulomas were confluent and had microscopic foci of necrosis. Subsequent reports extended the number of such cases and the 'entity' (termed necrotizing sarcoidosis) was generally categorized with the granulomatous vasculitides (Churg *et al.*, 1979; Koss *et al.*, 1980; Edwards, 1982; Cole *et al.*, 1983). The anatomical distribution of the lesions, the tendency of the granuloma to hyalinize and the overall good prognosis are features in common with sarcoidosis. Churg (1983) has presented a convincing analysis that this entity is really a variant of sarcoidosis. Other unusual manifestations of sarcoidosis include a cavitary sequela with a high risk for development of aspergilloma (Israel *et al.*, 1982) (Section 4.4.1), and a nodular varient which mimicks neoplasm (Rømer, 1977; Corsello *et al.*, 1983).

Histologically the differential diagnosis of sarcoid-like granulomas includes infectious granulomas (Section 6.5.2 and Chapter 4), chronic ber-

---

Fig. 8.4   Pulmonary sarcoidosis. (a) Bronchial biopsy with a group of well-circumscribed sarcoidal granulomas each encircled by a layer of fibrocytes. There are a few scattered lymphocytes. There is no evidence of necrosis. (× 180) (b) At higher magnification, the hyaline character is evident as the epithelioid cells blend together. (× 710) (Paraffin sections stained with hematoxylin and eosin.)

ylliosis (Section 6.5.4 and Section 5.8.4) (Carrington *et al.*, 1976) and hypersensitivity pneumonitis (Section 5.7) (König *et al.*, 1981). Because the diagnosis of sarcoidosis by the surgical pathologist frequently terminates clinical pursuit of the cause of pulmonary lesions, and because other entities (some of which are responsive to specific therapy) are difficult or even impossible to distinguish from sarcoid, there is an extra responsibility to rule out all other granulomatous diseases of known etiology. Furthermore, the pathologist should be sure that the clinical presentation and all other supportive evidence is consistent before making the diagnosis of sarcoidosis on bronchoscopic specimens (Williams, 1982). In a study of 30 patients with the clinical x-ray picture of sarcoidosis and noncaseating sarcoid-like granulomas in biopsies, Kent *et al.* (1970) were able to make another definitive diagnosis in 27 of the patients. Their analysis included culture, special histological stains for micro-organisms, chemical analysis and immunological studies.

For a thorough review of sarcoidosis readers are referred to the collective works edited by Williams and Davies (1980).

8.8   Wegener's granulomatosis

In 1936, followed by an additional report in 1939, Wegener described a granulomatous disease of the blood vessels in the respiratory system and kidneys. Wegener's granulomatosis is a necrotizing vasculitis in the upper and lower respiratory tree associated with glomerulonephritis. The patients may present with an apparent sinusitis, and on examination there are crusted ulcers of the nasal mucosa (Casuccio and Yanagisawa, 1981). In the lungs, lesions are multiple, bilateral and of varying size. Renal symptoms usually occur after those in the respiratory tract, but the glomerulonephritis is the most common cause of death. Cytotoxic drugs have produced some remissions in patients who without treatment have a very poor prognosis. In their series, Fauci *et al.* (1983) had a remission of 48 months. For current review see Cole *et al.* (1983) and Fauci *et al.* (1983).

The vasculitis involves both small arteries and veins with a mixed inflammatory cell infiltrate including macrophages, epithelioid cells and multinucleated giant cells (Fig. 8.5). Eosinophils are often present but not in large numbers. Necrosis is conspicuous and elastic stains demonstrate the fragmentation of the vascular lamina (Fig. 8.6). The granulomatous lesions expand in a radial fashion from around the vessels. The centers become necrotic and with increasing necrosis the angiomatous nature is obscured; however, adjacent vessels show the early type lesion. Fibroblast proliferation and collagen deposition may be found at the margins of the larger lesions. Small necrotizing granulomas are frequently present in the bronchial wall but diagnosis by bronchoscopic specimens is difficult since

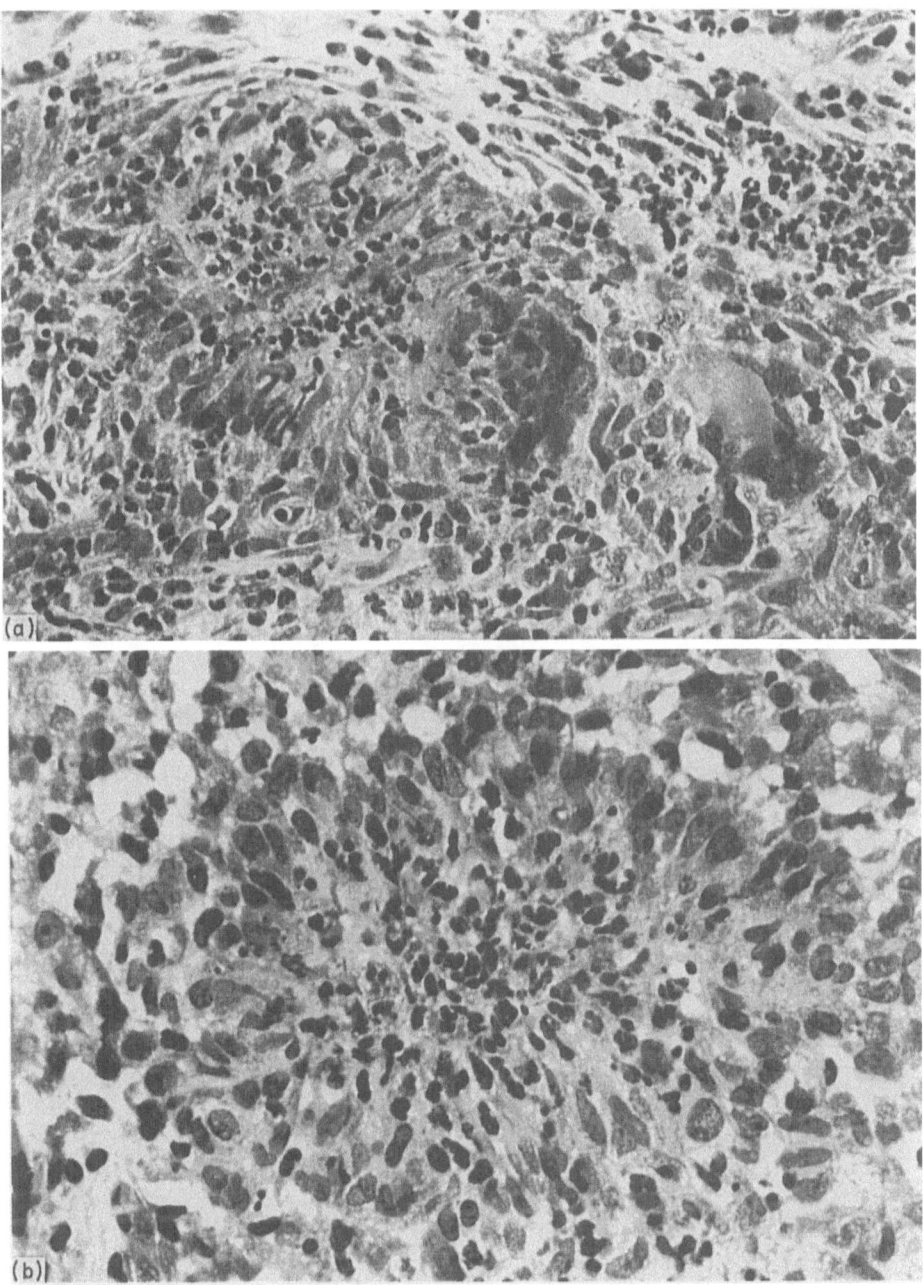

Fig. 8.5 Peribronchial biopsy, Wegener's granulomatosis. Necrotizing granulomas with numerous polymorphonuclear leukocytes and other inflammatory cells. The patient had a glomerulonephritis. (a) Somewhat disorganized reaction with several foci of necrosis, elongated epithelioid cells and multinucleated giant cells. (b) More organized granuloma, probably developing in the wall of a blood vessel (which has become obscured by the infiltrate). (Paraffin sections stained with hematoxylin and eosin: × 470.)

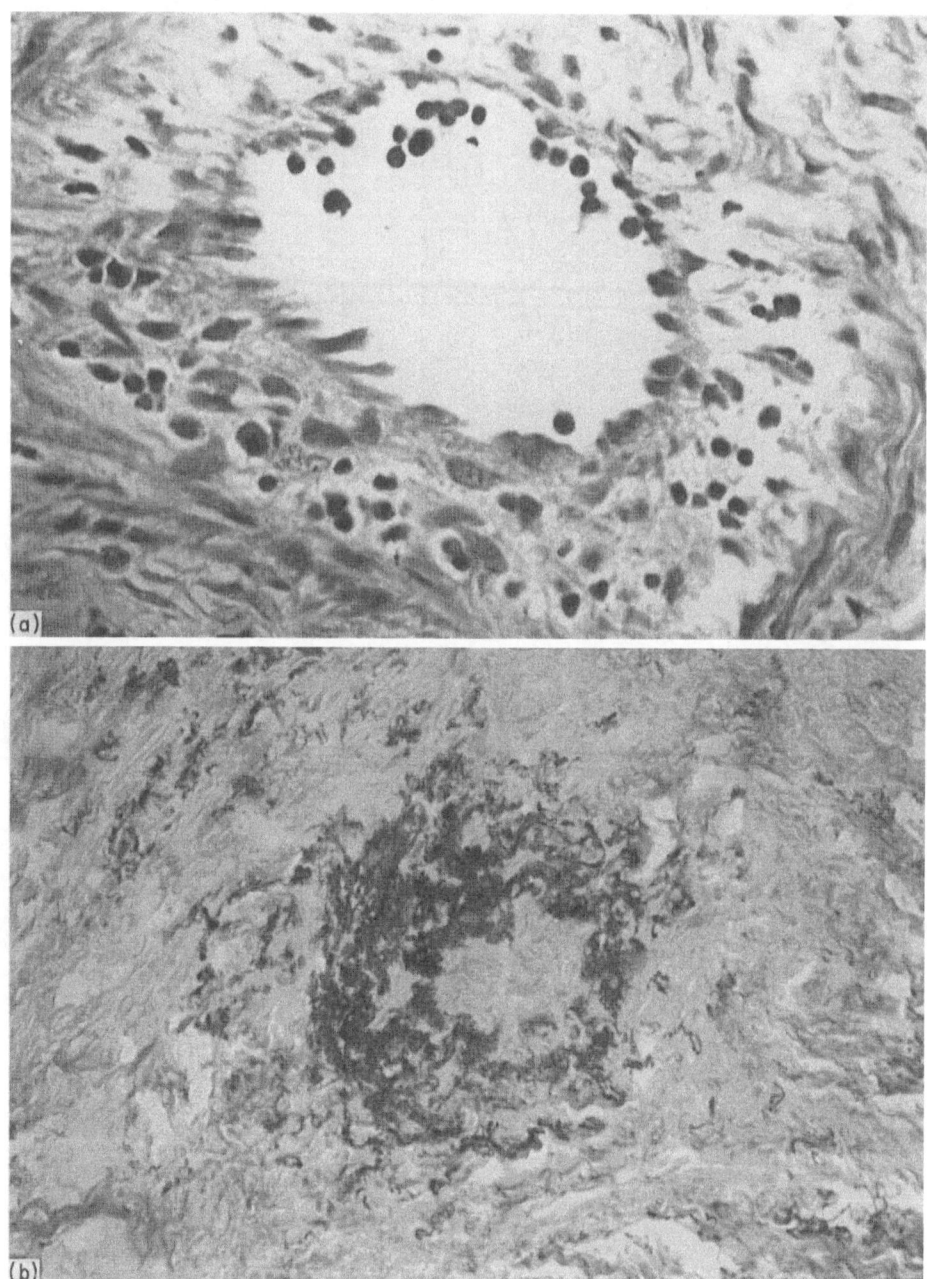

Fig. 8.6 Wegener's granulomatosis in lung. (a) Vessel somewhat distant from the adjacent necrotizing lesions but with acute inflammatory cell infiltrate within the wall. Hematoxylin and eosin stain. (b) Damaged artery with fragmented elastic lamina. Elastic stain. (Paraffin-embedded sections: × 470.)

a larger specimen is necessary to evaluate the overall process (Cole *et al.*, 1983; Fauci *et al.*, 1983).

The etiology of this disease is unknown at the present time. Circulating immune complexes have been reported and sporadic cases have demonstrated immunoglobulin deposition in lung lesions (Hui *et al.*, 1981; Shasby *et al.*, 1982). The vascular lesions are similar to those seen in hypersensitivity drug reactions (Cole *et al.*, 1983). However, these findings, although intriguing, have not been consistent or conclusive.

A limited form of Wegener's granulomatosis (that is, respiratory tract lesions without glomerulonephritis) was described by Carrington and Liebow (1966). It has been suggested that some of these cases may be necrotizing granulomas of unrecognized infectious etiology (Ulbright and Katzenstein, 1980; Churg, 1983) while in others the patients may not have developed their renal lesions at the time of diagnosis. Nevertheless, Cole *et al.* (1983) maintain that the limited form is histologically distinguishable and has a more favorable prognosis.

The differential diagnosis of necrotizing vasculitis with a granulomatous reaction includes infectious disease, hypersensitivity angitis (which usually has a significant number of eosinophils in the infiltrate), allergic granulomatous angitis of Churg-Strauss (associated with asthma and an eosinophilia), rheumatoid pulmonary nodules and so-called 'necrotizing sarcoidosis' (see Section 8.7) (Veevaete *et al.*, 1976; Koss *et al.*, 1980; Edwards, 1982; Kornblut *et al.*, 1982; Churg, 1983).

References

Abboud, R.T., Chase, W.H., Ballon, H.S., Grzybowski, S. and Magil, A. (1978), Goodpasture's syndrome: diagnosed by transbronchial lung biopsy. *Ann. Intern. Med.*, **89**, 635–8.

Armstrong, J.R., Radke, J.R., Eichenhorn, M.S., Kvale, P.A. and Popovich, J., Jr. (1981), Endoscopic findings in sarcoidosis. Characteristics and correlations with radiographic staging and bronchial mucosal biopsy yields. *Ann. Otol.*, **90**, 339–43.

Arnoux, A., Marsac, J., Stanislas-Leguern, G., Huchon, G. and Chretien, J. (1982), Broncho-alveolar lavage in sarcoidosis. Correlation between alveolar lymphocytosis and clinical data. *Pathol. Res. Pract.*, **175**, 62–79.

Attwood, H.D., Price, C.G. and Riddell, R.J. (1972), Primary diffuse tracheobronchial amyloidosis. *Thorax*, **27**, 620–4.

Balázs, M. (1983), Electron-microscopic examination of primary diffuse tracheobronchial amyloidosis. Role of fibroblasts in amyloid formation. *Virch. Arch. Pathol. Anat.*, **400**, 97–106.

Basset, F., Corrin, B., Spencer, H., Lacronique, J., Roth, C., Soler, P., Battesti, J-P., Georges, R. and Chrétien, J. (1978), Pulmonary histiocytosis X. *Am. Rev. Respir. Dis.*, **118**, 811–20.

Basset, F., Soler, P., Wyllie, L., Mazin, F. and Turiaf, J. (1976), Langerhans' cells and lung interstitium. *Ann. N.Y. Acad. Sci.*, **278**, 599–611.

Beechler, C.R., Enquist, R.W., Hunt, K.K., Ward, G.W. and Knieser, M.R. (1980),

Immunofluorescence of transbronchial biopsies in Goodpasture's syndrome. *Am. Rev. Respir. Dis.*, **121**, 869–72.

Benoit, F.L., Rulon, D.B., Theil, G.B., Doolan, P.D. and Watten, R.H. (1964), Goodpasture's syndrome. A clinicopathologic entity. *Am. J. Med.*, **37**, 424–44.

Bierny, J-P. (1978), Multinodular primary amyloidosis of the lung: diagnosis by needle biopsy. *Am. J. Roent.*, **131**, 1082–3.

Boucher, R.C., Knowles, M.R., Stutts, M.J. and Gatzy, J.T. (1983), Epithelial dysfunction in cystic fibrosis lung disease. *Lung*, **161**, 1–17.

Cantin, A., Bégin, R., Rola-Pleszczynski, M. and Boileau, R. (1983), Heterogeneity of bronchoalveolar lavage cellularity in state III pulmonary sarcoidosis. *Chest*, **83**, 485–6.

Caplan, A. (1953), Certain unusual radiological appearances in the chest of coal-miners suffering from rheumatoid arthritis. *Thorax*, **8**, 29–37.

Caplan, A., Payne, R.B. and Withey, J.L. (1962), A broader concept of Caplan's syndrome related to rheumatoid factors. *Thorax*, **17**, 205–12.

Carlson, R.A., Hattery, R.R., O'Connell, E.J. and Fontana, R.S. (1976), Pulmonary involvement by histiocytosis X in the pediatric age group. *Mayo Cl. Proc.*, **51**, 542–7.

Carrington, C.B., Gaensler, E.A., Mikus, J.P., Schachter, A.W., Burke, G.W. and Goff, A.M. (1976), Structure and function in sarcoidosis. *Ann. N.Y. Acad. Sci.*, **278**, 265–83.

Carrington, C.B. and Liebow, A.A. (1966), Limited forms of angitis and granulomatosis of Wegener's type. *Am. J. Med.*, **41**, 497–527.

Casuccio, J.R. and Yanagisawa, E. (1981), Disease of obscure etiology: sarcoidosis, Wegener's granulomatosis and midline granuloma. *Otolaryngol. Cl. No. Am.*, **14**, 331–45.

Celli, B.R., Rubinow, A., Cohen, A.S. and Brody, J.S. (1978), Patterns of pulmonary involvement in systemic amyloidosis. *Chest*, **74**, 543–7.

Cervantes-Perez, P., Toro-Perez, A.H. and Rodgriguez-Jurado, P. (1980), Pulmonary involvement in rheumatoid arthritis. *J. Am. Med. Assoc.*, **243**, 1715–19.

Churg, A. (1983), Pulmonary angiitis and granulomatosis revisited. *Human Pathol.*, **14**, 868–83.

Churg, A., Carrington, C.B. and Gupta, R. (1979), Necrotizing sarcoid granulomatosis. *Chest*, **76**, 406–13.

Colby, T.V. and Carrington, C.B. (1983), Lymphoreticular tumors and infiltrates of the lung. In *Pathology Annual 1983*, Part I (eds S.C. Sommers and P.P. Rosen), Appleton-Century-Crofts, Norwalk, Conn., pp. 27–70.

Cole, S.R., Johnson, K.J. and Ward, P.A. (1983), Pathology of sarcoidosis, granulomatous vasculitis, and other idiopathic granulomatous diseases of lung. In *Sarcoidosis and Other Granulomatous Diseases of the Lung* (ed. B.F. Fanburg), Marcel Dekker, New York, pp. 149–202.

Corsello, B.F., Lohaus, G.H. and Funahashi, A. (1983), Endobronchial mass lesion due to sarcoidosis: complete resolution with corticosteroids. *Thorax*, **38**, 157–8.

Crystal, R.G., Roberts, W.C., Hunninghake, G.W., Gadek, J.E., Fulmer, J.D. and Line, B.R. (1981), Pulmonary sarcoidosis: a disease characterized and perpetuated by activated lung T-lymphocytes. *Ann. Intern. Med.*, **94**, 73–94.

Darke, C., Wagner, M.M.F., Nuki, G. and Dyer, P.A. (1983), HLA-A, B and DR antigens and properdin factor B allotypes in Caplan's syndrome. *Brit. J. Dis. Chest*, **77**, 235–42.

Davies, B.H. (1983), Sarcoidosis--a gleam of light. *Thorax*, **38**, 165–7.

Davies, B.H., Williams, J.D., Smith, M.D., Jones-Williams, W. and Jones, K. (1982), Peripheral blood lymphocytes in sarcoidosis. *Pathol. Res. Pract.*, **175**, 97–109.

Davis, P.B., Hubbard, V.S., McCoy, K. and Taussig, L.M. (1983), Familial bronchiectasis. *J. Pediat.*, **102**, 177–85.

Desai, R.A., Mahajan, V.K., Benjamin, S., van Ordstrand, H.S. and Cordasco, E.M. (1979), Pulmonary amyloidoma and hilar adenopathy. *Chest*, **76**, 170–3.

Dines, D.E. (1979), To the editor. Lung biopsy in sarcoidosis. *Chest*, **75**, 411.

Edwards, C.W. (1982), Vasculitis and granulomatosis of the respiratory tract. *Thorax*, **37**, 81–7.

Fauci, A.S., Haynes, B.F., Costa, J., Katz, P. and Wolff, S.M. (1982), Lymphomatoid granulomatosis. Prospective clinical and therapeutic experience over 10 years. *New Engl. J. Med.*, **306**, 68–74.

Fauci, A.S., Haynes, B.F., Katz, P. and Wolff, S.M. (1983), Wegener's granulomatosis: prospective clinical and therapeutic experience with 85 patients for 21 years. *Ann. Intern. Med.*, **98**, 76–85.

Flemming, A.F.S., Fairfax, A.J., Arnold, A.G. and Lane, D.J. (1980), Treatment of endobronchial amyloidosis by intermittent bronchoscopic resection. *Brit. J. Dis. Chest*, **74**, 183–8.

Friedman, P.J., Liebow, A.A. and Sokoloff, J. (1981), Eosinophilic granuloma of lung. Clinical aspects of primary pulmonary histiocytosis in the adult. *Medicine*, **60**, 385–96.

Gilman, M.J. and Wang, K.P. (1980), Transbronchial lung biopsy in sarcoidosis. An approach to determine the optimal number of biopsies. *Am. Rev. Respir. Dis.*, **122**, 721–4.

Glenner, G.G. (1980), Amyloid deposits and amyloidosis. The β-fibrilloses. *New Engl. J. Med.*, **302**, 1283–92.

Godard, P., Clot, J., Jonquet, O., Bousquet, J. and Michell, F.B. (1981), Lymphocyte subpopulations in bronchoalveolar lavages of patients with sarcoidosis and hypersensitivity pneumonitis. *Chest*, **80**, 447–52.

Gottlieb, L.S. and Gold, W.M. (1972), Primary tracheobronchial amyloidosis. *Am. Rev. Respir. Dis.*, **105**, 425–9.

Gough, J., Rivers, D. and Seal, R.M.E. (1955), Pathological studies of modified pneumoconiosis in coal-miners with rheumatoid arthritis (Caplan's syndrome). *Thorax*, **10**, 9–18.

Greenberger, J.S., Crocker, A.C., Vawter, G., Jaffe, N. and Cassady, J.R. (1981), Results of treatment of 127 patients with systemic histiocytosis (Letterer-Siwe syndrome, Schüller-Christian syndrome and multifocal eosinophilic granuloma). *Medicine*, **60**, 311–38.

Groopman, J.E. and Golde, D.W. (1981), The histiocytic disorders: a pathophysiologic analysis. *Ann. Intern. Med.*, **94**, 95–107.

Huhn, D., König, G., Weig, J. and Schneller, W. (1981), Pulmonary histiocytosis X in adult patients. *Klin. Wochenschr.*, **59**, 377–84.

Hui, A.N., Ehresmann, G.R., Quismorio, F.P., Boylen, C.T., Mayberg, H. and Koss, M.N. (1981), Wegener's granulomatosis. Electron microscopic and immunofluoresenct studies. *Chest*, **80**, 753–6.

Hunninghake, G.W. and Crystal, R.G. (1981), Pulmonary sarcoidosis. A disorder mediated by excess helper T-lymphocyte activity at sites of disease activity. *New Engl. J. Med.*, **305**, 429–34.

Hunninghake, G.W. and Fauci, A.S. (1979), Pulmonary involvement in the collagen vascular diseases. *Am. Rev. Respir. Dis.*, **119**, 471–503.

Hunninghake, G.W., Fulmer, J.D., Young, R.C., Jr., Gadek, J.E. and Crystal, R.G. (1979a), Localization of the immune response in sarcoidosis. *Am. Rev. Respir. Dis.*, **120**, 49–57.

Hunninghake, G.W., Gadek, J.E., Kawanami, O., Ferrans, V.J. and Crystal, R.G.

(1979b), Inflammatory and immune processes in the human lung in health and disease: evaluation by bronchoalveolar lavage. *Am. J. Pathol.*, **97**, 149–206.

Israel, H.L., Lenchner, G.S. and Atkinson, G.W. (1982), Sarcoidosis and aspergilloma. The role of surgery. *Chest*, **82**, 430–2.

James, D.G. (1976), The centenary of sarcoidosis. *Ann. N.Y. Acad. Sci.*, **278**, 736–41.

James, D.G. and Neville, E. (1977), Pathobiology of sarcoidosis. In *Pathobiology Annual*, Vol. 7 (ed. H.L. Ioachim), Appleton-Century-Crofts, New York, pp. 31–62.

James, D.G., Neville, E., Siltzbach, L.E., Turiaf, J., Battesti, J.P., Sharma, O.P., Hosoda, Y., Mikami, R., Odaka, M., Villar, T.G., Djurič, B., Doulgas, A.C., Middleton, W., Karlish, A., Blasi, A., Olivieri, D. and Press, P. (1976a), Worldwide review of sarcoidosis. *Ann. N.Y. Acad. Sci.*, **278**, 321–34.

James, D.G., Turiaf, J., Hosada, Y., Williams, W.J., Israel, H.L., Douglas, A.C. and Siltzbach, L.E. (1976b), Description of sarcoidosis: report of the subcommittee on classification and definition. *Ann. N.Y. Acad. Sci.*, **278**, 742.

James, D.G. and Williams, W.J. (1982), Immunology of sarcoidosis. *Am. J. Med.*, **72**, 5–8.

Johnson, T.S., White, P., Weiss, S.T., Weiss, J.W. and Weinberger, S.E. (1982), Endobronchial necrobiotic nodule antedating rheumatoid arthritis. *Chest*, **82**, 199–200.

Kanada, D.J. and Sharma, O.P. (1979), Long term survival with diffuse interstitial pulmonary amyloidosis. *Am. J. Med.*, **67**, 879–82.

Kataria, Y.P., Shaw, R.A. and Campbell, P.B. (1982), Sarcoidosis: an overview II. *Clin. Notes Respir. Dis.*, **20**, No. 4, 3–15.

Kent, D.C., Houk, V.N., Elliott, R.C., Sokolowski, J.W., Jr., Baker, J.H. and Sorensen, K. (1970), The definitive evaluation of sarcoidosis. *Am. Rev. Respir. Dis.*, **101**, 721–7.

Kisilevsky, R. (1983), Biology of disease. Amyloidosis: a familiar problem in the light of current pathogenetic developments. *Lab. Invest.*, **49**, 381–90.

Koerner, S.K., Sakowitz, A.J., Appelman, R.I., Becker, N.H. and Schoenbaum, S.W. (1975), Transbronchial lung biopsy for the diagnosis of sarcoidosis. *New Engl. J. Med.*, **293**, 268–70.

Koffler, D., Sandson, J., Carr, R. and Kunkel, H.G. (1969), Immunologic studies concerning the pulmonary lesions in Goodpasture's syndrome. *Am. J. Pathol.*, **54**, 293–306.

Kollberg, H. (1982), Cystic fibrosis in adulthood. *Europ. J. Respir. Dis.* (suppl. 118), **63**, 101–9.

König, G., Baur, X. and Fruhmann, G. (1981), Sarcoidosis or extrinsic allergic alveolitis? *Respiration*, **42**, 150–4.

Koontz, C.H. (1978), Lung biopsy in sarcoidosis. *Chest*, **74**, 120–1.

Koontz, C.H. (1979), Lung biopsy in sarcoidosis. *Chest*, **75**, 411.

Koontz, C.H., Joyner, L.R. and Nelson, R.A. (1976), Transbronchial lung biopsy via the fiberoptic bronchoscope in sarcoidosis. *Ann. Intern. Med.*, **85**, 64–6.

Kornblut, A.D., deFries, H.O., Wolff, S.M. and Fauci, A.S. (1982), Wegener's granulomatosis. *Otolaryngol. Cl. No. Am.*, **15**, 673–83.

Koss, M.N., Hochholzer, L., Feigin, D.S., Garancis, J.C. and Ward, P.A. (1980), Necrotizing sarcoid-like granulomatosis: clinical, pathologic, and immunopathologic findings. *Human Pathol.*, **11**, 510–19.

Kradin, R.L. and Mark, E.J. (1983), Benign lymphoid disorders of the lung, with a theory regarding their development. *Human Pathol.*, **14**, 857–67.

Kullberg, F.C., Funahashi, A. and Siegesmund, K.A. (1982), Pulmonary eosinophilic granuloma: electron microscopic detection of x-bodies on lung lavage cells and transbronchoscopic lung biopsy in one patient. *Ann. Intern. Med.*, **96**, 188–9.

Kyle, R.A. and Bayrd, E.D. (1975), Amyloidosis: review of 236 cases. *Medicine*, **54**, 271–300.

Lee, S-C. and Johnson, H.A. (1975), Multiple nodular pulmonary amyloidosis. A case report and comparison with diffuse alveolar-septal pulmonary amyloidosis. *Thorax*, **30**, 178–85.

Lewis, J.G. (1964), Eosinophilic granuloma and its variants with special reference to lung involvement. A report of 12 patients. *Quart. J. Med.*, N.S., **33**, 337–59.

Lichtenstein, L. (1953), Histiocytosis X. Integration of eosinophilic granuloma of bone, 'Letterer-Siwe disease', and 'Schüller-Christian disease' as related to manifestations of a single nosologic entity. *Archiv. Pathol.*, **56**, 84–102.

Lieberman, J. (1976), The specificity and nature of serum-angiostensin-converting enzyme (serum ACE) elevations in sarcoidosis. *Ann. N.Y. Acad. Sci.*, **278**, 488–96.

Lieberman, P.H., Jones, C.R., Dargeon, H.W.K. and Begg, C.F. (1969), A reappraisal of eosinophilic granuloma of bone, Hand-Schüller-Christian syndrome and Letterer-Siwe syndrome. *Medicine*, **48**, 375–400.

Liebow, A.A. (1973), The J. Burns Amberson Lecture: pulmonary angiitis and granulomatosis. *Am. Rev. Respir. Dis.*, **108**, 1–18.

Liebow, A.A., Carrington, C.R.B. and Friedman, P.J. (1972), Lymphomatoid granulomatosis. *Human Pathol.*, **3**, 457–558.

Longcope, W.T. and Freiman, D.G. (1952), A study of sarcoidosis. Based on a combined investigation of 160 cases including 30 autopsies from the Johns Hopkins Hospital and Massachusetts General Hospital. *Medicine*, **31**, 1–132.

Macfarlane, J.D., Dieppe, P.A., Rigden, B.G. and Clark, T.J.H. (1978), Pulmonary and pleural lesions in rheumatoid disease. *Brit. J. Dis. Chest*, **72**, 288–300.

Mainwaring, A.R., Williams, G., Knight, E.O.W. and Bassett, H.F.M. (1969), Localized amyloidosis of the lower respiratory tract. *Thorax*, **24**, 441–5.

Mäkinen, J., Nickels, J. and Halttunen, P.E.A. (1977), Amyloid tumour of the lung. Report of a case and a short review of the literature. *Acta Path. Microbiol. Scand. Section A*, **85**, 907–10.

Mall, W. (1980), Transbronchoscopic lung biopsy in sarcoidosis. *Bronchopneum.*, **30**, 331–5.

Martin, W.J., II, Williams, D.E., Dines, D.E. and Sanderson, D.R. (1983), Interstitial lung disease. Assessment by bronchoalveolar lavage. *Mayo Cl. Proc.*, **58**, 751–7.

Mitchell, D.M., Mitchell, D.N., Collins, J.V. and Emerson, C.J. (1980), Transbronchial lung biopsy through fibreoptic bronchoscope in diagnosis of sarcoidosis. *Brit. Med. J.*, **280**, 679–81.

Mitchell, D.N. and Scadding, J.G. (1974), Sarcoidosis. *Am. Rev. Respir. Dis.*, **110**, 774–802.

Nessan, V.J., Malin, J. and Parks, S.D. (1981), Sarcoidosis: a clinical, roentgenographic and pathological survey. *West. J. Med.*, **135**, 353–9.

Parrish, R.W., Williams, J.D. and Davies, B.H. (1982), Serum beta-2-microglobulin and angiotensin-converting enzyme activity in sarcoidosis. *Thorax*, **37**, 936–40.

Petrie, G.R., Bloomfield, P., Grant, I.W.B. and Crompton, G.K. (1980), Upper lobe fibrosis and cavitation in rheumatoid disease. *Brit. J. Dis. Chest*, **74**, 263–7.

Pierard, G.E., Pierre, S., Damseaux, M., Bartsch, P. and Franchimont, C. (1982), The histological structure of Kveim tests parallels the evolution of pulmonary sarcoidosis. *Am. J. Dermatopathol.*, **4**, 17–23.

Poe, R.H., Israel, R.H., Utell, M.J. and Hall, W.J. (1979), Probability of a positive transbronchial lung biopsy result in sarcoidosis. *Arch. Intern. Med.*, **139**, 761–3.

Prowse, C.B. (1958), Amyloidosis of the lower respiratory tract. *Thorax*, **13**, 308–20.

Reed, C.E. and deShazo, R. (1982), Immunologic aspects of granulomatous and interstitial lung diseases. *J. Am. Med. Assoc.*, **248**, 2683–91.

Roethe, R.A., Fuller, P.B., Byrd, R.B. and Hafermann, D.R. (1980), Transbronchoscopic lung biopsy in sarcoidosis. Optimal number and sites for diagnosis. *Chest*, **77**, 400–2.

Rohatgi, P.K., Kuzmowych, T.V. and Delaney, M.D. (1981), Indications for transbronchial lung biopsy in the diagnosis of intrathoracic sarcoidosis. *Respiration*, **42**, 155–60.

Rømer, F.K. (1977), Sarcoidosis with large nodular lesions simulating pulmonary metastases. An analysis of 126 cases of intrathoracic sarcoidosis. *Scand. J. Resp. Dis.*, **58**, 11–16.

Roth, C., Huchon, G.J., Arnoux, A., Stanislas-Leguern, G., Marsac, J.H. and Chretien, J. (1981), Bronchoalveolar cells in advanced pulmonary sarcoidosis. *Am. Rev. Respir. Dis.*, **124**, 9–12.

Rubinow, A., Celli, B.R., Cohen, A.S., Rigden, B.G. and Brody, J.S. (1978), Localized amyloidosis of the lower respiratory tract. *Am. Rev. Respir. Dis.*, **118**, 603–11.

Saab, S.B., Burk, J., Hopeman, A. and Almond, C. (1974), Primary pulmonary amyloidosis. Report of two cases. *J. Thor. Cardiovasc. Surg.*, **67**, 301–7.

Sappington, S.W., Davie, J.H. and Horneff, J.A. (1942), Primary amyloidosis of the lungs. *J. Lab. Cl. Med.*, **27**, 882–9.

Schoen, F.J., Alexander, R.W., Hood, C.I. and Dunn, L.J. (1980), Nodular pulmonary amyloidosis. Description of a case with ultrastructure. *Arch. Pathol. Lab. Med.*, **104**, 66–9.

Schraufnagel, D.E., Knight, L., Ying, W.L. and Wang, N.S. (1980), Favourable outcome in a case of endobronchial amyloidosis. *Canad. Med. Assoc. J.*, **122**, 559–61.

Scott, D.G.I., Bacon, P.A. and Tribe, C.R. (1981), Systemic rheumatoid vasculitis: a clinical and laboratory study of 50 cases. *Medicine*, **60**, 288–97.

Selroos, O. (1981), The diagnosis of sarcoidosis. *Europ. J. Respir. Dis.*, **62**, 219–22.

Shasby, D.M., Schwarz, M.I., Forstot, J.Z., Theofilopoulos, A.N. and Kassan, S.S. (1982), Pulmonary immune complex deposition in Wegener's granulomatosis. *Chest*, **81**, 338–40.

Shelburne, J.D., Wisseman, C.L., Broda, K.R., Roggli, V.L. and Ingram, P. (1983), Lung--nonneoplastic conditions. In *Diagnostic Electron Microscopy*, Vol. 4 (eds B.F. Trump and R.T. Jones), Wiley, New York, pp. 475–538.

Silverberg-Sinakin, I., Baer, R.L. and Thorbecke, G.J. (1978), Langerhans' cells. A review of their nature with emphasis on their immunologic functions. *Prog. Allergy*, **24**, 268–94.

Smith, M., McCormack, L.J., van Ordstrand, H.S. and Mercer, R.D. (1974), 'Primary' pulmonary histiocytosis X. *Chest*, **65**, 176–80.

Smith, R.R.L., Hutchins, G.M., Moore, G.W. and Humphrey, R.L. (1979), Type and distribution of pulmonary parenchymal and vascular amyloid. Correlation with cardiac amyloidosis. *Am. J. Med.*, **66**, 96–104.

Soler, P., Basset, F., Bernaudin, J.F. and Chretien, J. (1976), Morphology and distribution of the cells of a sarcoid granuloma: ultrastructural study of serial sections. *Ann. N.Y. Acad. Sci.*, **278**, 147–58.

Sordillo, P.P., Epremian, B., Koziner, B., Lacher, M. and Lieberman, P. (1982),

Lymphomatoid granulomatosis. An analysis of clinical and immunologic characteristics. *Cancer*, **49**, 2070–6.

Tamaki, K., Stingl, G. and Katz, S.I. (1980), The origin of Langerhans' cells. *J. Invest. Derm.*, **74**, 309–11.

Teirstein, A.S., Chuang, M., Miller, A. and Siltzbach, L.E. (1976), Flexible-bronchoscope biopsy of lung and bronchial wall in intrathoracic sarcoidosis. *Ann. N.Y. Acad. Sci.*, **278**, 522–6.

Thompson, P.J. and Citron, K.M. (1983), Amyloid and the lower respiratory tract. *Thorax*, **38**, 84–7.

Thompson, P.J., Jewkes, J., Corrin, B. and Citron, K.M. (1983), Primary bronchopulmonary amyloid tumour with massive hilar lymphadenopathy. *Thorax*, **38**, 153–4.

Turner-Warwick, M. and Evans, R.C. (1977), Pulmonary manifestations of rheumatoid disease. *Cl. Rheum. Dis.*, **3**, 549–64.

Uehlinger, E. (1963), The sarcoid tissue reaction. The origin and significance of inclusion bodies. Differential diagnosis with particular delineation from tuberculosis. *Acta Medica Scand.*, (suppl.), **425**, 7–13.

Ulbright, T.M. and Katzenstein, A.A. (1980), Solitary necrotizing granulomas of the lung. *Am. J. Surg. Pathol.*, **4**, 13–28.

Valenti, S., Scordamaglia, A., Crimi, P. and Mereu, C. (1982), Bronchoalveolar lavage and transbronchial lung biopsy in sarcoidosis and extrinsic allergic alveolitis. *Europ. J. Respir. Dis.*, **63**, 564–9.

Veevaete, F., van der Straeten, M., del Vos, M. and Roels, H. (1976), Allergic granulomatous angiitis. *Scand. J. Respir. Dis.*, **59**, 287–96.

Verea-Hernando, H., Fontan-Bueso, J., Martin-Egana, M.T., Arnal-Monreal, F. and Canalejo, C.S.J. (1982), Langerhans' cells in bronchoalveolar lavage in the late stages of pulmonary histiocytosis X. *Chest*, **81**, 130.

Walker, W.C. and Wright, V. (1968), Pulmonary lesions and rheumatoid arthritis. *Medicine*, **47**, 501–20.

Wegener, F. (1936), Über generalisierte septische Gefäßerkrankungen. *Verh. Deut. Path. Ges.*, **29**, 202–10.

Wegener, F. (1939), III. Über eine eigen artige rhinogene Granulomatose mit besonderer Beteiligung des Arteriensystems und der Nieren. *Beitr. Pathol.*, **102**, 36–68.

Wester, S.M., Beabout, J.W., Unni, K.K. and Dahlin, D.C. (1982), Langerhans' cell granulomatosis (histiocytosis X) of bone in adults. *Am. J. Surg. Pathol.*, **6**, 413–26.

Williams, W.J. and Davies, B.H. (1980), *Proceedings of the 8th International Conference on Sarcoidosis and other Granulomatous Diseases*, Alpha and Omega Press, Cardiff.

Williams, W.J. (1982), Aetiology of sarcoidosis. *Pathol. Res. Pract.*, **175**, 1–12.

Wiman, L-G. and Hörnblad, Y. (1979), Transbronchial lung biopsy in sarcoidosis. *Brit. J. Dis. Chest*, **73**, 417.

Wood, R.E., Boat, T.F. and Doershuk, C.F. (1976), Cystic fibrosis. *Am. Rev. Respir. Dis.*, **113**, 833–78.

Wright, J.R. and Calkins, E. (1981), Clinico-pathologic differentiation of common amyloid syndromes. *Medicine*, **60**, 429–48.

9 Hyperplasia, metaplasia and carcinoma *in situ*

When the tracheobronchial epithelium is damaged, mucous cells and basal cells proliferate in response to the injury. Mucous cells appear to play the dominant proliferative role and, resulting from a marked increase in their mitotic rate, pathological lesions are produced which include 'goblet' cell hyperplasia, stratification and noncornifying and cornifying epidermoid (squamous) metaplasias. These lesions, although morphologically dissimilar, are brought about by the wide and varied spectrum of phenotypic expression of mucous cells. Depending on the nature and extent of the injury, one or more of these lesions may be expressed simultaneously in the same specimen, and one lesion may change into another.

The epithelium demonstrates a stereotyped response to diverse forms of injury. For example, epidermoid metaplasia occurs in man and animals in response to a variety of insults including mechanical and nutritional injuries (vitamin A deficiency), radiation injury, irritant gases, infectious agents and carcinogens, to name but a few (Francis and Stuart-Harris, 1938; Wong and Buck, 1971; Harris *et al.*, 1972; Asmundsson *et al.*, 1973; Nettesheim, 1976; Nettesheim and Griesemer, 1978; McDowell *et al.*, 1979; Wilson *et al.*, 1984). Moreover, combined epidermoid (well-developed keratin tonofilaments) and secretory specializations (mucous granules) are characteristic of the cells of these lesions irrespective of the cause.

When the insult and adverse environment are removed, the metaplastic lesions may reverse. Experiments in hamsters have shown that division of mucous cells, both metaplastic and normal columnar forms, provide for columnar mucous and preciliated cell progeny which restore the mucociliary state (Keenan *et al.*, 1982a, b, c, 1983). However, if the epithelial cells have been exposed to an initiating dose of carcinogen and promoting factors, lesions may progress towards carcinoma *in situ*, which in turn may lead to invasive carcinoma.

A working hypothesis will be developed throughout this chapter which emphasizes the pivotal role of mucous cells in the development, maintenance, and regeneration of the neoplastic state (Scheme 9.1). This hypothesis has been presented in more detail elsewhere (McDowell and Trump, 1983).

264

Scheme 9.1 Development, maintenance, regeneration and neoplasia of the mucociliary tracheobronchial epithelium: a working hypothesis.

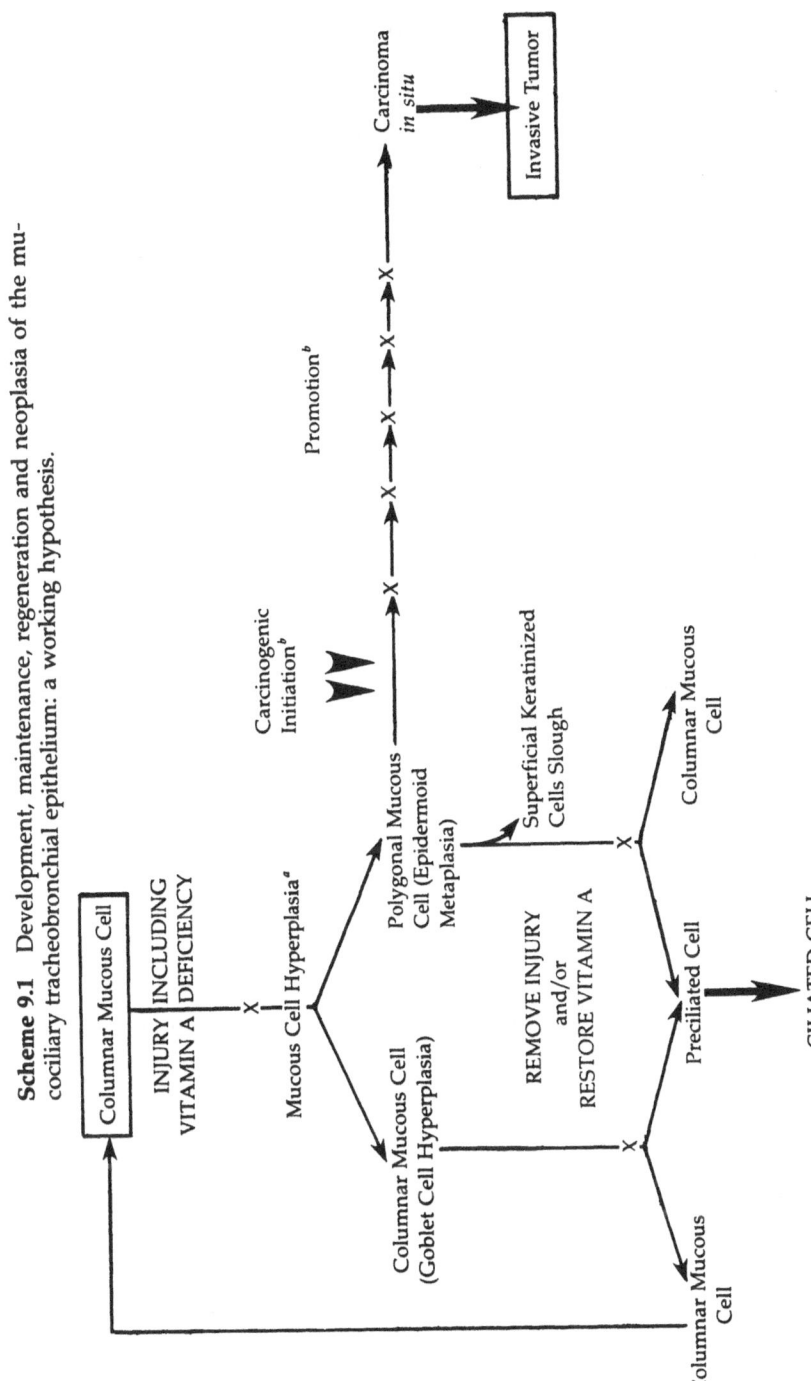

[a] Mucous cell hyperplasia is a late change in vitamin A deficiency, associated with death and sloughing of epithelial cells.
[b] Initiation and promotion may act on columnar and/or polygonal mucous cells.
X Mitotic division(s).

9.1   The hyperplastic response

Mitotic activity is very low in undisturbed tracheobronchial epithelium. Basal cells and mucous cells synthesize DNA and undergo mitosis; however, the extent to which each cell type normally participates to replace effete cells, thereby maintaining the mucociliary state, is not yet resolved in man or animals (Section 3.2.5). However, the proliferative potential of the progenitor cells is realized following diverse forms of injury, and analysis of epithelial lesions induced experimentally in the tracheobronchial epithelium of animals has been fundamental to understanding the histogenesis and morphogenesis of similar and related lesions in humans.

It is widely assumed that basal cells are the progenitor cells responsible for regeneration of the tracheobronchial epithelium following injury. However, this is not supported by results from several experiments in animals. For example, following mechanical injury to rat tracheal epithelium, large numbers of cells were stimulated to divide, and many of these were columnar cells (Condon, 1942; Wilhelm, 1953). In rats with chronic respiratory disease over 80% of all mitotic activity occurred in superficial cells, with less than 20% in basal cells (Wells, 1970). Recent experiments in hamsters, using 1–2 μm glycol methacrylate sections stained with PAS, showed that mucous cells accounted for about 80% of all mitotic activity in the regenerating tracheal epithelium following mechanical injury (Fig. 9.1a) (Keenan et al., 1982a, b, c).

9.1.1   Basal cell hyperplasia

Basal cells have a characteristic morphology in the normal epithelium. They rest on the basal lamina, to which they are attached by hemidesmosomes. They have a high nuclear to cytoplasmic ratio because their cytoplasm is very scant. The endoplasmic reticulum and Golgi apparatus

---

Fig. 9.1 (a) Hamster tracheal epithelium adjacent to a denuding wound made by mechanical injury 24 hours previously. The hamster was given colchicine to block mitosis at metaphase. Three mucous cells (m) are in division. Basal cells marked b. (Glycol methacrylate section, stained with PAS-lead hematoxylin: × 1500.) (b) Mucous 'goblet' cell hyperplasia. The mucous cells are columnar and most of them are distended with secretion product. Some cells appear dark and slender; these are mucous cells which have expelled secretions (arrows). The pseudostratified architecture is retained and some columnar cells reach from base to lumen. No ciliated cells are seen. (Paraffin section, stained with hematoxylin and eosin: × 350.) (c) Mucous 'goblet' cell hyperplasia in a ciliated epithelium. The mucous cells are columnar and most are distended with secretion. A slender mucous cell with scant secretion is present (arrow). Basal cells (marked b) form two or more layers focally and cover the basal lamina (from Trump et al., 1978). (Epon section, stained with toluidine blue: × 450.)

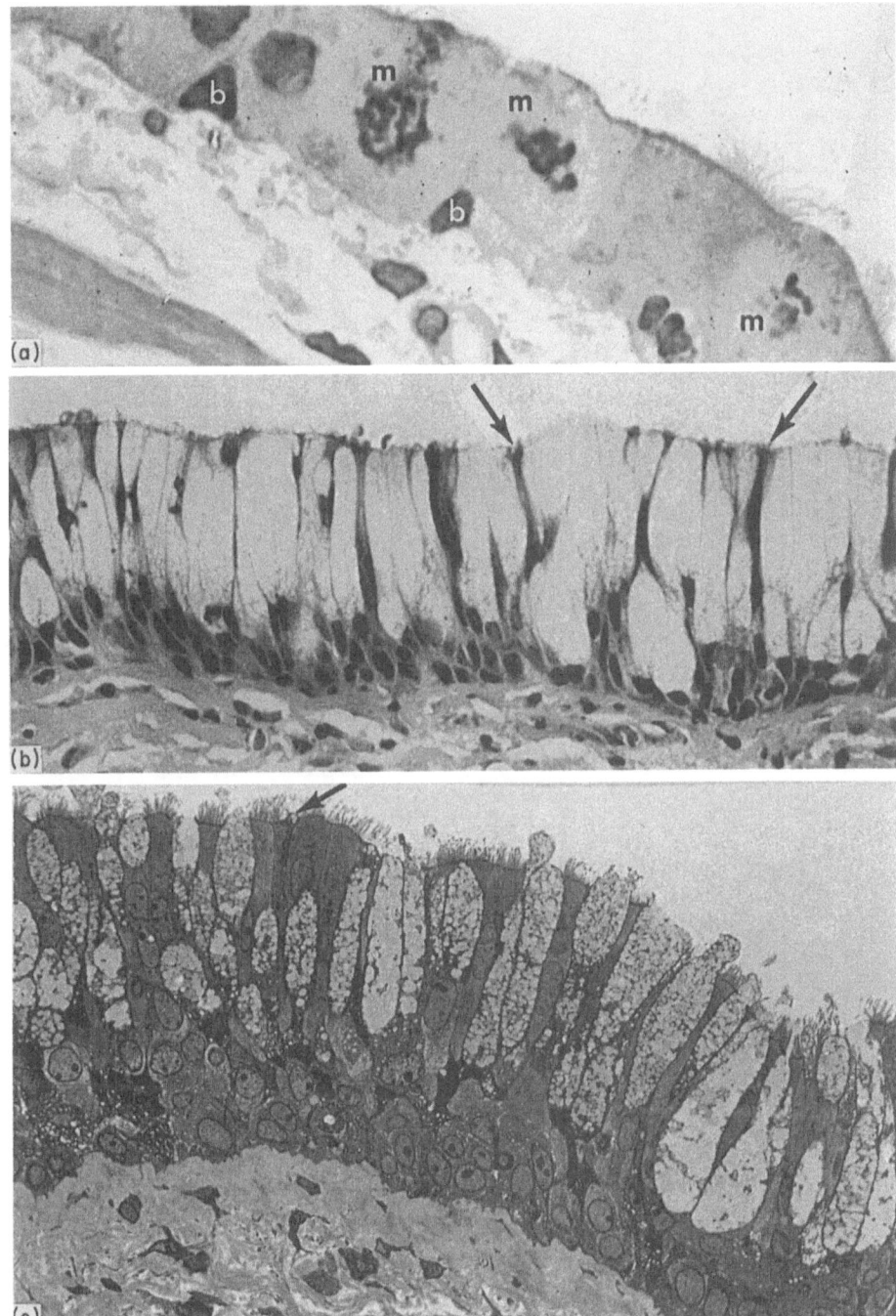

(a)

(b)

(c)

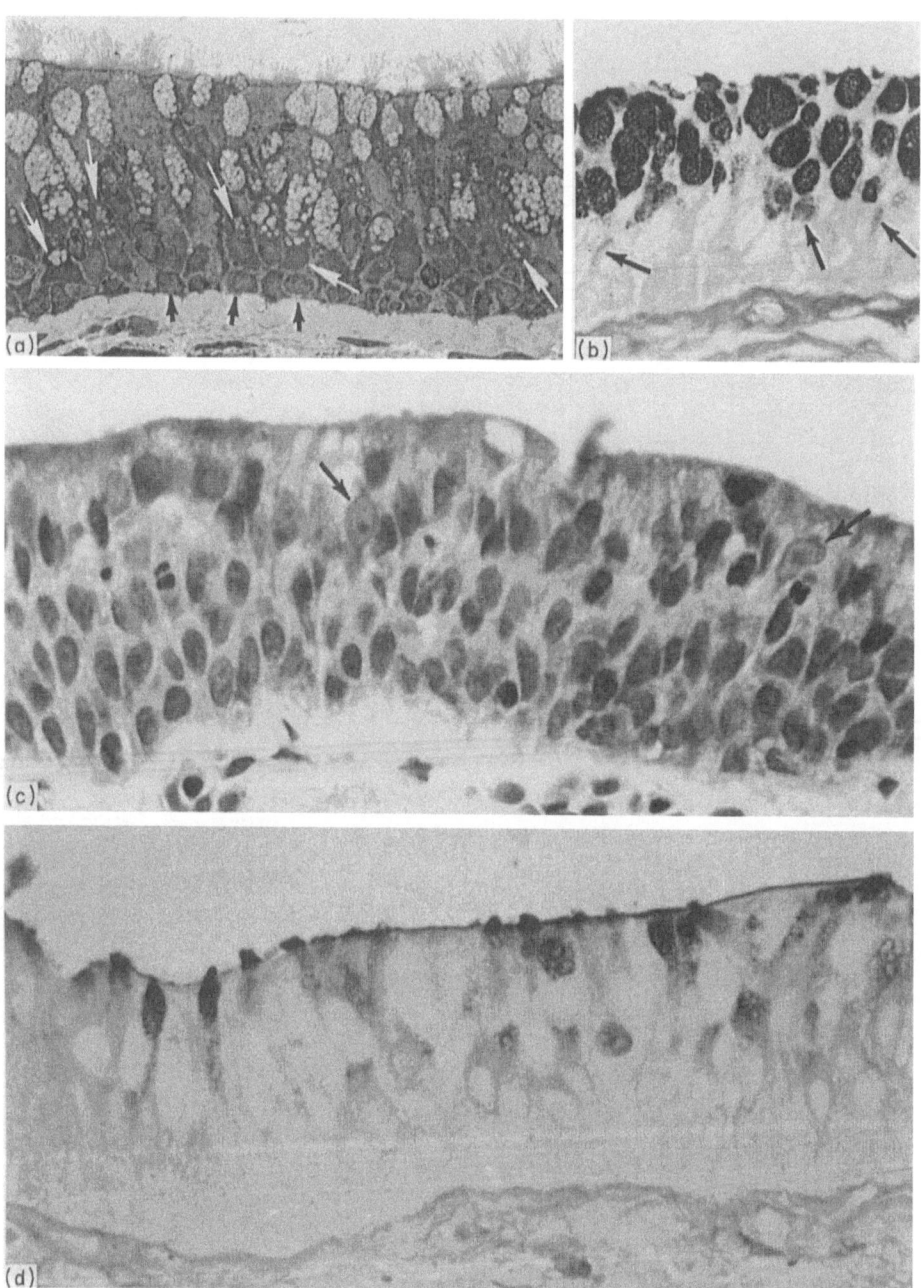

Fig. 9.2 (a) Mucous 'goblet' cell hyperplasia in a ciliated epithelium. The mucous
cells are cuboidal in shape and the epithelium is multilayered. Small basal cells
rest upon the basal lamina (black arrows) but mucous granules are present in some

are poorly developed and the cells do not synthesize mucus (Chapter 3; Fig. 3.8a). In the normal pseudostratified bronchial epithelium, basal cells do not form a continuous cell layer covering the basal lamina but are separated by the basal parts of the columnar cells (Chapter 3; Fig. 3.4; Fig. 9.1b). This architecture is not seen in many bronchial specimens obtained at biopsy and basal cells often appear to be contiguous, completely covering the basal lamina, sometimes forming more than one layer of cells (Fig. 9.1c). In the extensive study of Auerbach *et al.* (1961), the mucociliary epithelium was considered to be other than 'normal' if three or more rows of cells were found below the superficial columnar cells or if *any* atypical cells were observed.

It has been customary to consider that all polygonal or rounded cells in the basal and suprabasal layers are basal cells. However, this assumption is tenuous and it is not easy to say how many of these cells are of *true* basal cell type. In hyperplastic states many of the suprabasal cells, which superficially resemble basal cells by light microscopy, are in fact altered mucous cells (Fig. 9.2a, b). Various degrees of basal cell hyperplasia do occur but experimental evidence from studies in animals suggests that in many situations the hyperplastic response to injury is due mainly to proliferation of mucous cells.

9.1.2   *Mucous cell hyperplasia*

The classical experiments of Florey *et al.* (1932) demonstrated that hyperplasia of mucous cells was a stereotyped response--a defense mechanism against injury and irritants--and many experiments have since confirmed that mucous cell hyperplasia occurs following mechanical injury (see above), irritation from noncarcinogenic gases (Elmes and Bell, 1963; Asmundsson *et al.*, 1973) and following insults from potentially carcinogenic substances (Frasca *et al.*, 1968; Stenbäck, 1973; Becci *et al.*, 1978; Hayashi *et al.*, 1978).

The cell progeny which derive from division of mucous cells exhibit a wide range of phenotypic expressions and hence the morphology of the

---

cells of the next layer (white arrows). (Epon section, stained with toluidine blue: × 360.) (b) Epithelium similar to that in Fig. 9.2a. Note acidic mucosubstances (arrows) in all cell layers except the most basal layer. (Paraffin section, stained with Alcian blue-PAS: × 360.) (c) Stratification. The epithelium is composed of multiple layers of cuboidal and polygonal mucous cells. Most of the nuclei are of regular size and shape but a few are larger, indicative of mild atypia (arrows). From a patient with epidermoid carcinoma. (Paraffin section, stained with hematoxylin and eosin: × 450.) (d) Same specimen as Fig. 9.2c. Mucosubstances are present in many of the suprabasal cells. (Paraffin section, stained with Alcian blue-PAS: × 450.)

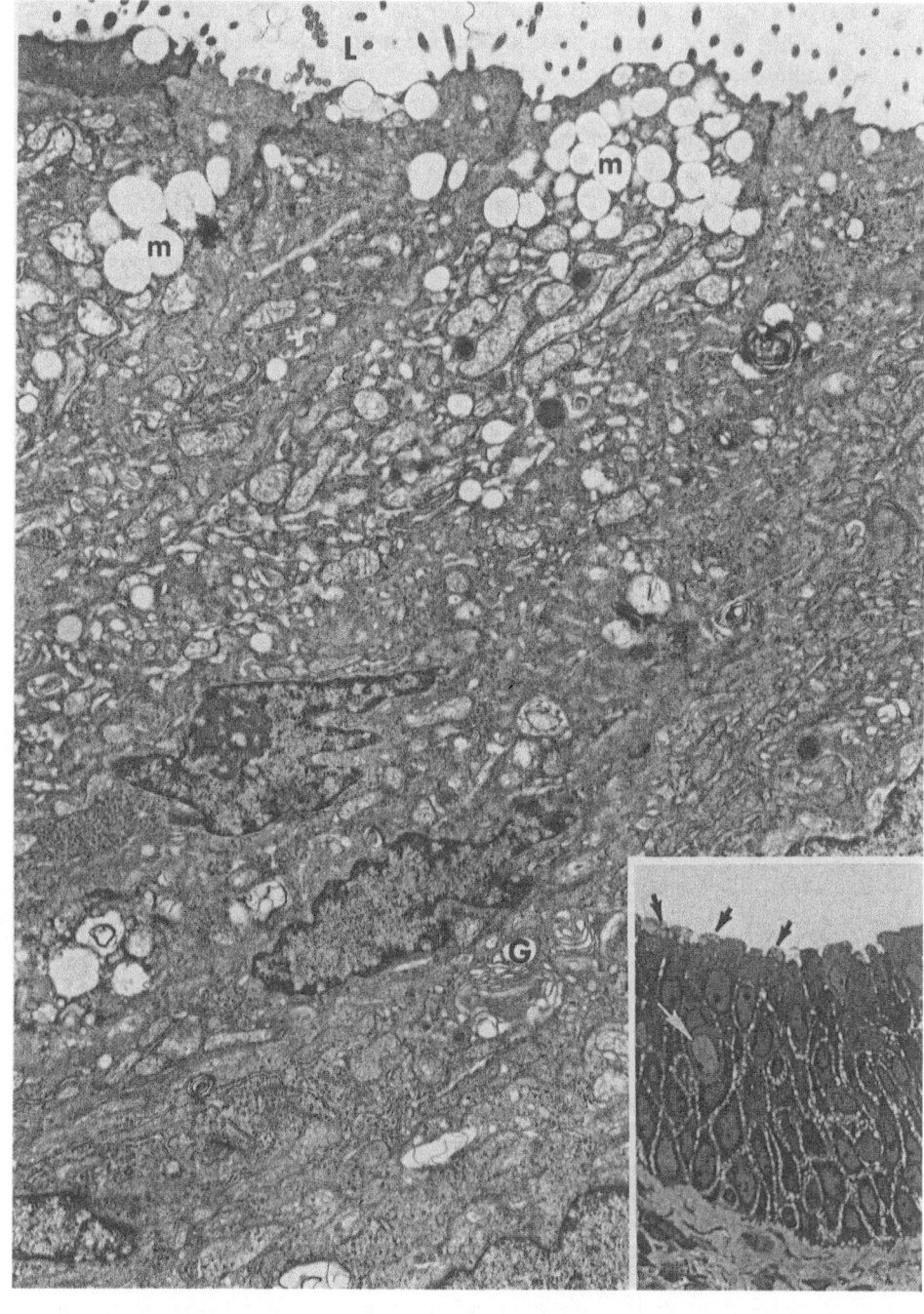

resultant pathological lesions may vary widely. If the daughter cells are mucous cells which retain columnar or cuboidal forms and synthesize copious amounts of mucosubstances, so-called 'goblet' cell hyperplasia results. If some of the columnar cells reach from base to lumen, the pseudostratified architecture is retained (Fig. 9.1b). The mucous cells are characteristically distended with secretions, but slender dark-staining cells are interspersed between them (Fig. 9.1b, c). The latter are thought to be mucous cells that have expelled their secretions (Chapter 3; Fig. 3.5a). Abundant secretions are seen in mucous cells soon after inhalation of irritants such as cigarette smoke and air pollutants. This is one of the earliest responses to injury (Kotin, 1968). The change is characteristic of chronic bronchitis in both the surface and submucosal glandular epithelium (Reid, 1954).

Often, in adjacent foci within the same specimen, the mucous cells are cuboidal and polygonal, piled up one upon the other, so that the epithelium is multilayered (Fig. 9.2a). A row of small cells without mucosubstances, the basal cells, rests upon the basal lamina but mucus is secreted by cells of the other layers, including some quite deep in the epithelium (Fig. 9.2a, b).

Varying numbers of ciliated cells may be intercalated between the mucous cells (Figs 9.1c, 9.2a) but ciliated cells may be much reduced or even focally absent (Fig. 9.1b). When an injury persists or is severe, ciliated cells, which are easily damaged, are lost from the epithelium. Ciliated cells are end-stage cells; they do not synthesize DNA, nor can they divide. They are not replaced in the regenerative process until after the adverse situation is terminated (Section 9.2). Loss of ciliated cells is an early response to many forms of injury (Frasca *et al.*, 1968; Stenbäck, 1973; Asmundsson *et al.*, 1973; McDowell *et al.*, 1979; Keenan *et al.*, 1982c). In Auerbach's study (Auerbach *et al.*, 1961), lesions without ciliated cells increased in proportion to the number of cigarettes smoked. Ciliated cells may also react to injury by internalizing their cilia, so that the cells are no longer recognizable as ciliated *per se* (McDowell *et al.*, 1979; Keenan *et al.*, 1983).

Fig. 9.3 Characteristic ultrastructure of stratified epithelium. The superficial mucous cells have well-developed Golgi apparatus (G) and contain many mucous granules (m). Airway lumen (L). (Electron micrograph: × 9000.) *Inset*: Light micrograph of similar area. Note mucous granules in superficial cells (black arrows). Intercellular spaces are widened and intercellular bridging is prominent. Some of the nuclei are enlarged (white arrow)--mild atypia. From a patient with epidermoid carcinoma. (Epon section, stained with toluidine blue: × 500.)

9.1.3 Stratification

Stratified lesions are composed of multiple layers of mucous cells (4 to 6 layers is not uncommon), overlying one or more layers of basal cells (Fig. 9.2c, d, Fig. 9.3 and inset). The cells are cuboidal or polygonal and sometimes flattened cells are seen at the surface. Ciliated cells are rare or absent. In some specimens the intercellular spaces are widened so that intercellular bridging is rather prominent (Fig. 9.3 inset).

Varying degrees of nuclear atypia may be associated with this change and cells with enlarged nuclei may be seen at any level within the epithelium (Fig. 9.2c). Nasiell (1963) observed this lesion, which he called transitional metaplasia, in 88% of specimens from patients with lung cancer. However, similar lesions are seen in the tracheal epithelium of animals following exposure to irritant substances such as dilute formalin (Florey *et al.*, 1932) or sulfur dioxide gas (Asmundsson *et al.*, 1973). In man and experimental animals, foci of 'goblet' cell hyperplasia, stratification and epidermoid metaplasia (see below) are often found blending with one another (Fig. 9.4a, b) and with more normal columnar mucociliary epithelium.

9.1.4 Epidermoid (squamous) metaplasia

The term metaplasia is derived from the Greek *meta* meaning change and *plasia* meaning modeling. It refers in pathology to a potentially reversible change in which one adult cell type is replaced by another adult cell type.

Fig. 9.4 (a) Areas of transition between columnar 'goblet' cell hyperplasia (at left), stratification (at center), and epidermoid metaplasia (at right). From 25-year-old male, following tracheal intubation. (Paraffin section, stained with hematoxylin and eosin: × 125.) (b) Higher power of same area of transition; 'goblet' cell hyperplasia (at left), stratification (center), epidermoid metaplasia (at right). Note mucosubstances in apices of the cells of all layers (except the two most basal layers) in all epithelial states. (Paraffin section, stained with Alcian blue-PAS: × 300.) (c) Epidermoid metaplasia. The epithelium is composed of multiple layers of polygonal hyalinized cells. The surface cells are flattened and desquamating; ciliated cells are absent. Note mitotic figure at mid-epithelium (arrow). From non cancer patient following tracheostomy. (Paraffin section, stained with hematoxylin and eosin: × 300.) *Inset*: Same case. Mucosubstances are absent from cells at the base of the epithelium but are present in the apices of cells of mid and superficial layers. (Paraffin section, stained with AB-PAS: × 300.) (d) Noncornifying epidermoid metaplasia. The epithelium is multilayered, composed of polygonal metaplastic cells. Some of the flattened surface cells are desquamating (top right). Dense-stained rings around the nuclei are indicative of cytoplasmic keratinization and some of the keratinized cells retain columnar forms (arrow). Intercellular bridges can be seen between some cells (left). (Epon section, stained with toluidine blue: × 500.)

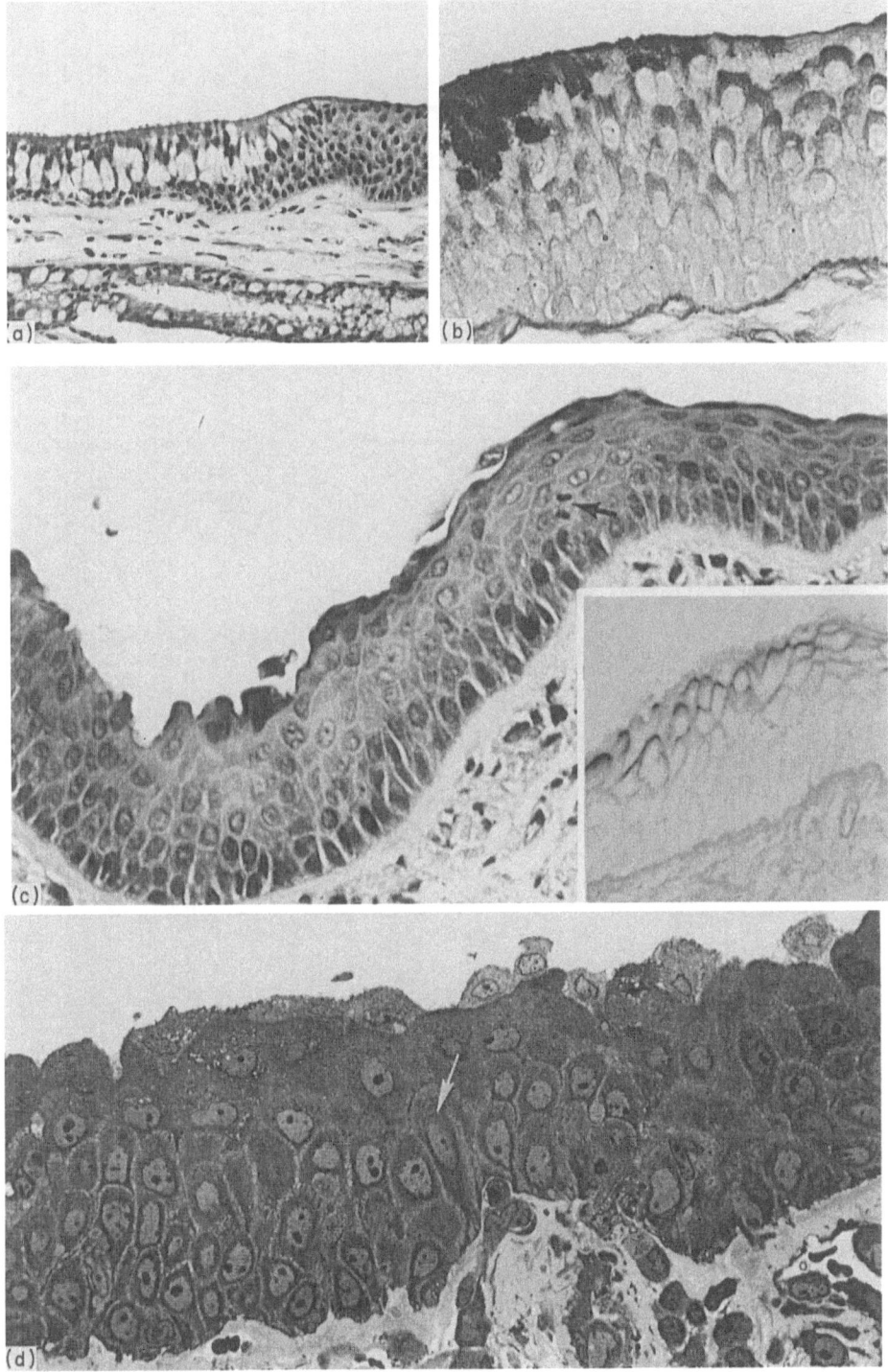

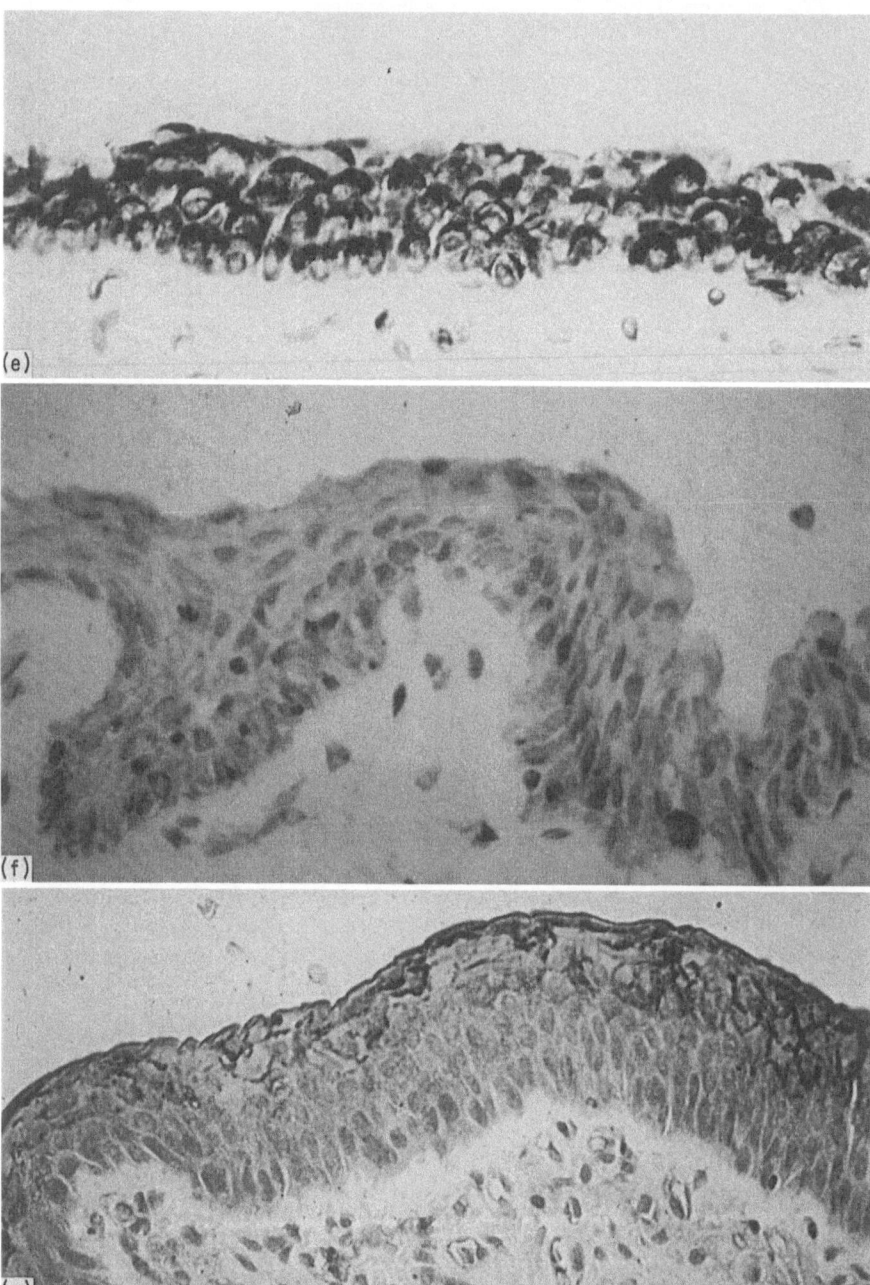

Fig. 9.4   (e) Regenerating hamster tracheal epithelium 48 hours after mechanical wounding. The multilayered metaplastic epidermoid cells stain strongly for keratin. Ethanol-fixed specimen, stained with anti-keratin antibody by the peroxidase-antiperoxidase method. (× 500) (f) Human bronchial epithelium showing epidermoid metaplasia. The epithelial cells stain for keratin but the stain is weak compared with Fig. 9.4e because the specimen was fixed in formaldehyde-glutaraldehyde, which partially inactivates the antigenicity of keratin proteins. Peroxidase-antiperoxidase method. (× 300) (g) Same specimen as in Fig. 9.4c, stained for carcinoembryonic antigen using the peroxidase-antiperoxidase method. The superficial metaplastic cells stain positively. (× 300)

The usual explanation given for this change is that the 'new' cell type has differentiated from a population of undifferentiated 'stem', reserve or basal cells. However, in the tracheobronchial epithelium, mucous cells, dividing in response to diverse forms of injury, give rise to progeny expressing combined epidermoid (skin-like) and mucus-secreting specializations, resulting in epidermoid metaplasia (Figs 9.4a–g, 9.5). The genesis of epidermoid metaplasia has been studied in detail in the hamster trachea following focal epithelial wounding (McDowell *et al.*, 1979; Keenan *et al.*, 1982a, b, c, 1983). Within a few hours following mechanical injury, viable mucous cells at the wound edge flatten to form squamous cells which migrate across the basal lamina to cover the wound site. These *flat mucous cells*, as well as columnar mucous cells and a few basal cells at the edge of the wound, divide to make an overtly keratinizing epidermoid metaplastic epithelium which is well developed by 48 hours (Fig. 9.4e). This lesion appears identical to epidermoid metaplasia seen in human bronchial epithelium following diverse forms of injury (Sections 5.9, 5.10).

Noncornifying epidermoid metaplasia is characterized by a stratified epithelium consisting of multiple layers of polygonal cells which are progressively flattened towards the epithelial surface (Figs 9.4c, d, 9.5). Ciliated cells are absent. The metaplastic cells are eosinophilic and appear hyalinized in sections stained with hematoxylin and eosin (Fig. 9.4c). The cells are joined by well-developed desmosomes which may be visible as intercellular bridges by light microscopy, if the spaces between the cells are widened (Fig. 9.4d). Keratin immunostaining (9.4e, f) is strong in many of the metaplastic cells (Gusterson *et al.*, 1982; Bejui-Thivolet *et al.*, 1982) and well-developed cytoplasmic tonofilament bundles are demonstrable by electron microscopy (Fig 9.5). Using a monoclonal antibody, keratin proteins characteristic of mucous cells have been demonstrated in some of the metaplastic cells (Ramaekers *et al.*, 1983). Mucus cannot be detected in cells of the most basal layers but is demonstrable in cells of the mid and superficial layers by light and electron microscopy (insets, Figs 9.4c, 9.5).

Carcinoembryonic antigen (CEA) is demonstrable by immunostaining in the superficial metaplastic cells and is increased above normal levels (Pascal *et al.*, 1977; Hill *et al.*, 1979; Boon *et al.*, 1982). Because CEA is increased in regular epidermoid metaplasia in patients without lung cancer, it should not be considered as a marker of neoplastic change. For example, the epithelium in Fig. 9.4c and inset, from a noncancer patient, stained strongly for CEA (Fig. 9.4g).

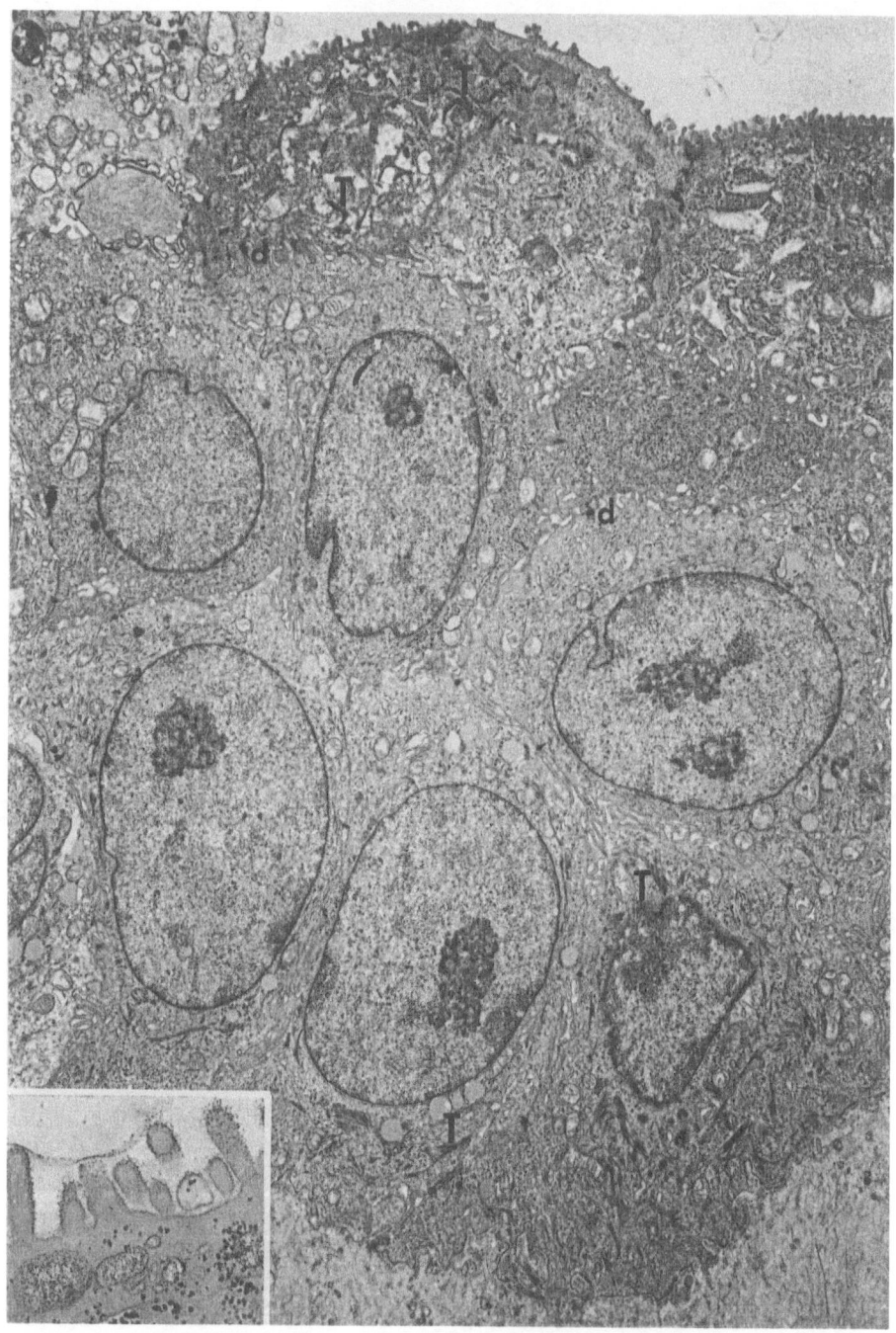

Fig. 9.5 Characteristic ultrastructure of noncornifying epidermoid metaplasia. Note tonofilament bundles (T) in basal and superficial cells. Cells are joined by well-developed desmosomes (d). From 22-year-old male, following tracheal intubation. (Electron micrograph: × 6000.) *Inset*: Fine deposits of silver in membrane-bounded granules indicate presence of mucosubstances in the apices of surface cells. Also note silver grains on the glycocalyx covering the microvilli. (PA-TCH-SP stain of Thiéry, 1967. Electron micrograph: × 25000.)

Epidermoid metaplasia may be widespread, or localized foci may occur together with areas of 'goblet' cell hyperplasia and/or stratification, so that the various lesions blend imperceptibly together (Fig. 9.4a). All types of lesions are common in bronchi of individuals who have undergone tracheal intubation and who have been maintained on respirators (Figs 9.4a, c, 9.5) (Sara, 1967; Sara and Reye, 1969; Rasche and Kuhns, 1972; Klainer *et al.*, 1975; Mithal and Emery, 1976; Trump *et al.*, 1978). It is apparent that foci of 'goblet' cell hyperplasia and stratification can become increasingly keratinized causing these lesions to progress into epidermoid metaplasia. As this change occurs, mucus secretions become very scant (Wang *et al.*, 1972; Trump *et al.*, 1978).

9.2 Reversal of the hyperplastic state and restoration of mucociliary epithelium

Very little is known about the reversal of hyperplastic and metaplastic lesions in human bronchi (Koss, 1979). However, results of animal experiments indicate that these lesions are at least potentially reversible, assuming that the injurious agent or adverse environment is removed and that the cells have not been initiated by a carcinogen. Following mechanical injury to hamster trachea, restoration of the normal mucociliary state occurs very rapidly. At 48 hours post-injury the epithelium is highly keratinized and metaplastic (Fig. 9.4e), yet within another two days the epithelium appears nearly normal. The return to normal is brought about by the genesis of columnar mucous and preciliated cells from division of metaplastic cells within the wound and from division of columnar mucous cells at the wound edges. Preciliated cells are larger than other epithelial cells (Fig. 9.6 and inset). They have an abundant pale-stained cytoplasm and fibrogranular areas and/or nascent basal bodies are seen in their apical cytoplasm, both prerequisites for ciliogenesis. Many preciliated cells contain apical mucous granules, apparently carried over from the parent mucous cell. The preciliated cells rapidly mature into ciliated cells by budding cilia from their apical surfaces (Keenan *et al.*, 1983). Mucous granules are often seen in the apices of human preciliated cells (Chapter 3; Fig. 3.7b, c), providing some evidence that similar processes occur during restoration and maintenance of the human mucociliary bronchial epithelium.

The regeneration of dense-cored granulated (DCG) cells has recently been studied in the cricoid epithelium of guinea pigs xenotransplanted into the subcutaneous tissues of nude mice by Di Augustine *et al.* (1984). The cricoid epithelium is especially suitable for studying these cells because they are more numerous here than elsewhere and make up 5% of the total epithelial population. By one week the epithelium was composed of

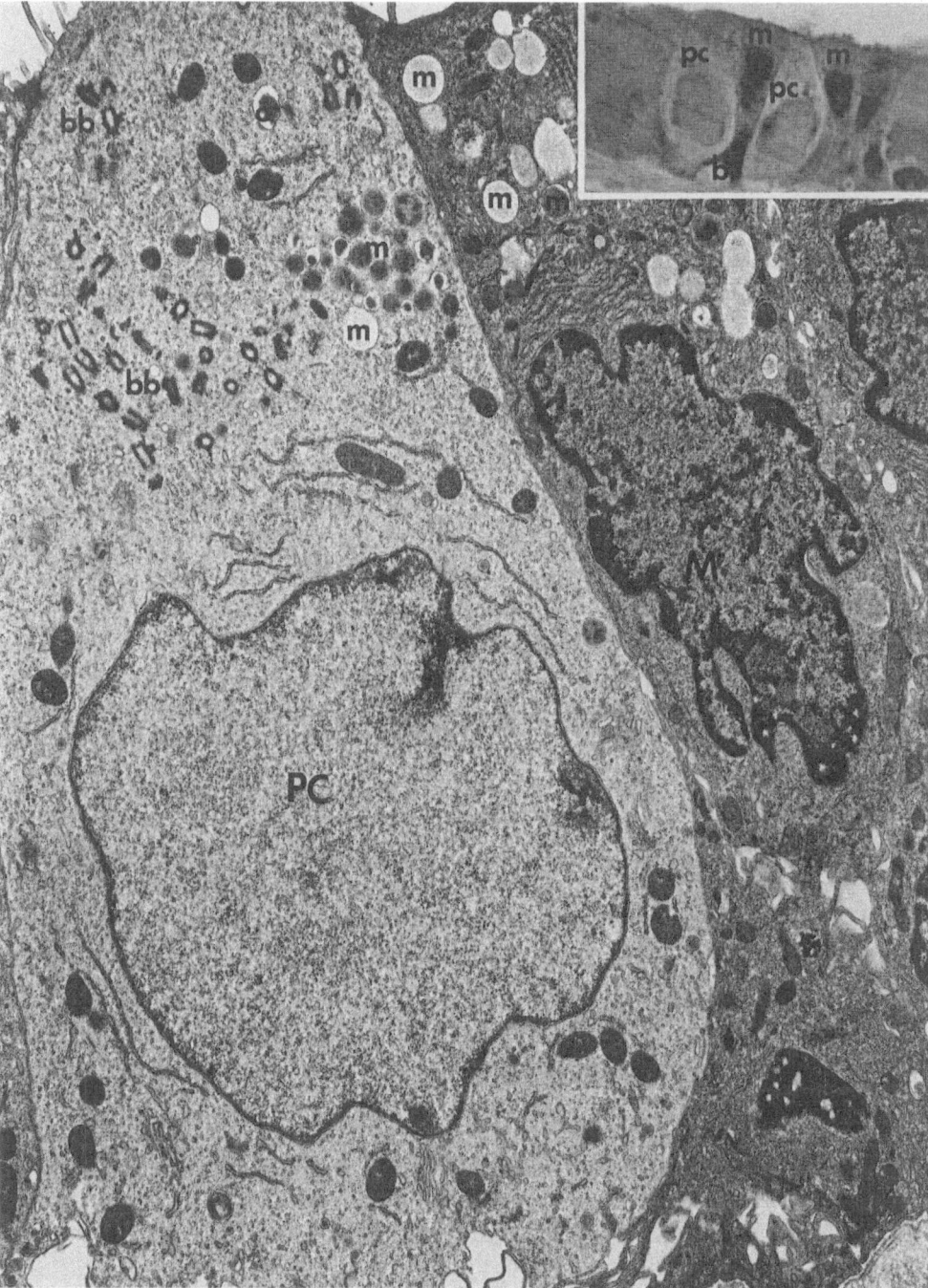

a single layer of flat cells and by two weeks the epithelium was stratified. By three weeks columnar mucous and ciliated cells were recognizable but DCG cells were extremely rare. However, by four weeks DCG cells were restored to about 5% in those areas showing normal maturation of mucous and ciliated cells. The late appearance of DCG cells in the regenerating grafts, together with additional evidence, suggests that these cells may arise from division of non-DCG precursor cells (Di Augustine and Sonstegard, 1984; Di Augustine *et al.*, 1984).

9.3 Similarities between development and regeneration

Animal experiments also point to there being striking similarities between the genesis of mucociliary epithelium in the fetus and restoration of the adult mucociliary epithelium following injury. Collective evidence indicates that the specialized cells are initially derived from primitive columnar cells (Chapter 3). Thereafter specialized basal and mucous cells undergo mitotic divisions, but the relative extents to which basal cells and mucous cells contribute to the development of the epithelium is presently unknown. Preliminary data derived from cell counts in young hamsters show that mitotic activity in mucous cells exceeds that in basal cells by about 4 to 1 and that nascent preciliated cells are derived from division of mucous cells (McDowell, unpublished). The preciliated cells contain mucous granules, presumably carried over from the parent cells, as appears to occur during regeneration of the adult epithelium (Fig. 9.6). Mucous granules have been described in cells undergoing ciliogenesis in tracheas of developing chicks (Kalnins and Porter, 1969), rats (Stockinger and Cireli, 1965; Cireli, 1966) and hamsters (Emura and Mohr, 1975). In chicks, mucous granules were present in cells where ciliogenesis had just begun, but granules were not seen in cells where ciliogenesis was advanced (Kalnins and Porter, 1969). A likely interpretation is that mucous granules in preciliated cells are inherited from parent mucous cells but are dissipated as ciliogenesis occurs.

Fig. 9.6 Restoration of the mucociliary state 72 hours following mechanical injury to hamster tracheal epithelium. A large pale-stained preciliated cell (PC) shows ciliogenesis in the apical cytoplasm. Numerous basal bodies (bb) are forming near to a group of mucous granules (m). Similar mucous granules are seen in the adjacent mucous cell (M). (Reprinted with permission from Keenan *et al.*, 1983). Compare with preciliated cell in human bronchus (Fig. 3.7b). (Electron micrograph: × 6000.) *Inset*: Preciliated (pc), mucous (m) and basal cells (b) as seen by light microscopy, 72 hours following epithelial injury. (Glycol methacrylate section stained with PAS-lead hematoxylin: × 900.)

9.4   Progression to neoplasia

Carcinogenesis is believed to occur in at least two major steps--initiation which involves exposure to a carcinogen, followed by promotion whereby 'neoplastic development', 'tumor formation' or 'cancer development' is accelerated or encouraged in a tissue that has been exposed for a relatively brief period to an initiating dose of a carcinogen (Farber, 1982). Promotion is the process whereby an initiated tissue or organ develops focal proliferations, one or more of which may act as precursors for subsequent steps in the carcinogenic process. Studies on initiation and promotion have been mainly performed on skin and liver. In the liver, cell proliferation is essential for initiation to occur, be it generated by a primary mitogenic stimulus, chemical mutagens, cell death or partial hepatectomy. At present little is known about either initiation or promotion in the respiratory tract or what effect wounding *per se* has on either process. However, the importance of injury and repair in promotion of the carcinogenic process in the lung has been emphasized and several studies have shown that tumorigenesis was enhanced if regeneration and repair were occurring at the site of action of a carcinogen (Kotin, 1968).

9.5   Histogenesis of bronchogenic neoplasms

It is widely accepted that bronchogenic neoplasms derive from pluripotent epithelial cells which display a continuum of phenotypic expression, but there is at present no consensus regarding the nature(s) of the progenitor cell(s). Only cells that can divide are potentially capable of hyperplastic, metaplastic and neoplastic change. In the bronchi, obvious candidates include mucous cells and basal cells, both of which divide in adult epithelium, and possibly DCG cells which divide in fetal airways but rarely if ever in the normal adult epithelium (Section 3.2.5). One hypothesis is that any one of these cell types may give rise to progeny which mature into *any* of the cell types of the mature epithelium, *irrespective of the nature of the parent cell*. Thus nascent cells from division of *either* mucous, basal or DCG cells might mature into basal cells, mucous cells, ciliated cells or DCG cells or into cells with mixed phenotypes such as DCG-ciliated, DCG-mucous, or even more complicated mosaics, under the influence of presently ill-defined microenvironmental factors (McDowell *et al.*, 1982). Furthermore, any one of the progeny has the capability to keratinize, thereby demonstrating an epidermoid phenotype, *in addition to and superimposed upon* the primary specialization. Thus, the hypothesis proposes that any cell capable of division has the potential to produce hyperplastic, metaplastic and neoplastic lesions composed of cells which may differ phenotypically from the parent cell(s). It follows that

Scheme 9.2 Postulated progression of changes towards invasive bronchogenic carcinoma.

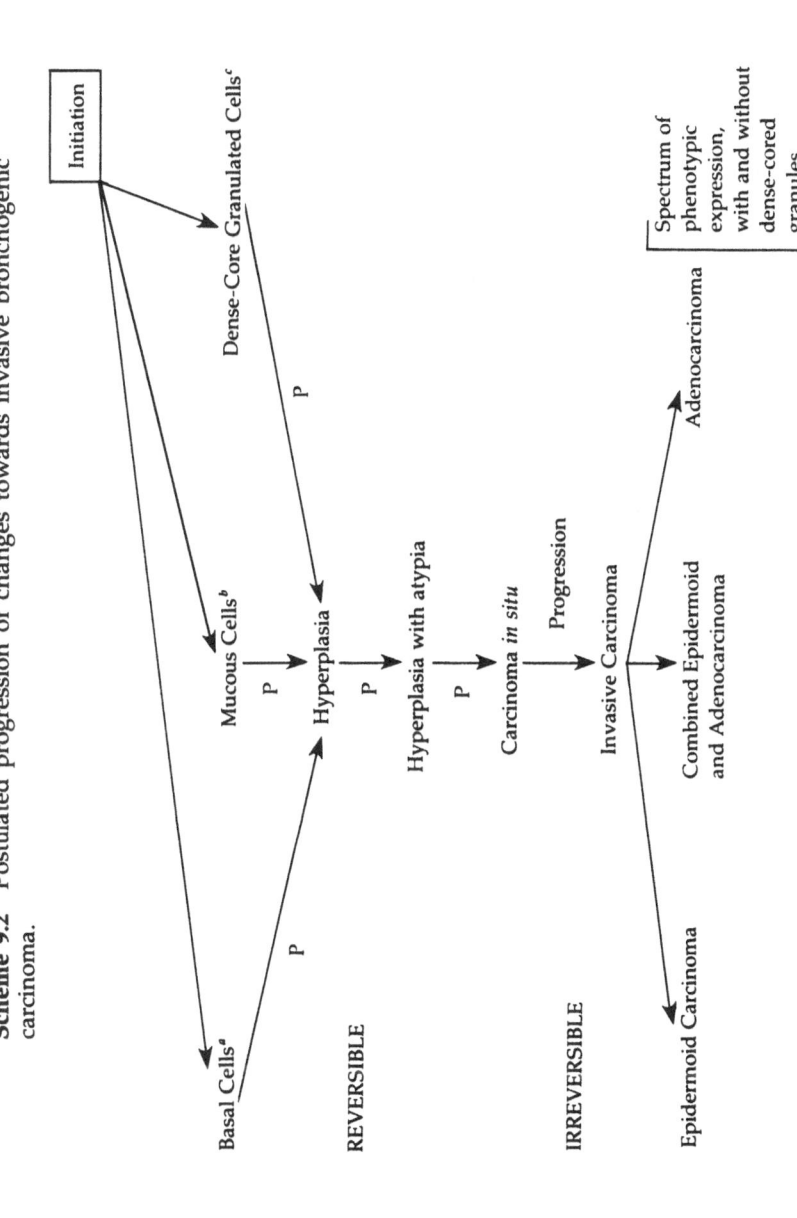

[a] Basal cells are absent from the bronchial submucosal glandular epithelium.

[b] Although basal cells and dense-core granulated cells are included as potential progenitor cells, mucous cells appear to be the progenitor cell for the majority of preneoplastic and neoplastic lesions in the tracheobronchial epithelium (see text).

[c] Collective data suggest that dense-core granulated cells divide infrequently or not at all in adult respiratory epithelium making this cell type an unlikely candidate for the initial source of hyperplastic cells (Di Augustine and Sonstegard, 1984).

P Promotion.

divisions of mucous cells could lead to hyperplastic, metaplastic and neoplastic foci of DCG cells or that divisions of DCG cells could lead to foci of mucous cells, with or without keratinization, or to complicated phenotypic mosaics showing mixed patterns of mucus secretion, keratin production and dense-cored granules.

The concept stresses that phenotypic specializations which occur within cells of a neoplasm are either glandular and secretory (adeno), or epidermoid and keratinizing, or combinations of both (Chapter 10). Secretory products include mucosubstances, both acidic and neutral, and hormones, certain of which are packaged in characteristic dense-cored granules.

Although this hypothesis presently includes basal cells, DCG cells and mucous cells, a personal (E.M. McDowell) bias is that mucous cells are the progenitor cell for the majority of bronchogenic neoplasms (Schemes 9.1 and 9.2).

9.6   Morphogenesis of epithelial neoplasms

The majority of primary carcinomas of the lung originate from the bronchial epithelium. Lesser numbers of neoplasms arise from the bronchiolar and alveolar linings, which fall outside the scope of this text. Studies which characterize any epithelial response to various types of injury have important implications regarding the morphogenesis of preneoplastic and neoplastic lesions. The histogenetic relationships between mucous cell hyperplasia, stratification and epidermoid metaplasia in tracheobronchial epithelium were discussed above. In the sections which follow the progression of epithelial lesions to invasive carcinomas will be described. The discussion will be limited to the genesis of four types of bronchogenic tumor: epidermoid carcinomas, adenocarcinomas, small cell carcinomas and carcinoid tumors.

9.6.1   Epidermoid carcinomas

Foci of epidermoid metaplasia are often present in the bronchi of patients with invasive epidermoid carcinoma (Black and Ackerman, 1952; Valentine, 1957; Auerbach et al., 1957, 1961; Nasiell, 1963, 1966, 1968 a, b). Epidermoid metaplasia per se is not committed to neoplasia and, assuming that carcinogenic initiation has not occurred and the adverse environment is removed, this lesion can potentially reverse (Section 9.2). However, several studies have stressed that the development of invasive carcinoma is preceded by stratification and epidermoid metaplasia, characterized by progressively increasing degrees of cellular and/or nuclei atypia, and correlations have been made between increasing atypia in metaplastic cells and the incidence of bronchogenic carcinoma (Black and Ackerman, 1952; Auerbach *et al.*, 1961; Nasiell, 1963, 1966, 1968 a, b). One of the striking findings of Auerbach's study was the marked increase in the number of atypical cells with the numbers of cigarettes smoked, emphasizing a direct causal relationship.

It is important to differentiate between metaplasia and atypia, although both changes often occur together in the same cells. In metaplasia, the phenotypic expression of the cells is changed, whereas in atypia the nuclear cytoplasmic (N/C) ratio is altered. Atypical nuclei are enlarged relative to the cytoplasm, so that the N/C ratio is increased. The enlarged nuclei may be abnormally shaped and hyperchromic with irregular chromatin patterns and prominent nucleoli. Nasiell *et al.* (1978) demonstrated good correlation between increasing degrees of nuclear atypia judged morphologically, with increasing degrees of aneuploidy, based upon increased DNA content.

Detailed morphological comparisons have been made of the progression of lesions in cytological and histological specimens (Nasiell, 1963, 1966, 1967, 1968a, b; Saccomanno *et al.*, 1970, 1974; Frost *et al.*, 1973; Schreiber *et al.*, 1974, 1979; Nasiell *et al.*, 1978; Konaka *et al.*, 1982; Frost *et al.*, 1983; Woolner, 1983). From these studies correlative cytologic and morphologic criteria of the spectrum of preneoplastic and neoplastic change have been characterized. Guidelines of the cytological morphologies of cells from normal epithelium, metaplastic epithelium (regular → mild atypia → moderate atypia → marked atypia), carcinoma *in situ* and invasive carcinoma, have been formulated. Descriptions of cytological specimens are beyond the scope of this book and readers are referred to specialized texts on cytology (Section 10.3.4). A summary of the morphological characteristics of cells found in sputum in each stage of development of epidermoid carcinoma was made by Saccomanno *et al.* (1974) (Table 9.1 and Fig. 9.7). The time of transition from moderate atypia to invasive carcinoma was estimated to be about 5 years. It is presently unknown what proportion of persons demonstrating foci of atypia or even carcinoma *in situ* eventually develop invasive carcinoma. Provided that the patient has received neither radio- nor chemotherapy, any epithelial abnormality that shows even mild nuclear abnormalities should be looked upon with suspicion. Furthermore, in a recent study in humans and dogs it was shown that *all* degrees of cellular atypia, including the cytological diagnosis of malignancy, may be consistent with reversible bronchial lesions, if the carcinogen and the promoting agents are removed (Auer *et al.*, 1982). Neither cytological methods nor DNA measurements provided distinction between cellular changes which were reversible (i.e., disap-

Table 9.1 Criteria of Cells Found in Sputum in each Stage of the Development of Carcinoma (from Saccomanno *et al.*, 1974)

Regular metaplasia

1. Cells are all of about same size.
2. Nuclei are of uniform size with normal nuclear/cytoplasmic ratio (N/C ratio).
3. Nuclear material is fine and powdery with rare chromocenters which are demonstrably smaller than nucleoli.
4. Cytoplasm is usually basophilic.
5. Cells usually occur in sheets, but may be single.

Metaplasia, mild atypia

1. Cells vary slightly in size.
2. Nuclei vary slightly in size; N/C ratio may vary slightly.
3. Nuclear material is fine and powdery with rare clusters of nuclear material near the nuclear membrane.
4. Cytoplasm may be acidophilic.
5. Cells usually occur in sheets, but may be found singly.

Metaplasia, moderate atypia

1. Cells vary moderately in size; some are smaller than in mild metaplasia.
2. Nuclei vary significantly in size.
3. N/C ratio varies moderately. It may be higher or lower than normal.
4. Nuclear material is fine and powdery in most areas, but nuclear masses are abundant, particularly along the nuclear membrane.
5. Nuclear lobulations, crevices, and nodules are present.
6. Cytoplasm may be basophilic, but acidophilia predominates.
7. Cells usually occur in sheets, but an increase in single cells is found.

Metaplasia, marked atypia

1. Cells vary markedly in size, but are generally larger than those in moderate atypia.
2. Nuclear pleomorphism is marked; nuclear material is coarse and sometimes clustered about nuclear membrane.
3. N/C ratio varies markedly. It may be higher or lower than normal.
4. Nucleoli are present, but are small and may be acidophilic.
5. Acidophilic cytoplasm predominates.
6. Single cells predominate.

Carcinoma *in situ*

1. Cells vary in size and may be double the size of those in metaplasia with marked atypia. Single cells are present, but clusters are more common than in invasive carcinoma.
2. Nuclear material is coarse and accumulated in large masses, but concentrations are not usually accumulated near membrane. Chromocenters are large, simulate nucleoli, but are not always acidophilic.
3. N/C ratio varies markedly. It may be higher or lower than normal.
4. Cannibalism and multinucleation may be present.
5. Acidophilic cytoplasm predominates.

Invasive carcinoma

1. Cells are usually larger than normal, but may be very pleomorphic and bizarre. They are usually single, but clusters are found.
2. Nuclear material is coarse and accumulated in masses. It is unevenly distributed adjacent to the nuclear membranes.
3. Nucleoli are large and acidophilic.
4. N/C ratio varies markedly. It may be higher or lower than normal.
5. Cannibalism and multinucleation are common.
6. Cytoplasm may be acidophilic and basophilic.

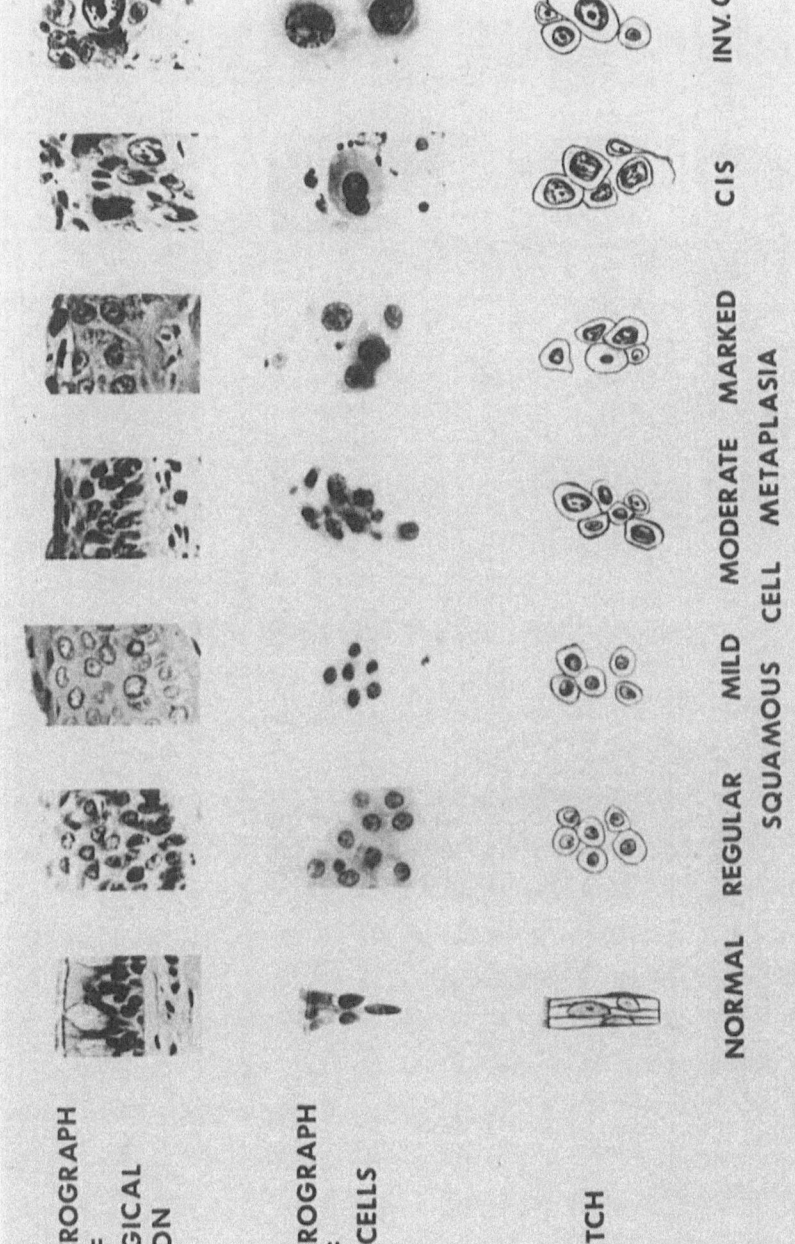

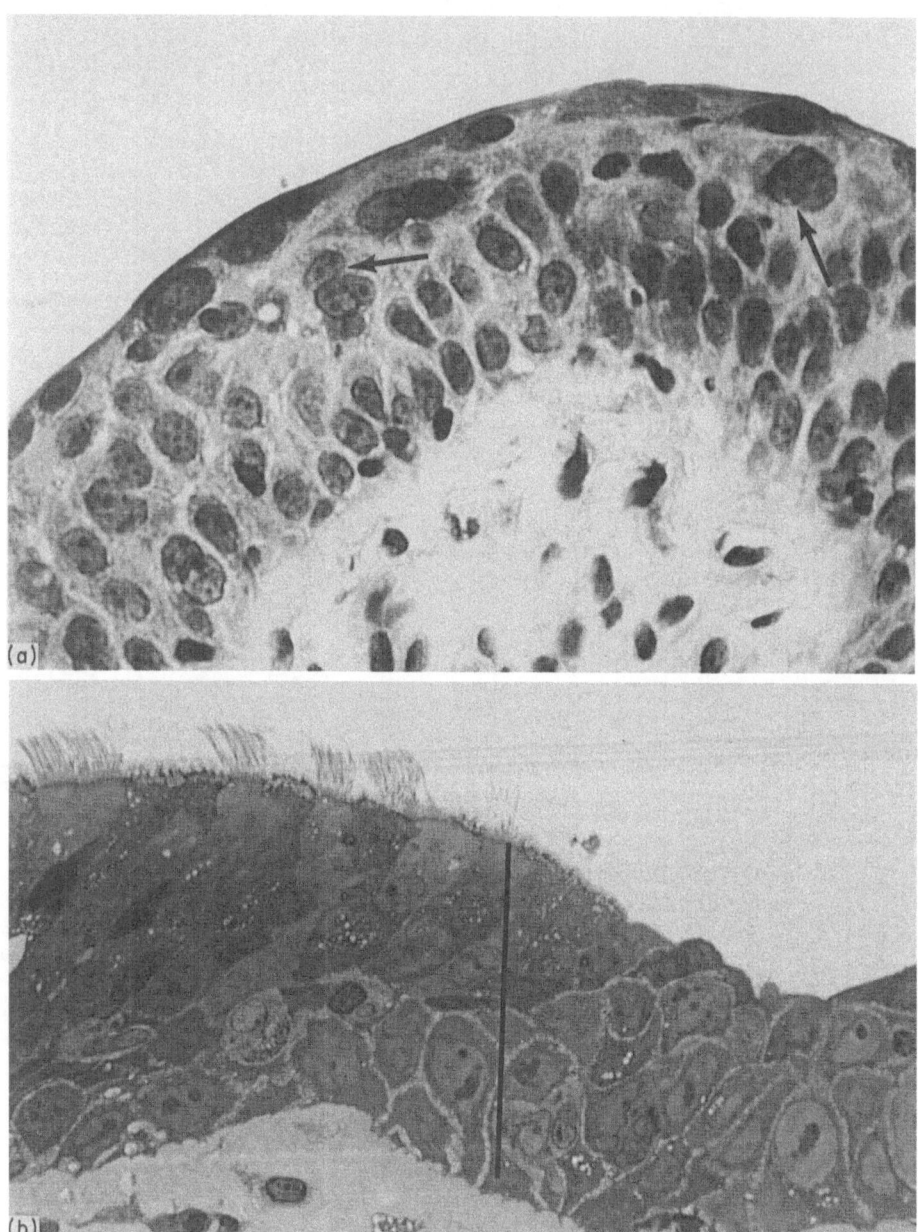

Fig. 9.8 (a) Noncornifying epidermoid metaplasia showing moderate nuclear atypia. Many of the nuclei are enlarged and hyperchromatic. The nucleoli are prominent and multiple. Some cells are multinucleated (arrows). From a patient with well-differentiated adenocarcinoma. (Paraffin section, stained with hematox-

peared after removal of the carcinogen) and irreversible changes that with time will progress to invasive cancer. Therefore, persons who smoke and who show any degree of cellular atypia should be strongly encouraged to stop smoking.

Mild atypia is characterized by cells and nuclei which vary slightly in size (Figs 9.2c, 9.3 inset). Accordingly the N/C ratios may vary slightly. Usually only a few cells are affected and there is no hyperchromasia. *Moderate atypia* shows more pronounced variations and the nuclei vary significantly in size. The nuclei are usually larger than normal and their outline may be crenated or lobulated; often the nucleoli are quite distinct. Some hyperchromasia is common and multinucleated cells may be present (Fig. 9.8a). Multinucleated cells have been observed following a variety of injuries such as bronchoscopy, x-ray therapy (Section 5.10), and exposure to fumes but their significance is unknown (Koss, 1979). Unfortunately it is impossible at present to distinguish between early morphological changes induced by noncarcinogenic or carcinogenic insults, and even relatively harmless interventions such as injections of water will cause cells to exhibit mild to moderate degrees of atypia (Konaka *et al.*, 1982).

In *marked or severe atypia* the cells and their nuclei vary markedly in size and are generally larger than those showing moderate change. Nuclear pleomorphism is marked and the N/C ratio varies greatly. Nucleoli may be very prominent (Fig. 9.8b). Experimentally, marked atypia is generally seen only in lesions induced by carcinogens (Konaka *et al.*, 1982). However, occasional nuclear enlargement, hyperchromasia and nucleolar prominence may occur in association with viral pneumonia. Furthermore, certain therapies, namely radiation and chemotherapy, may cause significant changes in epithelial cells, with degrees of atypia simulating malignancy (Sections 5.9, 5.10). For example, recently irradiated epithelium may show cells with very enlarged nuclei, nucleoli and chromatin granules. Some cells may be multinucleated. In rare instances the cells become very large, with enlarged nuclei and very prominent nucleoli. Such cells simulate bizarre giant cancer cells. Furthermore, chronic radiation injury may cause cellular change which ranges from mild atypia in otherwise normal columnar cells to epidermoid metaplasias with degrees of atypia

---

ylin and eosin: × 450.) (b) Noncornifying epidermoid metaplasia with marked nuclear atypia (right) blends abruptly with more normal mucociliary epithelium (left). At the epidermoid focus, metaplastic cells occupy the entire epithelium. If the section had been cut along the line shown, it would appear as if ciliated epithelium overlay the epidermoid cells. From a patient with epidermoid carcinoma (from Trump *et al.*, 1978). (Epon section stained with toluidine blue: × 900.)

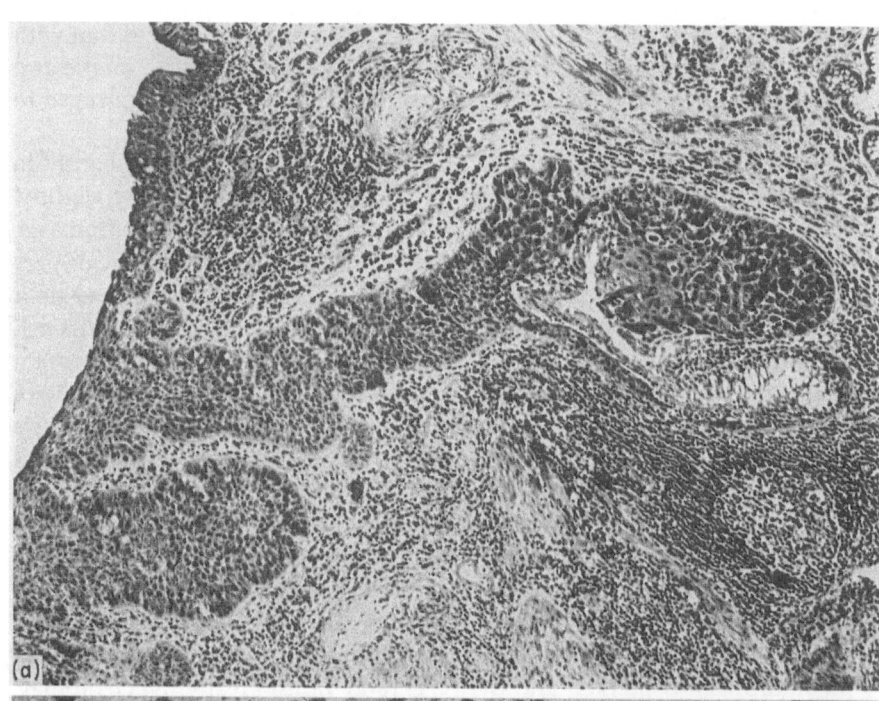

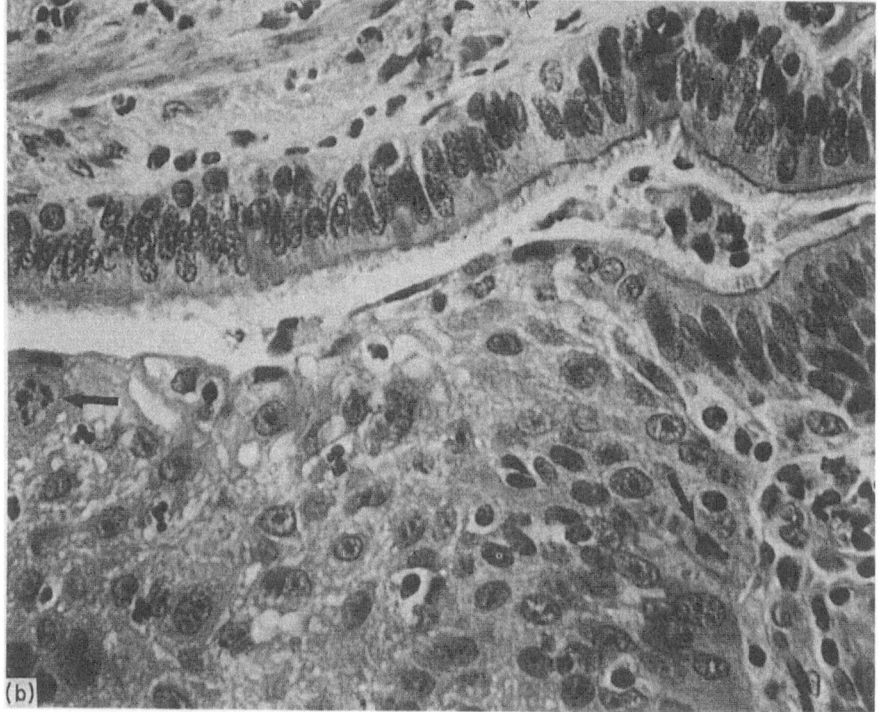

from mild to severe. Significant abnormalities may also occur in the bronchial epithelium of patients receiving alkylating agents and other anticancer chemotherapeutic drugs (Koss, 1979).

Foci of atypical epidermoid metaplasia may lie intercalated between more normal-appearing areas. When this occurs metaplastic and columnar cells interface with one another. Epidermoid metaplasia involves the full epithelial thickness, and the appearance of columnar mucociliary epithelium overlying groups of atypical epidermoid cells derives from fortuitous cuts through the periphery of a metaplastic focus, where the metaplastic epithelium undermines the mucociliary epithelium at the interfacing zone (Fig. 9.8b).

Epidermoid metaplasias demonstrating cellular and nuclear atypia are not necessarily confined to cells of the surface bronchial epithelium and may also be found in mucus-secreting cells which comprise the acini of the submucosal glands. Basal cells are absent from the bronchial glands but keratin is present in serous and mucous cells (Gusterson *et al.*, 1982; Blobel *et al.*, 1984).

Most epidermoid carcinomas arise in large to medium-sized bronchi, especially in the segmental branches and to a lesser extent in the lobar divisions (Black and Ackerman, 1952; Garland *et al.*, 1962; Lisa *et al.*, 1965; Carter *et al.*, 1976; Melamed *et al.*, 1977). Consequently, the predecessor of the invasive cancer, carcinoma *in situ*, is most commonly found at the same locations. Carcinoma *in situ* is characterized by an intact basement membrane and multiple layers of highly pleomorphic cells showing marked cytoplasmic and nuclear atypia (Figs 9.9a, b, 9.10a, b, 9.11, 9.12a, b). The morphology and arrangement of cells in carcinoma *in situ* is indistinguishable from invasive carcinoma, except of course for invasion (Melamed *et al.*, 1977). The nuclei are often more than twice the size of those of the normal epithelium (Figs 9.7, 9.9b, 9.10a, 9.12a). Mitotic figures are common and are seen at all levels throughout the epithelium (Fig. 9.9b). Carcinoma *in situ* may be composed of more cell layers than atypical metaplastic lesions and up to 38 cell layers have been reported, although the majority of lesions were only 5 cells thick (Auerbach *et al.*, 1961).

The dividing line between marked atypia and carcinoma *in situ* is not

---

Fig. 9.9 (a) Carcinoma *in situ* involving the surface epithelium and the neck of a submucosal gland. From a patient with epidermoid carcinoma. (Paraffin section stained with hematoxylin and eosin: × 80.) (b) Abrupt transition between normal columnar mucociliary epithelium and carcinoma *in situ*. The neoplastic nuclei are enlarged compared with the normal cells. Peripheral chromatin is clumped and nucleoli are prominent. Mitotic figures (arrows) are seen at all levels. From a patient with epidermoid carcinoma. (Paraffin section stained with hematoxylin and eosin: × 300.)

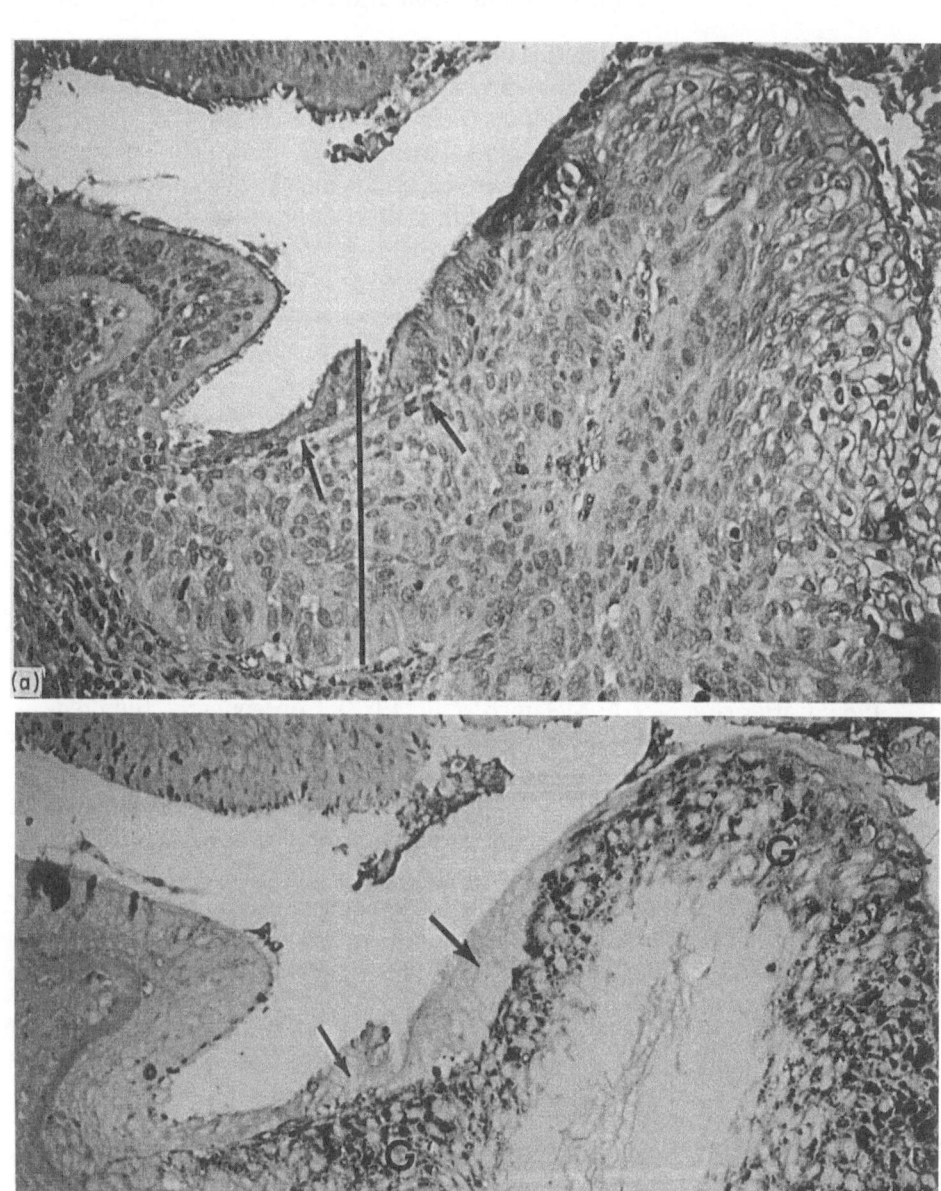

(a)

(b)

clear cut and separation of frankly malignant cells from severely atypical cells is not well defined. Overt cornification of epidermoid foci may help in the diagnosis of carcinoma *in situ*, for although cornification *per se* is not a marker for neoplasia (it occurs in vitamin A deficiency), it sometimes occurs in association with neoplastic change (Fig. 9.11) (Black and Ackerman, 1952; Trump *et al.*, 1978). Intraepithelial deposits of glycogen are frequently present in carcinoma *in situ* (Fig. 9.10b). CEA, although present in carcinomas *in situ* (Pascall *et al.*, 1977; Hill *et al.*, 1979; Boon *et al.*, 1982), cannot be considered a marker for neoplastic change because it is present in regular metaplasia as well as in lesions with varying degrees of atypia (Section 9.1.4).

An abrupt transition is often seen between carcinoma *in situ* and the more normal appearing columnar epithelium (Figs 9.9b, 9.10a) (Black and Ackerman, 1952; Lisa *et al.*, 1965; Rosenblatt *et al.*, 1967; Koss, 1979). As is sometimes the case with atypical lesions, it may appear that columnar mucociliary epithelium overlies and covers an area of carcinoma *in situ* (Fig. 9.10a). This appearance is due to fortuitous cuts through the periphery of the base of the neoplastic intraepithelial lesion, which undermines the adjacent non-neoplastic cells.

In situ lesions may extend proximal (Carlisle *et al.*, 1952; Carter *et al.*, 1976) or proximal and distal (Melamed *et al.*, 1977) from the site of invasion. At time of surgery the extent of the *in situ* lesion cannot be accurately determined and extension from segmental to lobar bronchi is to be anticipated. Moreover, several studies have described multifocal primary lesions (Black and Ackerman, 1952; Auerbach *et al.*, 1967; Suemasu *et al.*, 1974; Carter *et al.*, 1976; Melamed *et al.*, 1977). These factors caution that more functioning lung be removed at surgery than might at first seem desirable (Carter *et al.*, 1976).

It is widely supposed that carcinoma *in situ* and invasive epidermoid carcinoma are derived from neoplastic changes in basal cells. However, experimental studies in animals and careful examination of human lesions provide persuasive evidence that mucous cells are important progenitor cells (Trump *et al.*, 1978; Becci *et al.*, 1978). As in metaplastic lesions, combined epidermoid and mucus-secreting specializations are commonly

---

Fig. 9.10 (a) Carcinoma *in situ* undermines adjacent normal mucociliary columnar epithelium (arrows). At right, markedly atypical cells occupy the entire neoplastic epithelium. If the section had been cut along the line shown it would appear as if ciliated epithelium overlay the neoplastic cells (compare with Fig. 9.8b). From a patient with epidermoid carcinoma. (Paraffin section stained with hematoxylin and eosin: × 200.) (b) Adjacent section stained with AB-PAS. Glycogen deposits (G) are present in superficial cells of carcinoma *in situ* but glycogen is not seen in the overlying non-neoplastic epithelial cells (arrows). (× 200)

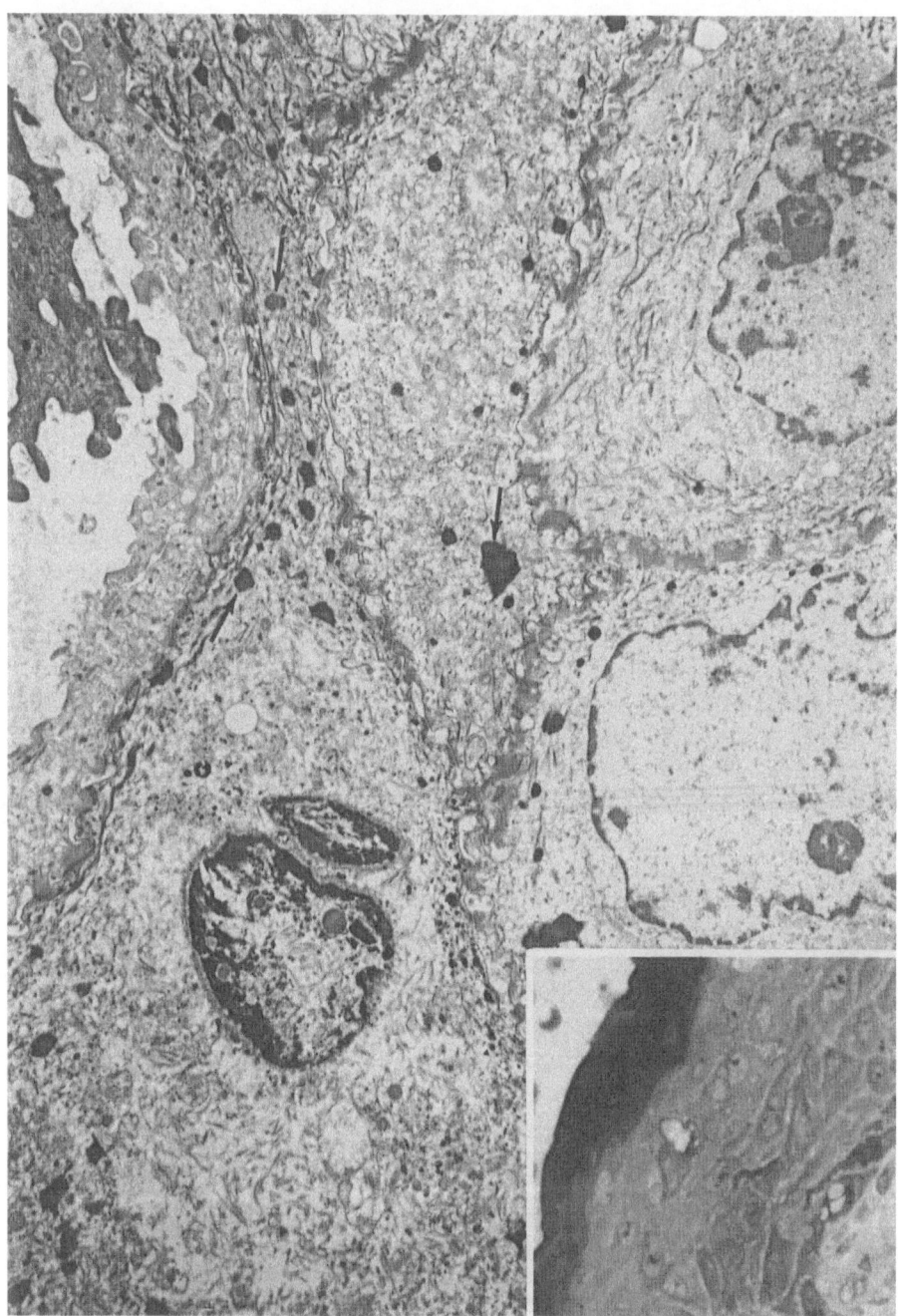

Fig. 9.11 Cornifying metaplastic epithelium. The superficial cells contain kera-
tohyalin granules (arrows). Cornified cells slough into the lumen (top left). From
a patient with epidermoid carcinoma. (Electron micrograph: × 6000.) *Inset*: Light
micrograph of same. The superficial cornified cells are dense stained. (Epon section
stained with toluidine blue: × 400.)

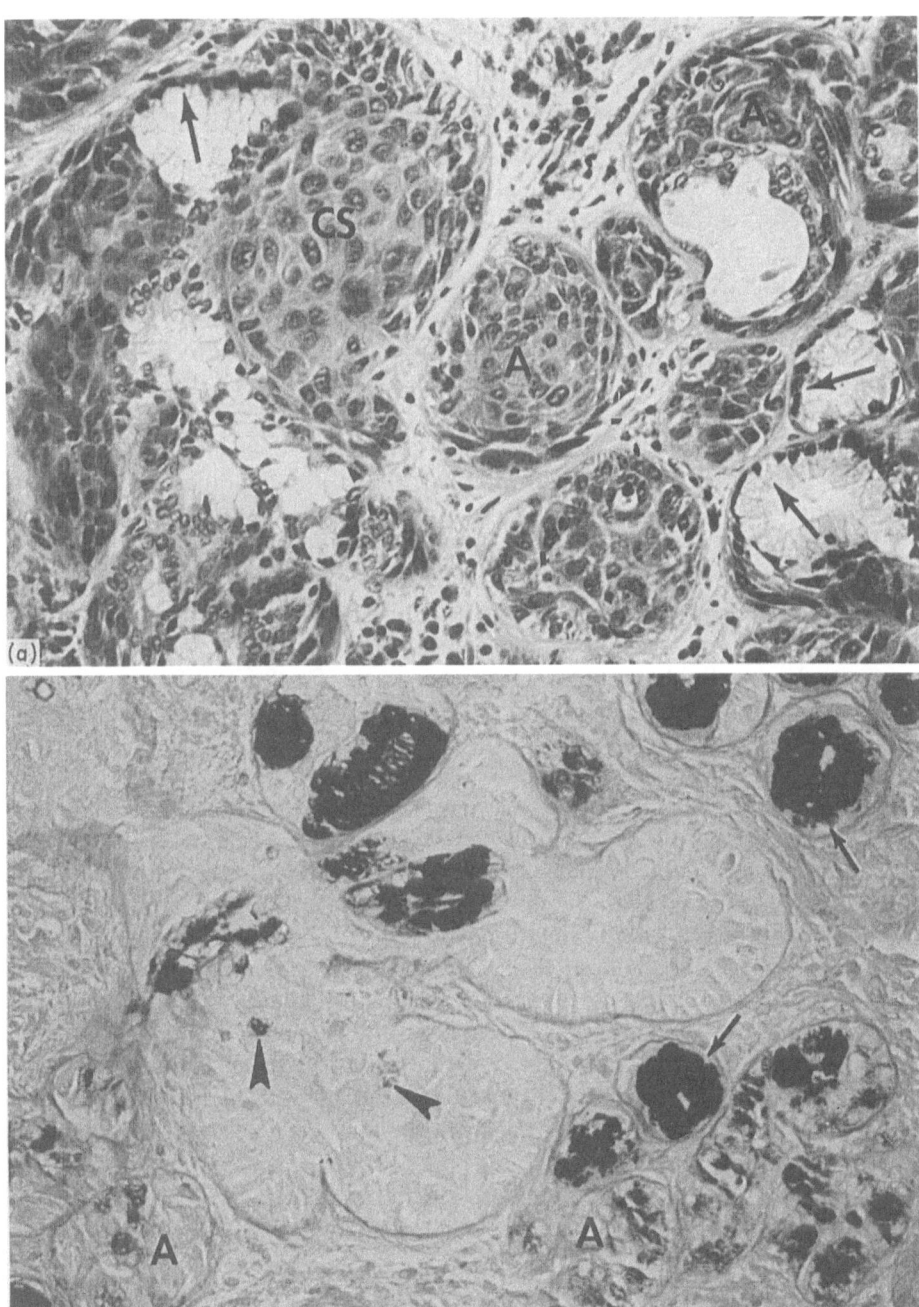

Fig. 9.12 (a) Marked atypia (A) and probable carcinoma *in situ* (CS) deep in the submucosal bronchial glands. Some mucous acini appear normal (arrows). From a patient with epidermoid carcinoma. (Paraffin section stained with hematoxylin and eosin: × 200.) (b) Adjacent section stained with Alcian blue-PAS. Abundant acidic mucosubstances are secreted by the normal cells (arrows). Mucosubstance secretion is diminished in aytpical cells (A) and is very sparse (arrowheads) in neoplastic foci. (× 200)

found in carcinoma *in situ* in man and experimental animals (Stenbäck, 1973; Trump *et al.*, 1978; Becci *et al.*, 1978; Klein-Szanto *et al.*, 1980) and mucosubstances can be demonstrated, even in the cornifying lesions (Trump *et al.*, 1978). Monoclonal antibodies for keratin are now available which distinguish keratin proteins of normal mucous cells and basal cells. Bronchial epidermoid (squamous) carcinomas stain variably positive for the glandular type of keratin, unlike tumors derived from stratified epithelium such as the skin, which are not stained (Ramaekers *et al.*, 1983; Blobel *et al.*, 1984). Furthermore, carcinoma *in situ* affects both the bronchial surface and glandular epithelium (Black and Ackerman, 1952; Valentine, 1957; Auerbach *et al.*, 1967; Suemasu *et al.*, 1974; Carter *et al.*, 1976; Melamed *et al.*, 1977). It has been questioned whether or not carcinoma *in situ* can arise primordially from the glandular epithelium, because serial sections may show continuities between lesions at the surface and in the glandular duct (Fig. 9.9a). However, evidence for a glandular origin is gained by observing lesions in glandular acini stained with a stain for mucus such as AB-PAS. It is clear that the mucus-secreting cells of the gland are involved and that their secretions are diminished as metaplasia with atypia progresses to neoplasia (Fig. 9.12a, b).

9.6.2 *Adenocarcinomas*

Adenocarcinomas of respiratory tract, with well-formed tubules and glands (Chapter 10), occur most commonly at the periphery of the lung. They derive from the epithelium of small bronchi, bronchioles and alveoli. Furthermore, some adenocarcinomas arise at the lung periphery associated with pre-existing lung scars (scar cancer). Raeburn and Spencer (1957) estimated that about a quarter of all lung cancers arose in association with pre-existing scars. Most of these were peripheral adenocarcinomas which arose from the regenerating bronchiolar and alveolar epithelium at the interface between fibrosed and undamaged lung. Only adenocarcinomas that arise from small bronchi are discussed in this and the following chapter because tumors that arise from the more distal airways lie outside the scope of this book.

Few studies have been made on the morphogenesis and site of origin of bronchogenic adenocarcinomas and relatively little is known compared

---

Fig. 9.13 (a) Focus of intraepithelial neoplasia in a small peripheral bronchus from a patient with a well-differentiated mucus-secreting adenocarcinoma (Figs 10.7a, b). The transition between neoplastic and non-neoplastic cells is abrupt; the neoplastic nuclei are hyperchromatic and enlarged. (Paraffin section stained with hematoxylin and eosin: × 220.) (b) Alcian blue-PAS staining of an adjacent section shows that some of the neoplastic cells are mucus secreting. (× 220)

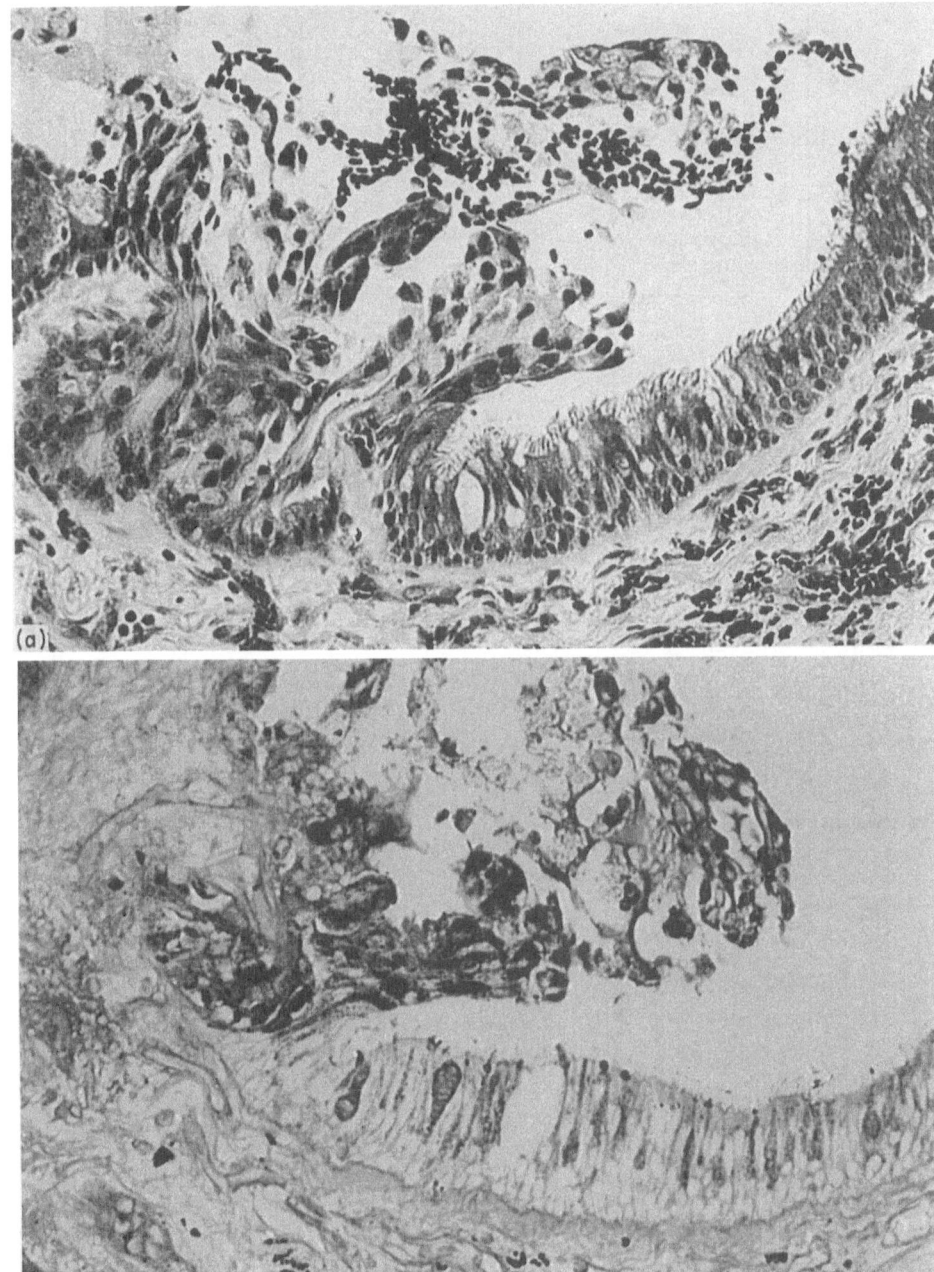

(a)

(b)

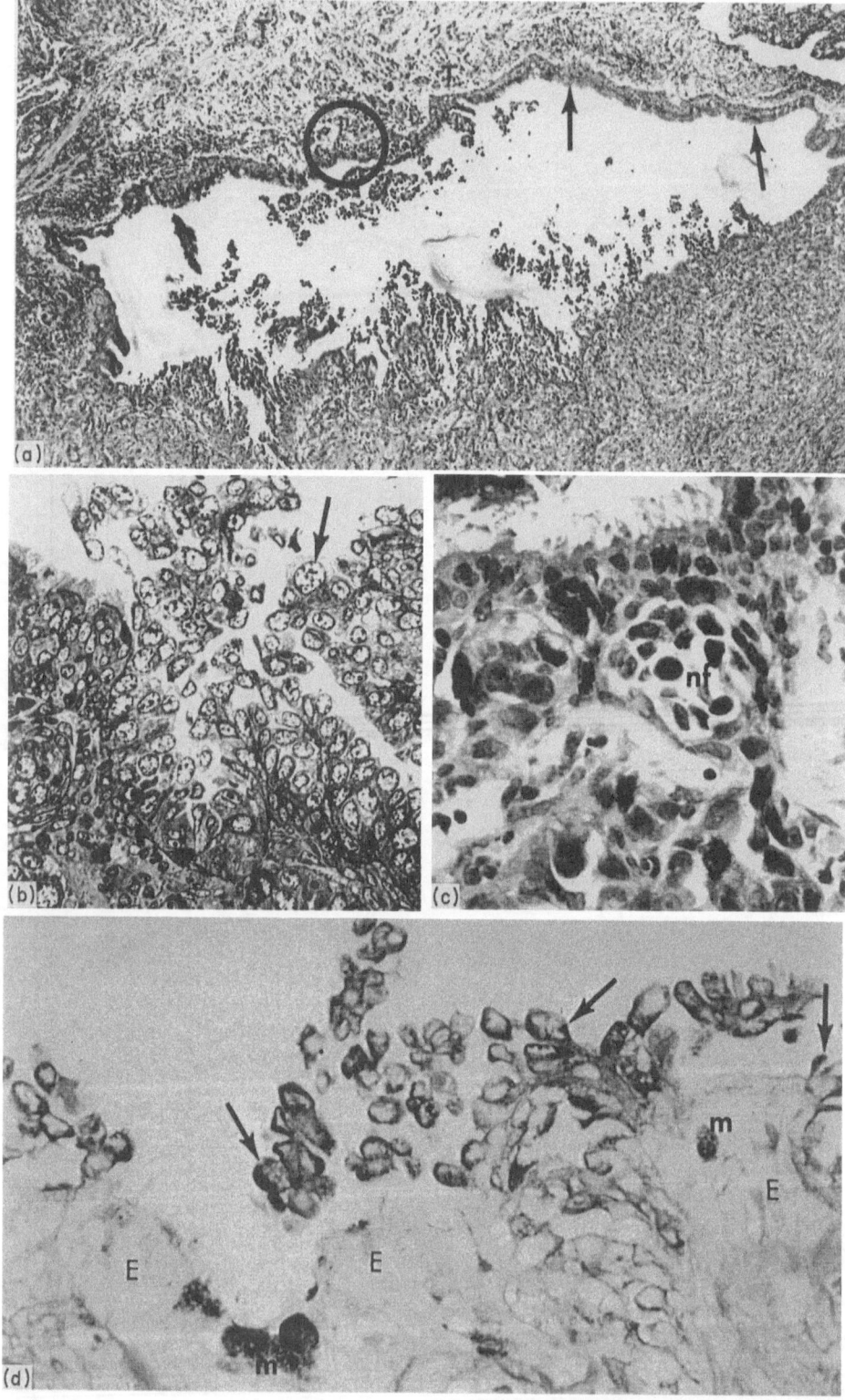

with that known about the type of carcinoma *in situ* that precedes epidermoid carcinomas. It is generally agreed that most bronchogenic adenocarcinomas arise from small peripheral bronchi (Walter and Pryce, 1955a, b; Lisa *et al.*, 1965; Rosenblatt *et al.*, 1967; Bennett *et al.*, 1969; Shimosato *et al.*, 1980). The evidence available suggests that mucous cells are the progenitors for these peripheral tumors. Adenocarcinomas stain positively with the monoclonal keratin antibody normally associated with mucous cells (Ramaekers *et al.*, 1983). In cases where the site of origin has been identified, the nonmalignant columnar epithelium of a small peripheral bronchus blended directly into atypical or malignant epithelium, from which the invasive cancer arose (Lisa *et al.*, 1965; Rosenblatt *et al.*, 1967; Bennett *et al.*, 1969; Shimosato, 1980).

Figures 9.13a, b show a focus of intraepithelial neoplasia in a small peripheral bronchus from a patient with a well-differentiated mucus-secreting adenocarcinoma (Chapter 10; Fig. 10.7a, b). This case shows similarity with one described by Rosenblatt *et al.* (1967). An abrupt transition is seen between the normal mucociliary epithelium of a small terminal bronchus and the malignant cells. Note that the neoplastic cells project as fronds into the bronchial lumen. The nuclei are hyperchromic and enlarged compared with nuclei of the adjacent normal epithelium.

Figures 9.14a–d show areas of intraepithelial neoplasia from a patient with a moderately well-differentiated (non-mucus-secreting) adenocarcinoma (Chapter 10; Fig. 10.6a, b). The neoplastic cells stream into the lumen from multiple foci, separated by areas of normal appearing mucociliary epithelium. The nuclei of the neoplastic cells are enlarged (Fig. 9.14b, c). Neoplastic cells are also observed penetrating the basal lamina, continuous with the underlying invasive tumor (Fig. 9.14c). Glycogen is demonstrable in the neoplastic cells (Fig. 9.14d).

Fig. 9.14 Areas of intraepithelial neoplasia associated with an invasive well-differentiated adenocarcinoma (Figs 10.6a, b). (a) Low power view of small peripheral bronchus. Fronds of neoplastic cells stream from the epithelium into the lumen. Much of the epithelium appears normal (arrows). Nests of tumor cells (T) are present in the surrounding connective tissue. The circled area is enlarged in Fig. 9.14c. (Paraffin section stained with hematoxylin and eosin: × 70.) (b) Abrupt junction between normal mucociliary epithelium (left) and a neoplastic focus. The neoplastic nuclei are enlarged (arrow) compared with those in normal cells. (Epon section stained with toluidine blue: × 300.) (c) Enlargement of circled area in Fig. 9.14a. Columnar mucociliary epithelium lies above a neoplastic focus (nf), which shows continuity with the underlying tumor. (Paraffin section stained with hematoxylin and eosin: × 480.) (d) The neoplastic cells (arrows) are rich in glycogen. Glycogen is not seen in the normal mucociliary epithelium (E) but mucous cells (M) contain acidic mucosubstances. (Paraffin section stained with Alcian blue-PAS: × 430.)

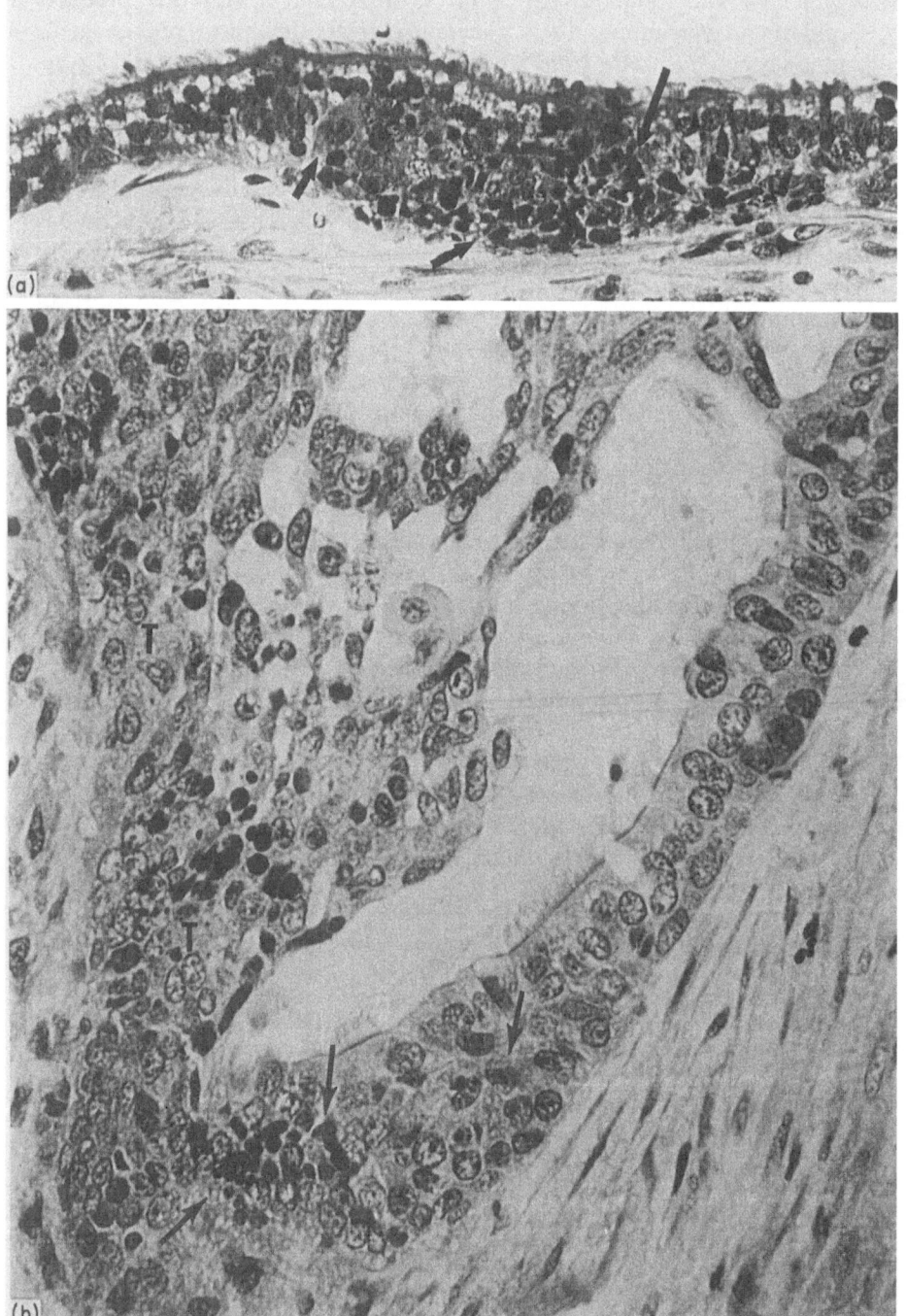

9.6.3 *Small cell carcinomas and carcinoid tumors*

Surprisingly few reports have been published which show the site of origin of small cell carcinomas or carcinoid tumors, although it is generally agreed that both types arise from the bronchial (and bronchiolar) epithelium. The cells of carcinoid tumors and of many small cell carcinomas contain dense-cored granules similar to those seen in normal DCG cells (Bensch *et al.*, 1965, 1968; Toker, 1966; Gmelich *et al.*, 1967; Hattori *et al.*, 1968, 1972; Hage, 1973; Bonikos *et al.*, 1968; McDowell *et al.*, 1976; Capella *et al.*, 1979). This has led to a long-held assumption that these types of tumors derive from DCG cells. However, several investigators are now questioning whether or not all (or any) of these tumors arise from pre-existing DCG cells (Yesner, 1980, 1981; Carter and Eggleston, 1980; Gazdar *et al.*, 1981; Sorokin *et al.*, 1981).

(a) Small cell carcinomas

These tumors may arise at all levels of the bronchial tree (Shimosato, 1980) but most arise centrally (Carter and Eggleston, 1980). An epithelial origin has been demonstrated and focal areas of hyperplastic cells, which resemble cells of the invasive tumor, are seen within the basal layers of the mucociliary epithelium (Fig. 9.15a) (Walter and Pryce, 1955a; Watson and Berg, 1962; Lisa *et al.*, 1965; Rosenblatt *et al.*, 1967; McDowell and Trump, 1981). Saccomanno *et al.* (1970) noted hyperplastic whorling of basally located small cells, below otherwise normal mucociliary epithelium, in *nonsmoking* uranium miners. This lesion appeared to be characteristic of radiation-induced injury and predominated in the bronchi of patients who developed small cell carcinoma. Small cell carcinoma has a particularly high incidence in uranium miners (Saccomanno *et al.*, 1971).

Hyperplastic foci at the base of the otherwise normal mucociliary epithelium contrast sharply with the histology of the type of carcinoma *in situ* which precedes epidermoid carcinoma in that the latter is characterized by metaplastic atypical cells throughout the epithelium and normal appearing columnar mucous and ciliated cells are absent (Section 9.6.1).

Fig. 9.15 From a patient with a small cell carcinoma (intermediate type). (Reprinted with permission from McDowell and Trump, 1981.) (a) A nest of basally situated cells, resembling tumor cells, lies below the normal appearing columnar mucociliary epithelium of a small peripheral bronchus (arrows). (Paraffin section stained with hematoxylin and eosin: × 380.) (b) The tumor streams from a small terminal bronchus. At right the epithelium appears normal. At the base of the micrograph the epithelium appears hypercellular in the basal area (arrows). This area is composed of cells identical to those of the tumor. At left this area is continuous with the tumor (T). (Paraffin section stained with hematoxylin and eosin: × 500.)

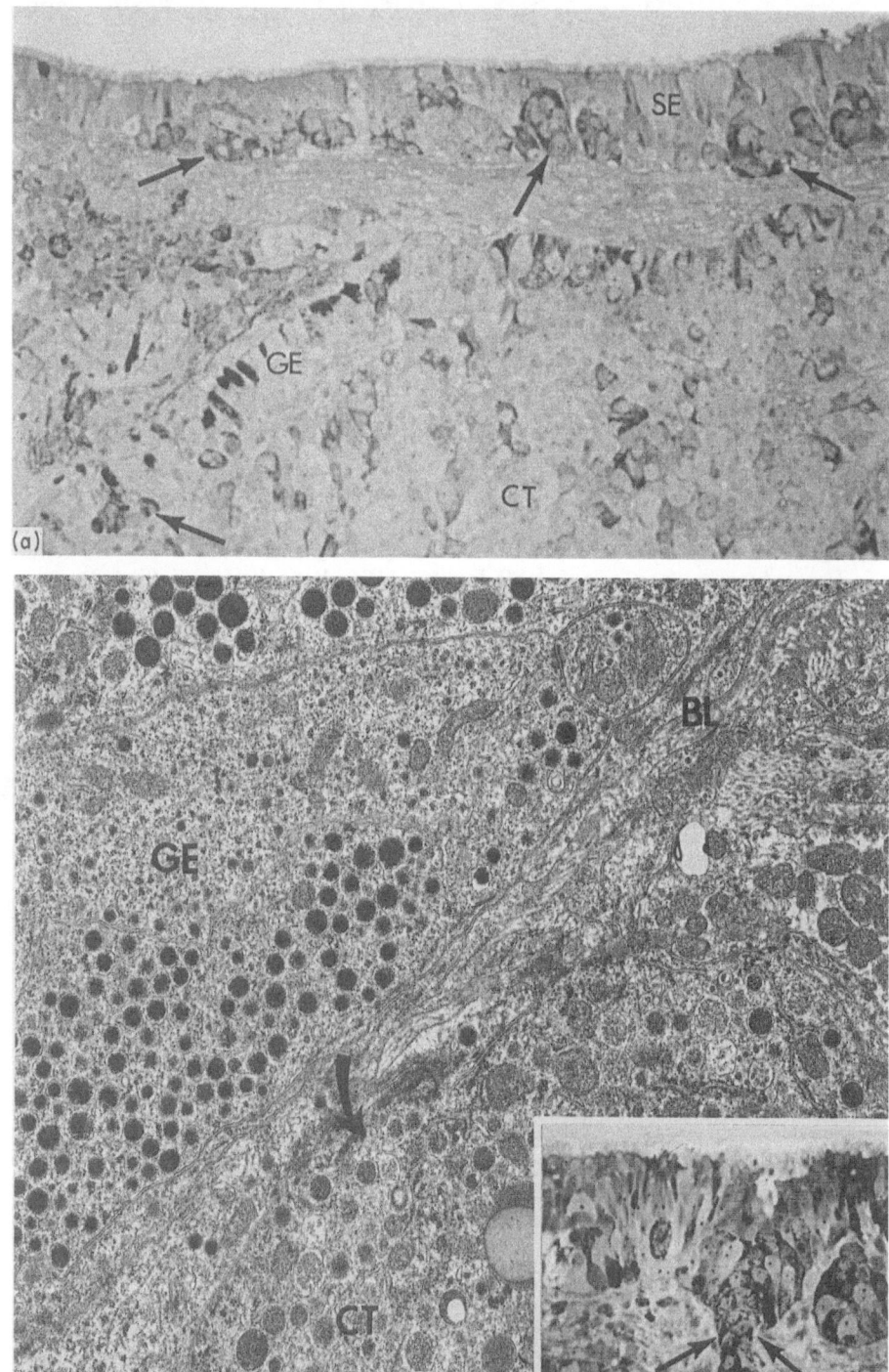

Small cell carcinomas are typically composed of small cells (hence their name) and, unlike epidermoid and adenocarcinomas, the tumor cells are similar in size or even smaller than those of the normal bronchial epithelium (Fig. 9.15a, b).

(b)   Carcinoid tumors

Carcinoid tumors may arise at all levels of the bronchial tree. Central carcinoids, arising from large bronchi, are most common (Carter and Eggleston, 1980). Carcinoid tumors, like small cell carcinomas, also appear to arise from neoplastic proliferations of cells at the epithelial base, which are overlaid by apparently normal mucociliary columnar cells (Kay *et al.*, 1958; Gmelich *et al.*, 1967; Salyer *et al.*, 1975). The abnormal cells and their nuclei are comparable in size to those of normal epithelial cells.

A rather unusual central carcinoid tumor was recently described which showed multiple continuities with clusters of abnormal endocrine cells, situated at the basal aspect of otherwise normal appearing bronchial surface and submucosal glandular epithelium (McDowell *et al.*, 1981; Sorokin *et al.*, 1981). Cells of the carcinoid tumor displayed a wide spectrum of DCG morphologies and histochemical staining characteristics, which were not shared by DCG cells of the normal epithelium. A similar abnormal spectrum was displayed by cells of the intraepithelial cell clusters (Fig. 9.16a, b). Some mucous cells and ciliated cells within these clusters also contained putative DCG. In addition to continuities with the underlying tumor mass (Fig. 9.16b and inset), some of the epithelial clusters were interconnected within the epithelium but a number of small clusters were clearly isolated from one another, as shown by serial sectioning (Sorokin *et al.*, 1981). The clusters represented hyperplastic foci, metaplastic foci and/or areas of carcinoma *in situ*, composed of abnormal DCG cells, some of which had mixed DCG-mucous and DCG-ciliated phenotypes.

In this case of carcinoid tumor, the population density of the intraepi-

---

Fig. 9.16   From a patient with a central carcinoid tumor. (a) Bronchial surface epithelium (SE), submucosal glandular epithelium (GE) and carcinoid tumor (CT). Note numerous basal clusters of DCG cells (arrows) which are overlaid by columnar mucociliary epithelium. (Reprinted with permission from McDowell *et al.*, 1982.) (Glycol methacrylate section stained with PAS-lead hematoxylin: × 180.) (b) A cluster of DCG cells in the submucosal glandular epithelium (GE) is continuous (arrow) with the underlying carcinoid tumor (CT). Basal lamina (BL). (Electron micrograph: × 10000.) *Inset*: Continuity (arrows) is seen between an abnormal cell cluster and the underlying tumor. (Reprinted with permission from McDowell *et al.*, 1981.) (Glycol methacrylate section stained with PAS-lead hematoxylin: × 350.)

thelial clusters far exceeded the normal distribution of DCG cells and thereby provided testimony favorable to the idea that these clusters and tumors such as this one can arise from phenotypic changes in pre-existing epithelial cells which do not contain DCG.

References

Asmundsson, T., Kilburn, K.H. and McKenzie, W.N. (1973), Injury and metaplasia of airway cells due to SO_2. *Lab. Invest.*, **29**, 41–53.

Auer, G., Ono, J., Nasiell, M., Caspersson, T., Kato, H., Konaka, C. and Hayata, Y. (1982), Reversibility of bronchial cell atypia. *Cancer Res.*, **42**, 4241–7.

Auerbach, O., Gere, B., Forman, J.B., *et al.* (1957), Changes in the bronchial epithelium in relation to smoking and cancer of the lung. Report of progress. *New Engl. J. Med.*, **256**, 97–104.

Auerbach, O., Stout, A.P., Hammond, E.C. and Garfinkel, L. (1961), Changes in bronchial epithelium in relation to cigarette smoking and in relation to lung cancer. *New Engl. J. Med.*, **256**, 253–67.

Auerbach, O., Stout, A.P., Hammond, E.C. and Garfinkel, L. (1967), Multiple primary bronchial carcinomas. *Cancer*, **20**, 699–705.

Becci, P.J., McDowell, E.M. and Trump, B.F. (1978), The respiratory epithelium. IV. Histogenesis of epidermoid metaplasia and carcinoma *in situ* in the hamster. *J. Natl Cancer Inst.*, **61**, 577–86.

Bejui-Thivolet, F., Viac, J., Thivolet, J. and Faure, M. (1982), Intracellular keratins in normal and pathological bronchial mucosa. *Virchows Arch. (Pathol. Anat.)*, **395**, 87–98.

Bennett, D.E., Sasser, W.F. and Ferguson, T.B. (1969), Adenocarcinoma of the lung in men. A clinicopathologic study of 100 cases. *Cancer*, **23**, 431–9.

Bensch, K.G., Corrin, B., Pariente, R. and Spencer, H. (1968), Oat cell carcinomas of the lung. Its origin and relationship to bronchial carcinoid. *Cancer*, **22**, 1163–72.

Bensch, K.G., Gordon, G.B. and Miller, L.R. (1965), Electron microscopic and biochemical studies on the bronchial carcinoid tumor. *Cancer*, **18**, 592–602.

Black, H. and Ackerman, L.V. (1952), The importance of epidermoid carcinoma *in situ* in the histogenesis of carcinoma of the lung. *Ann. Surg.*, **136**, 44–55.

Blobel, G.A., Moll, R., Franke, W.W. and Vogt-Moykopf, I. (1984), Cytokeratins in normal lung and lung carcinomas. *Virchows Arch. (Cell Pathol.)*, **45**, 407–29.

Bonikos, D.S., Bensch, K.G. and Jamplis, R.W. (1976), Peripheral pulmonary carcinoid tumors. *Cancer*, **37**, 1977–98.

Boon, M.E., Lindeman, J., Meeuwissen, A.L.J. and Otto, A.J. (1982), Carcinoembryonic antigen in sputum cytology. *Acta Cytol.*, **26**, 389–94.

Capella, C., Gabrielli, M., Polak, J.M., Buffa, R., Solcia, E. and Bordi, C. (1979), Ultrastructural and histological study of 11 bronchial carcinoids. Evidence for different types. *Virchows Arch. (Pathol. Anat.)*, **381**, 313–29.

Carlisle, J.C., McDonald, J.R. and Harrington, S.W. (1952), Bronchogenic squamous-cell carcinoma. *J. Thorac. Surg.*, **22**, 74–82.

Carter, D. and Eggleston, J.C. (1980), Tumors of the lower respiratory tract. *Atlas of Tumor Pathology*, 2nd series, fascicle 17. Armed Forces Institute of Pathology. Washington, DC.

Carter, D., Marsh, B.R., Robinson Baker, R., Erozan, Y.S. and Frost, J.K. (1976), Relationships of morphology to clinical presentation in ten cases of early squamous cell carcinoma of the lung. *Cancer*, **37**, 1389–96.

Cireli, E. (1966), Elektronenmikroskopiche Analyse der prä-und postnatalen Differenzierung des Epithels der oberen Luftwege der Ratte. *Z. Mikros. Anat. Forsch.*, **74**, 132–78.

Condon, W.B. (1942), Regeneration of tracheal and bronchial epithelium. *J. Thoracic Surg.*, **11**, 333–46.

Di Augustine, R.P., Jahnke, G.D. and Talley, F. (1984), Endocrine cells of the guinea-pig upper airways: morphology, distribution and disposition after xenotransplantation in the nude mouse. In *The Endocrine Lung in Health and Disease* (eds K.L. Becker and A.F. Gazdar), W. B. Saunders, Philadelphia, pp. 232–48.

Di Augustine, R.P. and Sonstegard, K.S. (1984), Neuroendocrine-like (small granule) epithelial cells in lung. *Environ. Health Perspec.*, **55**, 271–95.

Elmes, P.C. and Bell, D. (1963), The effects of chlorine gas on the lungs of rats with spontaneous pulmonary disease. *J. Path. Bact.*, **86**, 317–26.

Emura, M. and Mohr, U. (1975), Morphological studies on the development of tracheal epithelium in the Syrian golden hamster. I. Light microscopy. *Z. Versuchstierkd*, **17**, 14–26.

Farber, E. (1982), Chemical carcinogenesis. A biological perspective. *Am. J. Pathol.*, **106**, 271–96.

Florey, H., Carleton, H.M. and Wells, A.Q. (1932), Mucus secretion in the trachea. *Brit. J. Exp. Path.*, **13**, 269–84.

Francis, T. and Stuart-Harris, C.H. (1938), Studies on the nasal histology of epidemic influenza virus infection in the ferret. I. The development and repair of the nasal lesion. *J. Exp. Med.*, **68**, 789–802.

Frasca, J.M., Auerbach, O., Parks, V.R. and Jamieson, J.D. (1968), Electron microscopic observations on the bronchial epithelium of dogs. II. Smoking dogs. *Exp. Mol. Pathol.*, **9**, 380–99.

Frost, J.K., Erozan, Y.S., Gupta, P.K. and Carter, D. (1983), Cytopathology, Section 3. In *Atlas of Early Lung Cancer*, Igaku-Shoin, New York, Tokyo, pp. 39–76.

Frost, J.K., Gupta, P.K., Erozan, Y.S., Carter, D., Hollander, D.H., Levin, M.L. and Ball, W.C. (1973), Pulmonary cytologic alterations in toxic environmental inhalation. *Human Pathol.*, **4**, 521–36.

Garland, L.H., Beier, R.L., Coulson, W., Heald, J.H. and Stein, R.L. (1962), Apparent site of origin of carcinomas of the lung. *Radiology*, **78**, 1–11.

Gazdar, A.F., Carney, D.N., Guccion, J.C. and Baylin, S.B. (1981), Small cell carcinoma of the lung. Cellular origin and relationship to other pulmonary cancers. In *Small Cell Lung Cancer* (eds F.A. Greco, R.K. Oldham and P.A. Bunn), Grune and Stratton, New York, pp. 145–75.

Gmelich, J.T., Bensch, K.G. and Liebow, A.A. (1967), Cells of Kultschitzky type in bronchioles and their relation to the origin of peripheral carcinoid tumor. *Lab. Invest.*, **17**, 88–98.

Gusterson, B., Mitchell, D., Warburton, M. and Sloane, J. (1982), Immunohistochemical localization of keratin in human lung tumours. *Virchows Arch. (Pathol. Anat.)*, **304**, 269–77.

Hage, E. (1973), Histochemistry and fine structure of bronchial carcinoid tumors. *Virchows Arch. (Pathol. Anat.)*, **361**, 121–8.

Harris, C.C., Sporn, M.B., Kaufman, D.G., Smith, J.M., Jackson, F.E. and Saffiotti, U. (1972), Histogenesis of squamous metaplasia in the hamster tracheal epithelium caused by vitamin A deficiency or benzo(a)pyrene ferric oxide. *J. Natl Cancer Inst.*, **48**, 743–61.

Hattori, S., Matsuda, M., Tateishi, R., Nishihara, M. and Horai, T. (1972), Oat-cell carcinoma of the lung. Clinical and morphological studies in relation to its histogenesis. *Cancer*, **30**, 1014–24.

Hattori, S., Matsuda, M., Tateishi, R., Tatsumi, N. and Terazawa, T. (1968), Oat-cell carcinoma of the lung containing serotonin granules. *Gann*, **59**, 123–9.

Hayashi, M., Sornberger, C. and Huber, G.L. (1978), Differential response in the male and female tracheal epithelium following exposure to tobacco smoke. *Chest*, **73**, 515–8.

Hill, T.A., McDowell, E.M. and Trump, B.F. (1979), Localization of carcinoembryonic antigen (CEA) in normal, premalignant and malignant lung tissue. In *Carcinoembryonic Proteins*, Vol. II (ed. F.G. Lehmann), Elsevier/North-Holland, pp. 163–8.

Kalnins, V.I. and Porter, K.R. (1969), Centriole replication during ciliogenesis in the chick tracheal epithelium. *Z. Zellforsch Mikrosk. Anat.*, **100**, 1–30.

Kay, S. (1958), Histologic and histogenetic observations on the peripheral adenoma of the lung. *Arch. Pathol.*, **65**, 395–402.

Keenan, K.P., Combs, J.W. and McDowell, E.M. (1982a), Regeneration of hamster tracheal epithelium after mechanical injury. I. Focal lesions: quantitative morphologic study of cell proliferation. *Virchows Arch. B. (Cell Pathol.)*, **41**, 193–214.

Keenan, K.P., Combs, J.W. and McDowell, E.M. (1982b), Regeneration of hamster tracheal epithelium after mechanical injury. II. Multifocal lesions: stathmokinetic and autoradiographic studies of cell proliferation. *Virchows Arch. B. (Cell Pathol.)*, **41**, 215–29.

Keenan, K.P., Combs, J.W. and McDowell, E.M. (1982c), Regeneration of hamster tracheal epithelium after mechanical injury. III. Large and small lesions: comparative stathmokinetic and single pulse and continuous thymidine labeling autoradiographic studies. *Virchows Arch. B. (Cell Pathol.)*, **41**, 231–52.

Keenan, K.P., Wilson, T.S. and McDowell, E.M. (1983), Regeneration of hamster tracheal epithelium after mechanical injury. IV. Histochemical, immunocytochemical and ultrastructural studies. *Virchows Arch. B. (Cell Pathol.)*, **43**, 213–40.

Klainer, A.S., Turndorf, H., Wu, W.H., Maewal, H. and Allender, P. (1975), Surface alterations due to endotracheal intubation. *Am. J. Med.*, **58**, 674–83.

Klein-Szanto, A.J.P., Topping, D.C., Heckman, C.A. and Nettesheim, P. (1980), Ultrastructural characteristics of carcinogen-induced dysplastic changes in tracheal epithelium. *Am. J. Pathol.*, **98**, 83–100.

Konaka, C., Auer, G., Nasiell, M., Kato, H., Hayashi, N., Ono, J., Hayata, Y. and Caspersson, T.O. (1982), Pathogenesis of squamous bronchial carcinoma in 20-methylcholanthrene-treated beagle dogs. *Analyt. Quant. Cytol.*, **4**, 61–71.

Koss, L.G. (1979), The respiratory tract in the absence of cancer. In *Diagnostic Cytology and its Histopathologic Basis*, Vol. 2, J.B. Lippincott, Philadelphia, pp. 534–606.

Kotin, P. (1968), Carcinogenesis of the lung. Environmental and host factors. In *The Lung*, International Academy of Pathology Monograph, Williams and Wilkins, Baltimore, pp. 203–25.

Lisa, J.R., Salvador, T. and Rosenblatt, M.B. (1965), Site of origin, histogenesis, and cytostructure of bronchogenic carcinoma. *Am. J. Clin. Path.*, **44**, 375–84.

McDowell, E.M., Barrett, L.A. and Trump, B.F. (1976), Observations on small granule cells in adult human bronchial epithelium and in carcinoid and oat-cell tumors. *Lab. Invest.*, **34**, 202–6.

McDowell, E.M., Becci, P.J., Schürch, W. and Trump, B.F. (1979), The respiratory epithelium. VII. Epidermoid metaplasia of hamster tracheal epithelium during regeneration following mechanical injury. *J. Natl Cancer Inst.*, **62**, 995–1008.

McDowell, E.M., Harris, C.C. and Trump, B.F. (1982), Histogenesis and morphogenesis of bronchial neoplasms. In *Morphogenesis of Lung Cancer* (eds Y. Shimosato, M.R. Melamed and P. Nettesheim), CRC Press, Boca Raton, Florida, pp. 1–36.

McDowell, E.M., Sorokin, S.P., Hoyt, R.F. and Trump, B.F. (1981), An unusual bronchial carcinoid tumor. Light and electron microscopy. *Human Pathol.*, 12, 338–48.

McDowell, E.M. and Trump, B.F. (1981), Pulmonary small cell carcinoma showing tripartite differentiation in individual cells. *Human Pathol.*, 12, 286–94.

McDowell, E.M. and Trump, B.F. (1983), Histogenesis of preneoplastic and neoplastic lesions in tracheobronchial epithelium. *Surv. Synth. Path. Res.*, 2, 235–79.

Melamed, M.R., Zaman, M.B., Flehinger, B.J. and Martini, N. (1977), Radiologically occult *in situ* and incipient invasive epidermoid lung cancer. *Am. J. Surg. Path.*, 1, 5–16.

Mithal, A. and Emery, J.L. (1976), Squamous metaplasia of the tracheal epithelium in children. *Thorax*, 31, 167–71.

Nasiell, M. (1963), The general appearance of the bronchial epithelium in bronchial carcinoma: a histopathological study with some cytological viewpoints. *Acta Cytol.*, 7, 97–106.

Nasiell, M. (1966), Metaplasia and atypical metaplasia in the bronchial epithelium. A histopathologic and cytopathologic study. *Acta Cytol.*, 10, 421–7.

Nasiell, M. (1967), Abnormal columnar cell findings in bronchial epithelium. A cytologic and histologic study of lung cancer and non-cancer cases. *Acta Cytol.*, 11, 397–402.

Nasiell, M. (1968a), Comparative histological and sputum cytological studies of the bronchial epithelium in inflammatory and neoplastic lung disease. *Acta Pathol. Microbiol. Scand.*, 72, 501–18.

Nasiell, M. (1968b), Sputum--cytologic changes in smokers and nonsmokers in relation to chronic inflammatory lung diseases. *Acta Path. Microbiol. Scand.*, 74, 205–13.

Nasiell, M., Kato, H., Auer, G., Zetterberg, A., Roger, V. and Karlen, L. (1978), Cytomorphological grading and Feulgen DNA-analysis of metaplastic and neoplastic bronchial cells. *Cancer*, 41, 1511–21.

Nettesheim, P. (1976), Precursor lesions of bronchogenic carcinoma. *Cancer Res.*, 36, 2654–8.

Nettesheim, P. and Griesemer, R.A. (1978), Experimental models for studies of respiratory carcinogenesis. In *Pathogenesis and Therapy of Lung Cancer* (ed. C.C. Harris), Marcel Dekker, New York, pp. 75–188.

Pascal, R.R., Mesa-Tejada, R., Bennett, S.J., Garces, A. and Fenoglio, C.M. (1977), Carcinoembryonic antigen. Immunohistologic identification in invasive and intraepithelial carcinomas of the lung. *Arch. Pathol. Lab. Med.*, 101, 568–71.

Raeburn, C. and Spencer, H. (1957), Lung scar cancers. *Brit. J. Tuberc. Dis. Chest*, 51, 237–45.

Ramaekers, F., Huysmans, A., Moesker, O., Kant, A., Jap, P., Herman, C. and Vooijs, P. (1983), Monoclonal antibody to keratin filaments, specific for glandular epithelia and their tumors. Use in surgical pathology. *Lab. Invest.*, 49, 353–61.

Rasche, R.F. and Kuhns, L.R. (1972), Histopathologic changes in airway mucosa of infants after endotracheal intubation. *Pediatrics*, 50, 632–7.

Reid, L. (1954), Pathology of chronic bronchitis. *Lancet*, i, 275–8.

Rosenblatt, M.B., Lisa, J.R. and Collier, F. (1967), Criteria for the histologic diagnosis of bronchogenic carcinoma. *Dis. Chest*, 51, 587–95.

Saccomanno, G., Archer, V.E., Auerbach, O., Kuschner, M., Saunders, R.P. and

Klein, M.G. (1971), Histologic types of lung cancer among uranium miners. *Cancer*, **27**, 515–23.

Saccomanno, G., Archer, V.E., Auerbach, O., Saunders, R.P. and Brennan, L.M. (1974), Development of carcinoma of the lung as reflected in exfoliated cells. *Cancer*, **33**, 256–70.

Saccomanno, G., Saunders, R.P., Archer, V.E., Auerbach, O. and Brennan, L. (1970), Metaplasia to neoplasia. In *Morphology of Experimental Respiratory Carcinogenesis* (eds P. Nettesheim, M.G. Hanna and J.W. Deatherage), US Atomic Energy Commission, AEC Symposium Series no. 21, pp. 63–80.

Salyer, D.C., Salyer, W.R. and Eggleston, J.C. (1975), Bronchial carcinoid tumors. *Cancer*, **36**, 1522–37.

Sara, C.A. (1967), Histological changes in the trachea and bronchi with tracheostomy. *Med. J. Aust.*, **1**, 1174–7.

Sara, C.A. and Reye, R.D. (1969), Epithelial changes in the trachea of children. *Med. J. Aust.*, **2**, 328–31.

Schreiber, H., Bibbo, M., Wied, G.L., Saccomanno, G. and Nettesheim, P. (1979), Bronchial metaplasia as a benign or premalignant lesion. I. Cytologic and ultrastructural discrimination between acute carcinogen effects and toxin-induced changes. *Acta Cytol.*, **23**, 496–503.

Schreiber, H., Saccomanno, G., Martin, D.H. and Brennan, L. (1974), Sequential cytological changes during development of respiratory tract tumors induced in hamster by benzo(a)pyrene-ferric oxide. *Cancer Res.*, **34**, 689–98.

Shimosato, Y. (1980), Pathology of lung cancer. In *Lung Cancer 1980. Postgraduate Course*. II World Congress on Lung Cancer, Copenhagen, Denmark, 9–13 June (eds H.H. Hansen and M. Rørth), Excerpta Medica, Amsterdam, pp. 27–47.

Sorokin, S.P., Hoyt, R.F. and McDowell, E.M. (1981), An unusual bronchial carcinoid tumor analyzed by conjunctive staining. *Human Pathol.*, **12**, 302–13.

Stenbäck, F. (1973), Morphologic characteristics of experimentally induced lung tumors and their precursors in hamsters. *Acta Cytol.*, **17**, 476–86.

Stockinger, L. and Cireli, E. (1965), Eine Bisher ubekannte Art der Zentriolenvermehrung. *Z. Zellforsch Mikrosk. Anat.*, **68**, 733–40.

Suemasu, K., Shimosato, Y. and Ishikawa, S. (1974), Multiple minute cancers of major bronchi. A case report. *J. Thorac. Cardiovasc. Surg.*, **68**, 664–72.

Thiéry, J.P. (1967), Mise en évidence des polysaccharides dur coupes fines en microscopie électronique. *J. Microsc.*, **6**, 987–1018.

Toker, C. (1966), Observations on the ultrastructure of a bronchial adenoma (carcinoid type). *Cancer*, **19**, 1943–8.

Trump, B.F., McDowell, E.M., Glavin, F., Barrett, L.A., Becci, P.J., Schürch, W., Kaiser, H.E. and Harris, C.C. (1978), The respiratory epithelium. III. Histogenesis of epidermoid metaplasia and carcinoma *in situ* in the human. *J. Natl Cancer Inst.*, **61**, 563–75.

Valentine, E.H. (1975), Squamous metaplasia of the bronchus. A study of metaplastic changes occurring in the epithelium of the major bronchi in cancerous and non-cancerous cases. *Cancer*, **10**, 272–9.

Walter, J.B. and Pryce, D.M. (1955a), The histology of lung cancer. *Thorax*, **10**, 107–16.

Walter, J.B. and Pryce, D.M. (1955b), The site of origin of lung cancer and its relation to histological type. *Thorax*, **10**, 117–26.

Wang, N.S., Huang, S.N. and Thurlbeck, W.M. (1972), Squamous metaplasia of the opening of bronchial glands. *Am. J. Pathol.*, **67**, 571–86.

Watson, W.L. and Berg, J.W. (1962), Oat cell lung cancer. *Cancer*, **15**, 759–68.

Wells, A.B. (1970), The kinetics of cell proliferation in the tracheobronchial epithelia of rats with and without chronic respiratory disease. *Cell Tissue Kinet.*, **3**, 185–206.

Wilhelm, D.L. (1953), Regeneration of tracheal epithelium. *J. Pathol. Bact.*, **65**, 543–50.

Wilson, D.W., Plopper, C.G. and Dungworth, D.L. (1984), The response of the macaque tracheobronchial epithelium to acute ozone injury. A quantitative ultrastructural and autoradiographic study. *Amer. J. Pathol.*, **116**, 193–206.

Wong, Y.-C. and Buck, R.C. (1971), An electron microscopic study of metaplasia of the rat tracheal epithelium in vitamin A deficiency. *Lab. Invest.*, **24**, 55–66.

Woolner, L.B. (1983), Pathology of cancers detected cytologically, Section 5. In *Atlas of Early Lung Cancer*, Igaku-Shoin, New York, Tokyo, pp. 107–213.

Yesner, R. (1980), Are small-cell carcinomas of the lung derived from neural crest? *New Engl. J. Med.*, **303**, 51.

Yesner, R. (1981), The dynamic histopathologic spectrum of lung cancer. *Yale J. Biol. Med.*, **54**, 447–56.

10 Epithelial neoplasms

10.1 Tumor phenotypes—a histological spectrum

Characterization of the histological patterns and phenotypic expression of lung tumors is important because different phenotypes are linked to different risk factors (Fraumeni, 1975; Frank, 1978) and prognosis (Mountain, 1976; Mittman and Bruderman, 1977), and treatment varies according to tumor type (Straus, 1983). Furthermore, certain tumor histologies are more prevalant in some parts of the world than others, and even within continents tumor histologies may change during different eras (Vincent *et al.*, 1977; Valaitis *et al.*, 1981). However, it is well known that the morphology of lung tumors often differs widely in different areas of the same tumor and that the cells may bear little or no resemblance to the epithelium from which they arose. In fact, the majority of lung tumors showed two or more structural patterns when multiple histologic sections were examined (Reid and Carr, 1961; Reid, 1963; Roggli *et al.*, 1985). This is because lung tumors express multiple and complex phenotypes, which give rise to a wide and varied histological spectrum (McDowell *et al.*, 1978; Yesner, 1981). Willis (1961) stressed that the structural variants of bronchogenic carcinoma were manifestations of its pleomorphism; he fostered the idea that many or all epidermoid carcinomas could be considered as adenocarcinomas with extensive epidermoid metaplasia, and he argued that oat cell carcinomas with glandular differentiation were variants of adenocarcinomas.

The principal phenotypes presently recognized depend largely upon the synthetic product(s) of the tumor cells. For example, cells that accumulate large amounts of intermediate-sized keratin proteins (57 and 59 kd) in their cytosol and involucrin (a precursor of cross linked envelope protein) in their limiting membranes acquire an 'epidermoid' or 'squamous' phenotype (Said *et al.*, 1983a; Banks-Schlegel *et al.*, 1984), whereas cells that synthesize and package secretions for export, including mucosubstances and/or polypeptide hormones, demonstrate a glandular or 'adeno' phenotype. These pure phenotypes are shown in Table 10.1. However, expression of the 'pure' phenotype seldom if ever occurs and most tumors show various mixtures of the basic types. The phenotypic mosaics are

308

reflected in the numerous schemata of tumor classification (Sobin, 1972), including those based on histology such as the 1981 World Health Organization (WHO) classification (Table 10.2) and one which relies more specifically on phenotypic expression (Table 10.3).

Table 10.1 Pure phenotypes of bronchogenic carcinomas

	Involucrin	Keratin 57 and 59 kd proteins	Mucous granules	Dense-cored granules
Epidermoid (squamous) phenotype	present	abundant	absent	absent
Glandular phenotype				
Mucus-secretory type	absent	minimal	present	absent
Dense-core granulated type	absent	no information	absent	present

Table 10.2 WHO histological typing of malignant epithelial tumors

1. Squamous cell carcinoma (epidermoid carcinoma)
   Variant:
   a. Spindle cell (squamous) carcinoma
2. Small cell carcinoma
   a. Oat cell carcinoma
   b. Intermediate cell type
   c. Combined oat cell carcinoma
3. Adenocarcinoma
   a. Acinar adenocarcinoma
   b. Papillary adenocarcinoma[a]
   c. Bronchiolo-alveolar carcinoma[a]
   d. Solid carcinoma with mucus formation
4. Large cell carcinoma
   Variants:
   a. Giant cell carcinoma
   b. Clear cell carcinoma
5. Adenosquamous carcinoma
6. Carcinoid tumor
7. Bronchial gland carcinomas
   a. Adenoid cystic carcinoma
   b. Mucoepidermoid carcinoma
   c. Others
8. Others

Source: World Health Organization (1981).

[a] Papillary adenocarcinomas and bronchiolo-alveolar carcinomas are peripherally situated tumors and are the most frequent types of lung cancer found in relation to pulmonary scars. Because these tumors arise in terminal airways, distal to the bronchi, they are not discussed in detail in this text.

Table 10.3 Comparison of phenotypic and WHO (1981) tumor typing

Phenotypic	WHO
Tumors without dense-cored granules	
Epidermoid carcinoma (EC)	
Well, moderately differentiated	1. Squamous cell carcinoma
	5. Adenosquamous carcinoma[a]
Poorly differentiated	
Small cells	2. Small cell carcinoma
Large cells	4. Large cell carcinoma
Combined epidermoid and adenocarcinoma (CEAC)	
A. Epidermoid component, well differentiated; adeno component, well differentiated	7b. Mucoepidermoid carcinoma
B. Epidermoid component, well differentiated; adeno component, poorly differentiated	1. Squamous cell carcinoma
	5. Adenosquamous carcinoma[a]
C. Epidermoid component, poorly differentiated; adeno component, well differentiated	
I. Tubular glands present with or without mucus	3a. Acinar adenocarcinoma
II. Tubular glands minimal with mucus	3d. Solid carcinoma with mucus
D. Epidermoid component, poorly differentiated; adeno component, poorly differentiated	
Small cells	2. Small cell carcinoma
Large cells	4. Large cell carcinoma
Adenocarcinoma (AC)	
Well, moderately differentiated	
I. Tubular glands present with or without mucus	3a. Acinar adenocarcinoma
II. Tubular glands minimal with mucus	3d. Solid carcinoma with mucus
Poorly differentiated	
Tubular glands and mucus minimal	
Small cells	2. Small cell carcinoma
Large cells	4. Large cell carcinoma
Tumors with dense-cored granules	
Carcinoid tumor[b]	6. Carcinoid tumor
Small cell carcinoma[c]	2. Small cell carcinoma
Atypical endocrine carcinoma[c]	1. Squamous cell carcinoma
	3d. Solid carcinoma with mucus
	4. Large cell carcinoma

[a] Ducts lined by non-neoplastic Type II alveolar cells may be trapped in epidermoid cell nests giving the erroneous impression of adenosquamous carcinoma.

[b] Some carcinoid tumors are mucus secreting.

[c] Small cell carcinomas and atypical endocrine tumors may exhibit an epidermoid phenotype. Some tumors also secrete mucus. Small cell tumors with epidermization and/or mucus secretion are called combined oat cell carcinomas in the WHO classification.

10.1.1   Epidermoid specialization (Fig. 10.1)

The term squamous is used synonymously for well-differentiated epidermoid specialization, by which pathologists mean skin-like and forming abundant keratin. However, a truly squamous epithelium, such as lines blood vessels and the thin limbs of Henle, is composed of cells which are flat like a scale (Latin *squama*), whereas cells of so-called squamous cell carcinomas are, for the most part, polyhedral. Thus when tumors are typed by phenotype (Section 10.2.2), the term epidermoid seems to be more appropriate than squamous.

(a)   Light microscopy

In sections stained with H&E the cytoplasm appears glassy (hyalinized) and, in highly keratinized tumors, cornified cells at the center of the epithelial cell nests die and form keratin pearls (Fig. 10.1a). Intercellular bridges may sometimes be seen at light microscopic level. As mentioned above, epidermoid specialization is associated with the production of an abundance of intermediate-sized keratin proteins and involucrin. Moreover, the epidermoid phenotype is associated with an especially complex pattern of cytokeratins (Blobel *et al.*, 1984). A well-differentiated epidermoid carcinoma stained for keratin is shown in Fig. 10.1b.

(b)   Electron microscopy

Characteristic ultrastructural features include the presence of bundles of tonofilaments (keratin filaments). According to the degree of specialization, these bundles are well or moderately developed. Well developed desmosomes join adjacent cells, and tonofilament bundles are seen to insert into the desmosomal attachment points. Mitochondria tend to be small and sparse and the endoplasmic reticulum is poorly developed (Fig. 10.1c).

10.1.2   Glandular (adeno) specialization (Fig. 10.2)

The term gland (Latin *glans*) is used for cells or tissues that secrete substances to be used by or eliminated from the body. If the substances are secreted into a small duct (exocrine secretion), lumens are present within the glandular organ, but if the substances are secreted into the blood (as in endocrine glands), lumens are absent. The term adeno is derived from the Greek *adenos*, meaning a gland. Therefore, this prefix implies secretion. At the *cellular level*, glandular specialization involves synthesis and secretion of products from the cell. In the normal bronchial

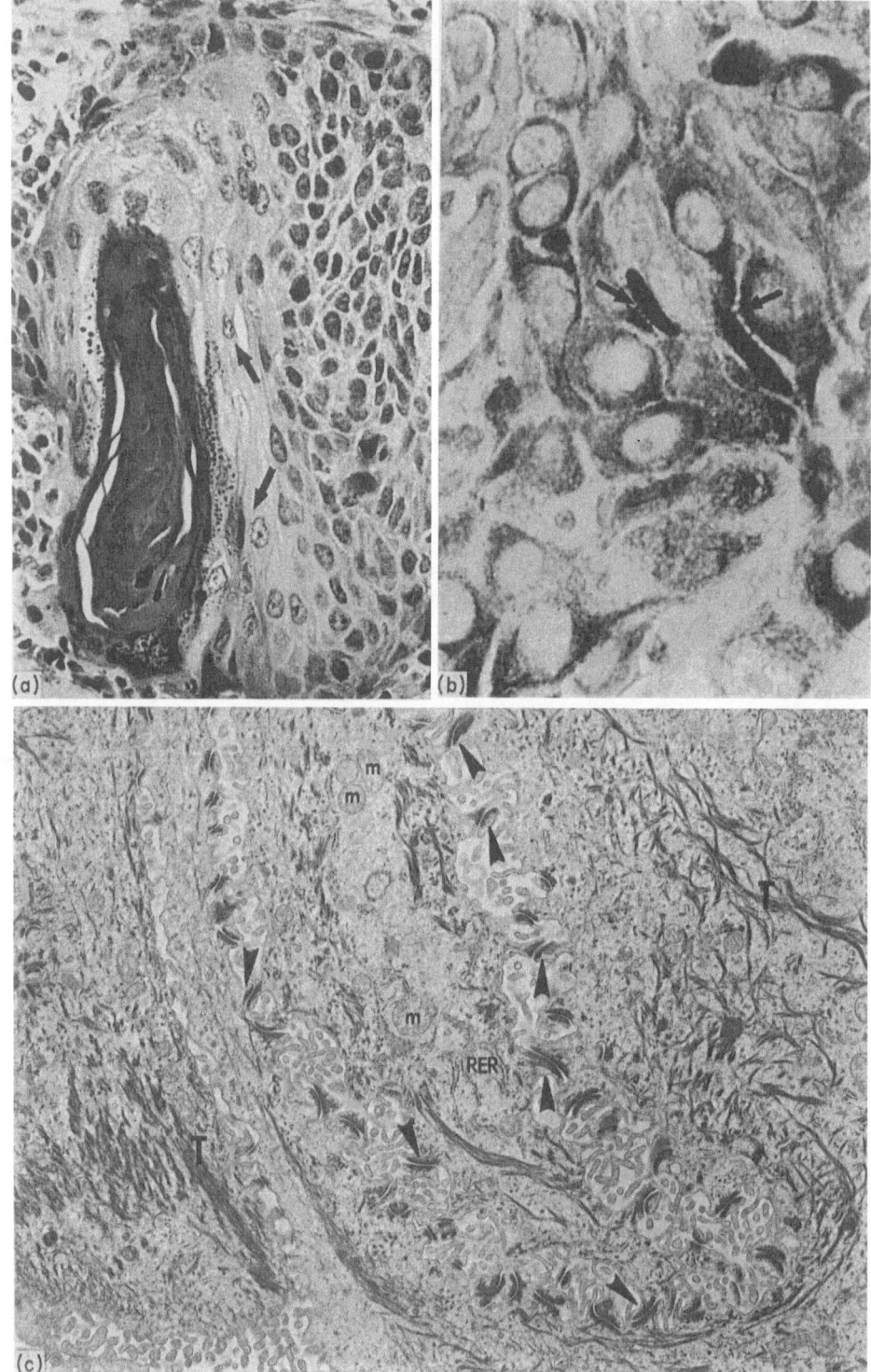

epithelium, mucous cells and dense-core granulated (DCG) cells can be considered as unicellular glands.

(a) Light microscopy

When tubules and acini are well developed the glandular phenotype is easily recognized in H&E-stained sections (Fig. 10.2a). However, tubules and acini are not essential for secretory specialization and the tumors may consist of solid nests of cells. Secretory specialization will pass unnoticed in solid tumors where tubular structures are minimal or absent, unless the secretion product(s) are specifically stained. Stains for neutral and acidic mucosubstances such as Alcian blue-PAS (AB-PAS) and stains for DCG are very useful in this regard. In both tubular and solid mucus-secreting tumors, glandular specialization at the *cellular level* may take the form of intracellular hollows filled with mucosubstances (Fig. 10.2a, b). Glandular specialization is associated with a characteristic pattern of keratin proteins. In particular, the 57 and 59 kd keratins are poorly developed (Banks-Schlegel *et al.*, 1984) and the keratin pattern is relatively simple (Blobel *et al.*, 1984).

(b) Electron microscopy

Ultrastructural features are those characteristically associated with secretion (Fig. 10.2c). These include well developed endoplasmic reticulum, well developed Golgi apparatus and fairly numerous mitochondria. Discrete secretion granules may be seen, such as mucous granules or DCG. The cells are joined laterally by small desmosomes. If the cells form tubules which surround central hollows (acinus formation), the cells are also joined apically by junctional complexes.

Fig. 10.1 Well-differentiated epidermoid specialization. (a) Epidermoid features include elongated hyalinized cells (arrows) and overt cornification at the center of a nest of tumor cells. (Paraffin section, H&E stain: × 340.) (b) Some cells of this epidermoid carcinoma are strongly stained for keratin. Note intercellular bridges (arrows), which also stain strongly. (Paraffin section stained for keratin by PAP: × 600.) (c) Electron micrograph of keratinizing cells similar to those at arrows in (a). The elongated cells contain well-developed tonofilament bundles (T) dispersed throughout the cytoplasm; rough endoplasmic reticulum (RER) is poorly developed and mitochondria (m) are small and sparse. The cells are joined by well-developed desmosomes (arrowheads) which span across the widened intercellular spaces and are equivalent to the intercellular bridges seen by light microscopy. (Electron micrograph: × 4000.)

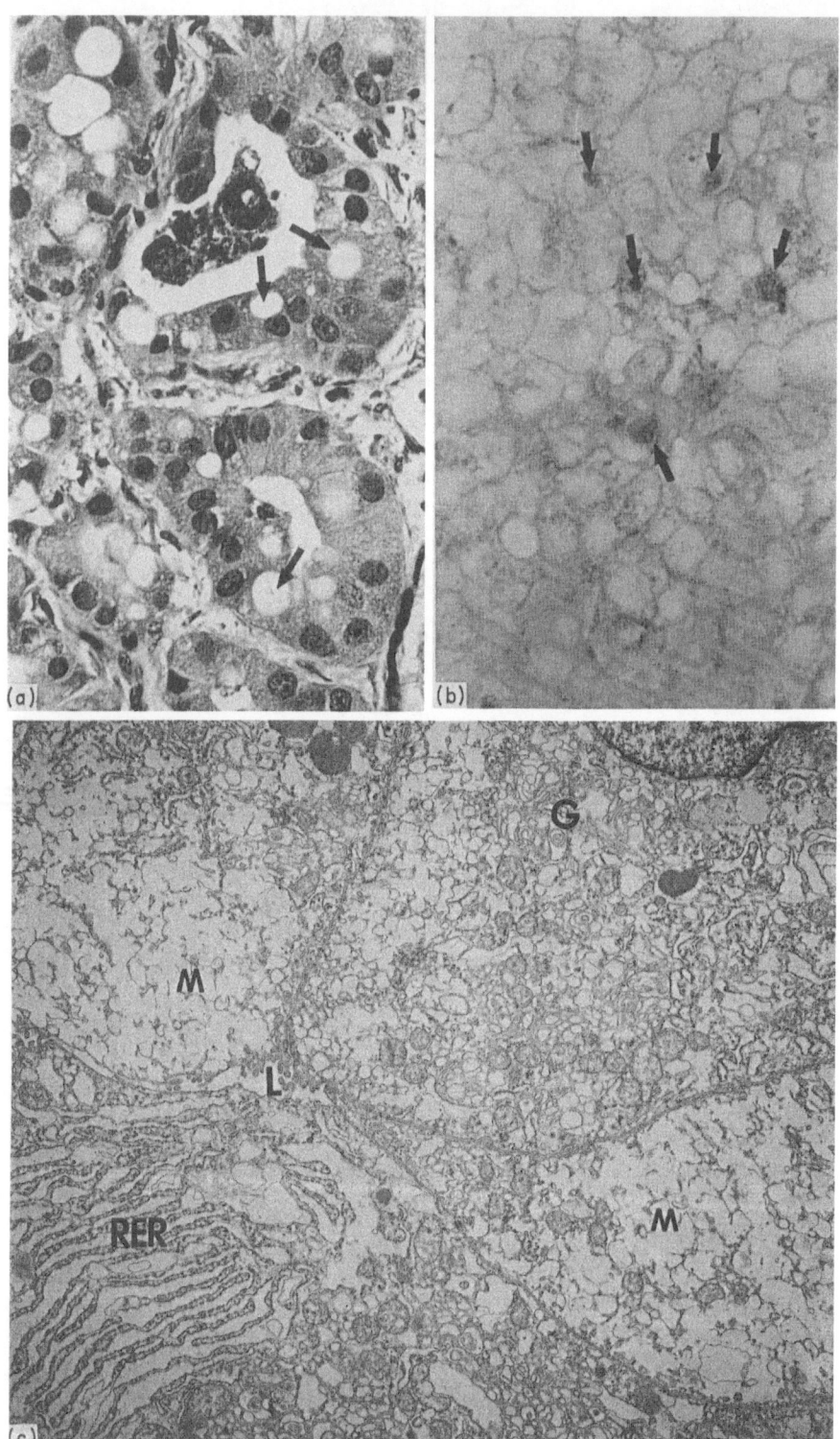

10.2   Classification of bronchogenic carcinomas

10.2.1   World Health Organization classification

Because numerous classifications have been used to type lung cancers, conflicting viewpoints on etiology, diagnosis, treatment and prognosis have arisen. Furthermore, interinstitutional comparisons are jeopardized unless standard criteria with reproducible results are used. To this end, there has been a steady increase in the number of pathologists who have accepted the WHO histologic classification of lung tumors, first published in 1967 and revised in 1981.

The WHO classification is histological and descriptive and is based upon morphologically identifiable cell types and growth patterns, seen by the light microscope. Hematoxylin and eosin staining, together with a mucin stain, are essential for complete typing. According to this classification, the majority of malignant bronchogenic tumors fall into 7 groups, each with one or more subtypes (Table 10.2). Group 1, *squamous cell (epidermoid) carcinomas*, are tumors with overt keratinization and/or intercellular bridges. Depending on the amount of keratinization visible in H&E-stained sections, these tumors are described as well, moderately or poorly differentiated. The presence of minute amounts of intracellular mucin should not exclude tumors from this category. Group 2, *small cell carcinomas*, are subtyped into oat cell carcinoma, intermediate cell type and combined oat cell carcinoma. Oat cell tumors are composed of uniform small lymphocyte-like cells with very scant cytoplasm, whereas the cells of intermediate cell type tumors have more abundant cytoplasm. Combined oat cell carcinomas are tumors where an oat cell component is mixed with squamous (epidermoid) and/or adenocarcinoma components. Group 3, *adenocarcinomas*, are malignant tumors with tubular, acinar or papillary growth patterns and/or mucus production by the tumor cells. Separate subtypes are recognized according to the site of origin. Most adenocarcinomas of bronchogenic origin are composed of tubular glands, so-called acinar adenocarcinomas. Solid tumors with mucus, which are poorly-differentiated adenocarcinomas, are included in this group. Group 4, *large cell carcinomas*, are composed of cells with large nuclei and abundant

---

Fig. 10.2   Well-differentiated glandular mucus-secreting specialization. (a) Characteristic tubular glands of an acinar adenocarcinoma. Intracellular mucus-filled hollows are also present in the tumor cells (arrows). (Paraffin section, H&E stain: × 340.) (b) Secretory specialization would pass unnoticed in this solid tumor if the intracellular mucus-filled hollows (arrows) had not been demonstrated by a mucus stain. (Paraffin section, AB-PAS stain: × 300.) (c) Same tumor as in (a). The RER and Golgi apparatus (G) are well developed. Mucus granules (M) are accumulated in the cell apices. Tubular lumen (L). (Electron micrograph: × 10700.)

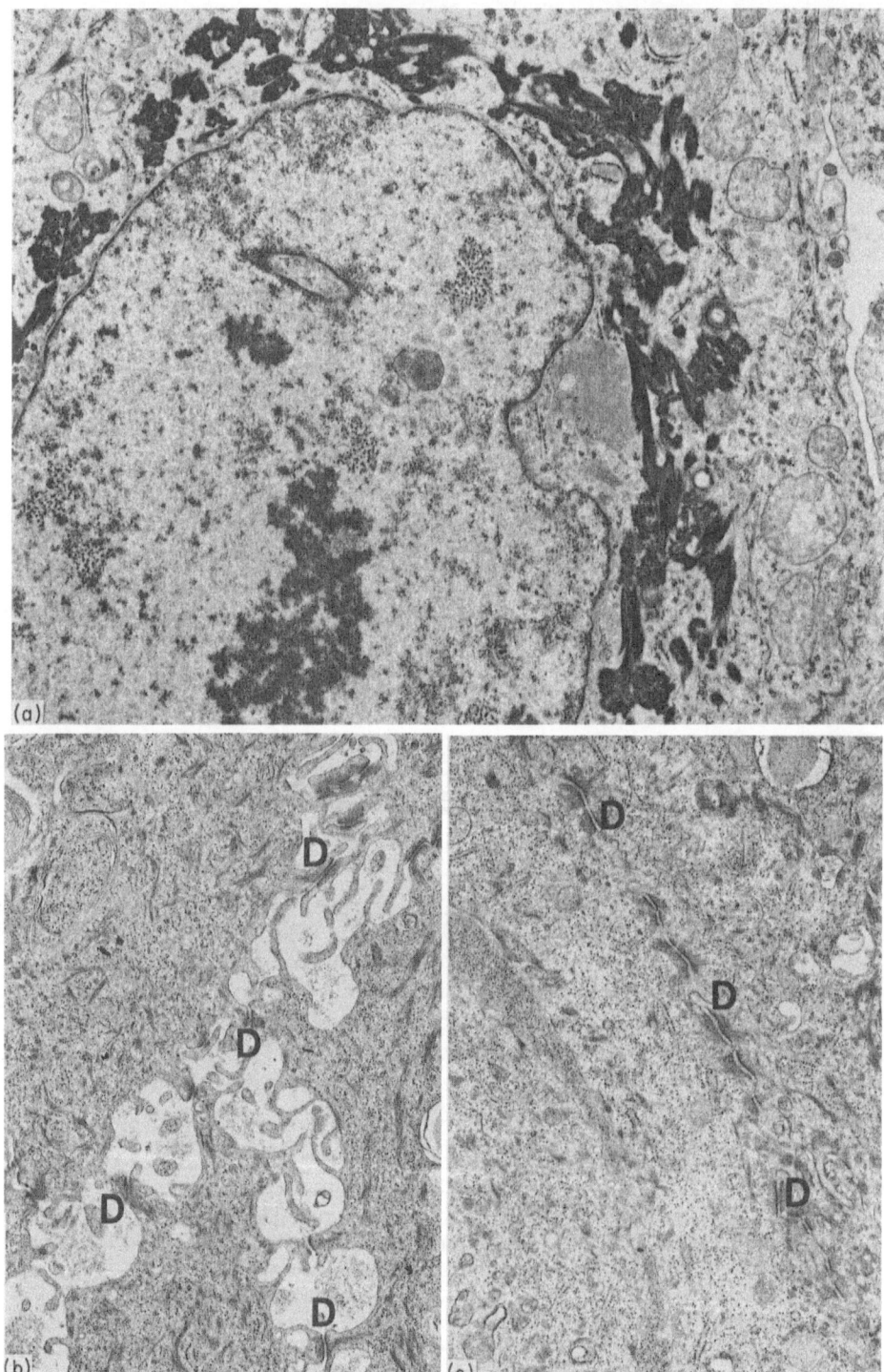

(a)

(b)

(c)

cytoplasm, without features of squamous, small cell or adenocarcinomas. Giant cell and clear cell carcinomas are recognized as variants of large cell carcinomas but tumors with squamous or adenocarcinoma features, which contain either giant cells or clear cells, are not included. Group 5, *adenosquamous carcinomas*, show both squamous (epidermoid) and adenocarcinomatous components. Group 6, *carcinoid tumors*, show a mosaic or trabecular arrangement of polygonal cells. These tumors may also have acinar structures and secrete mucin. Spindle-shaped cells may also occur, especially in peripheral tumors. The term atypical carcinoid is applied to carcinoid tumors demonstrating anaplasia. Group 7 includes adenoid cystic carcinomas and mucoepidermoid carcinomas, tumors which are thought to derive from bronchial glands. *Adenoid cystic carcinomas* are malignant tumors with a cribriform appearance. The tumor cells form small ducts or large masses, interspersed with cystic spaces, giving a lace-like pattern. The spaces are often filled with PAS-positive secretions. *Mucoepidermoid carcinomas* are characterized by the presence of squamous (epidermoid) cells, with recognizable intercellular bridges, mucus-secreting cells and cells with both features. These tumors are said to be less aggressive than the adenosquamous carcinomas of Group 5.

10.2.2 Typing by phenotype

The degree of differentiation designated to a tumor by a pathologist depends largely on the resolution of the diagnostic techniques that are used. World wide, the majority of tumors are classified using light microscopy, often with the use of H&E-stained sections alone. However, the use of more sophisticated methods including light microscopic immunocytochemistry and electron microscopy is rapidly increasing, and reports of new and sometimes unexpected observations are commonplace in the current literature. When paraffin sections are stained by H&E and a mucous stain (all that is required for WHO grouping), only tumors with overt keratinization, sufficient to cause cytoplasmic hyalinization, will be designated squamous cell (epidermoid) carcinoma using WHO criteria (Section 10.1.1). Moreover, tumors bearing DCG, but which do not demonstrate characteristic light microscopic carcinoid or small cell histologies, will inevitably be placed into other tumor categories not

---

Fig. 10.3 Well-differentiated epidermoid specialization. (a) Tonofilament bundles are aggregated into tight clusters which encircle the nucleus. This formation would appear as a perinuclear ring by light microscopy if keratin immunostaining was made. (Electron micrograph: × 6500.) (b) and (c) are from adjacent areas. Well-developed desmosomes (D) are present in both areas but intercellular bridges would be evident by light microscopy only if the intercellular spaces are widened, as in (b). (Electron micrographs: × 10500.)

generally associated with DCG. Few institutions have electron microscopes and those that do usually use them only on a proportion of cases, but the simplicity and relative low cost of light microscopic immunocytochemistry encourage widespread application and promise greater understanding of the complexity of tumor phenotypes in the near future.

Using these approaches, the once seemingly obvious and clear-cut distinction between epidermoid (squamous) carcinoma and adenocarcinoma has been narrowed by finding that some tumors with glands are composed of varying numbers of cells which reveal epidermoid features at immunocytochemical and ultrastructural levels and that many well-differentiated epidermoid carcinomas are mucus secreting and therefore glandular, at least in focal areas. In fact, several recent studies have revealed potential discrepancies between light and electron microscopic diagnoses, largely because the phenotypic expression(s) of tumors are more clearly discerned at higher resolution (McDowell *et al.*, 1978, 1981b; Churg, 1978; Mennemeyer *et al.*, 1979; Churg *et al.*, 1980; Shimosato, 1980; Li *et al.*, 1981; Horie and Ohta, 1981; Auerbach *et al.*, 1982; Bolen and Thorning, 1982; Leong, 1982; Said *et al.*, 1983b; Dingemans and Mooi, 1984; Warren *et al.*, 1984b).

When bronchogenic tumors are examined ultrastructurally some tumors bear DCG and some do not. The clinical significance of this is poorly understood at present (Section 10.3.2) but, for purposes of grouping by phenotype, tumors are presented here in two major groups--those with and those without DCG (Table 10.3). Tumors *with DCG* stain immunocytochemically for neuron specific enolase (NSE), whereas tumors *without DCG* are negative for this cytoplasmic enzyme (Section 10.3.3). Combined epidermoid and mucus-secreting adenocarcinoma phenotypes are commonly expressed in malignant tumors *without DCG*. The tumors range from those in which both epidermoid and adeno phenotypes are quantitatively well represented and neither component appears to be dominant,

---

Fig. 10.4 Combined epidermoid and adenocarcinoma where both phenotypes are well developed. (a) The tumor presents with a moderately-differentiated epidermoid component. There is a range of cell size and some giant nuclei are present. Some of the large cells are hyalinized (arrows). Note unstained circular hollows (arrowheads). (Paraffin section, H&E stain: × 340.) (b) Mucus is distributed diffusely within the cytoplasm of some cells (dark stain, top right), in small punctate intracellular hollows (arrow), and in a large extracellular hollow (arrowhead). The latter is comparable to the unstained hollows in (a) and to the structure in (c). (Paraffin section, AB-PAS stain: × 340.) (c) Cells with combined epidermoid (tonofilaments) and mucus-secreting specializations. Note many tiny mucous granules (M) in a cell apex which abuts an extracellular hollow. Widened intercellular spaces are bridged by well-developed desmosomes (D). (Electron micrograph: × 8300.)

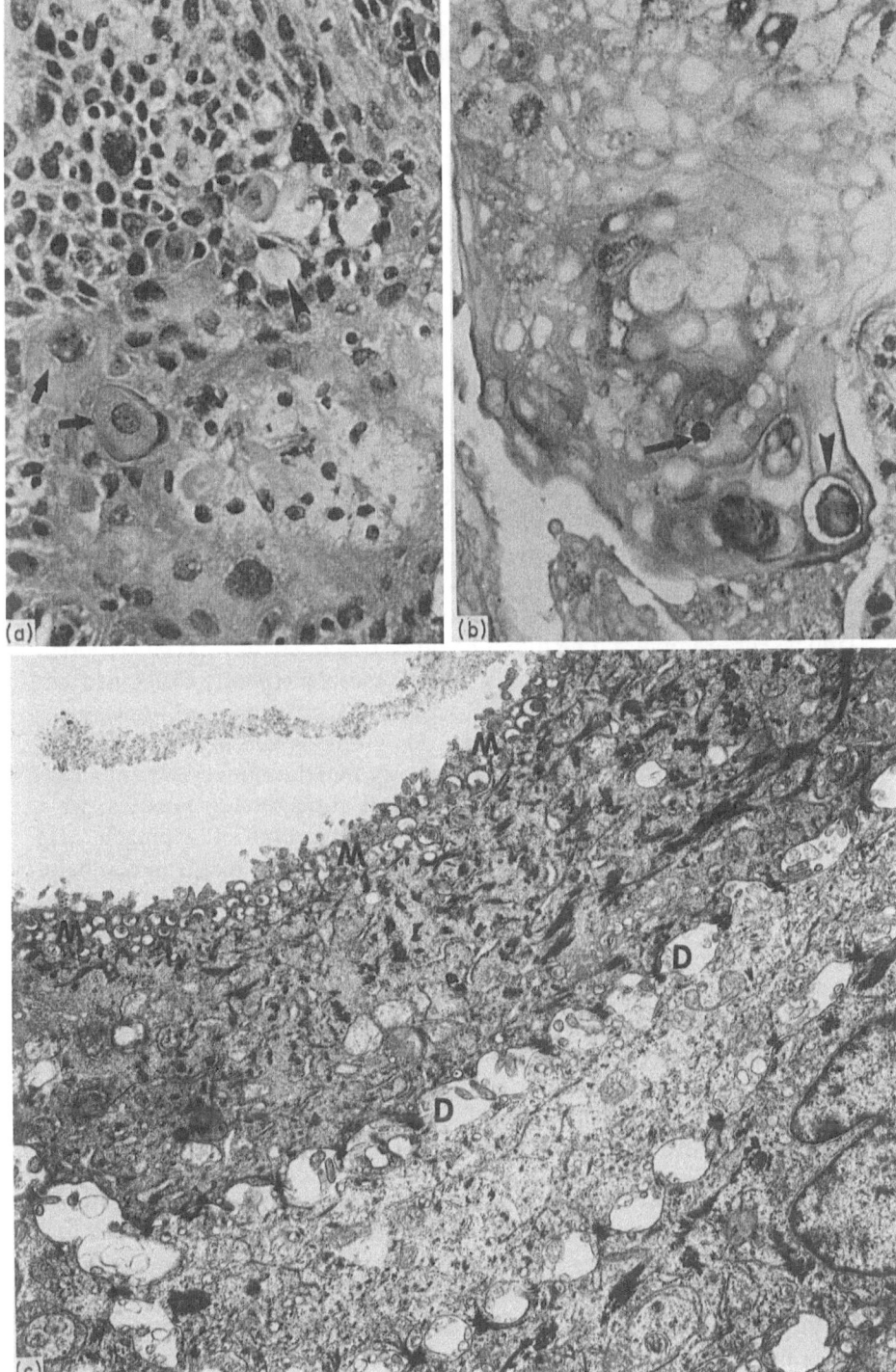

to tumors in which one phenotype is clearly dominant over the other. The phenotypic grouping of combined tumors depends not only on the relative amounts of the various differentiation patterns, but also on the degree of differentiation of each component (McDowell *et al.*, 1978, 1982). Tumors *with DCG* also commonly express complex phenotypes including epidermoid and mucus-secreting specializations (Section 10.3.2); however, a detailed breakdown is not shown in Table 10.3.

10.2.3   *The need for a double standard*

There is little doubt that the increasing use of sophisticated methods will change the pattern of tumor classification in the future. However, for the present and until the 'new' findings are specifically linked to etiological and prognostic yardsticks and to clinical behaviors and therapeutic protocols, caution must be exercised. Light microscopy, electron microscopy and immunocytochemistry are complementary techniques. We agree with Sobin's proposal (1983) for the use of a double standard; that is, results based on all these approaches should be reported in parallel to maintain precision in diagnosis while trying to obtain meaningful biological correlations. For example, a lung tumor could be described, using WHO criteria, as a solid carcinoma with mucus by light microscopy (poorly-differentiated adenocarcinoma) and by phenotypic criteria as containing well-developed tonofilament bundles, DCG and mucous granules (electron microscopy) and being positive for keratin, NSE and serotonin (immunocytochemistry). Such is the case with some of the atypical endocrine carcinomas (McDowell *et al.*, 1981b, Wilson *et al.*, 1985). This type of approach will encourage study of the biological significance of individual features, help to identify subsets of major categories, facilitate stratification of cases in clinical trials and enhance precision in statistical tabulation (Sobin, 1983).

Table 10.3 demonstrates how different tumor phenotypes compare with WHO histological typing and illustrates how light microscopic diagnoses made on routine H&E preparations may modify on immunocytochemical light microscopic or ultrastructural examination.

10.3   Diagnostic features of bronchogenic carcinomas

In this section the light and electron microscopic features of the various tumor types are illustrated. Most lung carcinomas arise from large, medium or small bronchi (Chapter 9). A lesser number, in particular some types of adenocarcinomas, arise from the terminal bronchiolo-alveolar epithelium or in relation to peripheral lung scars. Only bronchogenic tumors are described in this chapter because neoplastic changes in the lung periphery related to bronchioles and alveoli, and adenocarcinomas arising within peripheral lung scars, lie outside the scope of this book.

The concept of differentiation or functional specialization is used extensively in tumor description from any organ site. Full differentiation is used to describe the normal adult organ, whereas in tumors differentiation is impaired qualitatively and quantitatively to varying degrees (WHO, 1981). Tumors are described as well, moderately or poorly differentiated within a tumor type. The terms 'anaplastic' and 'undifferentiated' are often used to describe tumors in which functional specializations appear to be absent. These terms should be avoided because histochemistry, immunocyto-chemistry and electron microscopy demonstrate that some specializations are present, despite their apparent absence in routinely-stained light microscopic specimens. For example, so-called small cell 'anaplastic' carcinomas often bear DCG and synthesize bombesin and other hormonally active peptides which are markers of cell specialization (Section 10.3.2).

10.3.1 Tumors without dense-cored granules

(a) Epidermoid features well developed (Figs 10.1, 10.3, 10.4)

When carcinomas are grouped according to their phenotypes, well- to moderately-differentiated epidermoid carcinomas (EC) and certain combined epidermoid and adenocarcinomas (CEAC) demonstrate well-developed epidermoid features (Table 10.3: EC, CEAC.A, CEAC.B). Using WHO criteria, EC and CEAC.B are classified as squamous cell carcinomas, or sometimes incorrectly as adenosquamous carcinomas (see below), whereas CEAC.A may be classified as adenosquamous carcinomas or mucoepidermoid carcinomas, based on the presence of cells which show both overt keratinization and mucus secretion (Table 10.3). The WHO criteria specify that well-differentiated squamous cell carcinomas must show stratification, intercellular bridges and keratinization with pearl formation, whereas moderately-differentiated tumors must show overt keratinization without pearl formation. Most epidermoid carcinomas can be diagnosed by monitoring sputum cytology and about 60% can be biopsied by bronchoscopic techniques because of their favored central location (Yesner, 1974).

The epidermoid component is clearly recognizable in H&E-stained sections (Figs 10.1a, 10.4a). Polygonal-shaped cells are stratified to form solid nests. The cells appear eosinophilic and hyalinized due to their abundant keratin. Extensively hyalinized cells tend to be elongated and may coalesce at the center of cell nests to form keratin pearls. Nuclear sizes vary. The nuclear outline is sometimes irregular and the chromatin is clumped. Mitotic figures are common and may appear atypical. Occasional tumors have giant multilobulated nuclei, interspersed with small less irregular forms (Fig. 10.4a). Well-developed tonofilament bundles are often dispersed throughout the cytoplasm (Fig. 10.1c) but, in some cells, very highly-developed filaments lie close to and encircle the nucleus in tight aggregates (Fig. 10.3a). These filaments characteristically appear as perinuclear rings with keratin immunostaining. In some areas the cells become widely separated and the widened intercellular spaces are spanned by cytoplasmic processes which are joined by well-developed desmosomes (Figs 10.3b, 10.4c) forming the classical 'intercellular bridges', seen by light microscopy (Fig. 10.1b). However, bridging will not be evident by light microscopy if the cells are closely apposed (Fig. 10.1a), as is often the case, even when desmosomal junctions are well developed (Fig. 10.3c).

In CEAC.B, the epidermoid component clearly dominates and in most areas tumor cells show only epidermoid specialization, as described above. However, in focal areas, adeno specialization is well differentiated, and histochemical stains reveal mucus in intracellular and extracellular hollows. Small mucous granules may be seen throughout the cytoplasm in a few scattered cells. Ultrastructural examination reveals scattered foci composed of cells showing features typical of both epidermoid and adenocarcinoma differentiation (Dingemans and Mooi, 1984).

In CEAC.A, both epidermoid and adeno components are quantitatively well represented. Both phenotypes are readily demonstrated in paraffin sections stained with H&E and AB-PAS (Fig. 10.4a, b). The tumors are composed of nests of keratinizing polygonal cells. Numerous mucus-filled extracellular hollows lie within the epidermoid nests, and intracellular mucus, diffusely scattered in granules throughout the cytoplasm and/or in intracellular hollows, is often present in the keratinizing cells. Intercellular bridging may be prominent and keratin immunostaining and ultrastructural examination show that many individual tumor cells have highly specialized epidermoid *and* glandular components (Fig. 10.4c). Junctional complexes join the cell apices where they abut extracellular hollows.

Tumors with well- or moderately-differentiated epidermoid features characteristically produce a marked desmoplastic host response associated with lymphocytes, plasma cells and rarely eosinophils. The tumor cells may also elicit a foreign body giant cell reaction. It is not uncommon for

Fig. 10.5 Epidermoid (squamous) carcinoma that might be erroneously classified as an adenosquamous carcinoma. (a) Tubular elements are present within the epidermoid tumor nest. Note that the nuclei of the epidermoid cells are much larger than the nuclei of the tubules. (Paraffin section, H&E stain: × 340.) (b) Adjacent section stained with AB-PAS. Diastase-resistant neutral mucosubstances fill the tubular lumens. (Paraffin section: × 340.) (c) The tubular 'adeno' elements are normal-appearing Type II alveolar cells (at left), tumor cells (T). (Electron micrograph: × 6600.)

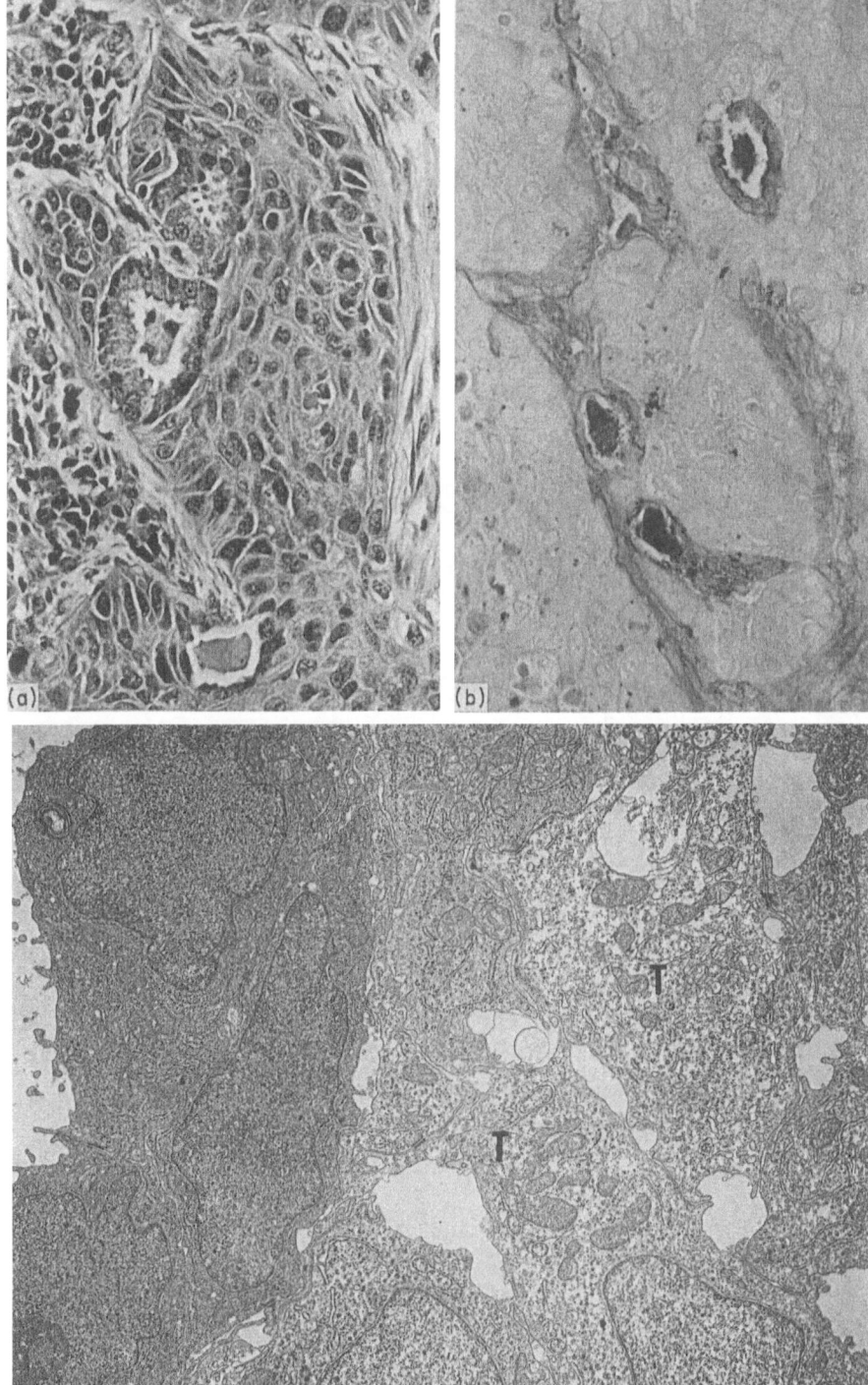

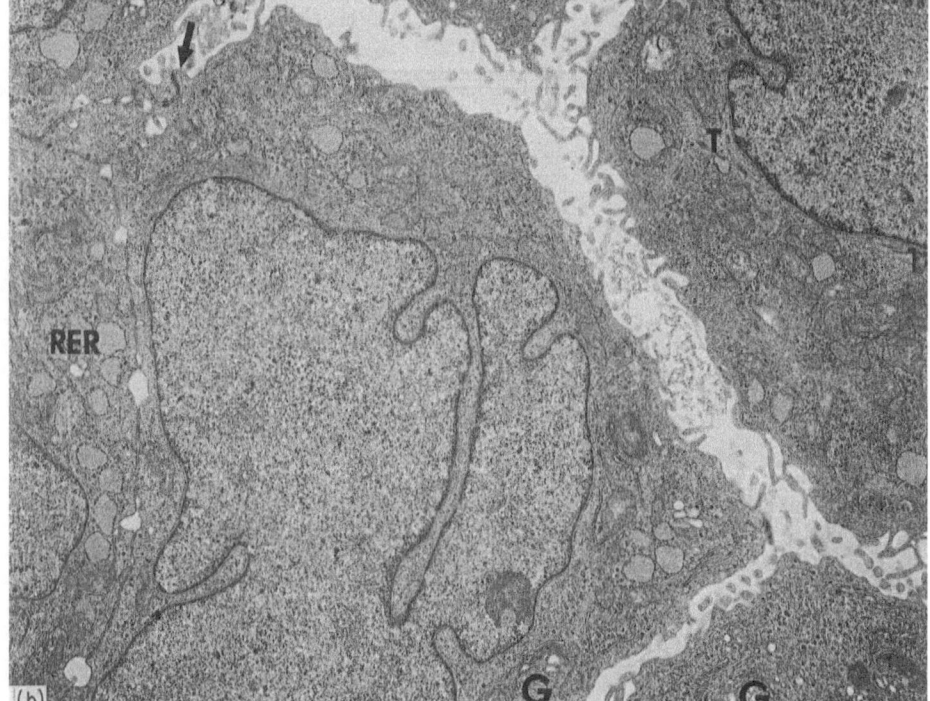

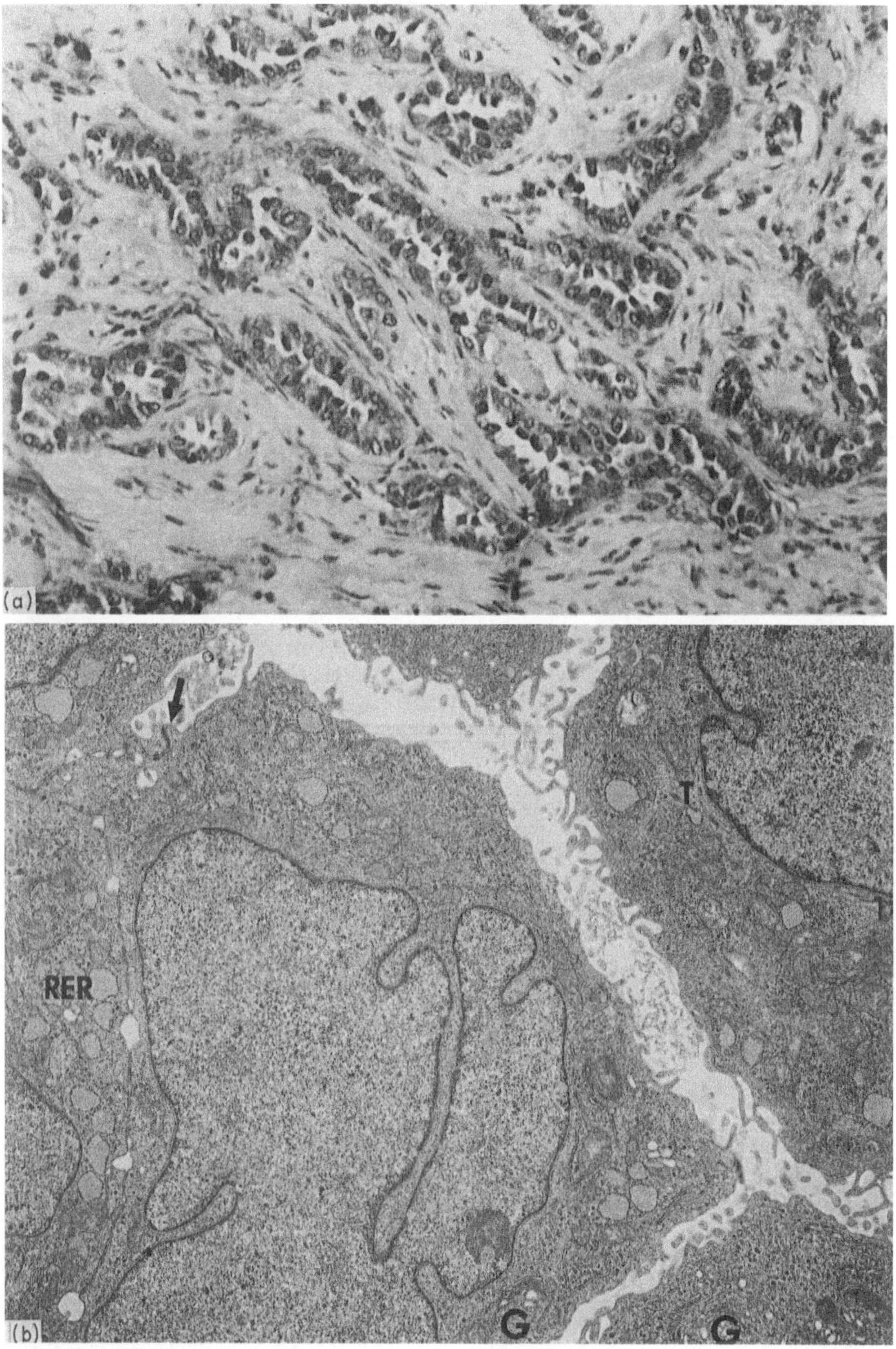

the centers of cell nests to become necrotic and the tumors may undergo massive cavitation. The tumors tend to be locally invasive and lesser numbers show extrathoracic extension (for detailed accounts of clinical behavior, see Matthews, 1976, and Matthews and Gordon, 1977). Differential diagnosis does not generally pose a problem; however, metastatic tumors from the pancreas may simulate bronchogenic epidermoid carcinoma (Rosenblatt *et al.*, 1966).

Spindle cell carcinomas are described in the WHO classification as variants of squamous cell cancers. These tumors have a biphasic appearance due to an epidermoid component and a spindle component, said to be derived from it. Carter and Eggleston (1980) consider these to be carcinomas with spindle metaplasia. They are easily confused with carcino-sarcomas (Section 10.4) and efforts to distinguish these lesions by ultrastructure have been unsuccessful.

Some tumors with an epidermoid phenotype may be classified incorrectly as adenosquamous carcinomas (WHO, Table 10.3). In such tumors, small tubules are present within the epidermoid cell nests and diastase-resistant, PAS-positive neutral mucosubstances are present within the tubular lumens (Fig. 10.5a, b). However, ultrastructural examination reveals that the glandular component is not neoplastic but is composed of normal appearing Type II alveolar cells which are surrounded by nests of tumor cells (Fig. 10.5c) (McDowell *et al.*, 1978; Alvarez-Fernandez, 1982; Dingemans and Mooi, 1984). This situation is similar to that described with some primary sarcomas, when the sarcomatous growth surrounds and traps pre-existing air spaces which are not part of the tumor (Carter and Eggleston, 1980).

(b) Glandular (adeno) features well developed (Figs 10.2, 10.6–10.9)

With the exception of CEAC.A described above, where both epidermoid and glandular phenotypes are well differentiated, adenocarcinomas tend to express epidermoid features that are focal and poorly differentiated (CEAC.C) or absent (AC) (Table 10.3). Specialization for secretion is present at the cellular level and endoplasmic reticulum and Golgi apparatus are well or moderately developed. Adenocarcinomas in phenotypic groups CEAC.C and AC fall into two subgroups, I and II, depending on the degree of tubular glandular organization, but there is no sharp dis-

---

Fig. 10.6 Light and electron micrographs of the bronchogenic adenocarcinoma, also shown in Fig. 9.14a–d. (a) Small cuboidal cells form tubular structures which are supported by a fibrous stroma. (Paraffin section, H&E stain: × 230.) (b) Although this tumor did not secrete mucus, the Golgi apparatus (G) is fairly well developed and RER is dilated. A few sparse tonofilament bundles (T) surround a nucleus. The cells are joined apically by junctional complexes (arrow). (Electron micrograph: × 10000.)

tinction between the two subgroups and most tumors are mixtures of tubular and solid areas in varying proportions. Because of their peripheral location these tumors are rarely biopsied by bronchoscopic techniques (Yesner, 1974) and are more frequently diagnosed by needle or open biopsy.

Adenocarcinomas may produce a desmoplastic response but rarely cavitate. The tumors commonly invade regional lymph nodes and pleura and distant metastases are common (Matthews, 1976; Matthews and Gordon, 1977).

(i) *Tubular glands present.* Tumors in the phenotypic subgroups CEAC.CI and ACI are classified as acinar adenocarcinomas according to the WHO scheme (Table 10.3). The tumors are composed of columnar or cuboidal epithelial cells arranged in palisade formation to form tubular acini, supported by a fibrous stroma (Figs 10.2a, 10.6a, 10.7a). The cells are joined at their luminal surfaces by junctional complexes and laterally by desmosomes. Tonofilament bundles may be present in the cells in varying amounts (Fig. 10.6b). Some tumors of this type are not mucus secreting, yet the endoplasmic reticulum and Golgi apparatus are generally well developed (Fig. 10.6b). Other tumors secrete mucosubstances and mucous granules accumulate in the apices of the tumor cells and mucus fills the tubular lumens (Fig. 10.7a, b). Mucus may also accumulate in intracellular hollows which appear as unstained vacuoles in H&E stained sections (Fig. 10.2a).

(ii) *Tubular glands minimal.* Tumors in the phenotypic subgroups CEAC.CII and AC II have predominantly solid growth patterns (Figs 10.8, 10.9). They are classified in the WHO scheme as solid carcinomas with mucus, which are mucus-secreting adenocarcinomas with solid growth patterns (Table 10.3). The cells, which usually have an abundant cytoplasm, large nuclei and prominent nucleoli, form solid nests. Sometimes the interior of the tumor nests undergoes necrosis. When small glandular acini are present the central lumens are oval (Fig. 10.8b) or slit-like (Fig. 10.8c), but because they are small they are not readily noticed in H&E-stained sections (Fig. 10.8a). These extracellular lumens, as well as mucus-filled intracellular hollows (Fig. 10.9b) and individual mucous granules

---

Fig. 10.7 Light and electron micrographs of the tumor which arose from a peripheral bronchus, also shown in Fig. 9.13a, b. (a) The cuboidal cells, filled with mucosubstances, form tubular structures which are supported by a delicate fibrous stroma. (Paraffin section, H&E stain: × 230.) (b) Mucous granules (M) are accumulated in the cell apices. Note irregular nucleus (N). (Electron micrograph: × 6000.)

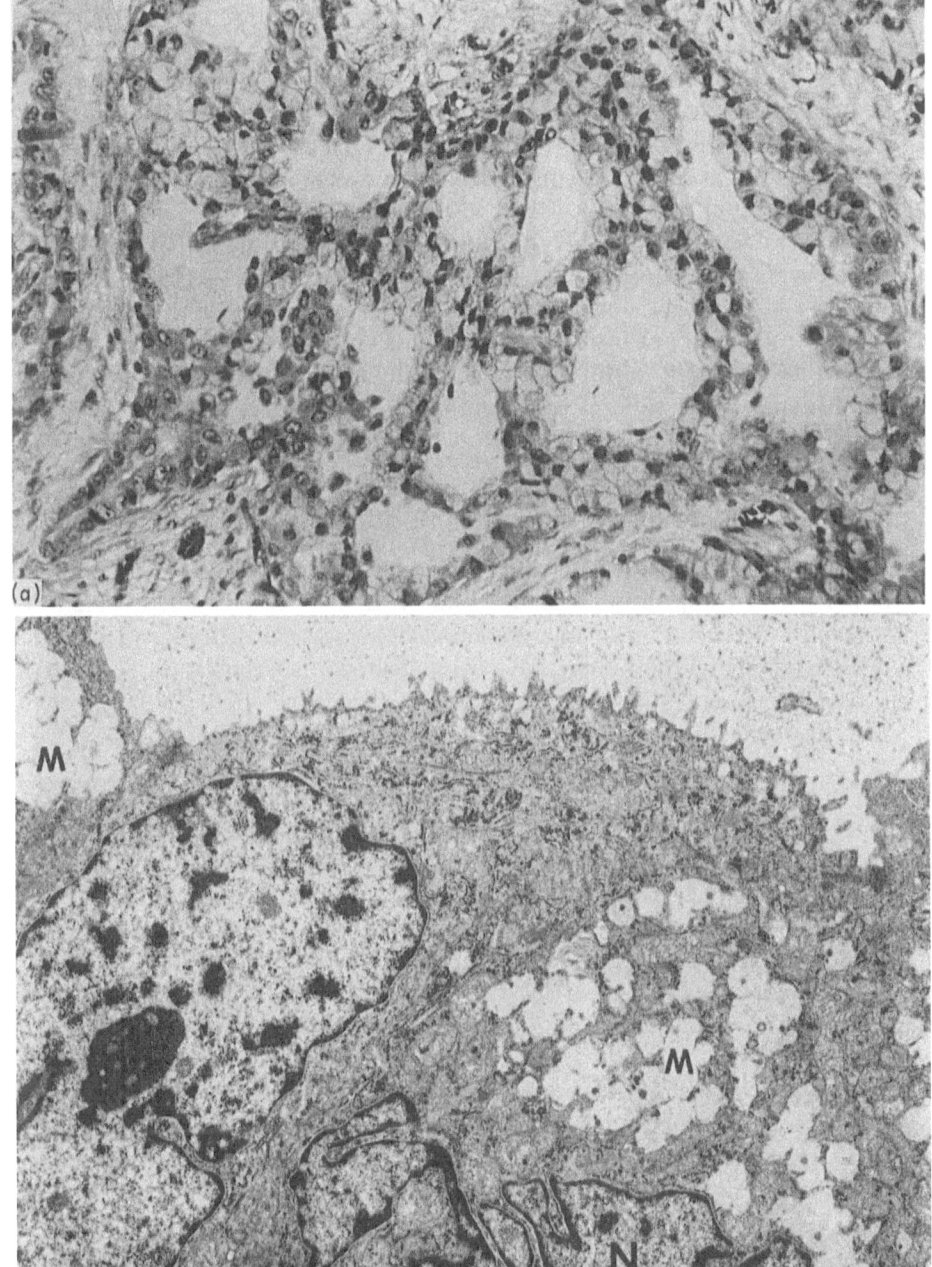

M

M

N

(Fig. 10.9c), are readily demonstrated in paraffin sections stained with AB-PAS (Fig. 10.2b, Fig. 10.9a inset).

Pleural mesotheliomas may closely resemble bronchogenic adenocarcinomas. A definitive diagnosis of mesothelioma is difficult but criteria that distinguish between mesothelioma and adenocarcinoma have been summarized (Table 10.4; Henderson, 1982). Appreciable amounts of diastase resistant PAS-positive mucosubstances, strong or moderate staining for carcino-embryonic antigen (CEA) (Section 10.3.3) and the absence of hyaluronic acid *exclude* the diagnosis of mesothelioma. Characteristic ultrastructural features also aid in the differential diagnosis (Table 10.4). Reactive hyperplastic changes in bronchial cells induced by mechanical injury (bronchoscope), inhalation of irritants and following radiation and/ or chemotherapeutic protocols may mimic adenocarcinoma. Moreover, the distinction between primary and metastatic adenocarcinoma may be rather difficult (Section 10.6).

(c)   Poorly-differentiated tumors (Figs 10.10, 10.11)

As already mentioned, the term 'undifferentiated' is still used to describe tumors which appear nondescript and without specialization by H&E staining. However, examination by more sophisticated methods invariably demonstrates that the tumors have some degree of specialization.

Poorly differentiated solid tumors, where mucus secretion is minimal or absent, are classified according to cell size in the WHO scheme. Large cell carcinomas are composed of large pleomorphic cells in solid nests. The nuclei are often enlarged and bizarre, with prominent nucleoli. Hemorrhage and necrosis may be prominent features (Fig. 10.10a). When phenotypic criteria are applied, the large cell carcinomas fall into the poorly-differentiated categories of epidermoid (EC) or combined tumors (CEAC.D) or into poorly-differentiated adenocarcinomas where secretory specialization (mucus secretion) is minimal at the cellular level (Table 10.3) (McDowell *et al.*, 1978; Churg, 1978; Mennemeyer *et al.*, 1979; Horie and Ohta, 1981; Auerbach *et al.*, 1982; Said *et al.*, 1983a, b). These poorly-differentiated carcinomas characteristically metastasize to distant sites (Matthews, 1976; Matthews and Gordon, 1977). When the tumors are composed of large glycogen-filled cells, the cells appear empty (clear) in H&E-stained sections (Fig. 10.11) (Katzenstein *et al.*, 1980). Such tumors are called 'clear cell' carcinomas in the WHO classification, where they are considered as a subset of the large cell group. Similar glycogen-filled 'clear' cells can also be seen in more differentiated tumors, particularly epidermoid carcinomas.

Large cell carcinomas may pose a difficult diagnostic problem, especially when the tumors are very poorly differentiated. Electron microscopy and

Table 10.4 Comparative histochemistry and ultrastructure of mesothelioma and mucin-secreting adenocarcinoma

	Mesothelioma[a]	Mucinous adenocarcinoma
Histochemistry		
Secretory products	Hyaluronic acid often present	Neutral mucosubstances
PAS-diastase	Negative	Positive
Alcian blue	Often positive	Positive
Alcian blue after hyaluroidase digestion	Negative	Positive
Carcinoembryonic antigen	Negative	Frequently positive
Ultrastructure		
Lamina externa	+	+
Desmosomes	+	+
Junctional.complexes	+	+
Acini	+	+
Intracytoplasmic crypts	+	+
Microvilli	Usually numerous, delicate and elongated	Fewer and shorter than those classically seen in mesotheliomas
Terminal filamentous web	Absent	Present
Intermediate (10 nm) filaments	+	+
Mucin-like granules	Typically absent	Present
Other granules and vesicles	Lysosomes, osmiophilic lamellar granules and vacuoles often present	Variable depending on pattern of cell differentiation
Glycogen granules	Often prominent	Variable
Other characteristics of infiltrating cells	May show microvilli interweaving with adjacent collagen fibres. Spectrum of appearances from epithelium-like cells to fibroblastoid cells, and sporadic epithelial features have been described even in predominantly fibrous mesothelioma. Myofibroblasts are also recorded, but are usually not conspicuous	Fibroblasts and myofibroblasts in stroma

Reproduced with permission from Henderson (1982) (see original article for references).

[a] In mesotheliomas only glycosaminoglycans associated with epithelial cell cytoplasm and/or acini have diagnostic significance, whereas their presence in sarcomatoid mesotheliomas (and in the stroma of carcinomas) lacks discriminant value. The ultrastructural appearances listed here also refer to epithelial cells unless stated otherwise; these features are most obvious in highly differentiated tumors and are depleted to varying degrees in poorly differentiated mesotheliomas.

immunocytochemistry are helpful in arriving at a definitive diagnosis. Antibodies against different types of intermediate filaments (Section 10.6) and against immunoglobulins and leucocyte common antigens are useful in the differential diagnosis of large cell carcinomas and lymphomas (Azar *et al.*, 1982; Lauder *et al.*, 1984).

Poorly-differentiated large cell carcinomas with numerous very en-larged, highly pleomorphic multinucleated cells are called *giant cell carci-nomas* (Table 10.2). These are highly malignant tumors associated with widespread lymphatic and vascular metastases. They are quite rare, form-ing less than 1% of lung cancers (Spencer, 1977). By light microscopy they may be confused with malignant fibrous histiocytomas or metastatic pleomorphic rhabdomyosarcomas. Electron microscopy and immunocy-tochemistry are helpful in making a differential diagnosis. The presence of desmosomes and/or keratin would confirm the epithelial nature of a giant cell tumor.

Measurement of tumor cell nuclear and cell diameters in poorly-differ-entiated lung carcinomas showed a continuum of cell size from large to small, with some overlap between carcinomas composed of primarily large or small cells (Vollmer, 1982; Said *et al.*, 1983b). Many tumors classified as small cell carcinomas using cell size and other specific light microscopic criteria contain DCG (Section 10.3.2). However, some small cell tumors apparently lack DCG, thereby falling into poorly-differentiated epider-moid, adeno- or combined epidermoid and adenocarcinoma categories without DCG, when the phenotypic criteria are applied (Table 10.3) (McDowell *et al.*, 1978; Mennemeyer *et al.*, 1979; Churg *et al.*, 1980; Shimosato, 1980; Li *et al.*, 1981; Bolen and Thorning, 1982; Leong, 1982). Nevertheless, despite considerable phenotypic heterogeneity, small cell carcinomas seem to share certain characteristic light microscopic features which are diagnostic and appear to be present irrespective of ultrastruc-tural phenotypes and whether or not the cells contain DCG. The light microscopic diagnostic features of small cell carcinoma, with and without DCG, are given in the following section.

Fig. 10.8 Mucus-secreting adenocarcinoma where tubular glands are minimal. (a) The tumor is composed of large cells which grow in a solid growth pattern. Note several unstained circular hollows (arrows). Mucus secretion passes unnoticed unless mucus stains are applied (compare with similar tumor in Fig. 10.2b). (Paraffin section, H&E stain: × 230.) (b) Ultrastructural examination reveals that some of the unstained circular hollows are extracellular lumens; note small cell junction (arrow). Intracellular hollows were also present in this tumor. (Electron micrograph: × 12000.) (c) Slit-like extracellular lumen. These structures are not readily seen by light microscopy. (Electron micrograph: × 5000.)

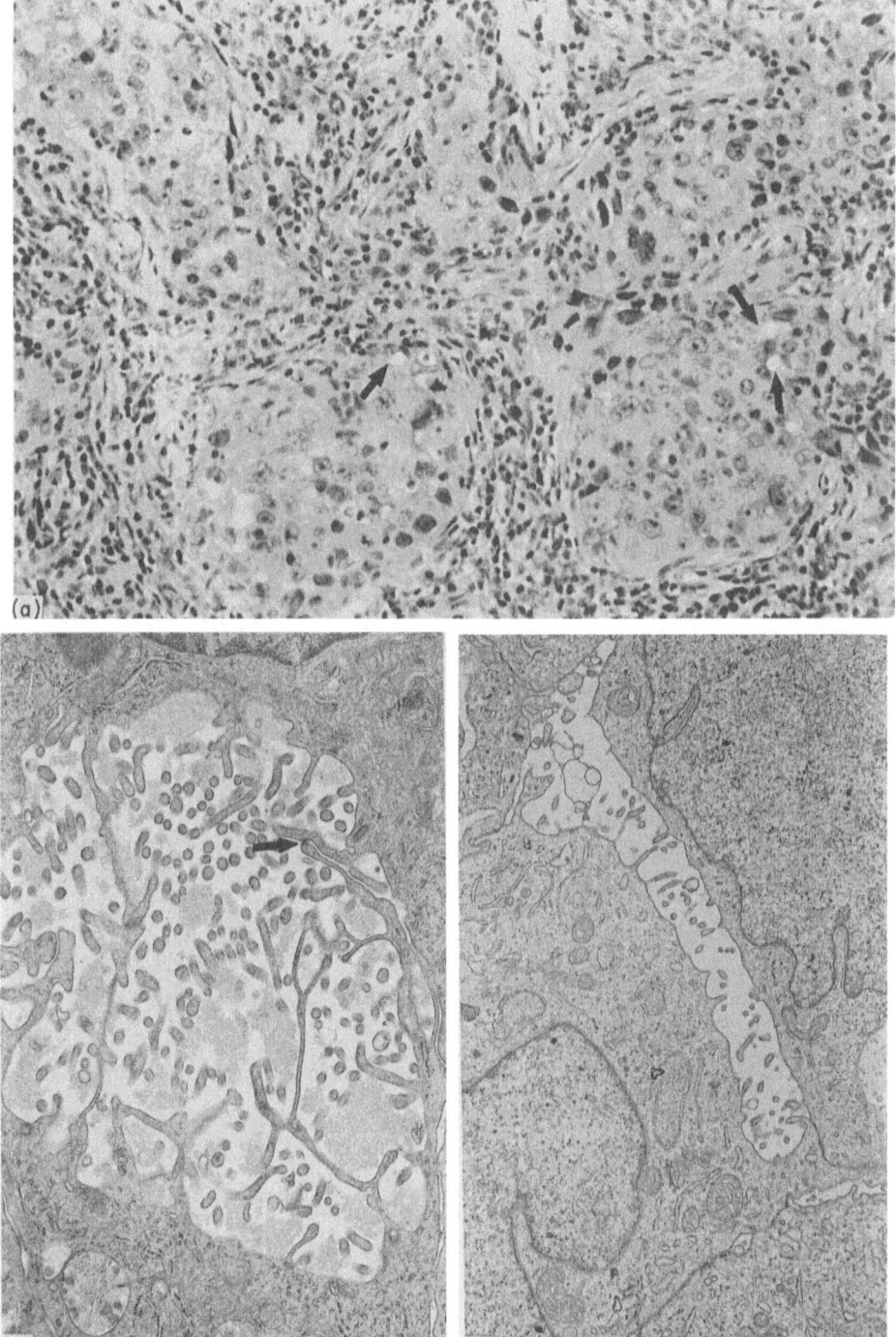

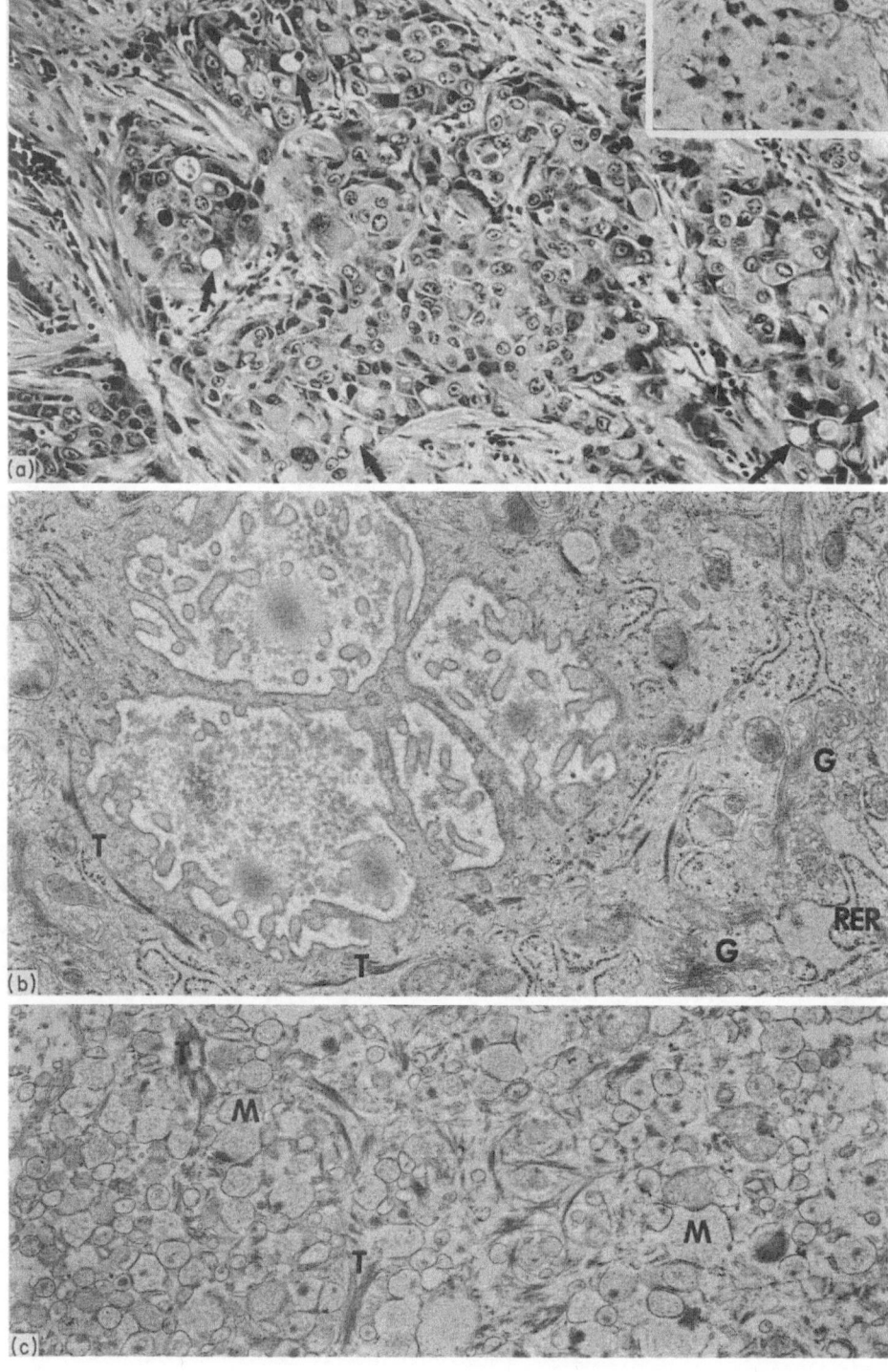

10.3.2 Tumors with dense-cored granules

The most sensitive diagnostic marker for tumors with DCG appears to be neuron-specific enolase (NSE), demonstrable by immunocytochemical staining (Tapia *et al.*, 1981). Carcinoid tumors, most small cell tumors with DCG (Fig. 10.17), and atypical endocrine tumors stain positively for NSE, whereas demonstration of other markers such as serotonin and/or calcitonin seems to be less reliable (Wick *et al.*, 1983; Sheppard *et al.*, 1984; Warren *et al.*, 1984a; Wilson *et al.*, 1985) (Section 10.3.3). Tumors with DCG also stain positively for gastrin-releasing peptide, the mammalian analog of bombesin (Bostwick *et al.*, 1984). Some tumors with DCG, in particular carcinoids, are argyrophilic when stained with the silver nitrate stain of Grimelius (1968). However, argyrophilia is notoriously capricious and even small cell carcinomas with numerous DCG may fail to stain (Tateishi *et al.*, 1978). Alcian blue staining after acid hydrolysis is a selective stain for DCG (Solcia *et al.*, 1968) and may be useful in the diagnosis of carcinoid tumors. Furthermore, if the specimen is embedded in glycol methacrylate, tumor cells with DCG can be stained using PAS-lead hematoxylin (Sorokin and Hoyt, 1978; Sorokin *et al.*, 1981).

For an up-to-date comprehensive account of the various types of bronchogenic tumors with DCG and of many other features of the endocrine lung, readers are referred to Becker and Gazdar (1984).

(a) Carcinoid tumors (Fig. 10.12, Fig. 10.17a)

Pulmonary carcinoid tumors are of low incidence, accounting for 1 to 2% of all lung tumors (Godwin, 1975; Carter and Eggleston, 1980). They are of low grade malignancy and only rarely metastasize beyond the thoracic lymph nodes. The tumors are usually small at diagnosis and are composed of moderate-sized polygonal cells which appear monotonously uniform in H&E-stained sections. Spindle-shaped cells have been described in peripheral carcinoids (Dube, 1970; Salyer *et al.*, 1975; Churg, 1977). Necrosis and mitotic figures are characteristically minimal or absent and the nuclei are of uniform size and round to oval in shape.

Centrally arising carcinoids may be composed of cells grouped in solid nests, in organoid patterns or arranged in trabeculae, tubules or rosettes.

Fig. 10.9 Mucus-secreting adenocarcinoma where tubular glands are minimal and an epidermoid component is present. (a) The tumor is composed of large cells which grow predominantly in a solid pattern. Note many unstained circular hollows (arrows). (Paraffin section, H&E stain: × 150.) *Inset*: Acidic mucosubstances fill the hollows. (Paraffin section, AB-PAS stain: × 150.) (b) Intracellular hollows are filled with mucosubstances. Note well-developed Golgi apparatus (G), RER and tonofilament bundles (T). (Electron micrograph: × 16500.) (c) Numerous mucous vacuoles (M) are dispersed in the cytoplasm, interspersed with well-developed tonofilament bundles (T). (Electron micrograph: × 10000.)

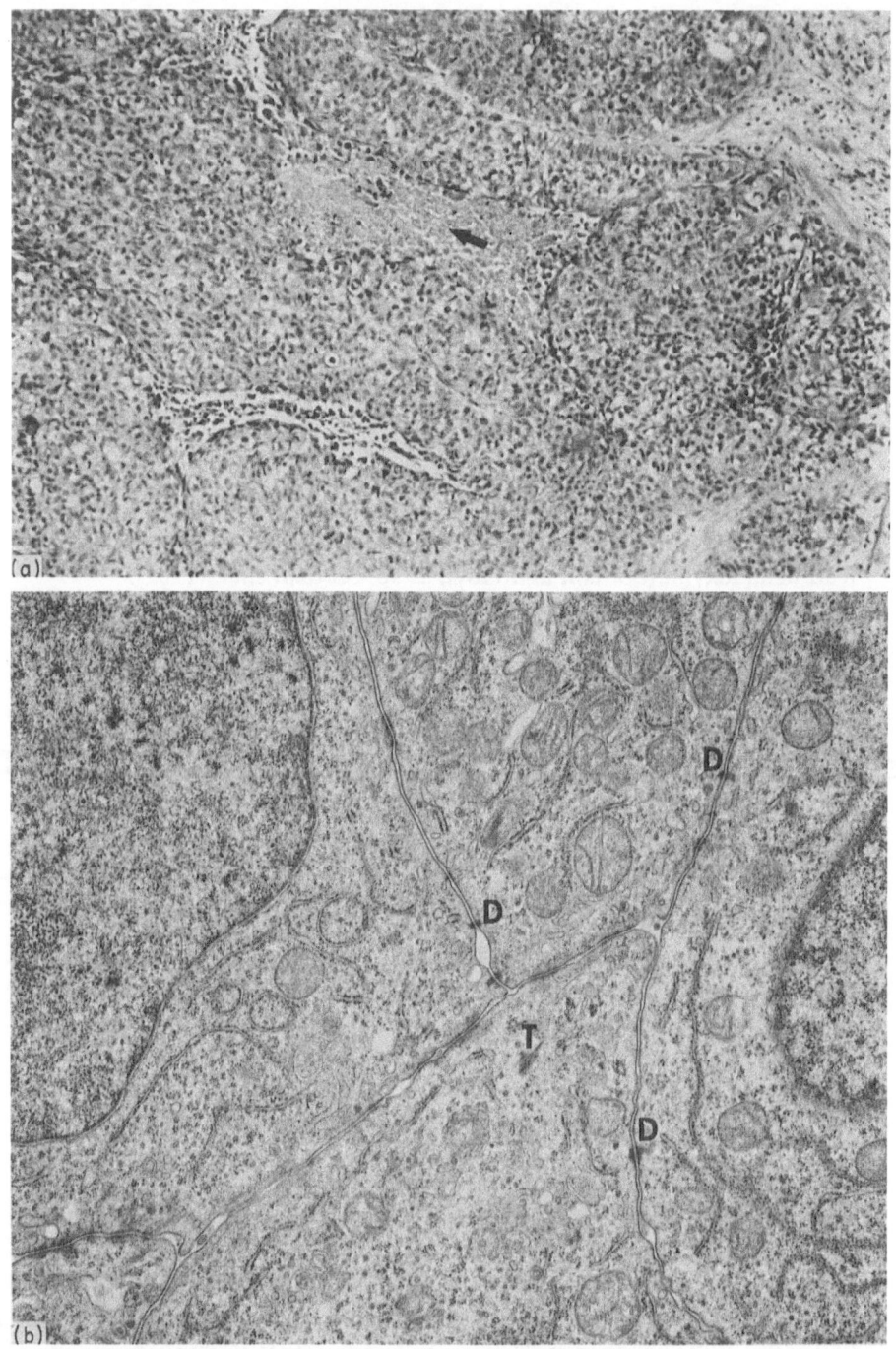

In three studies, the majority of carcinoid tumors showed mixtures of these various patterns (Salyer *et al.*, 1975; Jones and Dawson, 1977; Cooney *et al.*, 1979). A network of delicate vascular channels permeates between the tumor cells. Mark *et al.* (1981) emphasized the multiplicity of histologic patterns that carcinoid tumors may express and summarized their differential diagnoses. The very rare oncocytoma may be confused with a carcinoid tumor and some pleomorphic adenomas are composed of oncocyte-like cells which contain DCG (Section 10.5.2).

The ultrastructural characteristics of pulmonary carcinoid tumors have been described in detail (Bensch *et al.*, 1965, 1968; Gmelich *et al.*, 1967; Hage, 1973; McDowell *et al.*, 1976, 1981a; Capella *et al.*, 1979; Corrin, 1980; Mark *et al.*, 1981; Warren *et al.*, 1984a). The tumors are composed of polygonal cells, some of which have long cytoplasmic processes. The plasma membranes closely parallel each other so that intercellular spaces are minimal. The cytoplasm contains round to elongate mitochondria, a prominent Golgi complex, stacks of rough endoplasmic reticulum, and free ribosomes. Residual bodies containing lipofuscin are commonly observed.

The cells contain DCG but the number and types vary between tumors and sometimes even between cells of a single tumor. The majority of carcinoids contain small DCG (about 140 nm diameter), similar to those seen in DCG cells of the normal adult epithelium (reviewed by Capella *et al.*, 1979). However, polymorphic and large round granules have also been described (Hage, 1973). Tumors may be composed of cells with all three granule types, two types, or one type, but a single cell contains only one type of granule. The significance of these variations in granule morphology is not understood. The tumor shown in Fig. 10.12 was composed of cells bearing small, large or polymorphic DCG and was shown to have 10 distinct cytochemical staining patterns when conjunctive staining was applied to glycol methacrylate sections (McDowell *et al.*, 1981a; Sorokin *et al.*, 1981).

Some carcinoids present with areas of well-developed tubules and glands and secrete copious amounts of mucus. This may cause the tumors to be diagnosed as mucus-secreting adenocarcinomas (Sweeney and Cooney, 1978; Cooney *et al.*, 1979; Wise *et al.*, 1982). In fact, mucous granules and DCG may be found within a single cell (McDowell *et al.*, 1981a).

Fig. 10.10 Light and electron micrographs of a poorly-differentiated carcinoma which would be classified as a large cell carcinoma using WHO criteria. (a) The tumor is composed of solid nests of poorly-differentiated tumor cells. The center of the cell nest is necrotic (arrow). (Paraffin section, H&E stain: × 120.) (b) The cells contain sparse tonofilament (T) and are joined by small desmosomes (D). (Electron micrograph: × 10000.)

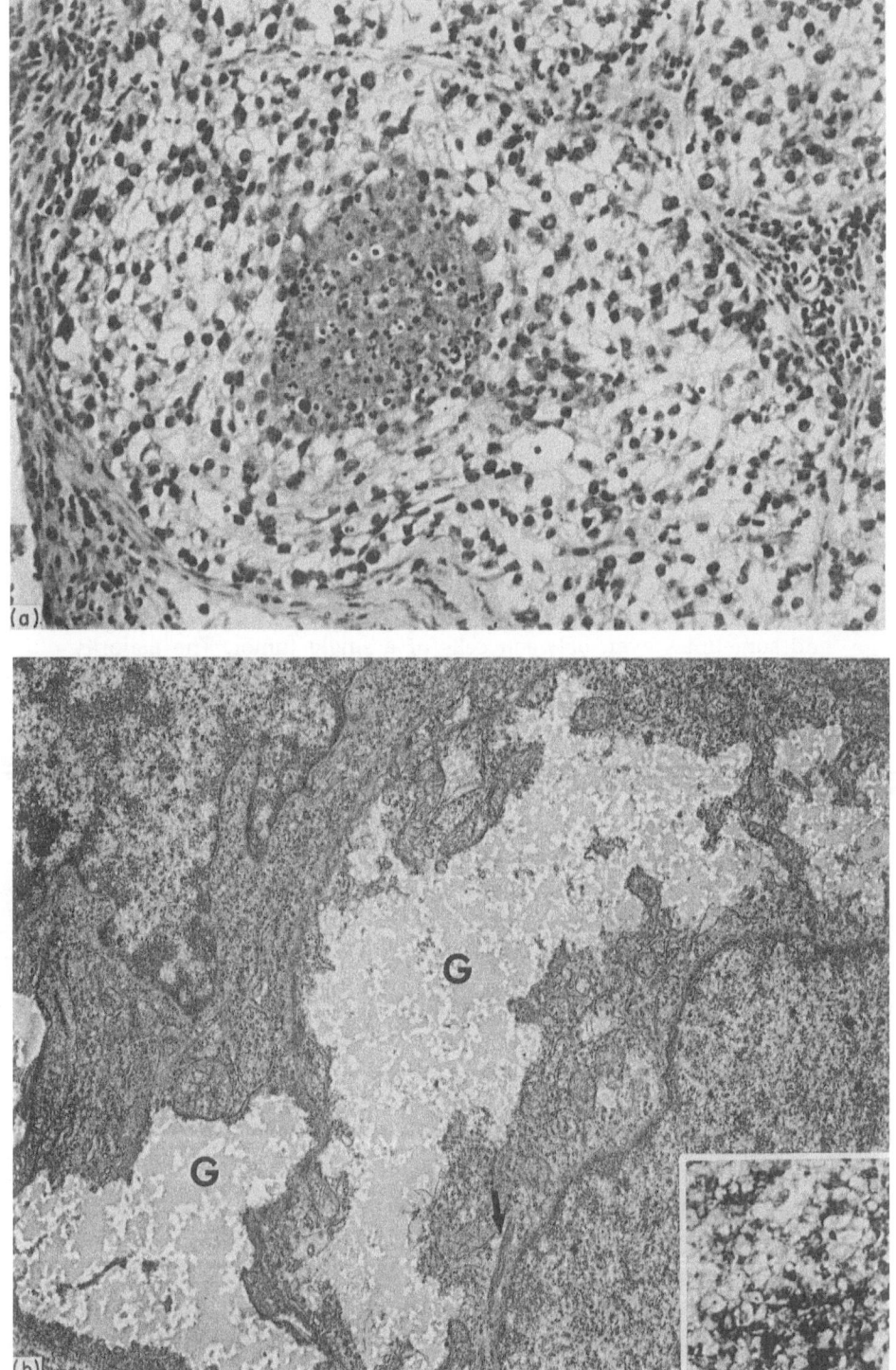

Furthermore, well-developed tonofilament bundles and keratin immuno-staining (Höfler and Denk, 1984; Warren *et al.*, 1984a) and fibrillary inclusions related to keratin (Berger *et al.*, 1984) have been described in some bronchial carcinoids. Involucrin has also been reported in isolated tumor cells (Said *et al.*, 1983a).

Although argentaffin stains are usually negative, many carcinoid tumors are argyrophilic when stained by the Grimelius procedure by light (Fig. 10.12a inset) or electron microscopy (Fig. 10.12b inset) and this can be helpful in their differential diagnosis (Cooney *et al.*, 1979; Capella *et al.*, 1979). However, the reaction may be focal and this must be borne in mind when dealing with small biopsy specimens (Blondal *et al.*, 1980).

Bone formation has been described in carcinoid tumors (Markel *et al.*, 1964; Okike *et al.*, 1976; Cooney *et al.*, 1979). The cause of ossification is unknown, but it has been speculated that local production of calcitonin by the tumor cells might be responsible for ossification of cartilage (Cooney *et al.*, 1979).

Although the majority of carcinoid tumors have a bland nuclear morphology and are clinically of low malignancy, more highly malignant *atypical carcinoids* occur (about 10% of all bronchial carcinoids), typified by cellular pleomorphism, nuclear atypia, mitotic figures and necrosis. These tumors, which may metastasize beyond the thoracic cavity, retain sufficient histologic features to allow their diagnosis as atypical variants of carcinoids (McBurney *et al.*, 1953; Goodner *et al.*, 1961; Abbey-Smith, 1969; Arrigoni *et al.*, 1972; Salyer *et al.*, 1975; Okike *et al.*, 1976; Mills *et al.*, 1982; Carter, 1983; DeCaro *et al.*, 1983).

(b)   Atypical endocrine tumors (Fig. 10.13)

The exact site of origin of these malignant tumors is presently unknown. Those recognized by McDowell *et al.* (1981b) were situated near the lung periphery. Using WHO criteria they may be classified as squamous cell carcinomas, solid carcinomas with mucus (poorly-differentiated adenocarcinomas) or as large cell carcinomas, because they do not show evidence by routine light microscopy of the characteristic carcinoidal or small cell histological patterns (Fig. 10.13a). Immunostaining for NSE, serotonin, β-HCG, somatostatin, and keratin was positive in the tumors studied to date

Fig. 10.11 Light and electron micrographs of a poorly-differentiated carcinoma which would be called a clear cell carcinoma using WHO criteria. (a) The tumor shows a solid growth pattern of large cells with a clear cytoplasm. The center of the cell nest is necrotic. (Paraffin section, H&E stain: × 230.) (b) The cells contain sparse tonofilaments (arrow). Much of the cytoplasm is filled with lakes of glycogen (G). (Electron micrograph: × 10000.) *Inset*: Paraffin section stained with PAS to demonstrate glycogen: × 230.)

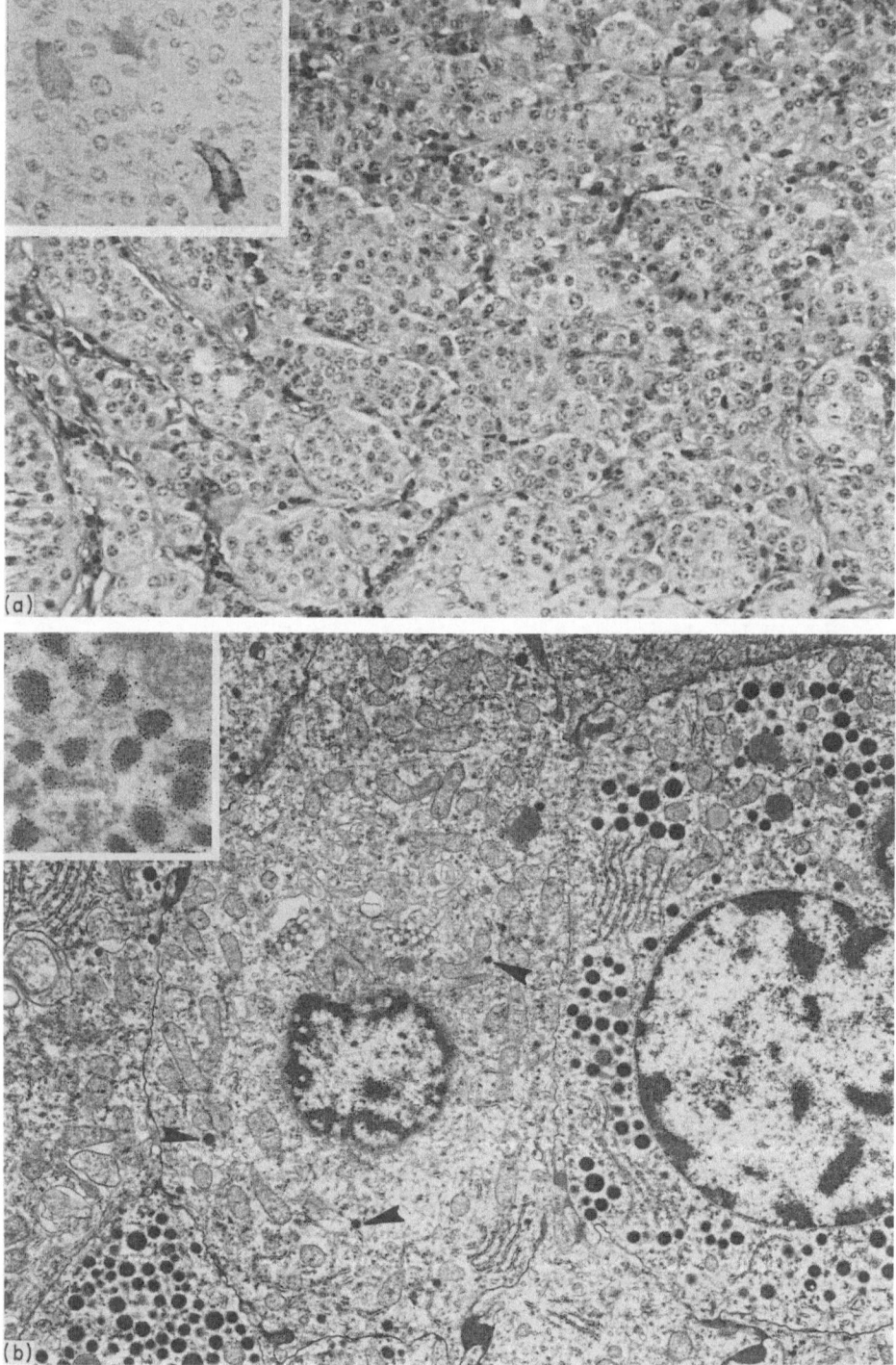

(Table 10.5). At ultrastructural level the cells bear DCG and tonofilament bundles (Fig. 10.13b and inset). The endoplasmic reticulum and Golgi apparatus are fairly well developed. In mucus-producing tumors, mucus is present in small intra- and extracellular hollows (Fig. 10.13a inset).

These tumors are being recognized with increasing frequency (Yesner, 1981; Leong, 1982; Azar *et al.*, 1982; Auerbach *et al.*, 1982; Kameya *et al.*, 1983; Chorba *et al.*, 1984; Pedraza *et al.*, 1984; Warren *et al.*, 1984b). For more details and reviews of the literature, readers are referred to McDowell *et al.* (1981b) and Warren *et al.* (1984b).

(c) Small cell carcinomas (Figs. 10.14–10.16, Fig. 10.17b)

Small cell carcinomas account for about 20% of all lung cancers. They are highly malignant tumors which metastasize widely and early (Matthews, 1976; Matthews and Gordon, 1977). About 50% of cases can be biopsied using a bronchoscope (Yesner, 1974). Accurate diagnosis is of paramount importance because some small cell carcinomas are particularly sensitive and responsive to intensive chemotherapy and radiotherapy. Although described here under tumors with DCG, there are several reports that tumors with characteristic light microscopic features of small cell carcinomas *may or may not bear DCG* (Hattori *et al.*, 1977; Tateishi *et al.*, 1978; Sidhu, 1979; Churg *et al.*, 1980; Shimosato, 1980; Gould *et al.*, 1981; Li *et al.*, 1981; Auerbach *et al.*, 1982; Bolen and Thorning, 1982; Said *et al.*, 1983b). Although the presence of DCG is a feature of glandular specialization (Section 10.1.2), small cell tumors with DCG are conventionally regarded as carcinomas rather than adenocarcinomas.

In spite of apparent heterogeneity regarding the presence or absence of DCG, it is established that small cell carcinoma of the lung can be reliably diagnosed with routine light microscopy using strict morphologic criteria. However, diagnostic problems may arise related to poor specimen preparation. A detailed account of the problems which may be encountered is given by Matthews and Hirsch (1981).

Fig. 10.12 Light and electron micrographs of a central carcinoid tumor. The same tumor is also shown in Fig. 9.16a, b. (a) In this area the carcinoid tumor shows an organoid pattern. The cells are very regular in size and shape. Nuclei are small and round and none is in mitosis. Small capillaries surround the cell nests. (Paraffin section, H&E stain: × 230.) *Inset*: Argyrophilia is demonstrated by the Grimelius stain in a few cells. (Paraffin section: × 400.) (b) The cell in the center has only a few small DCG (arrowheads) whereas cells at right and left contain numerous larger granules. This heterogeneity cannot be discerned by H&E staining (a) but may account for the scattered argyrophilic cells (a, inset). (Electron micrograph: × 6300.) *Inset*: The granules are argyrophilic (note silver grains) when stained by the Grimelius procedure. (Electron micrograph: × 25000.)

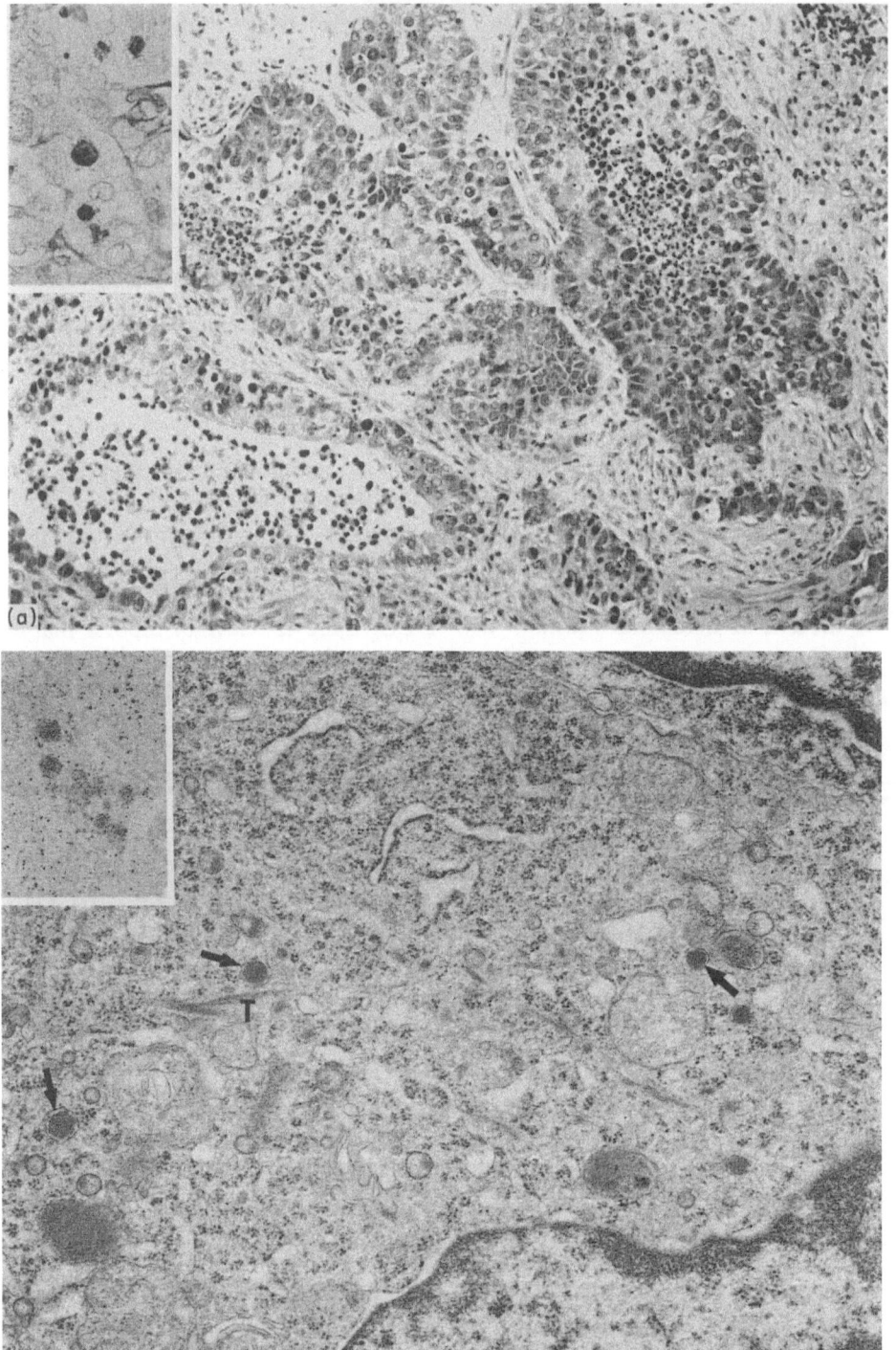

Three subtypes of small cell carcinoma are recognized in the WHO scheme: oat cell, intermediate cell and combined oat cell. *Oat cell carcinomas* consist of small cells with very scant cytoplasm resulting in molding and contouring of adjacent nuclei. The nuclei have a diffuse chromatin distribution and although the tumor cells are about twice the size of lymphocytes, they resemble them superficially (Figs 10.14a, 10.15a). Distortion due to 'crush artefact' often occurs, especially in biopsy specimens, in which case the cells are elongated and distorted and mitoses are difficult to interpret. Crush artefact, although not unique to oat cell carcinomas, should alert suspicion and precipitate a vigorous attempt to identify the tumor cells definitively. Nuclear detail is obscured because the nuclei are hyperchromatic (Fig. 10.14b). Ultrastructural examination indicates that nuclear hyperchromasia is a degenerative change.

Ultrastructurally oat cell tumors consist of small cells containing many free ribosomes; small desmosomes join adjacent cells (Fig. 10.14c). As discussed above it may not always be possible to find DCG; however, granules varying from 50 nm to 240 nm in diameter are frequently present. The polygonal tumor cells characteristically have irregular cell processes which extend between adjacent cells. Dense-cored granules are sometimes concentrated in these processes (Fig. 10.14c inset) (Hattori *et al.*, 1968, 1972; Bensch *et al.*, 1968). When oat cell tumors present with combinations of oat cell and squamous and/or adenocarcinomatous morphologies (Fig. 10.15) they are called *combined oat cell carcinomas*, using WHO terminology (WHO, 1981).

The *intermediate cell type* of small cell carcinoma consists of small cells which are a little larger than those of oat cell tumors because of a more abundant cytoplasm. The nuclear chromatin is dispersed in a more open pattern than in oat cell tumors. The cells may be polygonal or fusiform, often intermixed with smaller 'oat' type cells. A mucus-secreting small cell carcinoma (intermediate cell type) is shown in Fig. 10.16. The tumor shown in Fig. 9.15b is also characteristic of this tumor type. Combinations of small cell and large cell carcinomas are included in this subtype in the WHO scheme, but recent evidence suggests that tumors with mixed small

---

Fig. 10.13 Light and electron micrographs of an atypical endocrine tumor that might be classified as a solid carcinoma with mucus (poorly differentiated adenocarcinoma) using WHO criteria. (a) The tumor is composed of large cells which grow in solid nests. The centers of the cell nests are necrotic. (Paraffin section, H&E stain: × 150.) *Inset*: Acidic mucosubstances are demonstrated by the AB-PAS stain. (× 390) (b) Dense-cored granules (arrows) and sparse tonofilaments (T) are seen in the poorly-differentiated cells. (Electron micrograph: × 24500.) *Inset*: The granules are argyrophilic when stained with the Grimelius procedure. (Electron micrograph: × 30000.)

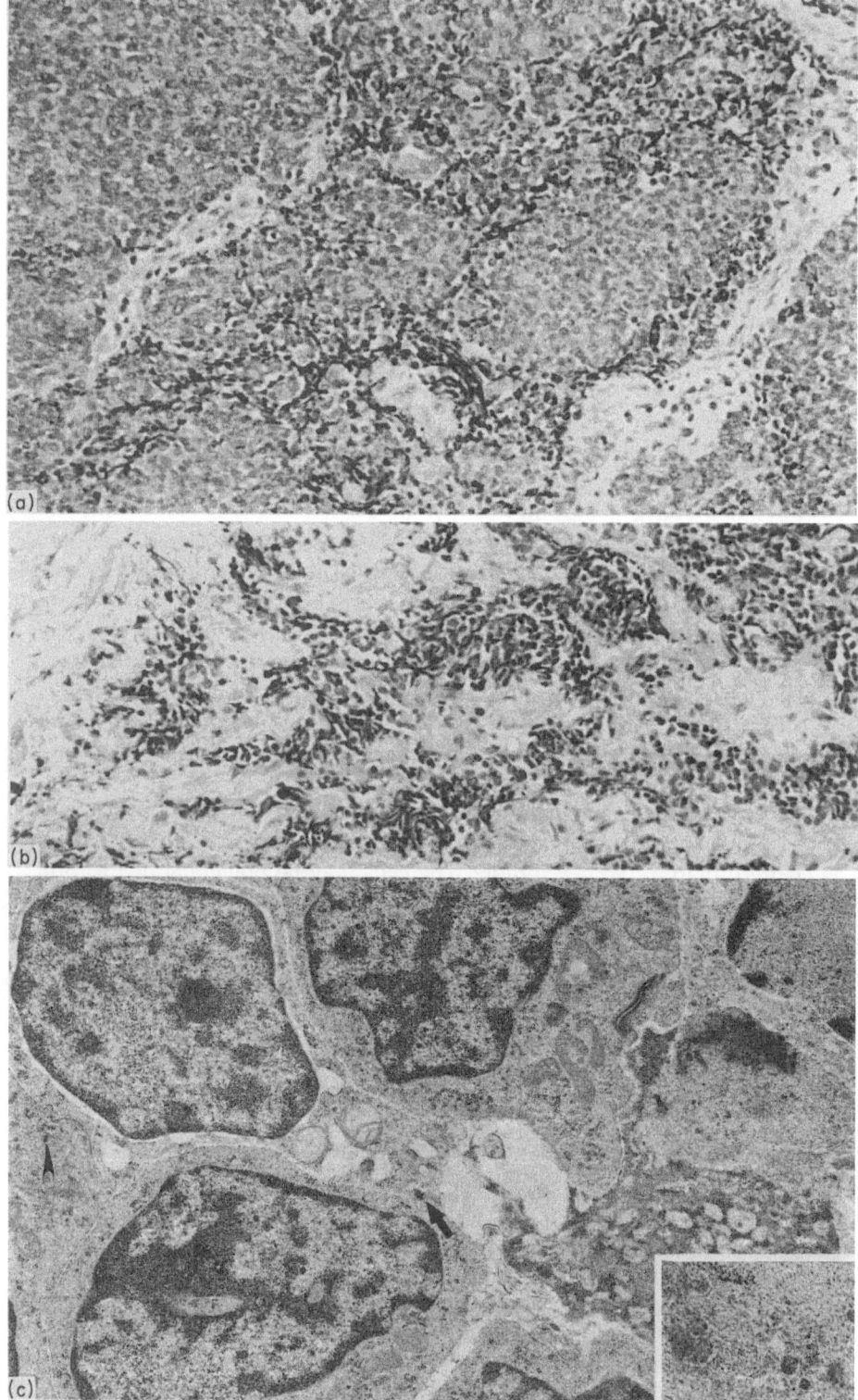

cell/large cell histologies should be considered distinct pathologic variants because patient survival was shorter than with oat cell or intermediate type small cell carcinoma (Radice *et al.*, 1982; Hirsch *et al.*, 1983).

If the tumor cells contain DCG, special stains are helpful in confirming the light microscopic diagnosis of small cell carcinoma. Although the cytoplasm is minimal, many small cell tumors stain positive for NSE (Sheppard *et al.*, 1984; Wilson, 1984). Furthermore, bombesin-like reactivity has been demonstrated immunocytochemically in tumors (Erisman *et al.*, 1982) and in extracts of cell lines derived from them (Moody *et al.*, 1981; Sorenson *et al.*, 1982). Bombesin-like reactivity is normally present in DCG cells of the fetal lung (Wharton *et al.*, 1978). The mammalian analog of bombesin, gastrin-releasing peptide, is present at variable levels in small cell carcinomas (Bostwick *et al.*, 1984). Argyrophilia, although positive in some small cell carcinomas, is generally not a reliable diagnostic aid even in tumors with DCG (Tateishi *et al.*, 1978; Steele, 1983; Yesner, 1983).

Interobserver variability may occur in the diagnosis of the WHO subtypes of small cell carcinoma (Hirsch *et al.*, 1982). However, unanimity in the diagnosis of small cell carcinoma as the main cell type is high. Three pathologists, two of which served on the advisory panel for the WHO classification, were in agreement on the following light microscopic criteria, irrespective of subtype. The following is abstracted directly from Hirsch *et al.* (1982).

Nuclear characteristics are considered the most significant diagnostic feature. Chromatin in these tumors is distributed in a uniform, fine or coarse stippled pattern throughout the entire nucleus. Nucleoli, for the most part, are small and inconspicuous. Size and shape of nuclei are of less significance. Nuclear details are obscure in cells with hyperchromatic nuclei.

The majority of the cells have meager cytoplasm, resulting in molding and contouring of adjoining nuclei. In some tumors, a moderate amount of cytoplasm may be identified.

Fig. 10.14 Light and electron micrographs of a small cell carcinoma, oat cell type. (a) The small 'oat' cells are in solid nests. Some of the cells, especially those at the peripheries of the nests, are very small with elongated and intensely hyperchromatic nuclei. (Paraffin section, H&E stain: × 230.) (b) Area of cells with hyperchromatic nuclei, streaming into the connective tissue. This appearance is typical of the so-called crush artefact, commonly seen in oat cell carcinomas. (Paraffin section, H&E stain: × 230.) (c) The small cells have a very scant cytoplasm and appear to be very poorly differentiated. A small desmosome (arrow) joins adjacent cells. One small dense-cored granule is seen (arrowhead). (Electron micrograph: × 9600.) *Inset*: Dense-cored granules were very rare in this tumor. This group of granules was present in a cytoplasmic process. (Electron micrograph: × 21000.)

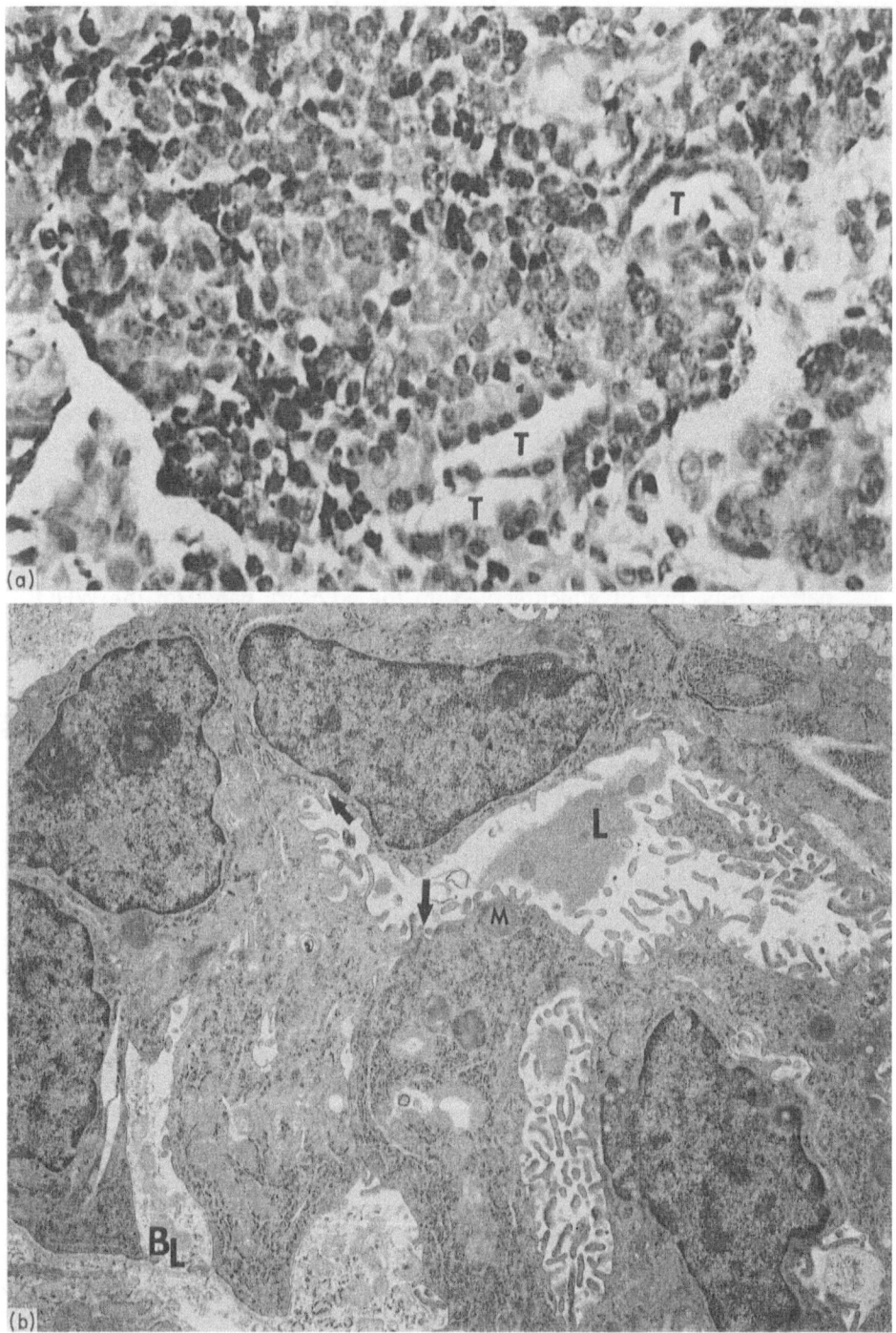

Mitoses may be numerous in well-preserved tumors but are usually difficult to appreciate in crushed biopsies and autopsy specimens, where nuclei tend to be hyperchromatic without distinct details.

The arrangement of cells may be variable. In some instances, neoplastic cells may be stratified or arranged in streams or ribbons along the fibrous stroma. Sometimes, the tumor cells may cuff thin walled blood vessels forming a perivascular mantle (pseudorosette). Occasional neoplastic cells form lumina, without polarization of the nuclei (rosettes), or occasional cuboidal or low columnar cells may form true tubules. The lumina may sometimes contain scanty mucin production. In a small percentage of tumors, a few discrete foci of squamous (epidermoid) differentiation or syncytial multinucleated giant cells may be identified.

The stroma is usually composed of thin fibrovascular elements; an inflammatory host response (lymphocytes and plasma cells) is most often minimal or absent.

As a group, small cell tumors are clinically aggressive and some are particularly sensitive to chemotherapy. Nuclear chromatin patterns may be a predictor of the response of small cell tumors to chemotherapy. It has been recently reported that tumors with fine chromatin distributions respond to chemotherapy better than those with more deeply-stained coarse chromatin distributions (Horai et al., 1981; Miyamoto et al., 1982).

There is growing appreciation that small cell carcinomas are of mixed phenotypes, with and without DCG (see above) and there are several ultrastructural reports of small cell carcinoma with DCG, coincident with epidermization and/or mucus-secreting specialization(s) (Figs 10.15, 10.16) (Sidhu, 1979; Hashimoto et al., 1979; Churg et al., 1980; Gazdar et al., 1981; Gould et al., 1981; Leong and Canny, 1981; Saba et al., 1981; Said et al., 1983a, b; Yesner, 1983). Moreover, individual tumor cells may contain tonofilament bundles (keratin), mucous granules and DCG (McDowell and Trump, 1981). Keratin has been demonstrated immuno-cytochemically in a proportion of cells in some small cell carcinomas (Gusterson et al., 1982; Said et al., 1983b) and keratin staining may be helpful in their differential diagnosis from lymphocytic infiltrates and

---

Fig. 10.15 Light and electron micrographs of a small cell carcinoma, oat cell type. Same case as in Fig. 10.14. (a) The small 'oat' cells resemble lymphocytes. Nuclear chromatin is finely dispersed and nucleoli are inconspicuous. Although most of the tumor has a solid pattern, some tubules (T) are seen. (Paraffin section, H&E stain: × 500.) (b) Ultrastructure of a tubular area. The small cells rest on a basal lamina (BL) and are joined apically by junctional complexes (arrows). Small mucous granules (M) are present at the cell apices. Mucosubstances are present in the tubular lumen (L). (Electron micrograph: × 8000.)

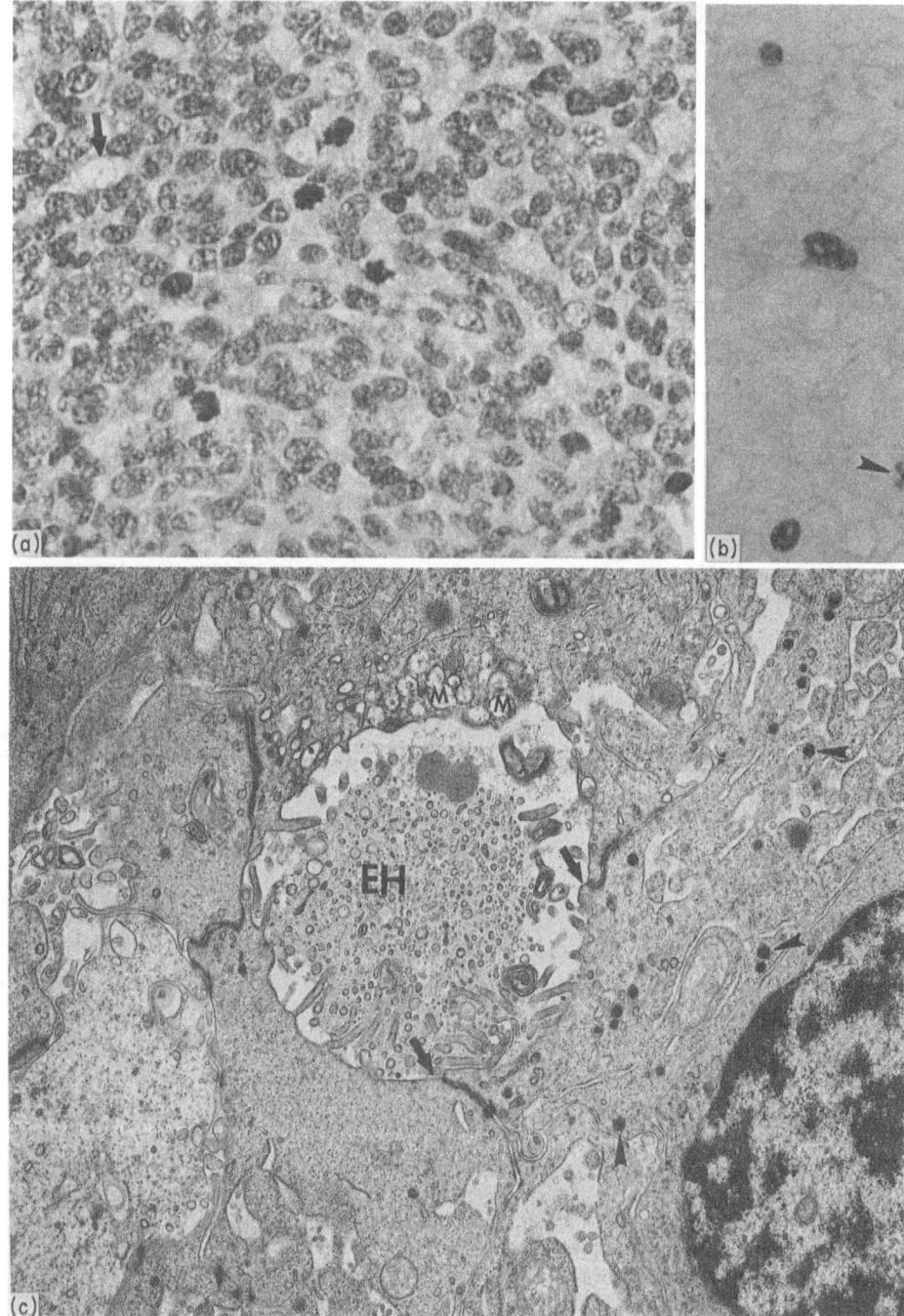

lymphomas. For example, Gabbiani *et al.* (1981) reported weak keratin staining in a lymph node biopsy initially diagnosed by frozen section as malignant lymphoma (keratin positivity is indicative of an epithelial origin, consistent with carcinoma). The patient died 6 months later and small cell carcinoma was present in the left lung.

Very little is presently known about clinical behavior and response to chemotherapy relative to the presence or absence of DCG or to the expression of other phenotypes such as epidermoid and mucus-secreting specializations (Hattori *et al.*, 1977; Li *et al.*, 1981; Bolen and Thorning, 1982). However, it has been shown that tumors with mixed small cell/large cell histologies are associated with lower response rates and shorter survival times than the 'pure' small cell subtypes (Radice *et al.*, 1982; Hirsch *et al.*, 1983). Much more work needs to be done relating clinical behaviors and response to therapy of small cell carcinomas to the nuances of their morphology. Furthermore, there is a growing awareness that radiotherapy and/or chemotherapy may effect changes in small cell tumor morphology so that tumors which recur following such treatments may convert partially or completely to another morphological type, including epidermoid carcinomas, adenocarcinomas and large cell carcinomas (Bates *et al.*, 1974; Bereton *et al.*, 1978; Bates, 1979; Abeloff *et al.*, 1979; Abeloff and Eggleston, 1981; Yesner, 1983). Giant cell formation has also been described (Bégin *et al.*, 1983; Steele, 1983).

10.3.3   *Immunocytochemical markers*

Bronchogenic neoplasms have been associated with numerous biochemical markers (Coombes *et al.*, 1978). With the advent of immunocytochemical methods which can be performed with relative ease on routinely-fixed paraffin-embedded specimens, considerable effort has been made in recent years to define the staining patterns of a number of markers in bronchogenic tumors (Nishiyama *et al.*, 1980; Harach *et al.*, 1983; Kameya *et al.*, 1983; Yang *et al.*, 1983; Wachner *et al.*, 1984; Warren *et al.*, 1984a; Wilson, 1984, Wilson *et al.*, 1985).

Fig. 10.16   Light and electron micrographs of a small cell carcinoma, intermediate cell type. (a) Cytoplasm is more abundant than in the oat cell tumor (Fig. 10.15a). The nuclear chromatin is less finely distributed and appears as aggregated clumps. Several mitotic figures are seen. Note the unstained hollow (arrow). (Paraffin section, H&E stain: × 500.) (b) When stained with AB-PAS, acidic mucosubstances are demonstrated in intra- (arrowhead) and larger extracellular hollows. (Paraffin section: × 500.) (c) Cells which contain numerous dense-cored granules (arrowheads) are joined apically by junctional complexes (arrows) to form a mucus-filled extracellular hollow (EH). Microvilli project into the hollow. Mucous granules (M) are present at the apex of one of the cells. (Electron micrograph: × 9600.)

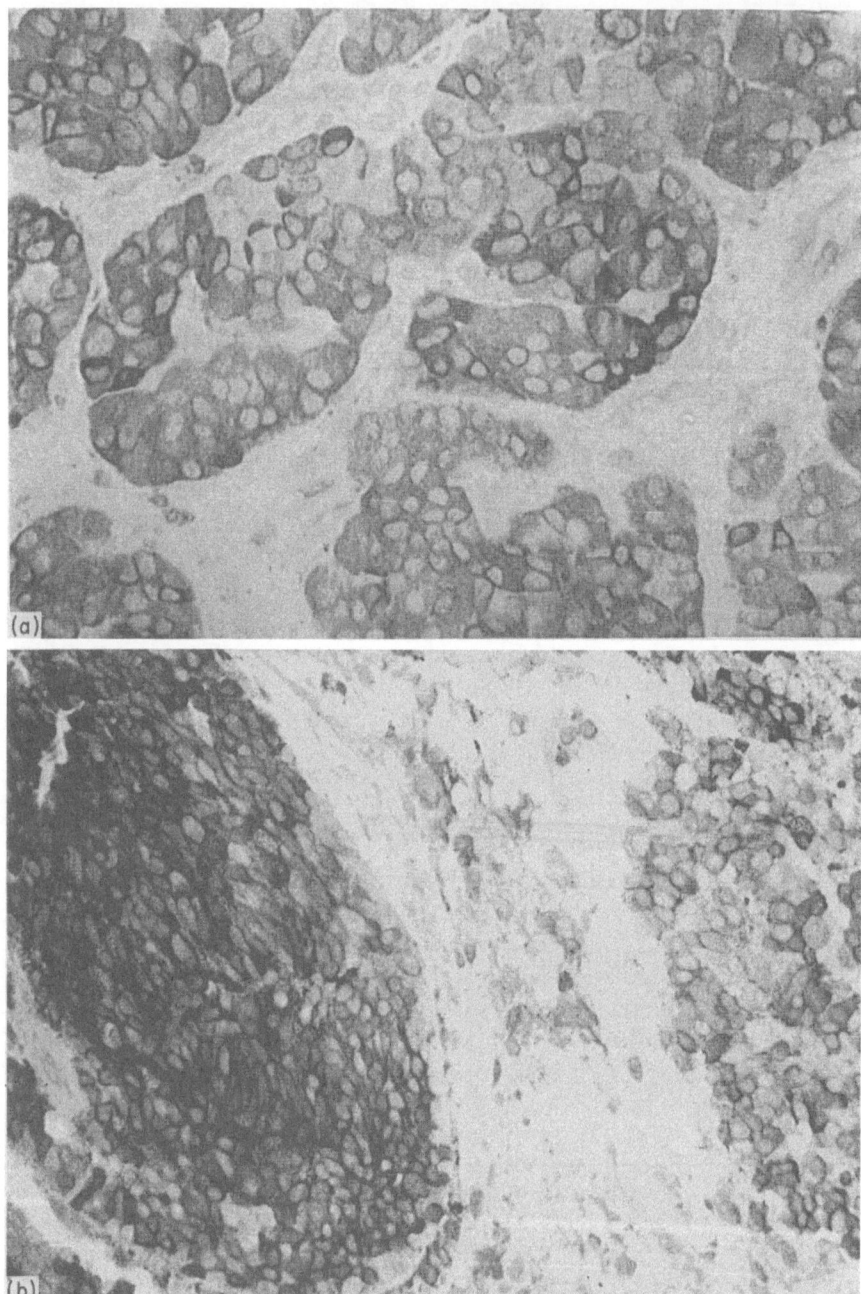

Fig. 10.17 Light micrographs of tumors with dense-cored granules, stained for neuron specific enolase (NSE). (Courtesy of Dr. Julia Polak, University of London.) (a) NSE-immunoreactive cells in a carcinoid tumor. Bouin's fixation, peroxidase-antiperoxidase method. (× 415) (b) NSE-immunoreactivity in a small cell carcinoma. Benzoquinone vapor fixation, peroxidase-antiperoxidase method. (× 330)

In a study of a large number of bronchogenic tumors, various markers were demonstrated by the PAP immunoperoxidase method (Table 10.5) and compared with tumor phenotype previously determined by routine H&E and AB-PAS staining and by electron microscopy (Wilson, 1984). The tumors had been fixed in 4% formaldehyde-1% glutaraldehyde and it now is well known that some antigenicity is destroyed by aldehydes. Therefore, the number of tumors stained for markers such as keratin, ACTH, and α-fetoprotein, which are sensitive to aldehyde fixation, were probably underestimated in this series.

Two major groups of bronchogenic tumors emerged depending on the presence or absence of NSE. All tumors *without* DCG failed to stain for NSE, whereas all those *with* DCG were stained positive. Furthermore, whereas serotonin was demonstrated in a proportion of tumors *with* DCG, all tumors *without* DCG failed to stain (Wilson *et al.*, 1985). Tumors *without* DCG include squamous cell carcinomas, adenocarcinomas, large cell carcinomas, adenosquamous and mucoepidermoid carcinomas; tumors *with* DCG include carcinoid, small cell and atypical endocrine tumors (Table 10.5).

Tumors without DCG: Staining for total keratin was generally strong in all well- to moderately-differentiated squamous cell carcinomas, including the adenosquamous tumors, although the staining intensity varied considerably between cells of a single tumor (Fig. 10.1b). Perinuclear keratin rings were a characteristic feature in strongly-stained cells. β-human chorionic gonadotropin (β-HCG) was demonstrated consistently, often associated with glycogen, and CEA was present in 90–100% of tumors, concentrated in the center of keratin pearls. Lesser numbers of poorly-differentiated squamous cell carcinomas stained for these markers. It is generally agreed that CEA is present in high incidence in epidermoid carcinomas but reports on the incidence of β-HCG in bronchogenic carcinomas of various types differ widely (Nishiyama *et al.*, 1980; Harach *et al.*, 1983; Wachner *et al.*, 1984).

Over 70% of adenocarcinomas stained for keratin, irrespective of their degree of glandular differentiation; the staining was generally weak and diffuse. Recent reports indicate that 100% of adenocarcinomas stain for keratin when fixed in ethanol or acetone (Ramaekers *et al.*, 1983; Blobel *et al.*, 1984). About 90% stained for β-HCG, which was higher than in other series (see above), and 100% stained for CEA. Several reports have described strong staining for CEA in adenocarcinomas (Pascal *et al.*, 1977; Hill *et al.*, 1979; Corson and Pinkus, 1982; Said *et al.*, 1983b; Wachner *et al.*, 1984). As mentioned above (Section 10.3.1), lack of CEA staining is helpful in the differential diagnosis of mesothelioma from other lung carcinomas (Wang *et al.*, 1979; Kwee *et al.*, 1982; Whitaker *et al.*, 1982). Whereas most adenocarcinomas stain strongly for CEA and weakly for

Table 10.5 Some immunocytochemical markers in bronchogenic carcinomas

	n	Keratin	β-HCG	CEA	ACTH	Somato-statin	Calcitonin	AFP	NSE	Serotonin
Tumors without dense-cored granules										
Adenosquamous/mucoepidermoid carcinoma	9	100%	100%	100% (n = 3)	78%	44%	22%	11%	0% (n = 6)	0%
Squamous cell carcinoma; well, moderately differentiated	20	100%	100%	90% (n = 19)	45%	70%	0%	0%	0% (n = 9)	0%
Squamous cell carcinoma; poorly differentiated	10	90%	90%	20% (n = 5)	50%	40%	20%	0%	0% (n = 4)	0%
Adenocarcinoma; well, moderately differentiated	23	74%	87%	100% (n = 19)	39%	39%	17%	4%	0% (n = 8)	0%
Solid carcinoma with mucus (poorly differentiated adenocarcinoma)	10	70%	90%	100% (n = 6)	50%	60%	40%	0%	0% (n = 11)	0%
Large cell carcinoma	16	75%	75%	61% (n = 13)	31%	25%	13%	6%	0% (n = 5)	0%
Tumors with dense-cored granules										
Carcinoid	2	0%	50%	NT	50%	50%	50%	0%	100%	50%
Small cell	10	30%	0%	100% (n = 3)	0%	20%	0%	0%	100%	10%
Atypical endocrine	7	100%	100%	NT	43%	100%	29%	0%	100%	100%

Data derived and modified from Hill *et al.* (1979) and Wilson (1984). Tumor typing according to WHO 1981, except for atypical endocrine tumors (McDowell *et al.*, 1981b). All tumors fixed in 4% formaldehyde–1% glutaraldehyde and embedded in paraffin.
NT: not tested.

n = number of tumors per group.

Percentages indicate proportion of tumors with any degree of immunoreactivity.

keratin, mesotheliomas tend to stain strongly for keratin but are weak or negative for CEA (Corson and Pinkus, 1982; Said *et al.*, 1983b). However, this is not absolute and stains for total keratin may not be discriminating (Holden and Churg, 1984).

Other markers such as ACTH, somatostatin, calcitonin and α-fetoprotein showed no consistent pattern for either squamous cell or adenocarcinomas. Calcitonin was demonstrated in 40% of solid carcinomas with mucus (poorly-differentiated adenocarcinomas). Keratin was demonstrated in 75% of large cell carcinomas. Some markers, β-HCG, CEA, ACTH and somatostatin, were demonstrated less frequently in the poorly-differentiated tumors than in those more highly differentiated (Table 10.5).

Tumors with DCG: Extensive immunocytochemical studies on bronchial tumors with DCG have been reported recently (Kameya *et al.*, 1983; Wick *et al.*, 1983; Yang *et al.*, 1983; Chorba *et al.*, 1984; Höfler and Denk, 1984; Sheppard *et al.*, 1984; Warren *et al.*, 1984a). The consensus of these studies is that NSE is a sensitive diagnostic marker (Fig. 10.17), confirming an earlier study (Tappia *et al.*, 1981).

With regard to other markers, different histological types of tumors with DCG show different staining patterns (Table 10.5). For example, none of the small cell carcinomas stained for β-HCG, ACTH, calcitonin or AFP but 30% stained for keratin and 20% for somatostatin. The lack of demonstrable ACTH and calcitonin was unexpected, as small cell tumors are often associated with elevated serum levels (Ratcliffe, 1982). Failure to demonstrate these markers in paraffin sections may reflect the very scant cytoplasm of the tumor cells. However, small cell tumors, or a proportion of them, do stain positive for CEA (Hill *et al.*, 1979; Sehested *et al.*, 1981; Goslin *et al.*, 1983; Said *et al.*, 1983b). On the other hand, all atypical endocrine tumors stained for keratin, β-HCG, somatostatin and serotonin and 43% for ACTH. Only two carcinoid tumors were tested in this series (Wilson, 1984).

10.3.4 Cytopathology

Some of the cytological features of epidermoid (squamous) carcinomas were summarized in Chapter 9 (Table 9.1 and Fig. 9.7). For detailed information on this and the cytological characteristics of other types of bronchogenic carcinoma, readers are referred to specialized cytological texts (Saccomanno, 1978; Koss, 1979; Johnston and Frable, 1979; Carter and Eggleston, 1980; Bonfiglio, 1983; Frost *et al.*, 1983; Kato *et al.*, 1983; Woolner, 1983).

Immunocytochemical stains can be applied as readily to cytological specimens as to histopathological sections, and this approach is now being used as a diagnostic tool (Nadji, 1980; Coleman *et al.*, 1981; Boon *et al.*, 1982; Kahn *et al.*, 1982; Walts and Said, 1983; Walts *et al.*, 1983; Springall *et al.*, 1984). Moreover, many of the phenotypic specializations described above (Sections 10.2, 10.3) can be recognized in ethanol-fixed Papanicolaou-stained cytology preparations. For example, sparse keratin filaments, not recognizable as such in paraffin sections stained with H&E, can be recognized in light microscopic cytology preparations as a hyalinized glassy appearing cytoplasm. For further details readers are referred to Hess *et al.* (1981a, b).

10.4   Carcino-sarcomas

Carcino-sarcomas are malignant neoplasms composed of malignant epithelial *and* mesenchymal elements. The epithelial component has been reported as epidermoid, adeno- and large cell carcinoma and the mesenchymal component as fibrosarcoma, chondrosarcoma, osteosarcoma and spindle cell sarcoma. Combinations of epidermoid carcinoma and fibrosarcoma or spindle cell sarcoma appear to be most common. These tumors can be easily confused with epidermoid carcinomas composed of spindle-shaped cells (Section 10.3.1).

To prove the existence of these tumors both elements must have metastasized (Carter and Eggleston, 1980). Prive *et al.* (1961) described pure deposits of epidermoid carcinoma and chondrosarcoma metastatic to the lymph nodes, and Chaudhuri (1971) described epidermoid carcinoma metastatic to hilar nodes and spindle cell sarcoma metastatic to the chest wall.

10.5   Low grade malignant and benign tumors

Carcinoid tumors are low grade malignant tumors. They are described above in Section 10.3.2. The other tumors described in this section are very rare but are included for completeness. Readers should refer to the references and to Spencer (1977) and Carter and Eggleston (1980) for illustrations.

10.5.1   Papillomas

These polypoid endobronchial tumors are rare; however, a wide spectrum exists from benign squamous cell papillomas to malignant papillary squamous (epidermoid) carcinomas, making it difficult to discern their true nature and to predict their clinical course (Spencer, 1977). Even in the absence of atypia these tumors may recur following resection and overt malignancy may supervene (WHO, 1981).

(a)   Squamous cell papillomas

These are very rare benign tumors composed of papillary processes with a core of fibrous tissue covered by stratified metaplastic epidermoid epithelium, sometimes with an admixture of columnar mucous cells. They are solitary or multiple. Further details of their morphology are given by Carter and Eggleston (1980). According to Spencer (1977), approximately 50% of solitary adult tumors become malignant with time.

(b)   Transitional papillomas

These are rare endobronchial papillary tumors which, by light microscopy, resemble transitional cell tumors of the urothelium. Areas of cuboidal, columnar and even ciliated epithelium and areas of epidermoid metaplasia may be present with or without mucus secretion (WHO, 1981). The tumors may be of multiple origin. Examination of one case with 'transitional' morphology by light microscopy (delicate branching stromal cores covered by a thick layer of transitional epithelium) showed only epidermoid characteristics when examined ultrastructurally and was considered to be a variant of epidermoid carcinoma (Smith and McClure, 1982). Spencer *et al.* (1980) consider these tumors to be papillary variants of carcinoma *in situ*.

10.5.2   *Adenomas*

These are very rare benign tumors that presumably arise from the cells that constitute the submucosal bronchial glands (Chapter 3).

(a)   Monomorphic adenomas

These are of three types: oncocytomas, mucous gland adenomas (cystadenomas) and acinic cell tumors. The three tumor types appear to arise from collecting duct cells, mucous cells and serous cells of the bronchial glands, respectively.

(i)   *Oncocytomas* (synonym, oxyphilic adenomas) are very rare tumors. The tumor cells resemble collecting duct cells of the bronchial gland. Collecting duct cells normally contain very numerous densely-packed large mitochondria, causing them to stain strongly eosinophilic with H&E (Chapter 3). Oncocytomas consist of collections of similar mitochondria-rich eosinophilic cells, with small hyperchromatic nuclei arranged in acinar patterns and solid clumps. The stroma is minimal and the tumor cells show no atypia (Spencer, 1979; Warter *et al.*, 1981). These tumors may be mistaken for carcinoid tumors, especially by light microscopy (Black,

1969). Electron microscopy should be employed to establish the definitive diagnosis. The absence of DCG and the presence of numerous tight-packed mitochondria would confirm a diagnosis of oncocytoma (see also the section on pleomorphic adenomas below).

(ii)   *Mucous gland adenomas*   (cystadenomas) appear to arise from mucous cells of the submucosal glands of large bronchi. They usually present as pedunculated polyps in the lumen. Their diagnosis can be established by bronchoscopy. Histologically, mucus-filled acini are lined by columnar or cuboidal mucous cells (Ramsey and Reimann, 1953; Gilman *et al.*, 1956; Kroe and Pitcock, 1967; Emory *et al.*, 1973; Allen *et al.*, 1974; Pritchett and Key, 1978; Spencer, 1979; Edwards and Matthews, 1981). These tumors are unequivocally benign.

(iii)   *Acinic cell tumors*   are thought to arise from serous cells of the bronchial glands. Only two cases have been reported (Fechner *et al.*, 1972; Katz and Bubis, 1976). The tumors, which are analogous to acinic tumors of the salivary glands, consist of sheets of clear tumor cells grouped in small nests, with occasional trabecular patterns.

(b)   Pleomorphic adenomas

Also called 'mixed' tumors, these are very rare tumors of the glands of the trachea and large bronchi, characterized by a pleomorphic appearance with recognizable epithelial tissue intermixed with mucoid, myxoid or chondroid elements. Sheets of myoepithelial cells may also be seen. The epithelial components may appear as sheets or strands, as ducts or as epidermoid structures (Payne *et al.*, 1965; Davis *et al.*, 1972; Spencer, 1979).

In addition, adenomas have been reported with diverse phenotypic expressions analogous to the situation described above for malignant tumors. For example, adenomas have been described composed of onco-cyte-like cells with numerous tightly-packed mitochondria, but also containing varying numbers of DCG (Fechner and Bentinck, 1973; Santoz-Briz *et al.*, 1977; Walter *et al.*, 1978; Sajjad *et al.*, 1980; Alvarez-Fernandez and Folque-Gomez, 1981; Scharifker and Marchevsky, 1981). A tumor described by Sklar *et al.* (1980) was composed of an admixture of oncocytes and cells containing DCG. There is also a report of a bronchial adenoma composed of oncocytes, mucous cells and serous cells (Akhtar *et al.*, 1974).

10.5.3   Low grade mucoepidermoid tumors

These tumors arise in large bronchi from both the metaplastic surface and submucosal glandular epithelium and project as polypoid masses into the bronchial lumen. As the tumors grow they compress the bronchial carti-lages. The tumors consist of cells expressing varying degrees of epidermoid and glandular mucus-secreting specializations. Single cells expressing both phenotypes are observed (Perrone and Dickersin, 1983) and morphologic forms intermediate between mucous cells, epidermoid cells and oncocytes have been described (Stafford et al., 1984). Some areas of the tumors consist of solid nests of epidermoid cells. Other areas show mixtures of mucus-secreting acini, surrounded by cells with abundant eosinophilic cytoplasm (Sniffen et al., 1958; Payne et al., 1959; Leonardi et al., 1978; Klacsmann et al., 1979; Mullins and Barnes, 1979; Spencer, 1979). The histology of the tumors is very similar to their malignant counterparts, except that low grade tumors are generally well circumscribed with little or no tendency to invade; their nuclei show minimal atypia with few mitotic figures (Conlan et al., 1978).

10.5.4   Adenoid cystic carcinomas (cylindromas)

Adenoid cystic carcinomas are low grade malignant tumors of the glands of the trachea and large bronchi. They rarely metastasize to distant sites but may invade the bronchial wall, resulting in cartilage destruction, and spread into the lung alveoli. They are very rare tumors, accounting for about one tenth of the small group of bronchial carcinoids and other low grade or benign bronchial tumors combined. They may be polypoid or annular. Histologically, they are identical to similar tumors of the salivary glands (Payne et al., 1959; Conlan et al., 1978; Hoshino and Yamamoto, 1970). The tumor cells may be arranged in clumps with a cribriform pattern enclosing cystic spaces filled with mucosubstances, in trabeculae, or in poorly-differentiated tumors in solid masses. Occasionally groups of cells show overt cornification.

At least two cell types have been identified in adenoid cystic carcinomas of the bronchus (Kodama et al., 1982). One type is fusiform and lies on the basement membrane which surrounds the cribriform or solid nests of cells. Because of a characteristic ultrastructure (myofilaments, dense plaques, hemidesmosomes, etc.) these cells are thought to be neoplastic myoepithelial cells. The second cell type is polyhedral and forms the bulk of the tumors. These small cells with round hyperchromatic nuclei and scant cytoplasm may contain tonofilament bundles and numerous ribo-somes; however, mitochondria, Golgi complexes and endoplasmic reticu-lum are poorly developed. Desmosomes join the cells and intercellular spaces may be wide and filled with flocculent material. Cells which line the cystic spaces are joined apically by junctional complexes; secretory granules are accumulated in the apical cytoplasm.

Because of its distinctive appearance this tumor is seldom confused with other types of lung cancer. However, the tumor cells are small and solid tumors may simulate small cell carcinomas. Usually mitotic activity is low in adenoid cystic tumors and the nuclei are vesicular with clumped chromatin, contrasting with the dispersed chromatin pattern typical of small cell carcinomas. These tumors may also simulate carcinoid tumors. In this case electron microscopical examination and a search for DCG are indicated. The stroma of adenoid cystic carcinomas is varied. In some tumors replicated hyaline basement membrane expands into dense sclerotic fibrous bands which separate the tumor cell nests, whereas in other tumors a loose myxomatous connective tissue stroma predominates (Spencer, 1979; Carter and Eggleston, 1980).

10.6 Metastatic carcinomas

About one third of all extrathoracic carcinomas metastasize to the lungs (Abrams et al., 1950; Trinidad et al., 1963). The secondary tumors may simulate primary bronchogenic carcinomas and metastatic carcinomas should always be included in the differential diagnosis (Greenberg and Young, 1958; Trinidad et al., 1963). Cavitation may occur in both primary and metastatic lung tumors (Chaudhuri, 1970). Differential diagnosis may be especially difficult if the metastases involve the bronchi (Rosenblatt et al., 1966; Braman and Whitcomb, 1975; King et al., 1979; Baumgartner and Mark, 1980; Cassiere et al., 1980). Primary tumors that most commonly produce endobronchial metastases include kidney, breast and colon; metastases have also been reported from cervix, uterus, ovary, pancreas, penis, bladder and thyroid (Nöu, 1981; Sheperd, 1982). Regardless of site of origin of the tumor, the histologic changes in the bronchi may be quite similar, involving permeation of the mucosal lymphatics with malignant cells. Groups of tumor cells coalesce within the swollen lymphatics to form solid tumors below the bronchial epithelium. Eventually the entire mucosal surface is replaced by malignant tissue which projects into the bronchial tumor, simulating a bronchogenic neoplasm to bronchoscopist and pathologist. Endobronchial metastases may also be confused with foreign bodies (Amer et al., 1981) and pieces of the metastatic tumor may be expectorated (Jariwalla et al., 1981). Metastases to the airways is said to occur in 2–5% of patients dying of extrathoracic malignancies.

Pulmonary metastases which may mimic bronchogenic carcinoma are common from colorectal, renal and pancreatic carcinomas. They may also arise from adrenal glands, breast, endometrium, prostate, stomach, thyroid, larynx, ovary and esophagus (Rosenblatt et al., 1966). Some of the features of metastatic renal and colorectal carcinomas are discussed by Katzenstein et al. (1978) and Berg et al. (1984), respectively. The role of electron microscopy in the diagnosis of metastatic neoplasms has been discussed recently (Herrera, et al., 1985). A special mucus stain may be useful in distinguishing metastases from adenocarcinomas of the colon (Culling et al., 1975).

Immunocytochemical techniques are of value in the diagnosis of metastatic tumors and may be helpful in tracing the origin of the primary tumor. Different classes of cells can be distinguished on the basis of their intermediate filament proteins (Gabbiani *et al.*, 1981; Altmannsberger *et al.*, 1981; Osborn and Weber, 1983). It is possible, using paraffin-embedded alcohol-fixed specimens, to differentiate between epithelial, mesenchymal and smooth muscle cells, both normal and neoplastic, based on the presence of keratin, vimentin and desmin proteins, respectively, which constitute the intermediate filaments of these classes of cells (Altmannsberger *et al.*, 1981). This is very helpful in diagnosis because the primary tumors, as well as their metastases, retain the protein typical of the tissue of origin. This provides a reliable way to differentiate between keratin-positive primary epithelial tumors and keratin-negative mesenchymal tumors (Espinoza and Azar, 1982) and aids in the differential diagnosis of malignant lymphomas and nodular metastases of poorly-differentiated carcinomas (Gabbiani *et al.*, 1981; Lauder *et al.*, 1984). It is without doubt that these types of approaches, including the use of various monoclonal antibodies, will provide increasing diagnostic accuracy in the future (Munro Neville *et al.*, 1982; Borowitz and Stein, 1984).

References

Abbey-Smith, R. (1969), Bronchial carcinoid tumors. *Thorax*, **24**, 43–50.

Abeloff, M.D. and Eggleston, J.C. (1981), Morphologic changes following therapy. In *Small Cell Cancer of the Lung* (eds F.A. Greco, R.K. Oldham and P.A. Bunn), Grune & Stratton, New York, pp. 235–58.

Abeloff, M.D., Eggleston, J.C., Mendelsohn, G., Ettinger, D.S. and Baylin, S.B. (1979), Changes in morphological and biochemical characteristics of small cell carcinoma of the lung. *Am. J. Med.*, **66**, 757–64.

Abrams, H.L., Spiro, R. and Goldstein, N. (1950), Metastases in carcinoma. Analysis of 1000 autopsied cases. *Cancer*, **3**, 74–85.

Akhtar, M., Young, I. and Reyes, F. (1974), Bronchial adenoma with polymorphous features. *Cancer*, **33**, 1572–6.

Allen, M.S., Marsh, W.L. and Geissinger, W.T. (1974), Mucus gland adenoma of the bronchus. *J. Thorac. Cardiovasc. Surg.*, **67**, 966–8.

Altmannsberger, M., Osborn, M., Schauer, A. and Weber, K. (1981), Antibodies to different intermediate filament proteins. Cell type-specific markers on paraffin-embedded human tissues. *Lab. Invest.*, **45**, 427–34.

Alvarez-Fernandez, E. (1982), Alveolar trapping in pulmonary carcinomas. *Diagnostic Histopathol.*, **5**, 59–64.

Alvarez-Fernandez, E. and Folque-Gomez, E. (1981), Atypical bronchial carcinoid with oncocytoid features. Its ultrastructure, with special reference to its granular content. *Arch. Path. Lab. Med.*, **105**, 428–31.

Amer, E., Guy, J. and Vaze, B. (1981), Endobronchial metastasis from renal adenocarcinoma simulating a foreign body. *Thorax*, **36**, 183–4.

Arrigoni, M.G., Woolner, L.B. and Bernatz, P.E. (1972), Atypical carcinoid tumors of the lung. *J. Thorac. Cardiovasc. Surg.*, **64**, 413–21.

Auerbach, O., Frasca, J.M., Parks, V.R. and Carter, H.W. (1982), A comparison of World Health Organization (WHO) classification of lung tumors by light and electron microscopy. *Cancer*, **50**, 2079–88.

Azar, H.A., Espinoza, C.G., Richman, A.V., Saba, S.R. and Wang, T.-Y. (1982), 'Undifferentiated' large cell malignancies: an ultrastructural and immunocyto-chemical study. *Human Pathol.*, **13**, 323–33.

Banks-Schlegel, S.P., McDowell, E.M., Wilson, T.S., Trump, B.F. and Harris, C.C. (1984), Keratin proteins in human lung carcinomas. Combined use of morphology, keratin immunocytochemistry, and keratin immunoprecipitation. *Amer. J. Pathol.*, **114**, 273–86.

Bates, H.R. (1979), Morphological variation in oat-cell carcinoma of the bronchus. *Lancet*, **i**, 1413.

Bates, M., Hurt, R., Levison, V. and Sutton, M. (1974), Treatment of oat-cell carcinoma of bronchus by preoperative radiotherapy and surgery. *Lancet*, **i**, 1134–5.

Baumgartner, W.A. and Mark, J.B.D. (1980), Metastatic malignancies from distant sites to the tracheobronchial tree. *J. Thorac. Cardiovasc. Surg.*, **79**, 499–503.

Becker, K.L. and Gazdar, A.F. (1984), *The Endocrine Lung in Health and Disease*, W.B. Saunders, Philadelphia and London.

Bégin, P., Sahai, S. and Wang, N.S. (1983), Giant cell formation in small cell carcinoma of the lung. *Cancer*, **52**, 1875–9.

Bensch, K.G., Corrin, B., Pariente, R. and Spencer, H. (1968), Oat cell carcinoma of the lung: its origin and relationship to bronchial carcinoid. *Cancer*, **22**, 1163–72.

Bensch, K.G., Gordon, G.B. and Miller, L.R. (1965), Electron microscopic and biochemical studies on the bronchial carcinoid tumor. *Cancer*, **18**, 592–602.

Bereton, H.D., Mathews, M.M., Costa, J., Kent, H. and Johnson, R.E. (1978), Mixed anaplastic small-cell and squamous cell carcinoma of the lung. *Ann. Int. Med.*, **88**, 805–6.

Berg, H.K., Petrelli, N.J., Herrera, L., Lopez, C. and Mittleman, A. (1984), Endobronchial metastasis from colorectal carcinoma. *Dis. Colon. Rectum.*, **27**, 745–8.

Berger, G., Berger, F., Bejui, F., Bouvier, R., Rochet, M. and Feroldi, J. (1984), Bronchial carcinoid with fibrillary inclusions related to cytokeratins: an immunohistochemical and ultrastructural study with subsequent investigation of 12 foregut APUDomas. *Histopathology*, **8**, 245–57.

Black, W.C. (1969), Pulmonary oncocytoma. *Cancer*, **23**, 1347–57.

Blobel, G.A., Moll, R., Franke, W.W. and Vogt-Moykopf, I. (1984), Cytokeratins in normal lung and lung carcinomas. *Virchows Arch. (Cell Pathol.)*, **45**, 407–29.

Blondal, T., Grimelius, L., Nöu, E., Wilander, E. and Aberg, T. (1980), Argyrophil carcinoid tumors of the lung. *Chest*, **78**, 840–4.

Bolen, J.W. and Thorning, D. (1982), Histogenetic classification of lung carcinomas. Small cell carcinomas studied by light and electron microscopy. *J. Submicrosc. Cytol.*, **14**, 499–514.

Bonofiglio, T.A. (1983), *Cytopathologic Interpretation of Transthoracic Fine-Needle Biopsies*, Masson Monographs in Diagnostic Cytopathology (ed. W.W. Johnston), Masson, New York.

Boon, M.E., Lindeman, J., Meeuwissen, A.L.J. and Otto, A.J. (1982), Carcinoembryonic antigen in sputum cytology. *Acta Cytol.*, **26**, 389–94.

Borowitz, M.J. and Stein, R.B. (1984), Diagnostic applications of monoclonal antibodies to human cancer. *Arch. Pathol. Lab. Med.*, **108**, 101–5.

Bostwick, D.G., Roth, K.A., Evans, C.J., Barchas, J.D. and Bensch, K.G. (1984), Gastrin-releasing peptide, a mammalian analog of bombesin, is present in human neuroendocrine lung tumors. *Amer. J. Pathol.*, **117**, 195–200.

Braman, S.S. and Whitcomb, M.E. (1975), Endobronchial metastasis. *Arch. Intern. Med.*, **135**, 543–7.

Capella, C., Gabrielli, M., Polak, J.M., Buffa, R., Solcia, E. and Bordi, C. (1979), Ultrastructural and histological study of 11 bronchial carcinoids. Evidence for different types. *Virchows Arch. (Pathol. Anat.)*, **381**, 313–29.

Carter, D. (1983) Small-cell carcinoma of the lung. *Amer. J. Surg. Path.*, **7**, 787–95.

Carter, D. and Eggleston, J.C. (1980), *Tumors of the Lower Respiratory Tract*, 2nd series, fascicle 17, Armed Forces Institute of Pathology, Washington, DC.

Cassiere, S.G., McLain, D.A., Emory, W.B. and Hatch, H.B. (1980), Metastatic carcinoma of the pancreas simulating primary bronchogenic carcinoma. *Cancer*, **46**, 2319–21.

Chaudhuri, M.R. (1970), Cavitary pulmonary metastases. *Thorax*, **25**, 375–81.

Chaudhuri, M.R. (1971), Bronchial carcinosarcoma. *J. Thorac. Cardiovasc. Surg.*, **61**, 319–23.

Chorba, T., Orenstein, J.M., Harisiadis, L., Moody, T., Burton, T. and Schulof, R.S. (1984), An atypical endocrine tumor of the lung responsive to radiation therapy and 5-fluorouracil-streptozotocin. *Cancer*, **53**, 2430–8.

Churg, A. (1977), Large spindle cell variant of peripheral bronchial carcinoid tumor. *Arch. Pathol. Lab. Med.*, **101**, 216–18.

Churg, A. (1978), The fine structure of large cell undifferentiated carcinoma of the lung. Evidence for its relation to squamous cell carcinomas and adenocarcinomas. *Human Pathol.*, **9**, 143–56.

Churg, A., Johnston, W.H. and Stulbarg, M. (1980), Small cell squamous and mixed small cell squamous-small cell anaplastic carcinomas of the lung. *Am. J. Surg. Path.*, **4**, 255–63.

Coleman, D.V., To, A., Ormerod, M.G. and Dearnaley, D.P. (1981), Immunoperoxidase staining in tumor marker distribution studies in cytologic specimens. *Acta Cytol.*, **25**, 205–6.

Conlan, A.A., Payne, W.S., Wollner, L.B. and Sanderson, D.R. (1978). Adenoid cystic carcinoma (cylindroma) and mucoepidermoid carcinoma of the bronchus. *J. Thorac. Cardiovasc. Surg.*, **76**, 369–77.

Coombes, R.C., Ellison, M.L. and Neville, A.M. (1978), Biochemical markers in bronchogenic carcinoma. Review article. *Br. J. Dis. Chest*, **72**, 263–87.

Cooney, T., Sweeney, E.C. and Luke, D. (1979), Pulmonary carcinoid tumours: a comparative regional study. *J. Clin. Pathol.*, **32**, 1100–9.

Corrin, B. (1980), Lung endocrine tumours. *Invest. Cell Pathol.*, **3**, 195–206.

Corson, J.M. and Pinkus, G.S. (1982), Mesothelioma: profile of keratin proteins and carcinoembryonic antigen. An immunoperoxidase study of 20 cases and comparison with pulmonary adenocarcinomas. *Amer. J. Pathol.*, **108**, 80–7.

Culling, C.F.A., Reid, P.E., Burton, J.D. and Dunn, W.L. (1975), A histochemical method of differentiating lower gastrointestinal tract mucin from other mucins in primary or metastatic tumours. *J. Clin. Path.*, **28**, 656–8.

Davis, P.W., Briggs, J.C., Seal, R.M.E. and Storring, F.K. (1972), Benign and malignant mixed tumours of the lung. *Thorax*, **27**, 657–73.

DeCaro, L.F., Paladugu, R., Benfield, J.R., Lovisatti, L., Pak, H. and Teplitz, R.L. (1983), Typical and atypical carcinoids within the pulmonary APUD tumor spectrum. *J. Thorac. Cardiovasc. Surg.*, **86**, 528–36.

Dingemans, K.P. and Mooi, W.J. (1984), Ultrastructure of squamous cell carcinoma of the lung. *Pathol. Ann.*, **19**, 249–73.

Dube, V.E. (1970), Peripheral bronchial carcinoid with a spindle-cell pattern. *Arch. Pathol.*, **89**, 374–7.

Edwards, C.W. and Matthews, H.R. (1981), Mucous gland adenoma of the bronchus. *Thorax*, **36**, 147–8.

Emory, W.B., Mitchell, W.T. and Hatch, H.B. (1973), Mucous gland adenoma of the bronchus. *Amer. Rev. Respir. Dis.*, **108**, 1407–10.

Erisman, M.D., Linnoila, R.I., Hernandez, O., *et al.* (1982), Human lung small-cell carcinoma contains bombesin. *Proc. Natl Acad. Sci.*, **79**, 2379–83.

Espinoza, C.G. and Azar, H.A. (1982), Immunohistochemical localization of keratin-type proteins in epithelial neoplasms. Correlation with electron microscopic findings. *Amer. J. Clin. Pathol.*, **78**, 500–7.

Fechner, R.E. and Bentinck, B.R. (1973), Ultrastructure of bronchial oncocytoma. *Cancer*, **31**, 1451–7.

Fechner, R.E., Bentinck, B.R. and Askew, J.B. (1972), Acinic cell tumor of the lung. A histologic and ultrastructural study. *Cancer*, **29**, 501–8.

Frank, A.L. (1978), Occupational lung cancer. In *Pathogenesis and Therapy of Lung Cancer* (ed. C.C. Harris), Marcel Dekker, New York, pp. 25–51.

Fraumeni, J.F. (1975), Respiratory carcinogenesis: an epidemiologic appraisal. *J. Natl Cancer Inst.*, **55**, 1039–46.

Frost, J.K., Erozan, Y.S., Gupta, P.K. and Carter, D. (1983), Cytopathology, Section 3. In *Atlas of Early Lung Cancer*, Igaku-Shoin, New York, Tokyo, pp. 39–76.

Gabbiani, G., Kapanci, Y., Barazzone, P. and Franke, W.W. (1981), Immunochemical identification of intermediate-sized filaments in human neoplastic cells. A diagnostic aid for the surgical pathologist. *Am. J. Pathol.*, **104**, 206–16.

Gazdar, A.F., Carney, D.N., Guccion, J.G. and Baylin, S.B. (1981), Small cell carcinoma of the lung. Cellular origin and relationship to other pulmonary cancers. In *Small Cell Lung Cancer* (eds F.A. Greco, R.K. Oldham and P.A. Bunn), Grune & Stratton, New York, pp. 145–75.

Gilman, R.A., Klassen, K.P. and Scarpelli, D.G. (1956), Mucous gland adenoma of bronchus. Report of a case with histochemical study of secretion. *Amer. J. Clin. Path.*, **26**, 151–4.

Gmelich, J.T., Bensch, K.G. and Liebow, A.A. (1967), Cells of Kultschitzky type in bronchioles and their relation to the origin of peripheral carcinoid tumor. *Lab. Invest.*, **17**, 88–98.

Godwin, J.D. (1975), Carcinoid tumors: an analysis of 2837 cases. *Cancer*, **36**, 560–9.

Goodner, J.T., Berg, J.W. and Watson, W.L. (1961), The nonbenign nature of bronchial carcinoids and cylindromas. *Cancer*, **14**, 539–46.

Goslin, R.H., O'Brien, M.J., Skarin, A.T. and Zamcheck, N. (1983), Immunocytochemical staining for CEA in small cell carcinoma of lung predicts clinical usefulness of the plasma assay. *Cancer*, **52**, 301–6.

Gould, V.E., Memoli, V.A. and Dardi, L.E. (1981), Multidirectional differentiation in human epithelial cancers. *J. Submicrosc. Cytol.*, **13**, 97–115.

Greenberg, B.E. and Young, J.M. (1958), Pulmonary metastasis from occult primary sites resembling bronchogenic carcinoma. *Dis. Chest*, **33**, 496–505.

Grimelius, L. (1968), A silver nitrate stain for α_2 cells in human pancreatic islets. *Acta. Soc. Med. Upsalien*, **73**, 243–70.

Gusterson, B., Mitchell, D., Warburton, M. and Sloane, J. (1982), Immunohistochemical localization of keratin in human lung tumours. *Virchows Arch. (Pathol. Anat.)*, **394**, 269–77.

Hage, E. (1973), Histochemistry and fine structure of bronchial carcinoid tumors. *Virchows Arch. (Pathol. Anat.)*, **361**, 121–8.

Harach, H.R., Skinner, M. and Gibbs, A.R. (1983), Biological markers in human lung carcinoma: an immunopathological study of six antigens. *Thorax*, **38**, 937–41.

Hashimoto, T., Fukuoka, M., Nagasawa, S., *et al.* (1979), Small cell carcinoma of the lung and its histological origin. *Am. J. Surg. Path.*, **3**, 343–51.

Hattori, S., Matsuda, M., Ikegami, H., Horai, T. and Takenaga, A. (1977), Small cell carcinoma of the lung: clinical and cytomorphological studies in relation to its response to chemotherapy. *Gann*, **68**, 321–31.

Hattori, S., Matsuda, M., Tateishi, R., Nishihara, H. and Horai, T. (1972), Oat cell carcinoma of the lung. Clinical and morphological studies in relation to its histogenesis. *Cancer*, **30**, 1014–24.

Hattori, S., Matsuda, M., Tateishi, R., Tatsumi, N. and Terazawa, T. (1968), Oat-cell carcinoma of the lung containing serotonin granules. *Gann*, **59**, 123–9.

Henderson, D.W. (1982), Editorial review. Asbestos-related pleuropulmonary diseases: asbestosis, mesothelioma and lung cancer. *Pathology*, **14**, 239–43.

Herrara, G.A., Alexander, C.B. and Jones, J.M. (1985) Ultra-structural characterization of pulmonary neoplasm. *Surv. Synth. Path. Res.*, **4**, 163–84.

Hess, F.G., McDowell, E.M., Resau, J.H. and Trump, B.F. (1981a), The respiratory epithelium. IX. Validity and reproducibility of revised cytologic criteria of human and hamster respiratory tract tumors. *Acta Cytol.*, **25**, 485–98.

Hess, F.G., McDowell, E.M. and Trump, B.F. (1981b), The respiratory epithelium. VIII. Interpretation of cytologic criteria for human and hamster respiratory tract tumors. *Acta Cytol.*, **25**, 111–34.

Hill, T.A., McDowell, E.M. and Trump, B.F. (1979), Localization of carcinoembryonic antigen (CEA) in normal, premalignant and malignant lung tissue. In *Carcino-Embryonic Proteins*, Vol. II (ed. F.G. Lehmann), Elsevier/North-Holland Biomedical Press, pp. 163–8.

Hirsch, F.R., Matthews, M.J. and Yesner, R. (1982), Histopathologic classification of small cell carcinoma of the lung. Comments based on an interobserver examination. *Cancer*, **50**, 1360–6.

Hirsch, F.R., Østerlind, K. and Hansen, H.H. (1983), The prognostic significance of histopathologic subtyping of small cell carcinoma of the lung according to the classification of the World Health Organization. *Cancer*, **52**, 2144–50.

Höfler, H. and Denk, H. (1984), Immunocytochemical demonstration of cytokeratin in gastrointestinal carcinoids and their probable precursor cells. *Virchows Arch. (Pathol. Anat.)*, **403**, 235–40.

Holden, J. and Churg, A. (1984), Immunohistochemical staining for keratin and carcinoembryonic antigen in the diagnosis of malignant mesothelioma. *Amer. J. Surg. Path.*, **8**, 277–9.

Horai, T., Sone, H., Takenaga, A., *et al.* (1981), Cytologic characteristics of oat cell carcinoma of the lung in relation to the effect of chemotherapy. *Cancer*, **47**, 22–6.

Horie, A. and Ohta, M. (1981), Ultrastructural features of large cell carcinoma of the lung with reference to the prognosis of patients. *Human Pathol.*, **12**, 423–32.

Hoshino, M. and Yamamoto, I. (1970), Ultrastructure of adenoid cystic carcinoma. *Cancer*, **25**, 186–98.

Jariwalla, A.G., Seaton, A., McCormack, R.J.M., Gibbs, A., Campbell, I.A. and Davies, B.H. (1981), Intrabronchial metastases from renal carcinoma with recurrent tumour expectoration. *Thorax*, **36**, 179–82.

Johnston, W.W. and Frable, W.J. (1979), *Diagnostic Respiratory Cytopathology*, Masson, New York.

Jones, R.A. and Dawson, I.M.P. (1977), Morphology and staining patterns of endocrine cell tumours of the gut, pancreas and bronchus and their possible significance. *Histopathology*, **1**, 137–50.

Kahn, H.J., Hanna, W., Yeger, H. and Baumal, R. (1982), Immunohistochemical localization of prekeratin filaments in benign and malignant cells in effusions. *Am. J. Pathol.*, **109**, 206–14.

Kameya, T., Shimosato, Y., Kodama, T., Tsumuraya, M., Koide, T., Yamaguchi, K. and Abe, K. (1983), Peptide hormone production by adenocarcinomas of the lung: its morphologic basis and histogenetic considerations. *Virchows Arch. (Pathol. Anat.)*, **400**, 245–57.

Kato, H., Konaka, C., Ono, J., Takahashi, M. and Hayata, Y. (1983), *Cytology of the Lung. Techniques and Interpretation*, Igaku-Shoin, Tokyo, New York.

Katz, D.R. and Bubis, J.J. (1976), Acinic cell tumor of the bronchus. *Cancer*, **38**, 830–2.

Katzenstein, A.A., Prioleau, P.G. and Askin, F.B. (1980), The histologic spectrum and significance of clear-cell change in lung carcinoma. *Cancer*, **45**, 943–7.

Katzenstein, A., Purvis, R., Gmelich, J. and Askin, F. (1978), Pulmonary resection for metastatic renal adenocarcinoma. Pathologic findings and therapeutic value. *Cancer*, **41**, 712–23.

King, T.E., Neff, T.A. and Ziporin, P. (1979), Endobronchial metastasis from the uterine cervix. Presentation as primary lung abscess. *J. Amer. Med. Assoc.*, **242**, 1651–2.

Klacsmann, P.G., Olson, J.L. and Eggleston, J.C. (1979), Mucoepidermoid carcinoma of the bronchus. An electron-microscopic study of low grade and the high grade variants. *Cancer*, **43**, 1720–33.

Kodama, T., Shimosato, Y. and Kameya, T. (1982), Histology and ultrastructure of bronchogenic and bronchial gland adenocarcinomas (including adenoid cystic and mucoepidermoid carcinomas) in relation to histogenesis. In *Morphogenesis of Lung Cancer*, Vol. 1 (eds Y. Shimosato, M.R. Melamed and P. Nettesheim), CRC Press, Boca Raton, Florida, pp. 147–65.

Koss, L.G. (1979), Cancer of the lung. In *Diagnostic Cytology and its Histopathologic Bases*, Vol. 2, 3rd edn, Lippincott, Philadelphia, pp. 607–86.

Kroe, D.J. and Pitcock, J.A. (1967), Benign mucous gland adenoma of the bronchus. *Arch. Path.*, **84**, 539–42.

Kwee, W.S., Veldhuizen, R.W., Golding, R.P., Mullink, H., Stam, J., Donner, R. and Boon, M.E. (1982), Histologic distinction between malignant mesothelioma, benign pleural lesion and carcinoma metastasis. *Virchows Arch. (Pathol. Anat.)*, **397**, 287–99.

Lauder, I., Holland, D., Mason, D.Y., Gowland, G. and Cunliffe, W.J. (1984), Identification of large cell undifferentiated tumours in lymph nodes using leucocyte common and keratin antibodies. *Histopathology*, **8**, 259–72.

Leonardi, H.K., Jung-Legg, Y., Legg, M.A. and Neptune, W.B. (1978), Tracheobronchial mucoepidermoid carcinoma. *J. Thorac. Cardiovasc. Surg.*, **76**, 431–8.

Leong, A. S.-Y. (1982), The relevance of ultrastructural examination in the classification of primary lung tumours. *Pathology*, **14**, 37–46.

Leong, A. S.-Y. and Canny, A.R. (1981), Small cell anaplastic carcinoma of the lung with glandular and squamous differentiation. *Am. J. Surg. Path.*, **5**, 307–9.

Li, W., Hammar, S.P., Jolly, P.C., Hill, L.D. and Anderson, R.P. (1981), Unpredictable course of small cell undifferentiated lung carcinoma. *J. Thorac. Cardiovasc. Surg.*, **81**, 34–43.

Mark, E.J., Quay, S.C. and Dickersin, G.R. (1981), Papillary carcinoid tumor of the lung. *Cancer*, **48**, 316–24.

Markel, S.F., Abell, M.R., Haight, C. and French, A.J. (1964), Neoplasms of bronchus commonly designated as adenomas. *Cancer*, **17**, 590–608.

Matthews, M.J. (1976), Problems in morphology and behavior of bronchopulmonary malignant disease. In *Lung Cancer. Natural History, Prognosis and Therapy* (eds L. Israel and A.P. Chahinian), Academic Press, New York, pp. 23–62.

Matthews, M.J. and Gordon, P.R. (1977), Morphology of pulmonary and pleural malignancies. In *Lung Cancer. Clinical Diagnosis and Treatment* (ed. M.J. Strauss), Grune & Stratton, New York, pp. 49–69.

Matthews, M.J. and Hirsch, F.R. (1981), Problems in the diagnosis of small cell carcinoma of the lung. In *Small Cell Lung Cancer* (eds F.A. Greco, R.K. Oldham and P.A. Bunn), Grune & Stratton, New York, pp. 35–50.

McBurney, R.P., Kirklin, J.W. and Woolner, L.B. (1953), Metastasizing bronchial adenomas. *Surg. Gynec. Obstet.*, **96**, 482–92.

McDowell, E.M., Barrett, L.A. and Trump, B.F. (1976), Observations on small granule cells in adult human bronchial epithelium and in carcinoid and oat cell tumors. *Lab. Invest.*, **34**, 202–6.

McDowell, E.M., Harris, C.C. and Trump, B.F. (1982), Histogenesis and morphogenesis of bronchial neoplasms. In *Morphogenesis of Lung Cancer*, Vol. 1 (eds Y. Shimosato, M.R. Melamed and P. Nettesheim), CRC Press, Boca Raton, Florida, pp. 1–36.

McDowell, E.M., McLaughlin, J.S., Merenyi, D.K., Kieffer, R.F., Harris, C.C. and Trump, B.F. (1978), The respiratory epithelium. V. Histogenesis of lung carcinomas in the human. *J. Natl Cancer Inst.*, **61**, 587–606.

McDowell, E.M., Sorokin, S.P., Hoyt, R.F. and Trump, B.F. (1981a), An unusual bronchial carcinoid tumor. Light and electron microscopy. *Human Pathol.*, **12**, 338–48.

McDowell, E.M. and Trump, B.F. (1981), Pulmonary small cell carcinoma showing tripartite differentiation in individual cells. *Human Pathol.*, **12**, 286–94.

McDowell, E.M., Wilson, T.S. and Trump, B.F. (1981b), Atypical endocrine tumors of the lung. *Arch. Pathol. Lab. Med.*, **105**, 20–8.

Mennemeyer, R., Hammar, S.P., Bauermeister, D.E., Wheelis, R.F., Jones, H.W. and Bartha, M. (1979), Cytologic, histologic and electron microscopic correlations in poorly differentiated primary lung carcinoma. A study of 43 cases. *Acta Cytol.*, **23**, 297–302.

Mills, S.E., Cooper, P.H., Walker, A.N. and Kron, I.L. (1982), Atypical carcinoid tumor of the lung. *Amer. J. Surg. Pathol.*, **6**, 643–54.

Mittman, C. and Bruderman, I. (1977), Lung cancer: to operate or not. State of the art. *Am. Rev. Resp. Dis.*, **116**, 477–96.

Miyamoto, H., Inoue, S., Abe, S., *et al.* (1982), Relationship between cytomorphologic features and prognosis in small cell carcinoma of the lung. *Acta Cytol.*, **26**, 429–33.

Moody, T.W., Pert, C.B., Gazdar, A.F., *et al.* (1981), High levels of intracellular bombesin characterize human small-cell lung cancer. *Science*, **214**, 1246–8.

Mountain, C.F. (1976), The relationship of prognosis to morphology and the anatomic extent of disease: studies of a new clinical staging system. In *Lung Cancer. Natural History, Prognosis and Therapy* (eds L. Israel and A.P. Chahinian), Academic Press, New York, pp. 107–40.

Mullins, J.D. and Barnes, R.P. (1979), Childhood bronchial mucoepidermoid tumors. *Cancer*, **44**, 315–22.

Munro Neville, A., Foster, C.S., Moshakis, V. and Gore, M. (1982), Monoclonal antibodies and human tumor pathology. *Human Pathol.*, **13**, 1067–81.

Nadji, M. (1980), The potential value of immunoperoxidase techniques in diagnostic cytology. *Acta Cytol.*, **24**, 442–7.

Nishiyama, T., Stolbach, L.L., Rule, A.H., DeLellis, R., Inglis, N.R. and Fishman, W.H. (1980), Expression of oncodevelopmental markers (Regan isozyme, β-HCG, CEA) in tumor tissues and uninvolved bronchial mucosa. An immunohistochemical study. *Acta Histochem. Cytochem.*, **13**, 245–53.

Nöu, E. (1981), Bronchial adenocarcinoma: the value of attempts to exclude other primary tumors for randomized studies in an epidemiologic material. *Cancer*, **48**, 2121–5.

Okike, N., Bernatz, P.E. and Woolner, L.B. (1976), Carcinoid tumors of the lung. *Ann. Thoracic Surg.*, **22**, 270–7.

Osborn, M. and Weber, K. (1983), Biology of disease. Tumor diagnosis by intermediate filament typing: a novel tool for surgical pathology. *Lab. Invest.*, **48**, 372–94.

Pascal, R.R., Mesa-Tejada, R., Bennett, S.J., Garces, A. and Fenoglio, C.M. (1977), Carcinoembryonic antigen. *Arch. Pathol. Lab. Med.*, **101**, 568–71.

Payne, W.S., Ellis, F.H., Woolner, L.B. and Moersch, H.J. (1959), The surgical treatment of cylindroma (adenoid cystic carcinoma) and mucoepidermoid tumours of the bronchus. *J. Thoracic. Cardiovasc. Surg.*, **38**, 709–26.

Payne, W.S., Schier, J. and Woolner, L.B. (1965), Mixed tumors of the bronchus (salivary gland type). *J. Thorac. Cardiovasc. Surg.*, **49**, 663–8.

Pedraza, M.A., Mason, D., Doslu, F.A., Marsh, R.A. and Hoffman, E. (1984), High resolution microscopy of lung and intrathoracic tumors. *Arch. Pathol. Lab. Med.*, **108**, 152–5.

Perrone, T.L. and Dickersin, G.R. (1983), Ultrastructure of a bronchial mucoepidermoid carcinoma. *Human Pathol.*, **14**, 1011–12.

Pritchett, P.S. and Key, B.M. (1978), Mucous gland adenoma of the bronchus: ultrastructural and histochemical studies. *Ala. J. Med. Sci.*, **15**, 43–8.

Prive, L., Tellem, M., Meranze, D.R. and Chodoff, R.D. (1961), Carcinosarcoma of the lung. *Arch. Path.*, **72**, 351–7.

Radice, P.A., Matthews, M.J., Ihde, D.C., *et al.* (1982), The clinical behavior of 'mixed' small cell/large cell bronchogenic carcinoma compared to 'pure' small cell subtypes. *Cancer*, **50**, 2894–902.

Ramaekers, F., Puts, J., Moesker, O., Kant, A., Jap, A. and Vooijs, P. (1983), Demonstration of keratin in human adenocarcinomas. *Amer. J. Pathol.*, **111**, 213–23.

Ramsey, J.H. and Reimann, D.L. (1953), Bronchial adenomas arising in mucous glands. Illustrative case. *Amer. J. Pathol.*, **29**, 339–51.

Ratcliffe, J.G. (1982), Hormone markers in lung cancer. In *Markers for Diagnosis and Monitoring of Human Cancer*, Vol. 46, Serono Symposia (eds M.I. Colnaghi, G.L. Buraggi and M. Ghione), Academic Press, New York, pp. 85–94.

Reid, J.D. (1963), The classification of lung cancer. *Aust. & New Zealand J. Surg.*, **32**, 239–43.

Reid, J.D. and Carr, A.H. (1961), The validity and value of histological and cytological classifications of lung cancer. *Cancer*, **14**, 673–98.

Roggli, V.L., Vollmer, R.T., Greenberg, S.D., McGavran, M.H., Spjut, H.J. and Yesner, R. (1985), Lung cancer heterogeneity: a blinded and randomized study of 100 consecutive cases. *Human Pathol.*, **16**, 569–579.

Rosenblatt, M.B., Lisa, J.R. and Trinidad, S. (1966), Pitfalls in the clinical and histologic diagnosis of bronchogenic carcinoma. *Dis. Chest*, **49**, 396–404.

Saba, S.R., Azar, H.A., Richman, A.V., *et al.* (1981), Dual differentiation in small cell carcinoma (oat cell carcinoma) of the lung. *Ultrastruct. Pathol.*, **2**, 131–8.

Saccomanno, G. (1978), *Diagnostic Pulmonary Cytology*, ASCP Press.

Said, J.W., Nash, G., Sassoon, A.F., Shintaku, I.P. and Banks-Schlegel, S.P. (1983a), Involucrin in lung tumors. A specific marker for squamous differentiation. *Lab. Invest.*, **49**, 563–8.

Said, J.W., Nash, G., Tepper, G. and Banks-Schlegel, S. (1983b), Keratin proteins and carcinoembryonic antigen in lung carcinoma. An immunoperoxidase study of fifty-four cases, with ultrastructural correlations. *Human Pathol.*, **14**, 70–6.

Sajjad, S.M., Mackay, B. and Lukeman, J.M. (1980), Oncocytic carcinoid tumor of the lung. *Ultrastruct. Pathol.*, **1**, 171–6.

Salyer, D.C., Salyer, W.R. and Eggleston, J.C. (1975), Bronchial carcinoid tumors. *Cancer*, **36**, 1522–37.

Santoz-Briz, A., Terrón, J., Sastre, R., Romero, L. and Valle, A. (1977), Oncocytoma of the lung. *Cancer*, **40**, 1330–6.

Scharifker, D. and Marchevsky, A. (1981), Oncocytic carcinoid of the lung. *Cancer*, **47**, 530–2.

Sehested, M., Hirsch, F.R. and Hou-Jensen, K. (1981), Immunoperoxidase staining for carcinoembryonic antigen in small cell carcinoma of the lung. *Europ. J. Cancer Oncol.*, **17**, 1125–31.

Shepherd, M.P. (1982), Endobronchial metastatic disease. *Thorax*, **37**, 362–5.

Sheppard, M.N., Corrin, B., Bennett, M.H., Marangos, P.J., Bloom, S.R. and Polak, J.M. (1984), Immunocytochemical localization of neuron specific enolase in small cell carcinomas and carcinoid tumours of the lung. *Histopathology*, **8**, 171–81.

Shimosato, Y. (1980), Pathology of lung cancer. In *Lung Cancer, 1980, II World Congress on Lung Cancer* (eds H.H. Hansen and M. Rørth), Excerpta Medica, Amsterdam, pp. 27–48.

Sidhu, G.S. (1979), The endodermal origin of digestive and respiratory tract APUD cells. *Am. J. Pathol.*, **96**, 5–20.

Sklar, J.L., Churg, A. and Bensch, K.G. (1980), Oncocytic carcinoid tumor of the lung. *Amer. J. Surg. Path.*, **4**, 287–92.

Smith, P.S. and McClure, J. (1982), A papillary endobronchial tumor with a transitional cell pattern. *Arch. Pathol. Lab. Med.*, **106**, 503–6.

Sniffen, R.C., Soutter, L. and Robbins, L.L. (1958), Muco-epidermoid tumors of the bronchus arising from surface epithelium. *Am. J. Pathol.*, **34**, 671–83.

Sobin, L.H. (1972), Multiplicity of lung tumour classifications. *Rec. Results Cancer Res.*, **39**, 29–35.

Sobin, L.H. (1983), The histologic classification of lung tumors. The need for a double standard. *Human Pathol.*, **14**, 1020–1.

Solcia, E., Vassallo, G. and Capella, C. (1968), Selective staining of endocrine cells by basic dyes after acid hydrolysis. *Stain Tech.*, **43**, 257–63.

Sorenson, G.D., Bloom, S.R., Ghatei, M.A., *et al.* (1982), Bombesin production by human small cell carcinoma of the lung. *Regulatory Peptides*, **4**, 59–66.

Sorokin, S.P. and Hoyt, R.F. (1978), PAS-lead hematoxylin as a stain for small-granule endocrine cell populations in the lungs, other pharyngeal derivatives and the gut. *Anat. Rec.*, **192**, 245–59.

Sorokin, S.P., Hoyt, R.F. and McDowell, E.M. (1981), An unusual bronchial carcinoid tumor analyzed by conjunctive staining. *Human Pathol.*, **12**, 302–13.

Spencer, H. (1977), *Pathology of the Lung*, Vol. 2, Pergamon Press, New York.

Spencer, H. (1979), Bronchial mucous gland tumours. *Virchows Arch. A Path. Anat.*, **383**, 101–15.

Spencer, H., Dail, D.H. and Arneaud, J. (1980), Non-invasive bronchial epithelial papillary tumors. *Cancer*, **45**, 1486–97.

Springall, D.R., Lackie, P., Levene, M.M., Marangos, P.J. and Polak, J.M. (1984), Immunostaining of neuron-specific enolase is a valuable aid to the cytological diagnosis of neuroendocrine tumours of the lung. *J. Pathol.*, **143**, 259–66.

Stafford, J.R., Pollock, W.J. and Wenzel, B.C. (1984), Oncocytic mucoepidermoid tumor of the bronchus. *Cancer*, **54**, 94–9.

Steele, R.H. (1983), Lung tumours: a personal review. *Diagn. Histopathol.*, **6**, 119–69.

Straus, M.J. (1983), *Lung Cancer. Clinical Diagnosis and Treatment*, 2nd edn (ed. M.J. Straus), Grune and Stratton, New York.

Sweeney, E.C. and Cooney, T. (1978), Mucin-producing atypical carcinoid. *J. Clin.*

Pathol., **31**, 1218–25.

Tapia, F.J., Polak, J.M., Barbosa, A.J.A., Bloom, S.R., Marangos, P.J., Dermody, C. and Pearse, A.G.E. (1981), Neuron specific enolase is produced by neuroendocrine tumours. *Lancet*, **i**, 808–11.

Tateishi, R., Horai, T. and Hattori, S. (1978) Demonstration of argyrophil granules in small cell carcinoma of the lung. *Virchows Arch. A Path. Anat.*, **377**, 203–10.

Trinidad, S., Lisa, J.R. and Rosenblatt, M.B. (1963), Bronchogenic carcinoma simulated by metastatic tumors. *Cancer*, **16**, 1521–9.

Valaitis, J., Warren, S. and Gamble, D. (1981), Increasing incidence of adenocarcinoma of the lung. *Cancer*, **47**, 1042–6.

Vincent, R.G., Pickren, J.W., Lane, W.W., Bross, I., Takita, H., Houten, L., Gutierrez, A.C. and Rzepka, T. (1977), The changing histopathology of lung cancer. A review of 1682 cases. *Cancer*, **39**, 1647–55.

Vollmer, R.T. (1982), The effect of cell size on the pathologic diagnosis of small and large cell carcinomas of the lung. *Cancer*, **50**, 1380–3.

Wachner, R., Wittekind, C. and von Kleist, S. (1984), Localisation of CEA, β-HCG, SP1, and keratin in the tissue of lung carcinomas. An immunohistochemical study. *Virchows Arch. (Pathol. Anat.)*, **402**, 415–23.

Walter, P., Warter, A. and Morand, G. (1978), Bronchial oncocytic carcinoid. Histological, histochemical and ultrastuctural study. *Virchows Arch. A Path. Anat.*, **379**, 85–97.

Walts, A.E. and Said, J.W. (1983), Specific tumor markers in diagnostic cytology. *Acta Cytol.*, **27**, 408–16.

Walts, A.E., Said, J.W. and Banks-Schlegel, S. (1983), Keratin and carcinoembryonic antigen in exfoliated mesothelial and malignant cells: an immunoperoxidase study. *Amer. J. Clin. Pathol.*, **80**, 671–6.

Wang, N.S., Huang, S.N. and Gold, P. (1979), Absence of carcinoembryonic antigen-like material in mesothelioma. An immunocytochemical differentiation from other lung cancers. *Cancer*, **44**, 937–43.

Warren, W.H., Memoli, V.A. and Gould, V.E. (1984a), Immunohistochemical and ultrastructural analysis of bronchopulmonary neuroendocrine neoplasms. I. Carcinoids. *Ultrastructural Path.*, **6**, 15–27.

Warren, W.H., Memoli, V.A., Kittle, C.F., Jensik, R.J., Farber, L.P. and Gould, V.E. (1984b), The biological implications of bronchial tumors. *J. Thorac. Cardiovasc. Surg.*, **87**, 274–82.

Warter, A., Walter, P., Sabountchi, M. and Jory, A. (1981), Oncocytic bronchial adenoma. Histological, histochemical and ultrastructural study. *Virchows Arch. (Pathol. Anat.)*, **392**, 231–9.

Wharton, J., Polak, J.M., Bloom, S.R., *et al.* (1978), Bombesin-like immunoreactivity in the lung. *Nature*, **273**, 769–70.

Whitaker, D., Sterrett, G.-F. and Shilkin, K.B. (1982), Detection of tissue CEA-like substance as an aid in the differential diagnosis of malignant mesothelioma. *Pathology*, **14**, 255–8.

Wick, M.R., Scheithauer, W. and Kovacs, K. (1983), Neuron-specific enolase in neuroendocrine tumors of the thymus, bronchus and skin. *Amer. J. Clin. Path.*, **79**, 703–7.

Willis, R.A. (1961), The incidence and histological types of pulmonary carcinoma, with comments on some fallacies and uncertainties. *Med. J. Aust.*, **1**, 433–40.

Wilson, T.S. (1984), Immunohistochemical studies of lung tumor markers. Ph.D. dissertation. University of Maryland, School of Medicine, Baltimore, USA.

Wilson, T.S., McDowell, E.M., Marangos, P.J. and Trump, B.F. (1985) Histochemical studies of dense-cone granulated tumors of the lung. *Arch. Pathol. Lab. Med.*, **109**, 613–20.

Wise, W.S., Bonder, D., Aikawa, M. and Hsieh, C.L. (1982), Carcinoid tumor of lung with varied histology. *Am. J. Surg. Path.*, **6**, 261–7.

Woolner, L.B. (1983), Pathology of cancers detected cytologically, Section 5. In *Atlas of Early Lung Cancer*, Igaku-Shoin, New York, Tokyo, pp. 107–213.

World Health Organization (1981), *Histological Typing of Lung Tumours*, 2nd edn. International Histological Classification of Tumours, no. 1, WHO, Geneva.

Yang, K., Ulich, T., Taylor, I., Cheng, L. and Lewin, K.J. (1983), Pulmonary carcinoids. Immunohistochemical demonstration of brain-gut peptides. *Cancer*, **52**, 819–23.

Yesner, R. (1974), Histologic typing of lung cancer with clinical implications. In *Front. Radiation Ther. Onc.*, Vol. 9, Karger, Basel, pp. 140–50.

Yesner, R. (1981), The dynamic histopathologic spectrum of lung cancer. *Yale J. Biol. Med.*, **54**, 447–86.

Yesner, R. (1983), Small cell tumors of the lung. *Amer. J. Surg. Path.*, **7**, 775–85.

11 Nonepithelial neoplasms

Nonepithelial neoplasms of the bronchi are rare. The histological appearance of these neoplasms does not differ from that of their more common extrapulmonary counterparts. Whimster (1983) has published a comprehensive annotated bibliography of the lower respiratory tract neoplasms, which includes listings of endobronchial cases and reviews. In this chapter the various nonepithelial neoplasms and some of the non-neoplastic lesions which may be confused with them will be discussed briefly.

Although fiberoptic bronchoscopy has increased the number of cases diagnosed by endobronchial biopsy (both by increasing the number of patients examined and by facilitation of the biopsy of lesions in the peripheral bronchi), the yield is not as good as it is with the epithelial neoplasms. Comments on bronchial biopsy findings were included in 108 of the case reports of endobronchial nonepithelial neoplasms reviewed for this chapter. Of these only 52 (48%) had diagnostic material in the biopsy. Two of these cases, which were interpreted as benign on bronchial biopsy, were eventually found to be malignant.

Essentially any neoplasm may be metastatic to lung and be included in bronchial biopsies or cytology smears. Some present as submucosal metastases and appear to the bronchoscopist as primary neoplasms. In these cases the recognition of the metastatic nature of the neoplasms must be based on clinical or radiological data and rarely is there a clue in the biopsy histopathology. Fortunately, the number of biopsies of metastatic neoplasms is very small. Albertini and Ekberg (1980) reported only 10 out of 1200 bronchoscopic biopsies were metastatic disease, and in a series of 90 patients with endobronchial metastases only 1 was a sarcoma (Shepherd, 1982).

The cytopathological diagnosis of nonepithelial neoplasms of the bronchus is reported, but difficult. Koss (1979) comments that identification of sarcoma cells in sputa is exceedingly rare and only occurs after the mucosa has ulcerated over the tumor. Takeda and Burechailo (1969) describe the potential pitfall of diagnosing exfoliated smooth muscle cells from an ulcerated bronchial wall as neoplastic.

368

11.1 Benign neoplasms

Endobronchial benign tumors are rarely encountered even in a large hospital practice (Arrigoni *et al.*, 1970; Roviaro *et al.*, 1981; Halttunen *et al.*, 1982). Whimster (1983) includes fibromas, hamartomas, histiocytomas, leiomyomas, lipomas, neurofibromas and teratomas. Cases present either with cough, wheezing, hemoptysis, signs and symptoms of distal lesions secondary to bronchial obstruction, or as incidental findings on chest x-ray (Miller, 1969). Treatment of benign endobronchial nonepithelial neoplasms is frequently endoscopical excision by multiple biopsies and follow-up for removal of recurrences. Halttunen *et al.* (1982) argue that more extensive surgical excision is warranted in some cases.

11.1.1 Fibromas

Halttunen *et al.* (1982) found reports of 22 cases of endobronchial fibroma. Engelman (1967) described one endobronchial fibroma, commenting that they tend to grow slowly as polypoid masses and that calcification is likely. Corona and Okeson (1974) report a case which was removed endoscopically, only to recur 5 months later necessitating a lobectomy. Normal respiratory epithelium usually covers the tumors.

11.1.2 Hamartomas

Miller (1969) found reports of 53 chondromatous hamartomas of endobronchial type. Arrigoni *et al.* (1970) and Roviaro *et al.* (1981) each had 3 in their experiences. The parenchymal chondromatous hamartoma is of course much more common than this and Bateson (1965 and 1973) makes a strong argument that the parenchymal form is actually of bronchial origin. This concept was subsequently supported by an analysis of 17 endobronchial cases (Tomashefski, 1982). Case reports of endobronchial 'chondromas' (Kaufman, 1969; Walsh and Healy, 1969; Brewster *et al.*, 1975) and 4 hamartomas which had adipose tissue as well as cartilage and epithelial cells (Butler and Kleinerman, 1969) point out the difficulty in classifying these lesions. Bronchial adenomas with ossification are also reported (Thomas and Morgan, 1958). Therefore, one person's adenoma may be another person's hamartoma or even a teratoma. There is a slight male predominance in the reported cases.

11.1.3 Histiocytomas

Pure tumors of 'histiocytes' must be remarkably rare. Bates *et al.* (1976) report an endobronchial polyp composed of spindle-shaped cells that they called histiocytes. In another case, a mass which obstructed a main bronchus of a 6-year-old boy was diagnosed by bronchoscopic biopsy. The boy was treated by pneumonectomy and was without recurrence 5 years later when he died of pneumonia (Bates and Hull, 1958). Katzenstein and Maurer (1979) describe a convincing case of parenchymal pure 'histiocytic' tumor. The endobronchial lesion described by Herczeg *et al.* (1978) may belong with these (although Liebow had interpreted the case as a plasma cell granuloma (Section 11.3.1). Herczeg *et al.* felt it was a form of inflammatory fibrous histiocytoma related to the group described by Kyriakos and Kempson (1976) as an aggressive fibrous histiocytoma.

11.1.4   *Leiomyoma*

Halttunen *et al.* (1982) included 21 cases of leiomyoma in their review. Shahian and MacEnany (1979) report a case arising from the wall of the left main bronchus which they were able to successfully treat with bronchoscopic forceps excision. Most of the recently reported cases have been treated with lobectomy (Laustela *et al.*, 1974; Vera-Román *et al.*, 1983) or bronchial resection (Halttunen *et al.*, 1982). Early reviews indicated a strong female predominance (Guida *et al.*, 1965); however, Vera-Román *et al.* (1983) caution that metastases from low grade leiomyosarcomas, misinterpreted as benign, could have caused this skew.

11.1.5   *Lipoma*

This is the most common benign soft tissue tumor of bronchus (Miller, 1969; Halttunen *et al.*, 1982). The review of Politis *et al.* (1979) which includes all intrathoracic lipomas is the most extensive. There is a strong male predominance (MacArthur *et al.*, 1977; Medelli *et al.*, 1980). Squamous (epidermoid) metaplasia of the overlying respiratory epithelium is very common (Hakimi *et al.*, 1975; Zafirakopoulos *et al.*, 1977; Guidice *et al.*, 1980; Farsad and Makoui, 1981; Ovil *et al.*, 1982), although not universal (Fig. 11.1). Crutcher *et al.* (1968) described a case in which the adipose tissue extended into the peribronchial tissues; nevertheless they recommended endobronchial removal and continued observation for recurrences. Bellin *et al.* (1971) report one case with 'metaplastic' cartilage in the tumor.

11.1.6   *Benign teratoma*

Bateson *et al.* (1968) and Jamieson and McGowan (1982) have each reported single cases of endobronchial teratomas. These were polypoid lesions with benign representatives of all embryonic cell lines. The tera-

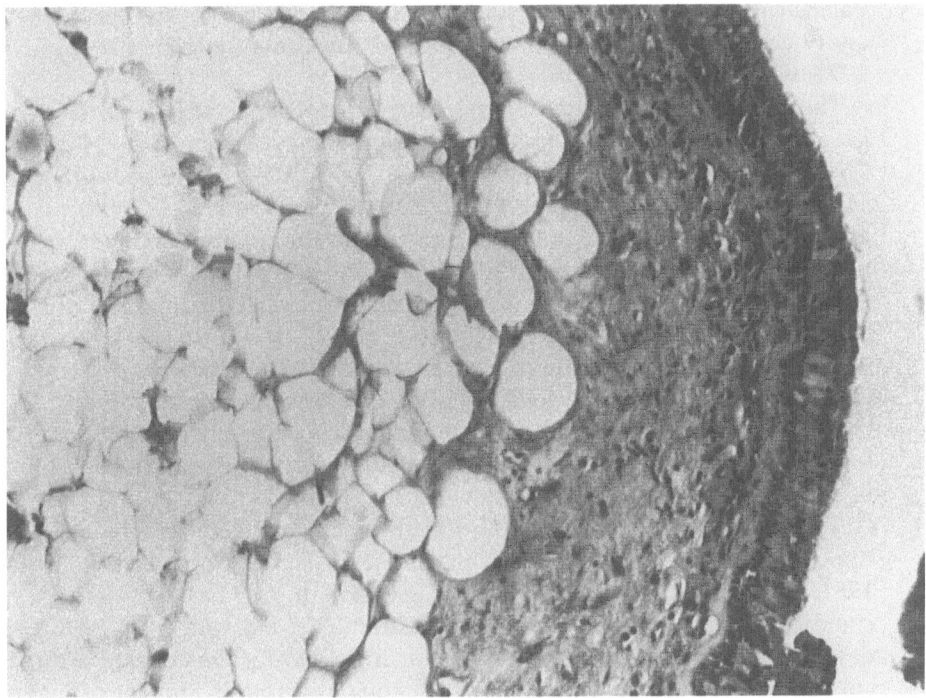

Fig. 11.1 Bronchial lipoma. Mucociliary respiratory epithelium covers this mass of mature adipose tissue. The tumor appeared as a smooth polypoid lesion on the wall of the bronchus and was removed with multiple forceps excision. (Paraffin section stained with hematoxylin and eosin: × 180.)

tomas were covered with respiratory epithelium. Both cases were treated with lobectomy.

11.1.7 Miscellaneous benign neoplasms

Sclerosing hemangiomas of the lung are well reviewed by Katzenstein *et al.* (1980). None has been endobronchial. Harding *et al.* (1978) describe a bronchial pedunculated capillary hemangioma. This lesion would be very difficult to distinguish from a pyogenic granuloma in bronchial biopsy (Section 5.14).

11.2 Granular cell tumor

Granular cell tumor (myoblastoma) is a condition found virtually at any site in the body (Sobel and Marquet, 1974). About 10% of the reported cases are associated with the tracheobronchial tree (DeClercq *et al.*, 1983).

Valenstein and Thurer (1978) found 47 bronchial cases in the literature and 9 additional cases have been reported subsequently (Dabouis *et al.*, 1979; Glant *et al.*, 1979).

The lesion is characterized by a proliferation of large, somewhat elongated cells with distinctly granular eosinophilic cytoplasm (Fig. 11.2a). The cytoplasm is filled with a heterogeneous population of inclusions (Fig. 11.2b) which are lysosomal and probably autophagosomal (Korompai *et al.*, 1974). These inclusions, which are responsible for the granular appearance by light microscopy, are PAS positive. The overlying epithelium is frequently metaplastic and pseudocarcinomatous hyperplasia of this epithelium is often prominent (Glant *et al.*, 1979).

One of the unusual features of these lesions is the tendency of some cases to be multifocal. Multifocal endobronchial lesions were described by Cooper and Arora (1982). Concurrent, bronchial, cutaneous and oral lesions were reported by Majmudar *et al.* (1981). Subsequent development of cutaneous granular cell tumors were described by Weitzner and Oser (1968) and Korompai *et al.* (1974). Extrathoracic malignant granular cell tumors have been reported with metastases in lung (Robertson *et al.*, 1981; Steffelaar *et al.*, 1982), emphasizing that multifocal bronchial lesions could be primary or metastatic from a distant site. Hurwitz *et al.* (1982) describe a case with granular cell tumor in left bronchus covered with epidermoid (squamous) pseudocarcinomatous hyperplasia and coexisting invasive epidermoid (squamous) carcinoma of the right bronchus.

Treatment of the benign bronchial granular cell tumors has been variable. Brown (1950) suggested bronchotomy which would allow inspection for extrabronchial extension. For the same reason Oparah and Subramanian (1976) suggested open surgical resection. In a thorough discussion of treatment in these cases Daniel *et al.* (1980) recommended a graded approach depending on the size of the lesion, the presence of parenchymal complications of bronchial obstruction, and multicentricity. Follow-up for local recurrences and subsequent lesions at other sites is clearly indicated in all cases.

Fig. 11.2   Granular cell tumor. (a) These plump, somewhat elongated cells accumulated in the submucosa and formed a slightly elevated mound, although they have been reported as flat or polypoid masses. The cytoplasm of the cells is abundant, granular and brightly eosinophilic. (Paraffin section stained with hematoxylin and eosin: × 710.) (b) The cytoplasmic characteristics are an expression of numerous pleomorphic lysosomal inclusions shown here in one small portion of the cell. The inclusions contain myelin figures, granules, microspherical particles and filamentous material. (Electron micrograph: × 8400.)

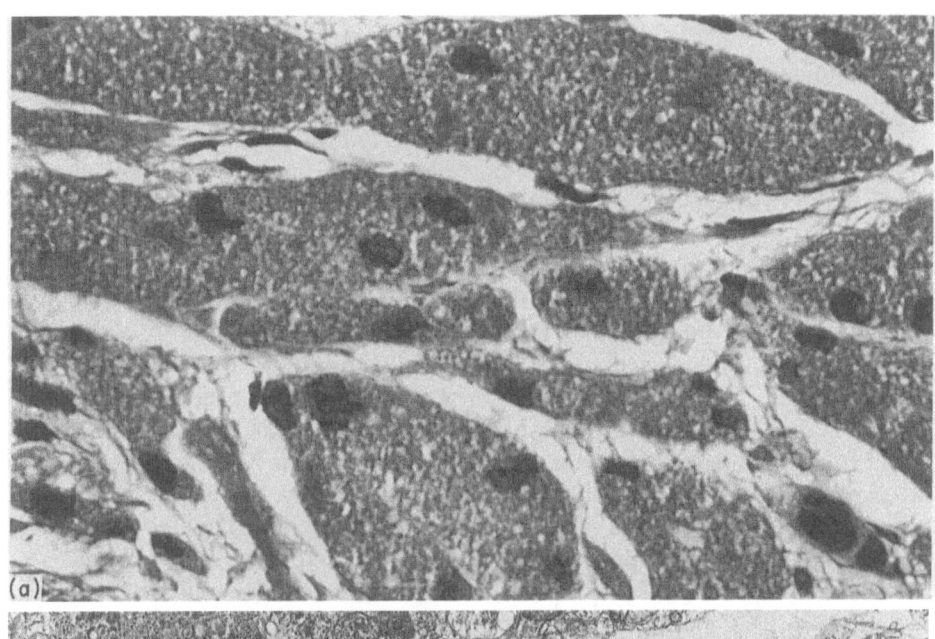

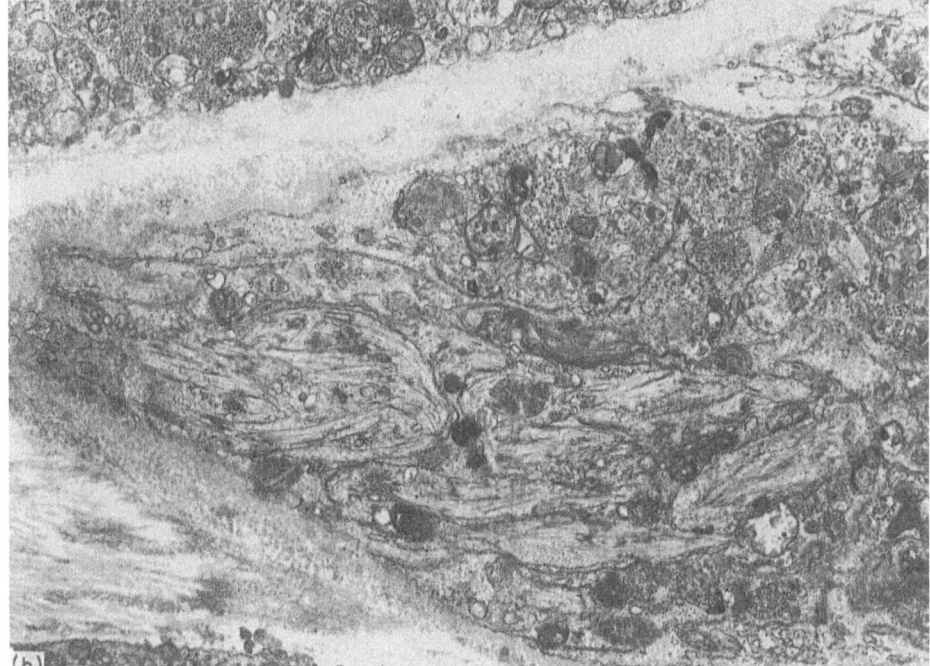

11.3   Lymphoma

Our understanding of cases of pulmonary lymphoid masses has progressed through three periods. Prior to 1963 mass lesions dominated by large numbers of lymphoid cells were classified as lymphomas. Saltzstein (1963) reviewed cases of primary lymphocytic tumors of the lung and concluded that the cases cited in the literature and his own cases were a mixture of true neoplasms and benign infiltrates. He chose to classify them as *pulmonary malignant lymphoma* and as *pseudolymphoma*. Others, concurring with the idea that the infiltrates were fundamentally different, joined in the attempt to distinguish the benign and malignant cases (Al-Saleem and Peale, 1969; Greenberg *et al.*, 1972; Julsrud *et al.*, 1978; Colby and Carrington, 1983a). Concepts centered on the monomorphous nature of the malignant cellular infiltrate versus the pleomorphic cellular character of the benign pseudolymphomas. The presence of true lymphoid germinal centers was considered definite evidence of benignity. Colby and Carrington (1983a) emphasized the peribronchial and perivascular (in the lymphatics) pattern of lymphomatous spread and the presence of scarring in pseudolymphomas. Lymph node involvement was generally acknowledged to be a manifestation of true lymphomas. One practical difficulty was the common finding of inflammatory reactions at the margins of expanding lymphomas. The literature during this period (1963–1981) becomes obscure, as some authors explain that prior reports of pseudolymphomas were undoubtedly true lymphomas and several reports included cases of pseudolymphoma which had 'progressed' to lymphoma (Greenberg *et al.*, 1972; Julsrud *et al.*, 1978; Richmond *et al.*, 1981).

Currently, our understanding results from the use of immunological markers to assess the cellular homogeneity of lymphomatous infiltrates, rather than relying solely on the histological patterns (Lipper *et al.*, 1980; Feoli *et al.*, 1981; Colby and Carrington, 1983b). As these immunohistological studies are more widely utilized we may resolve some of the diagnostic ambiguity of these lesions. The ultimate confusion arises from data which suggest that patients with pseudolymphoma of the lung may have a more progressive and rapidly fatal outcome than those patients with lymphocytic lymphoma (Al-Saleem and Peale, 1969; Gibbs and Seal, 1978; Marchevsky *et al.*, 1983).

11.3.1   *Non-neoplastic tumors of lymphoid cells*

Continued use of immunohistological methods on new cases will undoubtedly demonstrate that some lymphoid lesions, which present as bronchial masses, are truly non-neoplastic. Plasma cell granulomas, a term introduced by Bahadori and Liebow (1973), are occasionally bronchial in origin (Buell *et al.*, 1976). It may, however, be virtually impossible to preclude malignancy on the basis of bronchial biopsy specimens. Even polyclonal immunological patterns may reflect only the inflammatory margin of a deeper lymphoma.

11.3.2 Hodgkin's disease

Primary Hodgkin's lymphoma of lung is uncommon (Sternberg *et al.*, 1959; Kern *et al.*, 1961; Colby and Carrington, 1983a; Nelson *et al.*, 1983) and diagnosis by bronchoscopy is rare since most of the lesions are parenchymal.

Extension of Hodgkin's disease to the lung is common. Diagnosis by bronchial biopsy is usually in an attempt to identify the cause of radiologically detected pulmonary infiltrates in a patient with known Hodgkin's disease (Gribetz *et al.*, 1980; Nash, 1982; Canham *et al.*, 1983).

11.3.3 Non-Hodgkin's lymphoma

Primary lymphomas of the lung are rare. In their review in 1951, Beck and Reganis found 15 cases, only one of which had a diagnostic bronchoscopic biopsy. As pathologists sort through the cases of pulmonary nodular lymphocytic infiltrates (discussed in the introduction of Section 11.3), the frequency of primary lymphomas has apparently increased and current reviews include larger series (Greenberg *et al.*, 1972; Gibbs and Seal, 1978; Julsrud *et al.*, 1978; Colby and Carrington, 1983b; Marchevsky *et al.*, 1983). Most of these lymphomas are the well-differentiated lymphocytic type but plasmacytoid (Fig. 11.3) and poorly-differentiated forms are also seen. The bronchial wall is frequently involved, presumably in the lymphatics, but diagnosis by bronchial biopsy is uncommon. Extension of a monomorphous infiltrate of lymphoid cells into the bronchial cartilage is suggestive of lymphoma (Greenberg *et al.*, 1972).

Pulmonary involvement in generalized lymphoma is frequent and extension of lymphoma into the bronchial wall can be diagnosed during the work-up of patients with pulmonary infiltrates (Bank *et al.*, 1980; Philips *et al.*, 1980; Canham *et al.*, 1983; Gallagher *et al.*, 1983). Tenholder *et al.* (1982) reported a case of endobronchial metastatic plasmacytoma.

11.3.4 Lymphomatoid granulomatosis

Lymphomatoid granulomatosis has been discussed in Section 6.5.8 and Section 8.5. This lesion, originally thought to be inflammatory, is now considered to be an expression of malignant lymphoma, the lymphoproliferative process dominating or even obscuring the true lymphoma (Colby and Carrington, 1982; Fauci *et al.*, 1982; Churg, 1983; Colby and Carring-

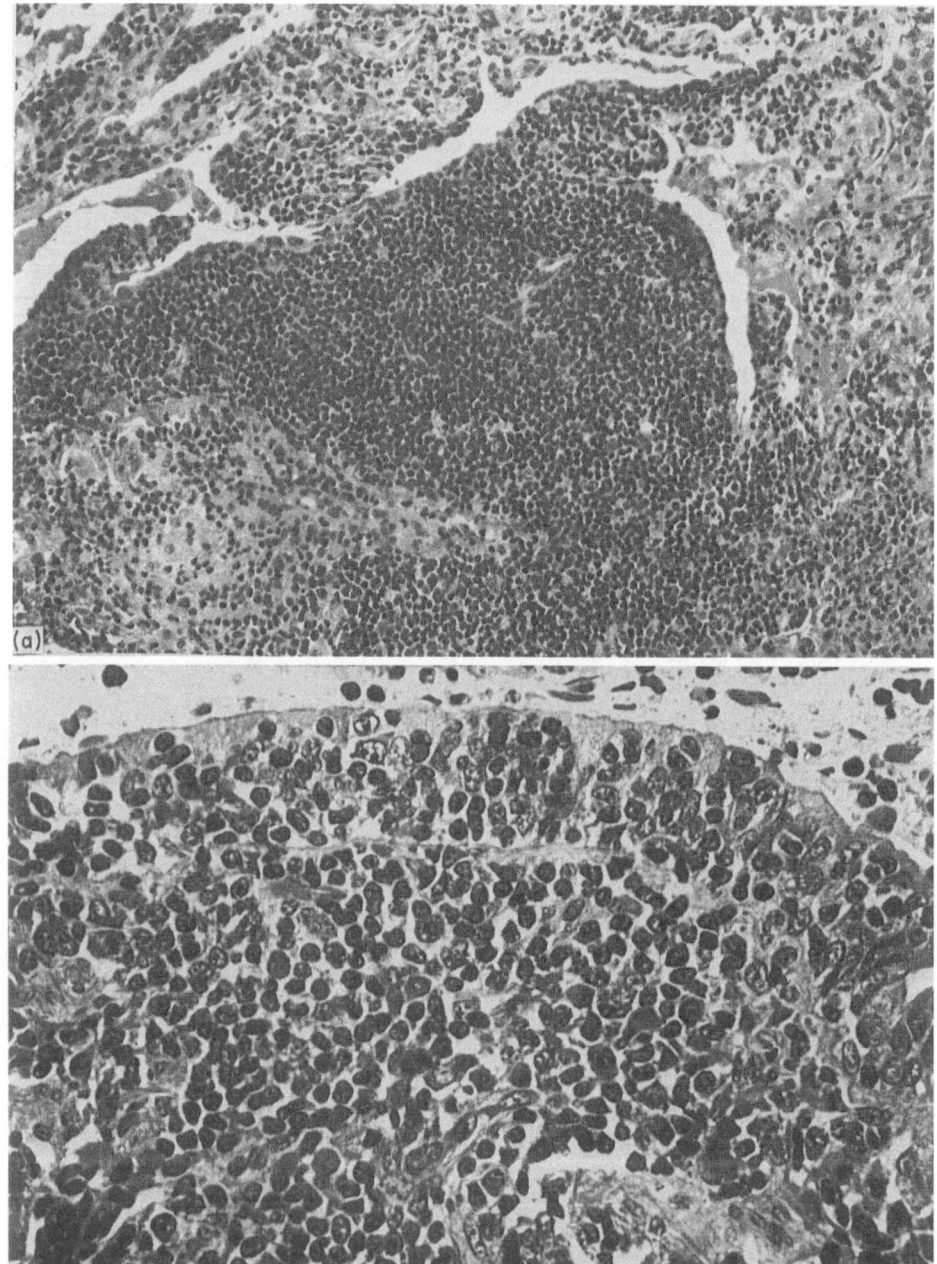

ton, 1983b). For a thorough clinicopathological review see Katzenstein *et al.* (1979).

11.4   Leukemic infiltrates

Pulmonary infiltrates with leukemic cells occur and diagnosis by bronchial biopsy is possible (Philips *et al.*, 1980; Canham *et al.*, 1983). In their series of 139 adult leukemics, Tenholder and Hooper (1980) had 8 cases which developed diffuse leukemic infiltrates in the lung. However, most of the patients with pulmonary lesions had an infectious etiology. Comparison of the cellular infiltrate with the patient's leukemic cells is very helpful in distinguishing leukemic from inflammatory infiltrates. Intravascular accumulations of leukemic cells can be seen in biopsies from patients with very high numbers of circulating cells (Colby and Carrington, 1983a).

11.5   Sarcomas

Primary pulmonary sarcomas are exceedingly rare. Hochberg and Crastnopol (1956) found 8 cases among 68404 surgical specimens and no cases in 2489 autopsies at one hospital in New York. Cameron (1975) found 9 cases in a series of 6000 bronchogenic carcinomas; of these only 2 were endobronchial. These lesions are more likely to be symptomatic than their benign counterparts, with cough, hemoptysis and weight loss frequently mentioned in the reports.

11.5.1   Fibrosarcoma

Fibrosarcoma is the most frequent form of pulmonary soft tissue malignancy (Cameron, 1975; Gebauer, 1982; Nascimento *et al.*, 1982) and the most likely to be bronchial in origin (Guccion and Rosen, 1972). These sarcomas may have a slower growth rate and behave less malignantly than the other forms of differentiation (Gebauer, 1982).

11.5.2   Leiomyosarcoma

Second only to fibrosarcoma in frequency, leiomyosarcomas are described in reviews by Gebauer (1982), Guccion and Rosen (1972), Cameron (1975),

---

Fig. 11.3   Pulmonary lymphoma. (a) Masses of lymphoid cells in the peribronchial tissue. The cells form a monotonous infiltrate. ($\times$ 180) (b) At higher magnification the lymphoid and plasmacytoid infiltrate extends into the overlying respiratory epithelium. Immunohistochemical studies on this biopsy gave a monoclonal pattern positive for lambda light chains. Thoracotomy confirmed a diffuse nodular process of the same infiltrate. ($\times$ 480) (Paraffin section stained with hematoxylin and eosin.)

and Nascimento *et al.* (1982). Eleven of the cases were endobronchial. As with the other sarcomas, leiomyosarcoma has a histological pattern in lung identical to that at other sites (Fig. 11.4). Case reports (Mylius and Aakhus, 1961; Morgan and Ball, 1980; Shoenfeld *et al.*, 1981; Gil-Zuricalday *et al.*, 1982) include 2 cases diagnosed by cytological smears (Fleming and Jove, 1975; Sawada *et al.*, 1977).

11.5.3   Liposarcoma

Unlike their benign counterpart, liposarcomas are very rare (Gebauer, 1982). Sawamura *et al.* (1982) reported a case which presented as a smooth surfaced polypoid endobronchial mass and was diagnosed by bronchial brushing cytology smears and biopsy.

11.5.4   Rhabdomyosarcoma

Five cases were found among the 230 reported sarcomas reviewed by Gebauer (1982). Bronchial biopsy was diagnostic in the case reported by

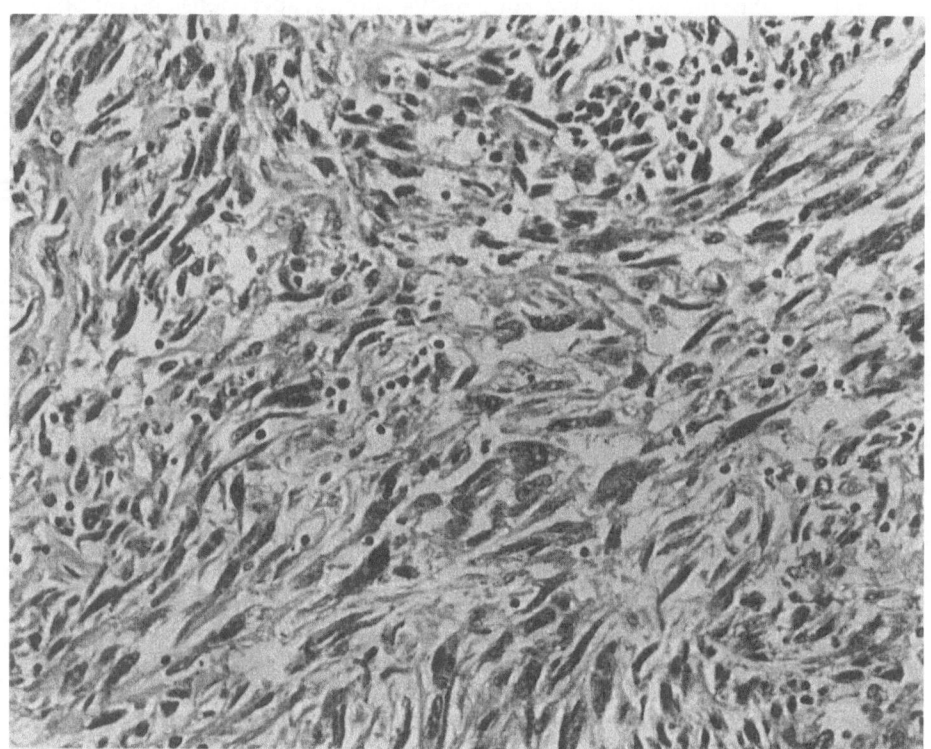

Fig. 11.4 Leiomyosarcoma. Autopsy specimen of mass in lung which encircled the bronchus. Ultrastructural analysis confirmed the smooth muscle differentiation of this sarcoma. (Paraffin section stained with hematoxylin and eosin: × 480.)

Fallon *et al.* (1971) but yielded only necrotic tissue in the case reported by Forbes (1955). Biopsy was not performed in the cases reported by Lee *et al.* (1981) and Eriksson *et al.* (1982). All 4 of these cases were endobronchial.

11.5.5   *Chondrosarcoma and osteogenic sarcoma*

These neoplasms are among the least frequent of the pulmonary sarcomas (Hochberg and Crastnopol, 1956; Cameron, 1975; Gebauer, 1982; Nascimento *et al.* (1982). The chondrosarcomas reported by Daniels *et al.* (1967) and Yellin *et al.* (1983) were both bronchial in origin. Both of these lesions contained foci of calcification and one contained metaplastic bone. Three case reports of pulmonary osteogenic sarcoma were parenchymal and not diagnosed bronchoscopically (Nosanchuk and Weatherbee, 1969; Reingold and Amromin, 1971).

11.5.6   *Malignant fibrous histiocytoma*

It is difficult to determine if any of the early reports of sarcomatous lesions in bronchi were malignant fibrous histiocytomas, since they were first recognized by Stout and Lattes in 1967. Five cases are reported in the current literature but none of these was diagnosed by bronchial biopsy, although the tumors were described as peribronchial (Bedrossian *et al.*, 1979; Kern *et al.*, 1979; Paulsen *et al.*, 1981; Silverman and Coalson, 1984). Lee *et al.* (1984) described an additional 5 cases, none described as bronchial and none diagnosed prior to thoracotomy.

The endobronchial tumor described by Herczeg *et al.* (1978) as an inflammatory fibrous histiocytoma was considered benign although it was aggressive in behavior. Katzenstein and Maurer (1979) described a tumor composed entirely of 'histiocytes' (macrophages). They interpreted the lesion as benign, cautioning that because the cells were very bizarre in appearance they might easily be interpreted as malignant. In their case there was no storiform pattern since there were no significant numbers of spindle-shaped cells.

11.5.7   *Others*

Kaposi's sarcoma can involve lung (Loring and Wolman, 1965; Dantzig *et al.*, 1974; Misra *et al.*, 1982) and was endobronchial in the case reported by Favera (1911). With the increased frequency of Kaposi's sarcoma associated with the acquired immune deficiency syndrome (AIDS), bronchial involvement may be expected to increase. Kornfeld and Axelrod (1983) report one such case with initial diagnosis suggested by a transbronchial biopsy.

Two cases of primary bronchial melanoma have been reported (Salm, 1963; Gephardt, 1981) with unsuccessful extensive search for any other possible primary site. The frequency of undetected primaries in metastatic melanoma would suggest that these cases are more likely metastatic.

Gebauer (1982) lists 19 cases of neurogenous sarcoma and 10 cases of angiosarcoma in his review of pulmonary sarcomas. Nascimento *et al.* (1982) have 3 cases of hemangiopericytoma in their series. It is not clear if any of these were endobronchial.

References

Albertini, R.E. and Ekberg, N.L. (1980), Endobronchial metastasis in breast cancer. *Thorax*, **35**, 435–40.

Al-Saleem, T. and Peale, A.R. (1969), Lymphocytic tumors and pseudotumors of the lung. Report of five cases with special emphasis on pathology. *Am. Rev. Respir. Dis.*, **99**, 767–72.

Arrigoni, M.G., Woolner, L.B., Bernatz, P.E., Miller, W.E. and Fontana, R.S. (1970), Benign tumors of the lung. A ten year surgical experience. *J. Thorac. Cardiovasc. Surg.*, **60**, 589–99.

Bahadori, M. and Liebow, A.A. (1973), Plasma cell granulomas of the lung. *Cancer*, **31**, 191–208.

Bank, D.E., Castellan, R.M. and Hendrick, D.J. (1980), Lymphocytic lymphoma recurring in multiple endobronchial sites. *Thorax*, **35**, 796–7.

Bates, H.R., Buis, L.J. and Johns, T.N.P. (1976), Endobronchial histiocytoma. *Chest*, **69**, 705–6.

Bates, T. and Hull, O.H. (1958), Histiocytoma of the bronchus. Report of a case in a six-year-old child. *Am. J. Dis. Child.*, **95**, 53–6.

Bateson, E.M. (1965), Relationship between intrapulmonary and endobronchial cartilage-containing tumours (so-called hamartomas). *Thorax*, **20**, 447–61.

Bateson, E.M. (1973), So-called hamartoma of the lung--a true neoplasm of fibrous connective tissue of the bronchi. *Cancer*, **31**, 1458–67.

Bateson, E.M., Hayes, J.A. and Woo-Ming, M. (1968), Endobronchial teratoma associated with bronchiectasis and bronchiolectasis. *Thorax*, **23**, 69–76.

Beck, W.C. and Reganis, J.C. (1951), Primary lymphoma of the lung. Review of the literature, report of one case, and addition of eight other cases. *J. Thorac. Surg.*, **22**, 323–8.

Bedrossian, C.W.M., Verani, R., Unger, K.M. and Salman, J. (1979), Pulmonary malignant fibrous histiocytoma. Light and electron microscopic studies of one case. *Chest*, **75**, 186–9.

Bellin, H.J., Libshitz, H.I. and Patchefsky, A.S. (1971), Bronchial lipoma. Report of two cases showing chondroitic metaplasia. *Arch. Pathol.*, **92**, 20–3.

Brewster, D.C., MacMillan, I.K.R. and Edwards, F.R. (1975), Chondroma of trachea. Report of a case and review of literature. *Ann. Thorac. Surg.*, **19**, 576–84.

Brown, A.L. (1950), Bronchial tumors: thoracobronchotomy. *Surg.*, **28**, 579–82.

Buell, R., Wang, N.-S., Seemayer, T.A. and Ahmed, M.N. (1976), Endobronchial plasma cell granuloma (xanthomatous pseudotumor). *Hum. Pathol.*, **7**, 411–26.

Butler, C., III and Kleinerman, J. (1969), Pulmonary hamartoma. *Arch. Pathol.*, **88**, 584–92.

Cameron, E.W.J. (1975), Primary sarcoma of the lung. *Thorax*, **30**, 516–20.

Canham, E.M., Kennedy, T.C. and Merrick, T.A. (1983), Unexplained pulmonary infiltrates in the compromised patient. An invasive investigation in a consecutive series. *Cancer*, **52**, 325–9.

Churg, A. (1983), Pulmonary angiitis and granulomatosis revisited. *Hum. Pathol.*, **14**, 868–83.

Colby, T.V. and Carrington, C.B. (1982), Pulmonary lymphomas simulating lymphomatoid granulomatosis. *Am. J. Surg. Pathol.*, **6**, 19–32.

Colby, T.V. and Carrington, C.B. (1983a), Lymphoreticular tumors and infiltrates of the lung. In *Pathology Annual 1983*, Part 1 (eds S.C. Sommers and P.P. Rosen), Appleton-Century-Crofts, Norwalk, Conn., pp. 27–70.

Colby, T.V. and Carrington, C.B. (1983b), Pulmonary lymphomas: current concepts. *Hum. Pathol.*, **14**, 884–7.

Cooper, J.A.D., Jr. and Arora, N.S. (1982), Multiple granular cell myoblastomas of the bronchial tree. *So. Med. J.*, **75**, 491–2.

Corona, F.E. and Okeson, G.C. (1974), Endobronchial fibroma. An unusual case of segmental atelectasis. *Am. Rev. Respir. Dis.*, **110**, 350–3.

Crutcher, R.R., Waltuch, T.L. and Ghosh, A.K. (1968), Bronchial lipoma. Report of a case and literature review. *J. Thorac. Cardiovasc. Surg.*, **55**, 422–5.

Dabouis, G., Nomballais, M.F., Maury, B., Peltier, P., Morineau, J.F. and Corroller, J. (1979), Tumeur d'Abrikossoff endobronchique. À propos de deux nouveaux cas associés à des tumeurs malignes. *Poumon*, **35**, 211–16.

Daniel, T.M., Smith, R.H., Faunce, H.F. and Sylvest, V.M. (1980), Transbronchoscopic versus surgical resection of tracheobronchial granular cell myoblastomas. *J. Thorac. Cardiovasc. Surg.*, **80**, 898–903.

Daniels, A.C., Conner, G.H. and Straus, F.H. (1967), Primary chondrosarcoma of the tracheobronchial tree. Report of a unique case and brief review. *Arch. Pathol.*, **84**, 615–24.

Dantzig, P.I., Richardson, D., Rayhanzadeh, S., Mauro, J. and Shoss, R. (1974), Thoracic involvement of non-African Kaposi's sarcoma. *Chest*, **66**, 522–5.

DeClercq, D., Van der Straeten, M. and Roels, H. (1983), Granular cell myoblastoma of the bronchus. *Europ. J. Respir. Dis.*, **64**, 72–6.

Engelman, R.M. (1967), Pulmonary fibroma: a rare benign tumor. *Am. Rev. Respir. Dis.*, **96**, 1242–5.

Eriksson, A., Thunell, M. and Lundqvist, G. (1982), Pendulating endobronchial rhabdomyosarcoma with fatal asphyxia. *Thorax*, **37**, 390–1.

Fallon, G., Schiller, M. and Kilman, J.W. (1971), Primary rhabdomyosarcoma of the bronchus. *Ann. Thorac. Surg.*, **12**, 650–4.

Farsad, G.R.H. and Makoui, C. (1981), Endobronchial lipoma. *Am. Surg.*, **47**, 236–8.

Fauci, A.S., Haynes, B.F., Costa, J., Katz, P. and Wolff, S.M. (1982), Lymphomatoid granulomatosis. Prospective clinical and therapeutic experience over 10 years. *New Engl. J. Med.*, **306**, 68–74.

Favera, G.B.D. (1911), Über das sog. Sarcoma idiop. multiplex haemorrhagieum (Kaposi). Klinische und histologische Beiträge. *Arch. Dermat. Res.*, **109**, 387–440.

Feoli, F., Carbone, A., Dina, M.A., Lauriola, L., Musiani, P. and Piantelli, M. (1981), Pseudolymphoma of the lung: lymphoid subsets in the lung mass and in peripheral blood. *Cancer*, **48**, 2218–22.

Fleming, W.H. and Jove, D.F. (1975), Primary leiomyosarcoma of the lung with positive sputum cytology. *Acta Cytol.*, **19**, 14–20.

Forbes, G.B. (1955), Rhabdomyosarcoma of bronchus. *J. Pathol. Bact.*, **70**, 427–31.

Gallagher, C.J., Knowles, G.K., Habeshaw, J.A., Green, M., Malpas, J.S. and Lister, T.A. (1983), Early involvement of the bronchi in patients with malignant lymphoma. *Brit. J. Cancer*, **48**, 777–81.

Gebauer, Chr. (1982), The postoperative prognosis of primary pulmonary sarcomas. A review with a comparison between the histological forms and the other endothoracal sarcomas based on 474 cases. *Scand. J. Thorac. Cardiovasc. Surg.*, **16**, 91–7.

Gephardt, G.N. (1981), Malignant melanoma of the bronchus. *Human Pathol.*, **12**, 671–2.

Gibbs, A.R. and Seal, R.M.E. (1978), Primary lymphoproliferative conditions of lung. *Thorax*, **33**, 140–52.

Gil-Zuricalday, C., Lor, F. and Gil-Turner, C. (1982), Primary pedunculated leiomyosarcoma of the lung. *Thorax*, **37**, 153–4.

Glant, M.D., Wall, R.W. and Ransburg, R. (1979), Endobronchial granular cell tumor. Cytology of a new case and review of the literature. *Acta Cytol.*, **23**, 477–82.

Greenberg, S.D., Heisler, J.G., Gyorkey, F. and Jenkins, D.E. (1972), Pulmonary lymphoma versus pseudolymphoma: a perplexing problem. *So. Med. J.*, **65**, 775–84.

Gribetz, A.R., Chuang, M.T. and Teirstein, A.S. (1980), Fiberoptic bronchoscopy in patient with Hodgkin's and non-Hodgkin's lymphomas. *Cancer*, **46**, 1476–8.

Guccion, J.G. and Rosen, S.H. (1972), Bronchopulmonary leiomyosarcoma and fibrosarcoma. A study of 32 cases and review of the literature. *Cancer*, **30**, 836–47.

Guida, P.M., Fulcher, T. and Moore, S.W. (1965), Leiomyoma of lung. Report of a case. *J. Thorac. Cardiovasc. Surg.*, **49**, 1058–64.

Guidice, J.C., Gordon, R. and Komansky, H.J. (1980), Endobronchial lipoma causing unilateral absence of pulmonary perfusion. *Chest*, **77**, 104–5.

Hakimi, M., Font-Soto, D., Gonzalez-Lavin, L. and Davila, J.C. (1975), Endobronchial lipoma associated with squamous metaplasia of bronchial mucosa. *Mich. Med.*, **74**, 129–39.

Halttunen, P., Meurala, H. and Standertskjöld-Nordenstam, C-G. (1982), Surgical treatment of benign endobronchial tumours. *Thorax*, **37**, 688–92.

Harding, J.R., Williams, J. and Seal, R.M.E. (1978), Pedunculated capillary haemangioma of the bronchus. *Brit. J. Dis. Chest*, **72**, 336–42.

Herczeg, E., Weissberg, D., Almog, C. and Pajewski, M. (1978), Inflammatory fibrous histiocytoma of the bronchus. *Chest*, **73**, 669–70.

Hochberg, L.A. and Crastnopol, P. (1956), Primary sarcoma of the bronchus and lung. *Arch. Surg.*, **73**, 74–98.

Hurwitz, S.S., Conlan, A.A., Gritzman, M.C.D. and Krut, L.H. (1982), Coexisting granular cell myoblastoma and squamous carcinoma of bronchus. *Thorax*, **37**, 392–3.

Jamieson, M.P.G. and McGowan, A.R. (1982), Endobronchial teratoma. *Thorax*, **37**, 157–9.

Julsrud, P.R., Brown, L.R., Li, C-Y., Rosenow, E.C., III and Crowe, J.K. (1978), Pulmonary processes of mature-appearing lymphocytes: pseudolymphoma, well-differentiated lymphocytic lymphoma, and lymphocytic interstitial pneumonitis. *Radiol.*, **127**, 289–96.

Katzenstein, A.-L.A., Carrington, C.B. and Liebow, A.A. (1979), Lymphomatoid granulomatosis. A clinicopathologic study of 152 cases. *Cancer*, **43**, 360–73.

Katzenstein, A.-L.A., Gmelich, J.T. and Carrington, C.B. (1980), Sclerosing hemangiomas of the lung. A clinicopathologic study of 51 cases. *Am. J. Surg. Pathol.*, **4**, 343–56.

Katzenstein, A.-L.A. and Maurer, J.J. (1979), Benign histiocytic tumor of lung. A light- and electron-microscopic study. *Am. J. Surg. Pathol.*, **3**, 61–8.

Kaufman, J. (1969), Endobronchial chondroma. Clinical and physiologic improvement following excision. *Am. Rev. Respir. Dis.*, **100**, 711–16.

Kern, W.H., Crepeau, A.G. and Jones, J.C. (1961), Primary Hodgkin's disease of the lung. Report of 4 cases and review of the literature. *Cancer*, **14**, 1151–65.

Kern, W.H., Hughes, R.K., Meyer, B.W. and Harley, D.P. (1979), Malignant fibrous histiocytoma of the lung. *Cancer*, **44**, 1793–1801.

Kornfeld, H. and Axelrod, J.L. (1983), Pulmonary presentation of Kaposi's sarcoma in a homosexual patient. *Am. Rev. Respir. Dis.*, **127**, 248–9.

Korompai, F.L., Awe, R.J., Beall, A.C. and Greenberg, S.D. (1974), Granular cell myoblastoma of the bronchus: a new case, 12-year follow up report, and review of the literature. *Chest*, **66**, 578–80.

Koss, L.G. (1979), In *Diagnostic Cytology and its Histopathologic Bases*, 3rd edn, J.B. Lippincott, Philadelphia, p. 673.

Kyriakos, M. and Kempson, R.L. (1976), Inflammatory fibrous histiocytoma. An aggressive and lethal lesion. *Cancer*, **37**, 1584–1606.

Laustela, E., Koshinen, R. and Ahlqvist, J. (1974), Leiomyoma of the bronchus. *Ann. Chir. Gync. Fenn.*, **63**, 346–50.

Lee, J.T., Shelburne, J.D. and Linder, J. (1984), Primary malignant fibrous histiocytoma of the lung: a clinicopathologic and ultrastructural study of five cases. *Cancer*, **53**, 1124–30.

Lee, S.H., Rengachary, S.S. and Paramesh, J. (1981), Primary pulmonary rhabdomyosarcoma: a case report and review of the literature. *Hum. Pathol.*, **12**, 92–6.

Lipper, S., Wheeler, M.S. and Jennette, C. (1980), Malignant pulmonary lymphoproliferative angiitis. A monoclonal neoplasm. *Cancer*, **46**, 1411–17.

Loring, W.E. and Wolman, S.R. (1965), Idiopathic multiple hemorrhagic sarcoma of lung (Kaposi's sarcoma). *N.Y. State J. Med.*, **65**, 668–76.

MacArthur, C.G.C., Cheung, D.L.C. and Spiro, S.G. (1977), Endobronchial lipoma: a review with four cases. *Brit. J. Dis. Chest*, **71**, 93–100.

Majmudar, B., Thomas, J., Gorelkin, L. and Symbas, P.N. (1981), Respiratory obstruction caused by a multicentric granular cell tumor of the laryngotracheobronchial tree. *Hum. Pathol.*, **12**, 283–6.

Marchevsky, A., Padilla, M., Kaneko, M. and Kleinerman, J. (1983), Localized lymphoid nodules of lung. A reappraisal of the lymphoma versus pseudolymphoma dilemma. *Cancer*, **51**, 2070–7.

Medelli, J., Abet, D., Bertoux, J.P., Vermynck, J.P., Giroulle, H., Pietri, J. and Goudot, B. (1980), Le lipome bronchique. À propos de quatre observations. *Ann. Chir.*, **34**, 327–31.

Miller, D.R. (1969), Benign tumors of lung and tracheobronchial tree. *Ann. Thorac. Surg.*, **8**, 542–60.

Misra, D.P., Sunderrajan, E.V., Hurst, D.J. and Maltby, J.D. (1982). Kaposi's sarcoma of the lung: radiography and pathology. *Thorax*, **37**, 155–6.

Morgan, P.G.M. and Ball, J. (1980), Pulmonary leiomyosarcomas. *Brit. J. Dis. Chest*, **74**, 245–52.

Mylius, E.A. and Aakhus, T. (1961), Primary pulmonary leiomyosarcoma. *Acta Pathol. Microbiol. Scand. Suppl.*, **148**, 149–60.

Nascimento, A.G., Unni, K.K. and Bernatz, P.E. (1982), Sarcomas of the lung. *Mayo Cl. Proc.*, **57**, 355–9.

Nash, G. (1982), Pathologic features of the lung in the immunocompromised host. *Hum. Pathol.*, **13**, 841–58.

Nelson, S., Price, D. and Terry, P. (1983), Primary Hodgkin's disease of the lung: case report. *Thorax*, **38**, 310–11.

Nosanchuk, J.S. and Weatherbee, L. (1969), Primary osteogenic sarcoma in lung.

J. Thor. Cardiovasc. Surg., **58**, 242–7.

Oparah, S.S. and Subramanian, V.A. (1976), Granular cell myoblastoma of the bronchus: report of 2 cases and review of the literature. *Ann. Thorac. Surg.*, **22**, 199–202.

Ovil, Y., Schachner, A., Schujman, E., Spitzer, S.A. and Levy, M.J. (1982), Benign endobronchial lipoma masquerading as recurrent pneumonia. *Europ. J. Respir. Dis.*, **63**, 481–3.

Paulsen, S.M., Egeblad, K. and Christensen, J. (1981), Malignant fibrous histiocytoma of the lung. *Virch. Arch. A (Path. Anat.)*, **394**, 167–76.

Philips, M.J., Knight, R.K. and Green, M. (1980), Fiberoptic bronchoscopy and diagnosis of pulmonary lesions in lymphoma and leukemia. *Thorax*, **35**, 19–25.

Politis, J., Funahashi, A., Gehlsen, J.A., DeCock, D., Stengel, B.F. and Choi, H. (1979), Intrathoracic lipomas. Report of three cases and review of the literature with emphasis on endobronchial lipoma. *J. Thorac. Cardiovasc. Surg.*, **77**, 550–6.

Reingold, I.M. and Amromin, G.D. (1971), Extraosseous osteosarcoma of the lung. *Cancer*, **28**, 491–8.

Richmond, J.M., Dawkins, R.L., Henderson, D.W. and Tan, N.T.S. (1981), Immunodeficiency, pulmonary lymphoreticular infiltration, paraproteinemia, and terminal lymphoma. *Cancer*, **47**, 2641–7.

Robertson, A.J., McIntosh, W., Lamont, P. and Guthrie, W. (1981), Malignant granular cell tumour (myoblastoma) of the vulva: report of a case and review of the literature. *Histopathol.*, **5**, 69–79.

Roviaro, G.C., Varoli, F. and Paganini, C.S. (1981), Is the solitary papilloma of the bronchus always a benign tumor? *ORL J. Otorhinollaryngol. Relat. Spec.*, **43**, 301–8.

Salm, R. (1963), A primary malignant melanoma of the bronchus. *J. Pathol. Bact.*, **85**, 121–6.

Saltzstein, S.L. (1963), Pulmonary malignant lymphomas and pseudolymphomas: classification, therapy and prognosis. *Cancer*, **16**, 928–55.

Sawada, K., Fukuma, S., Seki, Y., Tanaka, F., Ishida, I., Ikeda, H. and Tanaka, N. (1977), Cytologic features of primary leiomyoarcoma of the lung. Report of a case diagnosed by bronchial brushing procedure. *Acta Cytol.*, **21**, 770–3.

Sawamura, K., Hashimoto, T., Nanjo, S., Nakamura, K., Iioka, S., Mori, T., Furuse, K. and Shakudo, Y. (1982), Primary liposarcoma of the lung: report of a case. *J. Surg. Oncol.*, **19**, 243–6.

Shahian, D.M. and MacEnany, M.T. (1979), Complete endobronchial excision of leiomyoma of the bronchus. *J. Thorac. Cardiovasc. Surg.*, **77**, 87–91.

Shepherd, M.P. (1982), Endobronchial metastatic disease. *Thorax*, **37**, 362–5.

Shoenfeld, Y., Avidor, I., Liban, E., Levy, M.J. and Pinkhas, J. (1981), Primary leiomyosarcoma of the pulmonary artery. *Respiration*, **41**, 208–13.

Silverman, J.F. and Coalson, J.J. (1984), Primary malignant myxoid fibrous histiocytoma of the lung. Light and ultrastructural examination with review of the literature. *Arch. Pathol. Lab. Med.*, **108**, 49–54.

Sobel, H.J. and Marquet, E. (1974), Granular cells and granular lesions. In *Pathology Annual 1974* (ed. S.C. Sommers), Appleton-Century-Crofts, New York, pp. 43–79.

Steffelaar, J.W., Nap, M. and Von Haelst, U.J.G.M. (1982), Malignant granular cell tumor. Report of a case with special reference to carcinoembryonic antigen. *Am. J. Surg. Pathol.*, **6**, 665–72.

Sternberg, W.H., Sidransky, H. and Ochsner, S. (1959), Primary malignant lymphoms of the lung. *Cancer*, **12**, 806–19.

Stout, A.P. and Lattes, R. (1967), *Tumors of Soft Tissues, Atlas of Tumor Pathology*, 2nd series, fascicle 1, AFIP, Washington.

Takeda, M. and Burechailo, F.A. (1969), Smooth muscle cells in sputum. *Acta Cytol.*, **13**, 696–9.

Tenholder, M.F. and Hooper, R.G. (1980), Pulmonary infiltrates in leukemia. *Chest*, **78**, 468–73.

Tenholder, M.F., Scialla, S.J. and Weisbaum, G. (1982), Endobronchial metastatic plasmacytoma. *Cancer*, **49**, 1465–8.

Thomas, C.P. and Morgan, A.D. (1958), Ossifying bronchial adenoma. *Thorax*, **13**, 286–93.

Tomashefski, J.F., Jr. (1982), Benign endobronchial mesenchymal tumors. Their relationship to parenchymal pulmonary hamartomas. *Am. J. Surg. Pathol.*, **6**, 531–40.

Valenstein, S.L. and Thurer, R.J. (1978), Granular cell myoblastoma of the bronchus. Case report and literature review. *J. Thorac. Cardiovasc. Surg.*, **76**, 465–8.

Vera-Román, J.M., Sobonya, R.E., Gomez-Garcia, J.L., Sanz-Bondia, J.R. and Paris-Romeu, F. (1983), Leiomyoma of the lung. Literature review and case report. *Cancer*, **52**, 936–41.

Walsh, T.J. and Healy, T.M. (1969), Chondroma of the bronchus. *Thorax*, **24**, 327–9.

Weitzner, S. and Oser, J.F. (1968), Granular cell myoblastoma of bronchus. *Am. Rev. Respir. Dis.*, **97**, 923–30.

Whimster, W.F. (1983), Tumours of the trachea, bronchus, lung and pleura. In *Diagnostic Tumour Bibliographies*, Pitman, London, pp. 1–167.

Yellin, A., Schwartz, L., Hersho, E. and Lieberman, Y. (1983), Chondrosarcoma of the bronchus. Report of a case with resection and review of the literature. *Chest*, **84**, 224–6.

Zafirakopoulos, P., Zorbas, J., Creatsas, G. and Tosios, J. (1977), Intrabronchial lipoma. *Intern. Surg.*, **62**, 399–400.

Index

Figures in *italics* refer to pages with illustrations

387